Rehabilitation of Movement

Other titles in the Series

Rehabilitation of Movement

Theoretical Basis of Clinical Practice

Edited by

JUDITH PITT-BROOKE

Lecturer in Physiotherapy, School of Physiotherapy,
University of Nottingham, Nottingham

with

HEATHER REID

Lecturer in Physiotherapy, School of Physiotherapy,
University of Nottingham, Nottingham

JANE LOCKWOOD

Lecturer in Physiotherapy, School of Physiotherapy,
University of Nottingham, Nottingham

and

KATE KERR

Senior Lecturer in Physiotherapy, School of Physiotherapy,
University of Nottingham, Nottingham

WB Saunders Company Ltd

London • Philadelphia • Toronto • Sydney • Tokyo

WB Saunders Company Ltd   24–28 Oval Road
London NW1 7DX, UK

The Curtis Center
Independence Square West
Philadelphia, PA 19106–3399, USA

Harcourt Brace & Company
55 Horner Avenue
Toronto, Ontario M8Z 4X6, Canada

Harcourt Brace & Company, Australia
30–52 Smidmore Street
Marrickville, NSW 2204, Australia

Harcourt Brace & Company, Japan
Ichibancho Central Building, 22–1 Ichibancho
Chiyoda-ku, Tokyo 102, Japan

A catalogue record for this book is available from the British Library

✓ ISBN 0-7020-2157-1

Typeset by J&L Composition Ltd, Filey, North Yorkshire

Printed and bound in Great Britain by The Bath Press, Avon

Contents

A   FACTORS INFLUENCING MOVEMENT

B   EXAMINATION, ASSESSMENT AND MEASUREMENT TECHNIQUES

Contents

Contributors

Kevin Banks BA MCSP SRP
*Member of the International Maitland
Teachers Association
Rotherham
Yorkshire*

Louis Gifford MAppSc BSc MCSP SRP
*Falmouth Physiotherapy Clinic
Kestrel
Swanpool
Falmouth
Cornwall TRII 5BD*

Vicki Harding MCSP SRP
*Research Physiotherapist
INPUT
St Thomas' Hospital
London SEI 7EH*

Sue Hignett MSc MCSP EurErg
*Ergonomist
Nottingham City Hospital NHS Trust
Hucknall Road
Nottingham NG5 IPG*

Kate Kerr PhD BA MCSP SRP
*Post Grad DipHealthEd, CertEd
Senior Lecturer in Physiotherapy
School of Physiotherapy
University of Nottingham
Hucknall Road
Nottingham NG5 IPG*

Jane Lockwood MSc MCSP SRP
*Lecturer in Physiotherapy
School of Physiotherapy
University of Nottingham
Hucknall Road
Nottingham NG5 IPG*

The late Maureen Maxwell MA MCSP SRP
*University of Ulster Jordanstown
Department of Occupational Therapy and
Physiotherapy
Shore Road
Newtownabbey
County Antrim BT37 0QB*

Simon Mockett MPhil MCSP SRP
*Lecturer in Physiotherapy
School of Physiotherapy
University of Nottingham
Hucknall Road
Nottingham NG5 IPG*

Judith Pitt-Brooke MSc MCSP SRP CertEd
*Lecturer in Physiotherapy
School of Physiotherapy
University of Nottingham
Hucknall Road
Nottingham NG5 IPG
and East Midlands Physiotherapy Clinic
Wyverne House
107 Ashby Road
Loughborough
Leicestershire LEII 3AB*

Fran Polak MSc MCSP SRP
*Research Physiotherapist
The Bioengineering Research Centre
Derbyshire Royal Infirmary NHS Trust
London Road
Derby DEI 2QY
and East Midlands Physiotherapy Clinic
Wyverne House
107 Ashby Road
Loughborough
Leicestershire LEII 3AB*

Heather Reid MMedSci MCSP SRP CertEd
*Lecturer in Physiotherapy
School of Physiotherapy
University of Nottingham
Hucknall Road
Nottingham NG5 IPG*

Preface

This book was conceived at a time when pre-registration education in the therapy professions had just completed its transition from diploma status to degree status. There was a lack of research oriented texts which offered an introduction to a broad range of therapeutic rehabilitation interventions. Whilst there has been a rapid increase in the number of more specialized texts which offer more focused attention to a specific skill, or intervention area, the general introductory texts which support the development of skills in the movement studies and musculoskeletal rehabilitation fields have, to date, lacked substance. In particular, clear identification of the extent and limitations of the scientific background which underpins therapy in some areas has been lacking.

The aim of this book is to provide a literature-based introduction to contemporary approaches in musculoskeletal physiotherapy and to encourage students and therapists to recognize the extent and limitations of the evidence provided by scientific findings, which underpins these approaches. It is hoped that recognition of the scientific 'state of the art' at this general level, by both students and therapists, will help to create a focus and appetite for further research through practice. This currently still evades the therapy professions to an extent. With increasing demand for physiotherapy intervention in the management of painful musculoskeletal conditions and increasing pressure to produce positive outcomes speedily, it is imperative that therapy interventions are appropriately focused. This requires a

sound, broad, research-based knowledge of the principles underpinning therapeutic interventions, rather than the 'recipe book' therapy approach which has been a feature indirectly implied by the followers of therapy 'gurus' in the recent past.

Therapists are and should be expected to be more questioning in their approach to study and to clinical practice. This questioning must be encouraged to linger well beyond undergraduate studies into postgraduate continuing development. Students should be encouraged to guard against the often persuasive explanations of the effectiveness of particular therapies often by those with considerable clinical experience, but which are often based on anecdotal evidence and unsubstantiated by scientific scrutiny. There is a need to rise to the challenge of research if only by constantly asking for evidence or searching for the science behind the 'magical therapies' which are sometimes offered to us.

There has been a deliberate attempt within this book to minimize reviewing specific 'named' approaches, but rather to review the principles on which groups of therapies are based. These reviews are therefore necessarily generalized, but, most importantly, there has been an attempt to expose some of the myths which have pervaded some areas of therapeutic interventions by providing an up to date critical literature-based assessment of contemporary areas of practice. This review is set in the context of the underpinning knowledge which students require in order to develop the sophisticated clinical reasoning skills now demanded of them.

This book is not intended as a comprehensive manual of physiotherapeutic interventions for the management of musculoskeletal conditions. Rather, it is a text which introduces the reader to the current scientific background to many of the contemporary approaches in this field. The material presented is comprehensively referenced and each chapter offers suggested learning objectives and summarizes key points. To encourage the reader to integrate and make full use of the information within the book, it is divided into sections which are preceded by a diagrammatic representation of its content. An example of this is given below. This pictorial representation attempts to help the reader to approach the information being presented in a logical, reasoned manner and, together with 'practical applications' and 'key points' within each chapter, to facilitate interaction with the material.

The contributors to this text have all entered into this project with the same philosophy and the same opinions of the need for such a text. It is hoped that we have gone some way to developing the style of basic textbook material to that which is more appropriate in the current climate of evidence-based practice. I would like to extend my sincere thanks to all the contributors to this book and to those who have supported them. I pay tribute to their determination to develop the approach offered here. I hope it will have been of value to us all and more importantly that the approach and the material presented in this

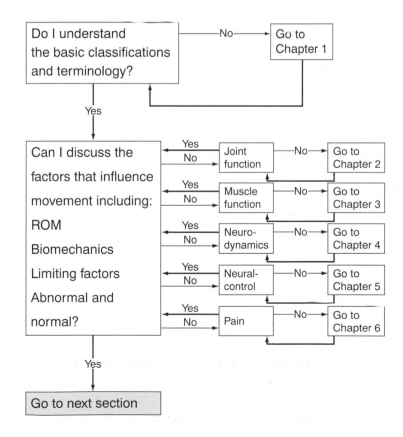

book will prove useful to students at undergraduate level and beyond.

On a final and sad note, one of the contributors, Maureen Maxwell, died during the preparation of this text. Her contribution had been completed prior to her sudden illness and is included as a tribute to her substantial contribution, particularly in the field of communication studies within physiotherapy during the course of her career. On behalf of all involved in the production of this book, I would like to thank Maureen's husband for his permission to include her work, which will be of considerable continuing value to those who read this text.

Judith Pitt-Brooke

A

Factors Influencing Movement

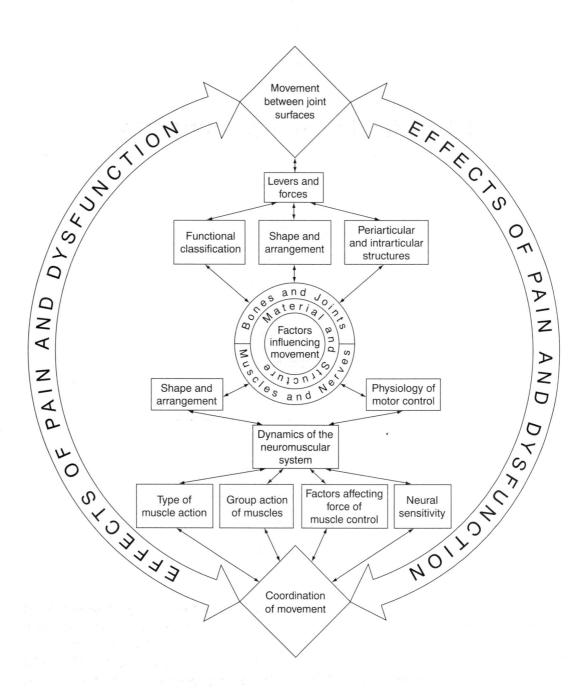

1

Classification and Terminology

JANE LOCKWOOD

Introduction

The study of the rehabilitation of normal movement requires an introduction to some of the standard terminology used when describing and analysing movement. This provides us with a common language, preventing ambiguity and misunderstanding between colleagues. In addition to this common language, there are some important basic mechanical principles affecting movement which require some consideration. This chapter will provide an overview of these two areas and for those who want to delve deeper, the recommended texts listed at the end of this chapter will provide more detailed discussion of biomechanics.

Chapter Objectives

At the end of this chapter you should have a basic understanding of the following:

- The terminology used to describe the aspects and areas of the body;
- The terminology used to describe the axes and planes of movement;
- The terminology used to describe movements of the body;
- The principles to be considered for kinematic and kinetic analysis of movement;
- An overview of the effect of external and internal forces on movement.

How is Movement Described?

Movement can be described both in terms of direction and force. The study of movement which includes its 'direction' is called *kinematics*, whereas the study of movement which analyses the forces affecting movement is called *kinetics*. Before we consider these in more detail we shall define some basic anatomical terminology.

Anatomical Terminology

All terminology is with reference to the anatomical position (Figure 1.1). This position is: standing, with the head facing forwards, feet flat on the floor (*plantigrade*) and slightly apart, with the arms down by the side and palms facing forwards. This position is the reference for describing all surfaces, postures and movements of the body irrespective of the actual starting position.

Aspects of the Body

The terms *anterior* or *ventral* indicate the surface facing forwards and their opposites are *posterior* or *dorsal*. The terms *medial* and *lateral* locate surfaces or structures relative to the midline of the body. For example, the skin on the *lateral* aspect of the upper limb is a strip from the tip of the shoulder down to the 'thumb side' of the hand and the *medial* digit of the hand is the little finger and the *lateral* digit is the thumb.

Superior or *cephalic* are terms used for the upper part or surface, and *inferior* or *caudal* are their opposites, describing the lower part or surface. Alternative terms for describing structures in relation to each other, commonly used when referring to the limbs, are *distal* and *proximal*. If something is distal in a limb it lies furthest away from the midpoint of the body (think *distal = distance*). If a structure is proximal it is close to the midline (think *proximal = close proximity*). For example, the wrist is distal to the elbow and the shoulder is proximal to the elbow.

Distal and proximal can also be used to indicate direction, for example arterial blood flows in a proximal (the heart) to distal (the capillaries) direction whereas the venous blood flows in a distal to proximal direction.

Using these terms, along with other anatomical landmarks such as bony points, helps in accurately describing a specific area/surface. This is important when recording the location of a tender area or the distribution of pain during patient assessment. However, in clinical practice these written records are usually supplemented by diagrams and body charts.

Figure 1.1 The anatomical position and terminology used to describe aspects and relationships in the body.

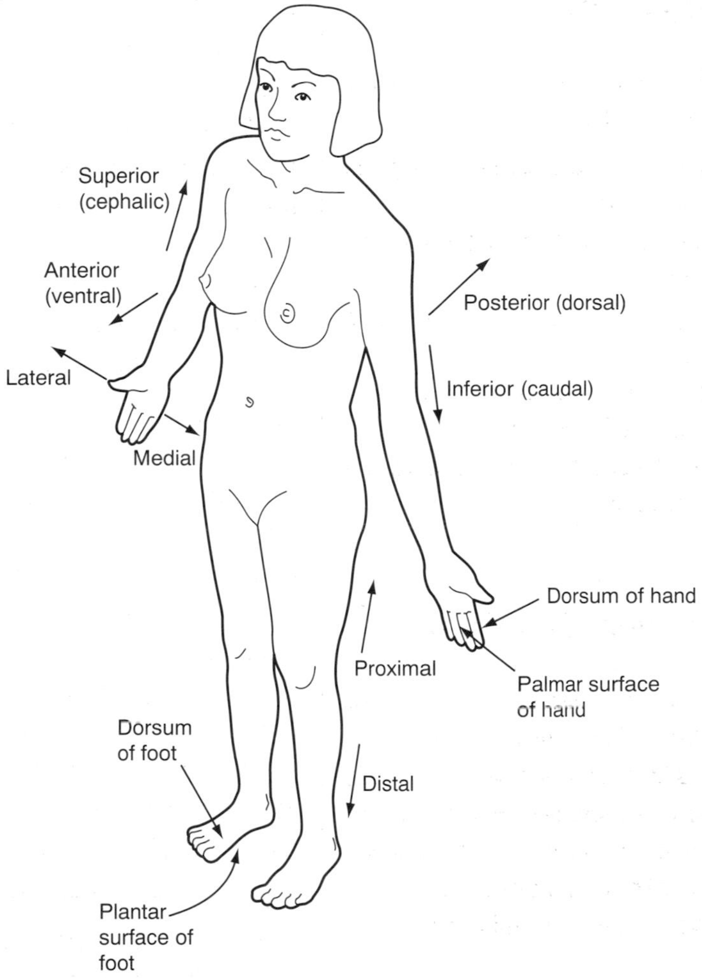

Superior (cephalic)

Anterior (ventral)

Lateral

Medial

Posterior (dorsal)

Inferior (caudal)

Dorsum of hand

Proximal

Palmar surface of hand

Dorsum of foot

Distal

Plantar surface of foot

Practical Task

On a partner indicate the following:

- *The distal part of the humerus;*
- *The anterior aspect of the forearm;*
- *The medial aspect of the leg (the 'leg' is the part of the limb distal to the knee);*
- *The proximal part of the thumb;*
- *The posterior aspect of the thigh;*
- *The lateral aspect of the knee joint.*

Terminology Used in Kinematics

In clinical practice the recording of movement frequently relies on a written description and angular measurements of joint range supplemented by diagrams. Other methods include Benesh notation (McGuiness-Scott, 1980), which records the patient's posture using symbols on musical score sheets. This is commonly used by choreographers but only a few physiotherapists.

Recording movement as a written description is not particularly accurate and some departments now have access to a human performance laboratory with specialist equipment linked to computer software. These allow more accurate and detailed quantitative measurements to be recorded and stored as a permanent record. They may then provide reliable data that can be used as a base-line for comparison with repeat measurements taken following treatment. (See Chapters 7 and 8 on measurement techniques.)

Whichever method is used to record movement, some basic terminology is required to describe the 'bending' and 'twisting' movements of our limbs. It is the combination of these movements which, when produced at more than one joint, allows the limbs to be shortened, lengthened and positioned in space, all of which are required for normal movement and function.

Axes and Planes

All angular movement can be said to occur around a particular axis and in a particular plane. Initially some find this a difficult concept when describing movements at a joint. It may help to think of a simple mechanical example such as a bicycle wheel (Figure 1.2). The strut or axle connecting the wheel to the fork of the frame is the **axis**. The space through which it is turning is the

plane. When cycling down a road, the axis is parallel to the surface of the road – so it can be further described as being a *horizontal axis*, and the wheel is turning through a plane which is perpendicular to the road, that is in a *vertical plane*. You might also wish to provide further detail on the orientation of the axis and plane. This could be done by points of the compass, for example, if travelling north, the wheels will be passing through a plane that runs in a 'north–south' direction, and the axis will be in an 'east–west' direction. *Note that the direction of the plane is always at right angles to that of the axis*. Remember this rule as it will help when thinking of the direction of the axes and planes of movements at the joints.

> Practical Task
>
> *There are many examples of everyday objects that have axes. Here are some; for each think about the direction of its axis then the direction of the plane of the moving part:*
>
> - *Opening a book which is lying flat on a desk;*
> - *Scissors cutting paper;*
> - *A door on its hinges;*
> - *A swivel seat of an office chair.*

In the above examples, as for most mechanical equipment, the axis is a fixed strut or pin which is often visible. This makes it somewhat easier to work out the direction of the axis and the plane of the associated movement. However, the axes of the joints in the body have to be imagined and, from experience, some students have difficulty with this concept. It might help to take a sheet of paper and a pencil. Use the pencil to make a

Figure 1.2   A bicycle wheel as an example of a simple mechanical axis and plane of movement.

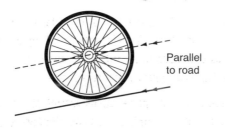

Parallel
to road

Figure 1.3   Pencil and paper — the pencil indicates the axis and the paper the plane of the movement.

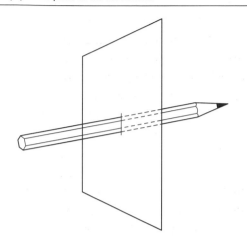

Although this terminology is standard there are acceptable alternatives.

The frontal plane can also be called the coronal plane, named after the suture by that name in the skull. The direction of this plane is from side to side and divides the body into posterior and anterior sections.

The sagittal plane is also named after a suture found in the skull. This is found between the right and left occipital bones. It divides the body into right and left parts. Yet another alternative for the sagittal plane is the *median* plane, again through the midpoint of the body, or *paramedian* if passing from front to back but not in the midline.

hole in the middle of the paper and leave the pencil passing through the paper, the pencil represents the axis and the paper, which can turn around the pencil, the plane of movement (Figure 1.3). Keep this to hand as you read the next section.

Strictly speaking, the coronal and sagittal planes divide the body into equal halves (anterior/ posterior and left/right). These are then the true *cardinal planes of the body*, but when we describe movement we usually use these terms more generally, and they can describe any plane that is parallel to the cardinal planes. If we were to be precise we should use *parasagittal* and *paracoronal*.

Planes and Axes of the Body

PLANES

The three major planes of movement pass from side to side, from anterior to posterior and from superior to inferior. They are called the frontal, sagittal and transverse planes respectively (see Figure 1.4).

AXES

We have already said that the plane of a movement is always perpendicular to its axis. Therefore if you know one you can deduce the other (Figure 1.4). However, to appreciate this let us take each plane in turn and, using the pencil and paper, name the axis of the movement.

Practical Task

Using the 'visual aid' you made earlier! Put the paper in each plane and spin it around the pencil. Note the direction of the pencil, this shows the axis of the movement for each plane. It will always be perpendicular to the plane of the movement.

Frontal plane The paper turns around the pencil in side to side plane. Therefore it is turning around an axis that runs in an anterior/posterior direction. This is a *sagittal (or median) axis*.

Sagittal plane The paper turns around the pencil lying in a plane running in an anterior/posterior

Figure 1.4 Axes and planes.

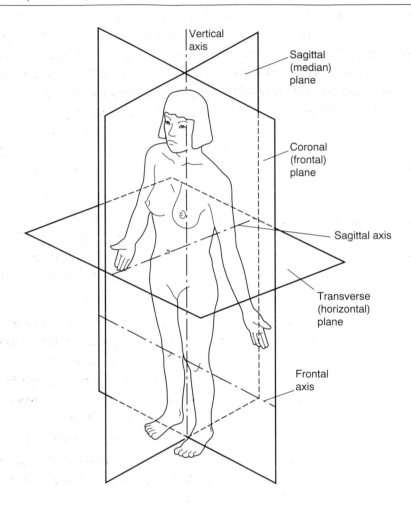

direction. Therefore the axis is passing in side to side direction. This is a *frontal (or coronal) axis.*

(Note that frontal and sagittal axes are parallel to the ground and so could also be described as being 'horizontal'.)

Horizontal plane The paper is turning in a plane parallel to the ground. This is called the *horizontal or transverse plane,* the axis of movement passes up through the paper and is described as a *vertical axis.*

Describing Movement

It is important to understand that the axis and plane of a movement that occurs at a joint are somewhat simplified descriptions. These movements do not have a fixed axis as there are no rigid pins connecting the bones. If that were so, we would have an extremely limited range of movement – rather like the joints of the skeletons hanging on stands in our classrooms! In reality the axis of a movement continually shifts when passing through a full range of movement. The amount of alteration or shift in the position of the axis will depend on the type of joint and the movement taking place. The position of the axis and how it shifts can be identified throughout the range. The position at any one point is called the *instant axis of rotation*. Although these axes are very important when determining the position of the bones and the support from ligaments, when assessing joint range we usually take the axis to be an approximate mean of all of the instant axes of rotation. It is this shifting of the axis during movement that makes a joint 'multiaxial', and movement occurs in many planes which lie between the three planes described earlier.

FREEDOM OF MOVEMENT

A joint is usually described as having one, two or three degrees of movement. These relate to the three (major) planes of movement available at a joint. These movements will now be described with reference to the axis and plane of the movement (Figure 1.5).

Flexion is the bending of a joint and usually indicates an approximation of two skin surfaces and the effective shortening of the limb. Flexion normally occurs around a frontal axis and in a sagittal plane.

Extension is the opposite movement to flexion. It is the straightening of a joint, and has the effect of lengthening the limb. This normally occurs around a frontal axis and in a sagittal plane.

Side or lateral flexion occurs in the joints of the spine. It is a sideways bend and occurs around an axis lying in the true cardinal sagittal direction, i.e. the midline, and the movement of the body is in the frontal plane. Further descriptors of 'left' and 'right' can be used to indicate the precise direction.

Dorsiflexion is the term used to describe extension at the joints of the ankle, mid-foot and toes. The angle between the dorsal or superior surface of the foot and the anterior surface of the leg (shin) is decreased. Dorsiflexion is also used as an alternative term for describing extension at the wrist, midcarpal and finger joints. Here the posterior/dorsal surface of the wrist moves towards the posterior surface of the forearm. Dorsiflexion in both the lower and upper limb occurs around a frontal axis in a sagittal plane.

Plantarflexion is the reverse of dorsiflexion, and occurs when pointing the toes. The opposite in the wrist and hand is called *palmarflexion*. These movements also take place around a frontal axis and in a sagittal plane.

Abduction is the movement that occurs at a joint when a limb is moved away from the midline of the body. (Remember if you abduct something or someone you take them away!) In the case of the fingers and toes the reference point is not the midline of the body. It is an imaginary line dissecting the second toe in the case of the foot and the middle finger in the case of the hand. Abduction occurs around a sagittal axis in the frontal plane.

Adduction is the opposite movement to abduction. It is bringing the limb or digit back to the midline. It too will occur around a sagittal axis and in a frontal plane.

Abduction and adduction at the wrist are commonly referred to as *radial deviation* and *ulnar deviation* respectively.

There is an exception to every rule and this is true for the above definitions. When describing the movements occurring at the carpometacarpal, metacarpophalangeal and interphalangeal joints

Figure 1.5   Movement of the body: (a) in the sagittal plane; (b) in the frontal plane; (c) in the transverse plane.

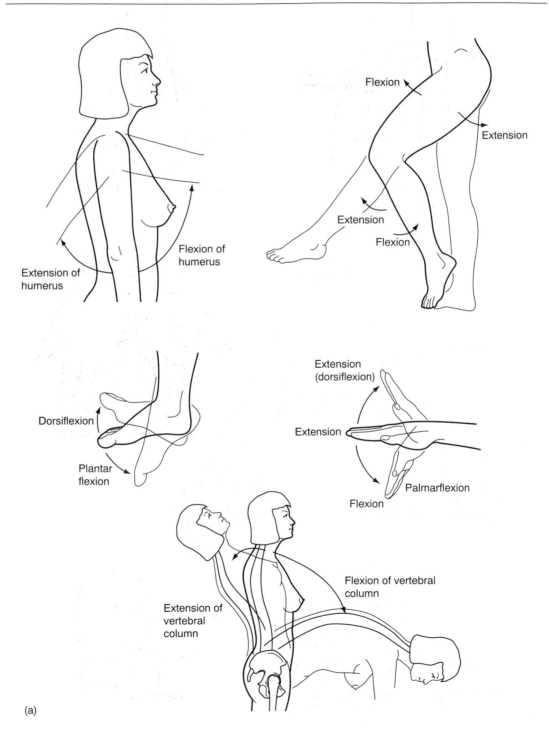

(a)

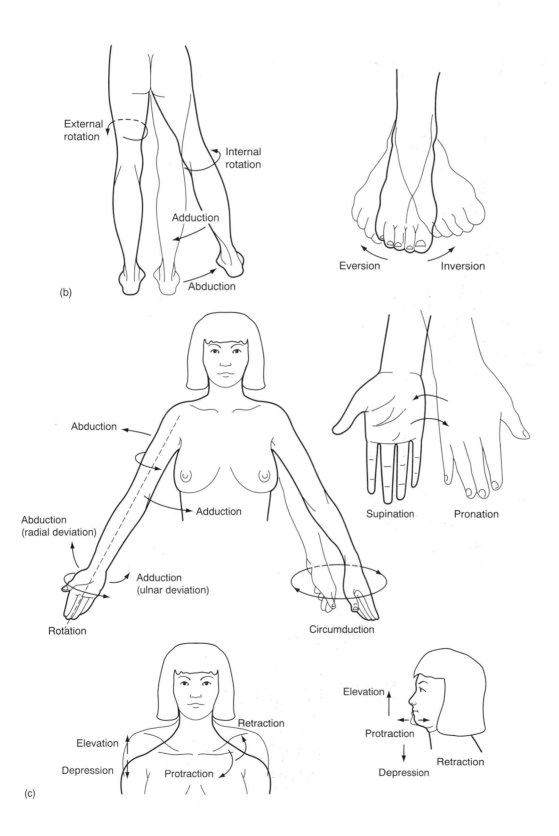

External rotation

Internal rotation

Adduction

Abduction

(b)

Eversion   Inversion

Abduction

Abduction (radial deviation)

Adduction

Adduction (ulnar deviation)

Rotation

Supination   Pronation

Circumduction

Retraction

Elevation

Depression   Protraction

(c)

Elevation

Protraction

Depression

Retraction

Figure 1.6   Movements of the thumb.

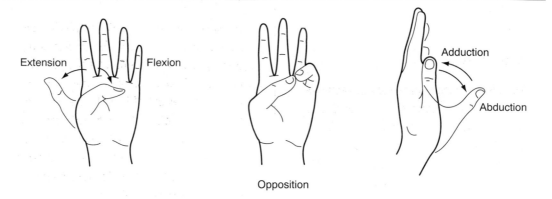

of the thumb they do not fall into the directions given (Figure 1.6).

> Practical Task
>
> *Look at your thumb in the relaxed position and note that the palmar surface, or pad, of the thumb lies in the sagittal plane; compare this to the pads of the fingers which lie in the frontal plane. This is due to the orientation of the carpometacarpal joint (the joint between the trapezium and the first metacarpal bone). It is rotated through 90° compared to the other four carpometacarpal joints in the hand.*

This results in a variation of the above description as follows.

Abduction/adduction of the thumb occurs around a frontal axis in a sagittal plane (compare to the axis and plane of flexion of the fingers). Abduction moves the thumb away from the palm and adduction into the palm.

Flexion/extension of the thumb takes the digit across the palm and then back across to the lateral side of the hand. These are around a sagittal axis and in a frontal plane (again compare this to the axis and plane of abduction and adduction of the fingers).

Opposition is a movement peculiar to the thumb and in particular to the first carpometacarpal joint. It is a combination of movements, starting from extension and abduction and passing into flexion and adduction with a simultaneous medial rotation of the first metacarpal. It is therefore a multiaxial movement passing through many planes.

It is an important movement as it brings the pad of the thumb into contact with the pad of any of the four fingers, producing *a pinch grip*. It is this ability to oppose and form a pinch grip that provides humans with the potential for fine manipulatory skill – no other animal has this high level of manual dexterity.

Rotation is turning the trunk, the head or a limb. Rotations of the head and trunk are described as rotation to the left or right – determined by the turning direction of the face or anterior surface. Rotation of the limbs is described as medial/internal or lateral/external. This depends on whether the anterior aspect is passing towards or away from the midline of the body. Rotation occurs around a vertical axis and in a transverse or horizontal plane.

Practical Task

The axis and plane of rotatory movements seem to cause some students problems when describing or analysing them. If the 'pencil and paper' method fails, think of the 'plane' as the undersurface of the chin or a transverse 'slice' of the limb. The axis then passes vertically through the head or middle of the 'slice' (like a skewer!), and rotation takes place around this axis.

Specific Types of rotation occur in the forearm and are called supination and pronation.

Supination of the forearm is the movement that turns the palm of the hand and the forearm to face anteriorly.

Pronation is the opposite of supination, and is the turning of the palm and forearm to face posteriorly.

Pronation and supination take place between the radius and ulna bones of the forearm, and occur around a vertical axis in a horizontal plane. In the anatomical position it is difficult to isolate these movements to the radioulnar joints. Try it yourself and you will find that supination naturally occurs with lateral rotation of the humerus at the shoulder joint. Similarly medial rotation tends to occur with pronation. It is for this reason that the range of movement of pronation and supination are usually tested with the elbow flexed to a right angle and tucked into the waist. This helps to prevent any rotation at the shoulder joint.

Practical Task

An aide-mémoire for supination is that it is an essential movement for eating soup politely! Take a spoonful of soup to your mouth. Without changing your hold on the spoon repeat this with the forearm fixed in pronation. You will find that it is virtually impossible, without excessive abduction at the shoulder joint, and you would then poke your neighbouring diner in the eye with your elbow!

Loss of either full pronation or supination is functionally very debilitating. To minimize this the forearm is usually immobilized in the 'mid prone' position (thumb pointing superiorly). If for some reason normal range of movement is not regained, at least the radioulnar joints will be 'fixed' in a relatively functional position, and the other joints of the upper limb can compensate.

The main exception to rotation occurring around a vertical axis and in a transverse plane is the complex rotatory movement that occurs as part of the combined movements in the foot and ankle. Here the axis is predominantly in a sagittal direction and the movement occurs mainly in a frontal plane. The movements are called *inversion* and *eversion*.

Inversion is when the sole of the foot is turned in towards the midline of the body. It is a combination of movements which include adduction and medial rotation of the foot (also called supination) and plantarflexion at the ankle joint (Williams and Warwick, 1990).

Eversion is the opposite movement, and is a

combination of abduction and lateral rotation of the foot (also called pronation) and dorsiflexion at the ankle joint.

The description of the combined movements which occur at the foot and ankle is an area where differences in use and meaning can lead to confusion. The differences concern both the specific movements that contribute to the combined movement, and also the name given to the combined movement. These are outlined below.

The first area of difference is the individual movements that contribute to inversion and eversion. Williams and Warwick (1980) in *Gray's Anatomy* associate *plantarflexion* with inversion and *dorsiflexion* with eversion; Kapandji (1985) on the other hand links *dorsiflexion* with inversion and *plantarflexion* with eversion. The former is the most frequently used.

The second area for confusion is the interchanging of terminology. Some texts, in particular those written for podiatrists, use the term *supination* for the composite movement we describe as inversion. They then call eversion *pronation*. Most traditional anatomy texts still use inversion and eversion for the combined movements of the foot and ankle complex, whereas texts and journals with a bias towards sports medicine often use the more contemporary terminology of pronation and supination. The only advice given here is to recognize that these terms are sometimes used interchangeably and with slightly different meanings, and to bear this in mind when reading the literature.

Circumduction is another composite movement, which can include all the above movements. It only occurs in a joint with many degrees of freedom and thus capable of multiaxial movement, such as a ball and socket joint. It is the movement that occurs when the hand or foot inscribes a large circle. If the circle is the base of a cone, the shoulder joint or hip joint is the apex. The axis is constantly shifting and the movement takes place in many planes.

Protraction/retraction is a forward/backward movement. The scapula protracts and retracts as it moves forwards and back around the rib cage. This movement also occurs at the jaw, in protraction the lower jaw moves forwards. The plane of movement is predominantly a sagittal one; the axis, although frontal, shifts throughout the movement.

Elevation and *depression* are also movements of the scapula and jaw. In the former they result in a 'shrug' and 'droop' of the shoulders, and in the latter they produce closing and opening of the mouth.

To reinforce some of these terms let us consider how they are used in a kinematic analysis of simple movement.

Kinematics

Definition: Kinematics is a description of the location, type, direction and magnitude of the movement.

To illustrate this we shall analyse the movement of knee extension, when sitting. Do this with your knee as you read the description, to help reinforce your understanding.

A kinematic analysis should include information on the following aspects of the movement.

The Location of the Movement

This is the identification and naming of the joint/s and the body segment/s involved in

Figure 1.7   Kinematic analysis of knee extension. (a) Movement occurring in the sagittal plane around a frontal axis; (b) the slide, roll and spin between the joint surfaces; (c) the range of movement.

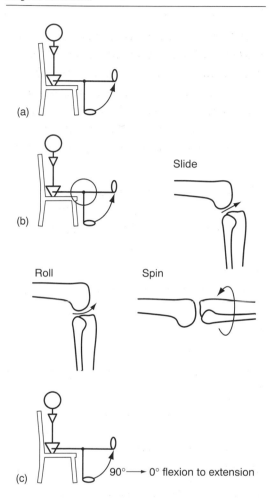

the action, and the plane/s in which the movement occurs.

Our example: The major joint involved is the knee joint, and the moving segment is the leg. Extension is in the sagittal plane around a frontal axis (Figure 1.7a).

The Type of Joint Movement

This includes a description of the movement occurring between the articular (joint) surfaces (*arthrokinematics*), and a description of the movement of the moving body segment (*osteokinematics*). We shall consider these two terms further.

ARTHROKINEMATICS

Arthrokinematics describes the movement between the articular surfaces. These are described as spins/rotations, glides/translations and rolls and occur in varying combinations throughout the full range of movement between two bones. These movements are dependent on the anatomy of the joint and surrounding musculature and this will be considered in more detail in Chapter 2.

> *Our example*: Here there is a combination of gliding and rolling between the bones throughout the movement with a pronounced spin between the lateral condyles of the tibia and femur just before full extension is reached (Figure 1.7b).

OSTEOKINEMATICS

The movements of the body segment usually take the form of an *'angular rotation'* around the joint axis (Norkin and Levangie, 1992). Williams and Warwick (1980), however, describe this movement as a *'swing'*. You will find that using the term swing avoids confusion with the rotation or spin described above which occurs between joint surfaces in arthrokinematic description.

> *Our example*: Here the leg (tibia and fibula) is the bony lever and the movement is in the form of a 'swing' around the axis at the knee joint (Figure 1.7c).

In our example the lever swings around a relatively fixed axis. However, this is not always so — the movement may be along a linear path. An example of this is the movement of the forearm when reaching forwards, as if to pick a pen off a desk.

Figure 1.8   Kinematic motion along a linear path, illustrated by the movement of the forearm when elongating the upper limb – any 'swing' component is from the flexion at the shoulder joint.

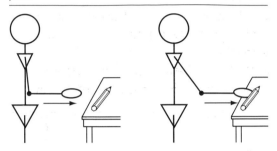

This movement produces an elongation of the upper limb (Figure 1.8)

The Direction of the Movement

The direction of the movement is described using the terms of flexion/extension, abduction/adduction etc. described earlier.

> *Our example*: The direction of the major movement is described as extension; further clarification may be given by describing it as 'extension from flexion' and the range of movement travelled stated as described below.

The Magnitude of the Movement

The amount or range of movement is an important factor when assessing function. This is done by measuring angular movement and linear movement.

ANGULAR MOVEMENT

Angular movement, or the amount of 'swing' about an axis of a joint, is measured in degrees. To do this physiotherapists use instruments called goniometers. These range from relatively inexpensive plastic protractors to more sophisticated electrogoniometers often used with computer programs to record and analyse joint movement. (See Chapters 7 and 8 for further discussion on the use and limitations of some of these instruments.)

> *Our example*: Full extension of the knee is usually considered to be 0°, although there may be movement beyond this, passing into *hyperextension*. (Hyperextension is usually expressed as a 'minus' quantity, e.g. −5°.) In our example the magnitude of movement might be 90°–0° (90° flexion to full extension) (see Figure 1.7c).

Alternatively, another unit used to measure angular movement is the *radian*. These tend to be used by engineers and mathematicians. They indicate the ratio of a length of the arc of movement to its radius. They are not used clinically, but may be encountered during further reading in literature relating to biomechanics. It is sufficient to know that **1 radian = 57.3°**.

As well as the range of movement we may also require information on the speed. This is expressed as degrees per second ($x°/s$). If we include the direction of movement then information regarding velocity is obtained, as *velocity is speed plus direction*.

LINEAR MOVEMENT

Linear movement is measured in metres. If speed is required it is recorded as metres per second (m/s).

> *Our example*: We might describe the knee extension as occurring at a speed of ten degrees per second (10°/s). However, to obtain accurate information of this type, specialized isokinetic equipment capable of measuring range of movement and calculating the speed needs to be used. It cannot be done by eye alone. (For a review of isokinetic equipment and measurement see Dvir (1995).)

The above outlines the information required to perform a kinematic analysis of a movement.

However, we often require more information on factors involved in producing, modifying or resisting the movement. The analysis of these factors is called a *kinetic analyis* of movement.

Kinetics

Definition: Kinetics is the analysis of the forces which will either resist or assist the movement.

The two major forces to be considered when analysing movement are, on the one hand, forces resisting movement, such as gravity, and on the other hand, forces producing movement, such as muscle contraction. However, there are many other factors which affect these, for example the position of the limb, the joint angle, the angle of pull from the muscle attachment. These and other influences must be considered when analysing normal movement.

In our example of knee extension, there are many factors which might affect the movement (see Figure 1.9). These can be classed as forces that resist the movement and those which assist or produce the movement:

The forces resisting the movement are:

- The 'weight' of the leg, produced by the effect of gravity;
- Additional external resistance from the weight of shoes and socks etc.;
- Inertia;
- The friction between the joint surfaces;
- The resistance from opposing soft tissues.

The forces assisting or producing the movement are:

- The force generated by the muscle;
- The elastic recoil of the intra- (within) and inter- (between/around) muscular connective tissue and the tendons.

Knee extension, in sitting, is against gravity. However, do remember that sometimes gravity is assisting the movement. In fact this is the case when, in sitting, the knee is taken back into flexion.

Generally, during day-to-day patient management, an accurate assessment of these forces is not required. However, the contribution they make to assisting or resisting movement must always be a consideration when assessing musculoskeletal function and especially when planning a suitable rehabilitation programme.

Figure 1.9   The major forces to be considered as part of a kinetic analysis extension at the knee joint. Forces assisting the movement are shown above the diagram; forces resisting the movement are shown below.

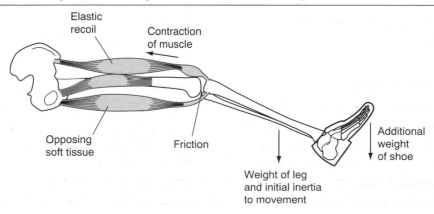

The factors identified will vary depending on the range of the movement. This is due to the variation in, for example, the direction of applied forces, the length of contracting muscles, the contact between joint surfaces and the extensibility of opposing soft tissues. These are discussed further in the next section which outlines some basic mechanical principles affecting movement. They will also be referred to again in Chapter 2, when the musculoskeletal system is reviewed with particular emphasis on how it meets the requirements for normal function.

Mechanical Principles Affecting Movement

We shall now consider how different forces, both internal and external, may affect range and quality of movement. For each, there will be a definition and brief explanation, followed by examples of the relevance to normal movement and / or the application of therapeutic skills.

The level and depth of the definitions and explanations is purposely limited to what is clinically essential and helpful. For those whose interest is stimulated, biomechanics can be studied in more detail in specialist texts, some of which are listed at the end of the chapter.

All units used are those recognized by the International Organization for Standardization (ISO), known as SI units.

Mass

Definition: The mass of a body is the quantity of matter it contains and the SI unit of mass is the kilogram (kg).

Weight

Definition: The weight of a body is the force it exerts on a surface that supports it and the SI unit of weight is the kilogram force (kgf).

All objects have mass, and this mass then has 'weight'. The density of the mass determines its size or volume and this will remain constant, but the weight may vary. The weight of an object is produced by the effect of the force of gravity pulling the object towards the earth's surface. Theoretically, this varies depending on its position on the earth's surface in relation to the centre of the earth. Perhaps in the future if physiotherapists are required to treat patients in outer space, the variability of weight due to less or no gravity will be an important issue. However, for our purposes we can usually ignore this — the variation is small and repeated measurements of weight, when used by physiotherapists, normally take place in approximately the same location!

Force

Definition: A force denotes either a push (a compression force) or a pull or stretch (a tensile force). It either produces movement and / or some internal deformation of the object. The force is often referred to as *stress* and the deformation is referred to as the *strain*. The SI unit of force is the newton (N).

A newton is a specific measure of force:

Definition: A newton is the force which produces an acceleration of one metre per second per second (1 m/s/s) when it acts on a mass of 1 kg (Force = Mass × Acceleration, F=MA). **1 kg = 9.81 N** (9.81 is the rate of acceleration of an object due to gravity).

Forces will produce movement; they can also

prevent movement and change the direction and speed (direction plus speed = *velocity*) of movement. Sir Isaac Newton is famous for his three laws of motion, which apply to both objects in motion and stationary objects. Although physiotherapists do not require a detailed knowledge of Newtonian physics, an understanding and working application of the principles of these three laws is important. You will find that they are fundamental to all aspects of normal movement and the analysis of movement, and so to physiotherapy.

Newton's Three Laws of Motion

Newton's First Law states that an object will remain in a constant state unless it is acted upon by an applied force. The tendency of an object to remain in a 'constant state' is called *inertia* and the constant state may be either stationary or a state of uniform motion.

Inertia is an important factor to consider when treating patients — the initiation of movement requires more force or effort than the continuation of the movement at the same speed and in the same direction. This means that a muscle must generate more force at the beginning of the movement, so if a muscle/muscle group is particularly weak, assistance may be needed to start the movement. This may be provided by '*active assisted exercise*', whereby the therapist provides manual assistance, which is gradually reduced as the performance of the muscle improves. Inertia is only one of many factors that influence muscle efficiency throughout the available range of movement. Some of these, such as muscle length and position, will be referred to later.

Newton's Second Law states that when a force is applied and an object does change its 'state', the amount of change of its velocity is dependent upon the force applied, the direction of the force and the mass of the object. This is also called the *law of acceleration*.

This can be applied to movement, for example the force from the contraction of the biceps brachii in the arm. A more forceful contraction of the biceps will produce faster flexion at the elbow, provided that the resistance remains the same.

The second law also states that the direction of the force affects the direction of the movement of the object — put simply, if you push someone from behind they will fall forwards! An example more specific to physiotherapy might be when applying passive manual techniques to the joints. The direction of the pressure applied during these techniques will govern the passive movement produced between the joint surfaces. This will also depend on other factors such as the shape of the articular surfaces, the ligaments and the type of joint.

Newton's Third Law states that for every action there is an equal and opposite reaction. For example during gait (walking) the force produced by the heel on contact with the ground is equal to the force transmitted up the leg from the ground — this force is known as the *ground reaction force*. If one force is increased then the opposing force must also increase. If, for example, you jump off a metre-high wall onto one heel, the force from contact between the heel and the ground increases (remember that Force = Mass × Acceleration) as does the risk of injury!

Practical Task

Imagine that two of your patients are a heavy gentleman weighing 90 kgf and a frail lady weighing 50 kgf. For ease of description we shall call them Mr Large and Mrs Little.

You must transport both patients from Ward 8 to the physiotherapy department in an identical wheelchair – and you are only allowed 5 minutes for this!

Let us now consider how we can apply Sir Isaac's laws to this task, taking each law in turn.

Newton's first law states that the patients and their wheelchairs will remain stationary until you start pushing them. When you do push, the force or effort required to overcome the inertia and move the wheelchair will be much greater for Mr Large than for Mrs Little.

Now consider **Newton's second law** of acceleration. Remember this links velocity to the mass of the object, the applied force and the direction of the force. If you only have five minutes to wheel each of them from the ward to the department, then the 'acceleration' has to be the same for each. However, we know that acceleration is inversely proportional to mass. So, if we applied the same force to each, Mr Large would have less acceleration., therefore a greater force is required to push Mr Large at the same rate as Mrs Little. (The amount of change of velocity is dependent on the force applied.) Finally, for the wheelchair to move forwards the force should also be applied in that direction, so, stating the obvious, to move the wheelchair forwards you apply a 'push' force from behind. The specific direction, obviously, would be towards the physiotherapy department!

Newton's third law states that there is an equal and opposite force acting against any other force. For example, if we consider the 'push' force on the wheelchair. This force is in a forward direction, so the opposing force will be in a backwards direction. This 'equal and opposite force' is from the weight of the patient, the wheelchair and some friction force between the tyres and the floor. All of these have to be overcome for the wheelchair to move forwards.

This 'equal and opposite' force will be greater when pushing Mr Large than when pushing Mrs Little.

The above example may seem a little trite – yet the important thing is that we remember that all movement is affected by these principles and the effects of inertia, direction, speed and resistance should all be considered when choosing appropriate exercises, applying manual resistance and assistance to regain function.

Gravity

Gravity is an invisible force that attracts or pulls all objects to the centre of the earth. The gravitational force exerted by the earth's *gravitational field* causes all objects to fall to the ground at a speed of 9.81 metres (32 feet) per second per second (9.81 m/s/s). This means that at the end of the first second of freefall the object would be dropping at a speed of 9.81 m/s but at the end of the next second it would have a speed of 19.62

m/s (9.81 + 9.81), at the end of the third second it would be falling at 29.43 m/s. The calculation of the exact speed is not always important to the physiotherapist in the clinical field. However, it is important to realize that if an object (for example a patient!), falls from a high treatment couch he will be travelling faster when he hits the floor than a patient on a lower couch. Remember, the height of the couch affects the speed, but the weight of the patients does not. So a heavier patient will travel at exactly the same 'speed' if dropped from the same height as a lighter patient. However, as he weighs more and has greater mass, he will hit the ground with more force – and so possibly do more damage to himself!

Practical Task

Consider how gravity affects the movement of the body. In the normal upright posture there are groups of muscle which tend to work against gravity most of the time, which are collectively called antigravity muscles. *For example, take your hand to your mouth, as when eating a biscuit. The muscles flexing the elbow and shoulder are, for the most part of the movement, working against gravity as it is a force resisting the movement.*

Now, crouch down on your haunches and then stand up again. Repeat this and feel the muscles on the anterior aspect of the thigh (the quadriceps femoris). You will find that the same group are working both when going down and standing up again. To bring you up again they must extend the knees against the force of gravity and so are actively shortening. This is called concentric muscle work. However, when crouching down, gravity

would actually produce the movement, but too quickly. In this case the same muscles are gradually lengthening to control the movement. This is eccentric muscle work. These different types of muscle work will be discussed further in Chapter 2.

Centre of Gravity

Definition: The centre of gravity is an imaginary point in the centre of an object's mass. It is the point of application of the resultant force from the earth's attraction.

This is also referred to as the *centre of mass,* and if an object is suspended or supported from that particular point it will be balanced. The centre of gravity for symmetrical objects is easy to find, for example, the centre of gravity of a metre rule held horizontally would be the 50 cm mark. Unfortunately, many objects, such as the human body, are not symmetrical, and although it is possible to calculate the precise centre of mass for each individual, in practice we usually rely on a good approximation. Normally we discourage the use of 'generalizations' for 'normal' individuals because there are very few people with a 'normal' body to match these generalized measurements. However sometimes, for simplification, it is acceptable to use some approximations. Studies have shown that there are points that indicate the centre of mass of the body or a segment/part of the body. The centre of mass of the body as a whole is in the midline, slightly anterior to the second sacral vertebra. Variations of this are from differences in the distribution of the 'mass' making up the body; for example there may be a difference in the ratio of muscle to fat in the lower limbs of one person compared to another. As muscle, per unit volume, has greater mass than fat, this will affect the overall distribution of the mass and so will shift the exact position off the centre of mass. The centre of mass for the person with more muscle in the lower limbs will move distally, or down towards the feet. Men usually have greater body mass in the upper part of the trunk than women. This is due to broader shoulders, larger bones and increased muscle bulk, and shifts the centre of mass slightly superiorly.

The 'normal' or average centre of mass for individual body segments have been calculated and they are usually said to be at the junction between the proximal 2/5th (40%) and the distal 3/5th (60%) of the limb or part of a limb. This is shown in Figure 1.10. (For further information refer to Low and Reed (1996) or LeVeau (1992).)

The position of the centre of mass is important in determining the stability of an object. To maintain a stable position the centre of mass must lie above

Figure 1.10   The approximate centres of mass of the body segments. (Adapted from Low and Reed, 1996, *Basic Biomechanics Explained*. Butterworth Heinneman Ltd, Oxford.)

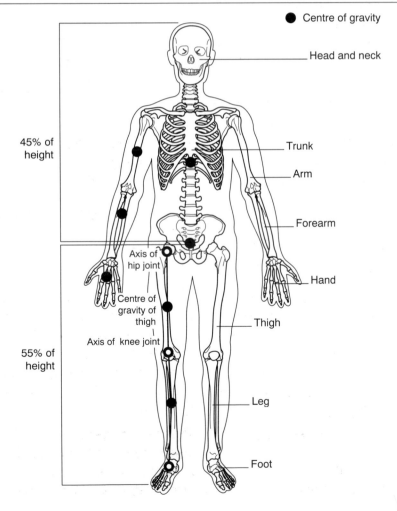

the base of support, otherwise the object will be unstable and fall over.

The Line of Gravity

Definition: The line of gravity is an imaginary line dropped vertically from the centre of mass of an object to its supporting surface.

Definition: The base of support is the contact area of the supporting surfaces plus any area that lies between these points of contact.

It is important to remember that the area between the supporting surfaces is included and so increases the base of support. For example, the base of support of a chair is where the chair legs make contact with the floor and the area of the floor between.

The body has a small base of support when standing with the feet close together. To increase this the feet can be placed further apart as when taking a long step or standing astride.

An object is most stable when its centre of mass is low and the line of gravity falls at the centre of its base of support, for example a cone or pyramidal structure. In this case the object is said to be in *stable equilibrium*. However, if the cone is inverted and balanced on a very small base with a high centre of mass, the object is very unstable and the line of gravity easily falls outside the base of support. In this case it is said to be in *unstable equilibrium*. If the object can be moved and yet the line of gravity still falls within the base, for example a rolling ball, it is then said to be in *neutral equilibrium* (Figure 1.11).

In summary an object is most stable with:

1 A large base of support;
2 A low centre of mass / gravity;

Figure 1.11   Objects in stable, unstable and neutral equilibrium.

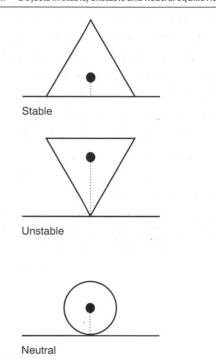

Stable

Unstable

Neutral

3 A line of gravity which falls in the middle of the base of support;
4 A symmetrical shape.

(See Practical Example and Practical Task on pages 24 and 25.)

Friction

Definition: Friction is the force that resists movement between two surfaces. It is measured in a unit called the coefficient of friction represented by the Greek letter mu (μ). A low coefficient of friction indicates that the surfaces will slide easily against each other.

There are two types of friction. There is *static* or *limiting friction*, which resists the start of any movement between two surfaces. The second type is *dynamic friction*, which resists the

Jane Lockwood

Practical Example

Think how the base of support alters over a lifespan.

A newborn baby lies on his back for most of the time, which provides a large base of support and a low centre of mass. In this position it is impossible for the line of gravity to fall outside the base – even when rolling! Therefore the baby is in neutral equilibrium. The next stage is when he begins to crawl, by first raising up onto hands and knees. The base of support is now between the four contact points of the hands and knees/legs. This is a position of fairly stable equilibrium, yet the baby can fall over, frequently to one side. The next stage is upright yet gaining additional support from furniture or push-along toys. We then progress to walking unaided, feet wide apart (to maintain a relatively large base) and taking small steps (to limit the length of time when the base is only the supporting foot).

As balance and coordination improve the final progression is walking and then running. Running has a phase when there is no base of support – the body is flying through the air and the support on landing is for a very short time with the line of gravity often falling in front of the base of support! The body is then – for a short time – in a state of unstable equilibrium, until the other foot moves forwards.

Consider too the need for greater support and increased size of base as we get older. This may result from loss of movement at the joints, with or without some loss of the balance mechanisms due to, for example, inner ear, neurological or musculoskeletal problems. In response to this, physiotherapists supply and instruct patients in the use of walking aids such as sticks, crutches and zimmer frames. All of these, if used correctly, will increase the number of contact points with the ground and so increase the size of the base of support (Figure 1.12).

Figure 1.12   The base of support in (a) standing, and the increase in the area when standing with (b) crutches or (c) a walking frame.

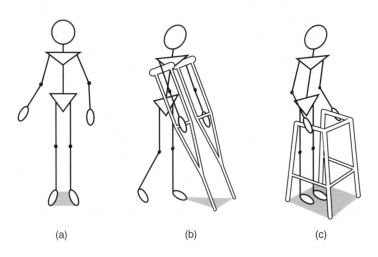

(a)   (b)   (c)

Practical Task

Although the position of the body's centre of mass can be approximated, it is continually shifting as we perform everyday activities

Try this, ideally in front of a mirror or watch someone else:

Pick up a bag full of books with your right hand.

What immediate effect does this have on the centre of mass?

It will shift across to the right and inferiorly.

Now look at yourself in the mirror (or your 'model'). Can you work out how the body adjusts to ensure that the centre of mass stays above your base — that is your feet? You might detect that your upper trunk has compensated by side-flexing to the left.

The above shows how the body adapts to an alteration in the distribution of the total mass. In this example the increase in mass is from the bag, so this postural adaptation is only temporary and normal posture is resumed once the bag is put down. However, sometimes the change is more long term, such as in the late stage of pregnancy. The weight of the baby within the uterus shifts the centre of mass forwards and slightly superiorly. A typical posture (not to be encouraged) is to lean backwards by extending the hips and lumbar spine. This does have the desired effect of shifting the centre of mass posteriorly, but some areas of the lumbar spine and hip joints are subject to increased stress, which can lead to tissue damage. A posture that creates a more even distribution of this increase in mass should be encouraged. The expectant mother should be encouraged to shift the centre of mass backwards, using the hip extensors and anterior abdominal muscles and thereby avoiding 'resting on', and stretching, the anterior ligaments of the hip joint and lumbar spine. Towards the latter part of pregnancy this is not always possible, so the best advice is to avoid having to stand for long periods of time.

Again, this alteration in the body mass is temporary. However, with patients who have had part of a limb amputated, it is important to re-educate them gradually to their 'new' distribution of weight. This is also an important consideration when supplying an artificial limb. A prosthetic limb which is as heavy as the natural one would require a huge amount of energy to move. However the body is thrown off balance if it is too light, so, there is a compromise when deciding the weight of the prosthesis. It should maintain low energy requirements yet still encourage a more normal weight distribution.

movement once it has started. Dynamic friction can be subdivided into either *sliding* or *rolling friction*. As their names suggest, these resist either a sliding motion between two surfaces or a rolling motion between one object and the surface over which it is rolling. It is important to remember that static friction is always greater than dynamic friction and sliding friction is greater than rolling friction. Like gravity, friction is an invisible force that continually has an effect on our activities. Even the air around us produces friction which we call air resistance.

The force required to overcome friction from air resistance is minimal and can be 'disregarded' in the clinical situation. However, there may be times when it can have a significant effect. Consider the effort required by a patient who may be short of breath and who has only a small energy reserve, trying to walk into a prevailing wind. The required increase in effort might be the difference between just being able do the shopping or not.

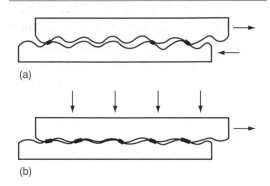

Figure 1.13 Friction: (a) Contact between asperities (on even relatively smooth surfaces) produce friction; (b) Increase in vertical pressure will flatten asperities and increase the true contact area. True contact area is shown by heavier line.

So what makes some surfaces 'non-slip' and others like ice? There are various factors to be considered:

- The true contact area between the surfaces;
- The composition and properties of the surface materials;
- The adhesion between the surfaces.

TRUE AND APPARENT CONTACT AREA

If the surface of an object is inspected by eye alone it may appear to be smooth. You might expect a smooth surface to produce less friction.. However this macroscopic appearance only informs us as to the size of the *apparent contact area*. This, however, does not tell us the actual area of contact between the surfaces. Even a smooth surface, when examined under a microscope, has many depressions and elevations, and these humps and bumps are called *asperities* (Figure 1.13a). It is the contact between the asperities of the surfaces which provide the *true contact area*, and increases the friction. The greater the true contact area then the greater the frictional force.

COMPOSITION OF THE SURFACE MATERIAL

Related to this is the hardness of the material. If the material is relatively malleable and deforms easily then the asperities will flatten when in contact with another surface (Figure 1.13b), thus increasing the true contact area. Also linked to this can be the amount of force that presses the two surfaces together: the greater the force the more the asperities flatten producing a larger true contact area and thus greater friction. This is applicable for materials of similar hardness. However, if one surface is softer than the other then the harder material will plough grooves into the softer surface, which will also increase the amount of friction.

There is another factor to consider and this is the 'stickiness' of the surfaces, producing a phenomenon called *adhesion*.

ADHESION

This is the attraction of the surface molecules to each other. Some surfaces have greater adhesive properties than others, i.e. are more 'sticky'. Each time a surface makes contact with another some 'adhesion' occurs. For movement to occur between the surfaces this adhesive bond has to be broken. It is this continual forming and breaking of the bond as the surfaces move against each other that contributes to the frictional force. These bonds occur between asperities and each time they 'break' there is some resultant wearing away of the surface. As you would expect a softer surface will wear faster than a hard one.

Practical Examples

We often think of friction as a force-resisting movement and so requiring increased effort to overcome its effect. However, remember that some friction is essential for normal movement. We need friction between the feet and the ground in order to propel ourselves forward when walking. Without friction our feet would slide backwards when we attempt to 'push off' during walking — and we would probably fall forwards!

Remember too, that it is the surfaces that are making contact that are important, so if the ward floor is wet, and the soles of the shoes/slippers become wet, then both contact surfaces are water — the water on the floor against the film of water on the sole of the shoes — a hazardous situation! Similarly if there is dust or other debris between the surfaces this can also alter the contact surface and affects the amount of friction. The water and dust will act as lubricants and so reduce friction creating a slippery surface. Lubricants are

used by physiotherapists to intentionally reduce friction between two surfaces. For example, the use of oil when massaging a patient, or applying talcum powder to make a 'sliding board' more slippery so reducing the effort required to move the limb across the board.

Excessive friction can be harmful. Friction between the skin and bedclothes can lead to a breakdown in the skin and underlying tissues, i.e. a 'pressure sore', and the risk of a pressure sore is increased as the coefficient of friction increases. In this situation friction is increased if the sheets are damp due to incontinence or perspiration, and also by the weight and position of the patient. Poor positioning and inappropriate or badly executed handling techniques may result in a breakdown of the skin and tissues in contact with the bed.

The examples in the box relate to friction affecting movement of the body and they are all external, but frictional forces also exist within the body. Examples of these are found between articular surfaces, tendons and underlying bone and even from the roughened scarred surfaces of previously damaged soft tissues. This can lead to wearing and inflammation of the tissues, and when it occurs between tendon and bone it causes an inflammatory condition called tendinitis. To reduce friction the body provides its own lubrication in the joints and around tendons, a lubricant called *synovial fluid*. This is considered further in Chapter 2.

We have seen that friction increases when the true contact area increases, and that true contact area increases when the asperities are flattened.

Therefore it is reasonable to suppose that as the weight of an object increases then the force applied to the supporting surface also increases, asperities are further flattened thereby increasing the true contact area. However, this not only depends on the 'weight' of the object, it is also related to the area of contact between the object and its supporting surface. These two factors influence the amount of *pressure*.

Pressure

Definition: Pressure is the force, acting perpendicularly, per unit area. The SI unit of pressure is 1 newton per metre square (N/m^2), also called a pascal (Pa).

$$Pressure = \frac{Force}{Area}$$

We have defined force which is measured in kilograms, and this tells us the total force applied to an object but does not indicate the size of the contact area receiving the force. Therefore we also require information on the *amount of force per unit area*, or the *pressure* being exerted on a particular contact point. High levels of pressure can lead to tissue damage. Physiotherapists should remember this when handling their patients. Manual resistance applied with a flat hand is less damaging, and uncomfortable, than a pinching grip.

Practical Example

Consider a person either standing or lying down. In each position the body weight remains the same, but the pressure from the skin in contact with the supporting surface will differ. In standing, the contact area is restricted to the soles of the feet, whereas in lying the weight is distributed over a large surface area. Hence the pressure is greater in standing. This is important to the physiotherapist. The application of force on a small area produces peaks of pressure which can cause considerable damage to the skin and underlying tissues. Patients who are overweight or underweight have an increased risk of developing the pressure sores mentioned when discussing friction. The areas particularly prone to this are where bony protuberances are taking most of the weight. In lying these are commonly the scapulae, the sacrum, the heels and elbows, whereas in sitting the ischial tuberosities take the majority of the weight. This means that particular care should be taken to minimize the effects of pressure on these vulnerable areas. This can be done by encouraging or assisting the patient to move around to relieve the pressure and/or by the use of special cushions which help to distribute the weight more evenly. Obviously there are some areas of the body — such as the soles of the feet — which are specially adapted for sustaining high pressures. In this case there is a thickening of the skin and pads of fat act as cushions between weight-bearing bones and the skin.

Analysis of Forces

The forces which must be considered during a kinetic analysis of movement are multidirectional. For example, gravity, friction and the force from muscle contraction can all act simultaneously in different directions and with different magnitude; collectively these are known as *force systems*. Force systems can be described with reference to magnitude, direction, point of application and resultant effect of the forces involved.

Magnitude This is the amount of force applied, in kilograms. This may be from the weight of the limb or moving body part, with any additional resistance applied as part of an exercise programme.

Direction This is described generally in terms such as 'vertical', or 'horizontal', or there may be more specific parameters such as '45° south' etc. The direction of the force is indicated by the direction of an action line with an arrow at the tip. To assist in the analysis of forces, the diagram should have a scale, so that the magnitude of the applied force can be represented by the length of the action line; for example, 1 cm = 1 kg.

Point of application This is the point where the applied force makes contact with the object. Remember, if this is a small area then there will be increased pressure.

Resultant effect This is the effect a force has on an object. It may be that the force moves the object, for example, when pushing the wheelchair down the ward, or applying passive movements. If movement does occur, the description should include both the direction and magnitude of the movement. However, force does not always produce movement – the effect may be internal, causing compression or tension. For example, the force of the body weight acting in standing will cause compression of the tissues on the plantar surface of the feet, and a muscle pulling on its attachment will produce a tensile force within the tendon and bone.

A general understanding of how forces act together is essential for the physiotherapist. Force systems can be categorized according to the position and direction of the forces:

- Coplanar forces;
- Colinear forces;
- Concurrent forces.

Coplanar Forces

These act in the same plane, either in the same or opposite directions.

An example of coplanar forces acting in the same direction is pushing a wheelchair. Each hand on the wheelchair handles provides a separate but parallel force acting in the same direction. If the force provided by each hand is equal then the wheelchair continues in a linear direction straight ahead – think back to Newton's second law! However, if more force were applied by the left handle,

Figure 1.14   Coplanar forces. (a) When forces of equal magnitude are applied the resultant force will follow the same path. (b) When 'push' forces of unequal magnitude are applied the resultant force is away from the greater force.

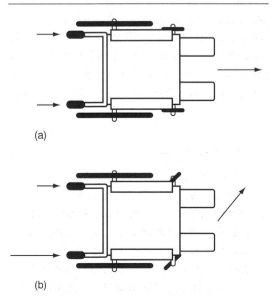

(a)

(b)

but still directed forwards, the resultant force would turn the wheelchair more to the left (Figure 1.14). Individual muscles within a group often act as coplanar forces, to assist in the overall strength and/or to modify the direction of the movement.

Practical Example

An example of coplanar forces within the body is the contraction of the right and left rectus abdominus. These two muscles pass from the ribs to the pelvis on the anterior aspect of the trunk and working together they flex the trunk. However, consider what would happen if there was an imbalance in the force produced by each – for instance the right rectus produced a greater force than the left. In this case the flexion would veer towards one side – the side that produced the greatest shortening of the muscle; in our example this would be the right (Figure 1.15a). Obviously these muscles do sometimes work in this manner intentionally and produce a controlled right side-flexion of the trunk, but this is voluntary. If the difference in the force of their contractions is not intentional normal function may be limited.

Coplanar forces may be applied to a rigid bar or lever which has a fixed axis along its length. If the forces are applied to the lever in the same direction but either side of the axis, they will produce a turning effect or a state of equilibrium. Let us

Figure 1.15 (a) Unequal coplanar forces producing rotation of a lever around its axis; (b) coplanar forces in the body. The two rectus abdominus muscles when working together with equal force will flex the trunk in the sagittal plane. If the right rectus is producing a greater 'pull' force then trunk flexion will deviate towards the same side.

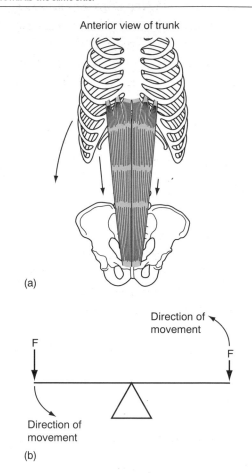

consider these in turn. If force A equals that of B, they will produce a state of balance or equilibrium and no movement will occur. If, however force A is greater than that of B (Figure 1.15b), then A will move downwards and B upwards.

Practical Example

Coplanar forces applied in the same direction to a 'bar' which is fixed at an axis can be illustrated by the simple seesaw. If two children, one at each end of the seesaw, weigh the same then the beam will be balanced. If the child on the left is heavier then the beam will go down on the left and up on the right.

In the body muscles often work together in this way. An example is those muscles which attach to the anterior (hip flexors) and posterior (hip extensors) surfaces of the pelvis. The hip flexors will rotate the pelvis anteriorly and the hip extensors will rotate the pelvis posteriorly – the axis is a frontal axis running through the hip joints. However, much of the time the pelvis is required to be balanced – thus the posterior and anterior forces should be equal (Figure 1.16).

Figure 1.17   A mechanical example of a 'force couple': a steering wheel.

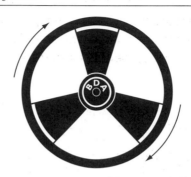

Another example of how forces may act on a lever with a fixed fulcrum, yet with a different resultant effect is when coplanar forces act in *parallel* yet are applied in *opposite* directions. This system is known as a *force couple*, and an everyday example is a car steering wheel. To turn the steering wheel to the right, there is force directed downwards on the right and one directed upwards on the left. That is, the right hand pulls down and the left hand pushes up and the wheel turns around its axis or steering column. In the body the forces produced by muscles on either side of the fulcrum produce a turning effect around a joint (Figure 1.17).

Figure 1.16   Anatomical example of coplanar forces from the hip flexors and extensors, together balancing the anteroposterior rotation of the pelvis on the lower limb.

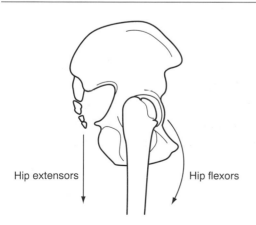

Hip extensors   Hip flexors

Anatomical Examples

There are many anatomical examples of muscles acting as force couples, as a turning or rotary effect is often required. The muscles controlling the turning of the scapula is one example. The trapezius is a large triangular muscle with its proximal, broad attachment to the vertebral column. Its lower fibres pass to the medial end of the spine of the scapula and its upper fibres to the lateral end. When both these sets of fibres contract the resultant movement is rotation of the scapula, its inferior angle being rotated laterally (Figure 1.18). Note that although the scapula has no mechanically 'fixed' axis like the centre of a steering wheel, it is stabilized by the action of surrounding muscles.

Colinear Forces

These are a specialized form of coplanar force systems. They are not only acting in the same plane, but also along the same lie of action. This may be in the same or the opposite directions. When acting in the same direction colinear forces will summate to produce a greater pushing or pulling force on the object. Colinear forces acting

Figure 1.18   An anatomical example of a force couple. The lower and upper fibres of trapezius working together to laterally rotate the scapula. Black area = approximate position of axis.

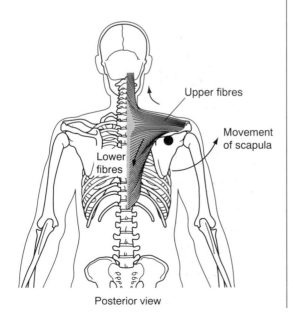

Upper fibres

Movement of scapula

Lower fibres

Posterior view

Figure 1.19   Colinear forces (a) acting together the forces summate; (b) acting in opposite directions to produce a compression stress; (c) acting in opposite directions to produce tensile stress.

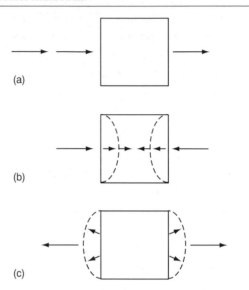

(a)

(b)

(c)

in opposite directions will oppose each other and produce either a compression force (e.g. squashing a ball), or distraction/tensile force (e.g. stretching a rubber band), within the object (Figure 1.19).

Practical Examples

A mechanical example of colinear force systems is a tug of war competition. The combined effort of the members of each team illustrate colinear forces acting in the same direction, all attempting to pull the other team towards the line. However the opposing forces produced by the two teams, each pulling in the opposite direction illustrate how when forces are in opposition they produce tensile or distractive forces within the rope.

Anatomical examples of true colinear forces, acting along the same action line are not common, but again we could refer to the rectus abdominus (Figure 1.17). This muscle has sections of muscle fibres separated by noncontractile tendinous tissue. These sections lie in series and therefore the resultant force of the muscle contraction will be from the sum of the forces of each section.

Another example is seen when studying the principles of muscle contraction. This is produced by the contraction of many individual sarcomeres, all lying in series. It is the combined force of all these working together, drawing the extremities of the muscle fibre and its attachments together.

Joints are continually subject to compression or tension/distraction forces. In standing the hip joint is compressed by the weight of the upper body acting in a downward direction and the ground reaction force acting up through the leg (remember Newton's third law?). Yet the glenohumeral joint at the shoulder tends to be subject to forces that produce distraction of the joint surfaces. The weight of the upper limb will produce a downwards force and the muscles holding the scapula in place will counterbalance this with an upwards force. Hence there will be a tendency for the head of the humerus to move away from its socket (the glenoid fossa). Note that the lower limb is a predominantly weight-bearing limb in contrast with the functions of the upper limb, therefore the forces described here are typical for joints of the upper and lower limbs.

Concurrent Forces

These have the same point of application but do not have the same action line. The resultant single force is a compromise. This is an important concept as many muscles in the body share attachments at one insertion yet arise from different origins; the different origins mean that the action lines lie in varying directions. This can also be applied to the arrangement of the fibres in individual muscles, for example the deltoid muscle on the superior aspect of the shoulder. This has three main groups of fibres, the anterior, middle and posterior, and their action lines all meet at the common attachment on the lateral surface of the humerus. The anterior fibres alone will assist flexion of the arm. Similarly the posterior fibres will assist extension. However, working together they produce abduction of the arm (Figure 1.20).

Figure 1.20   Concurrent forces at the shoulder joint. The deltoid has three distinct groups of fibres. The anterior produce flexion, the posterior extension and the middle abduction. When the anterior and posterior work together they produce and assist in abduction.

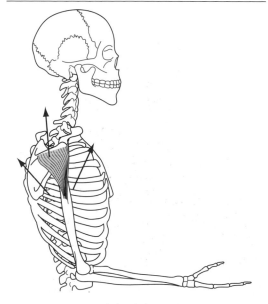

Lateral view

Composition of Forces

There is often a need to calculate the resultant force produced by a force system. If the forces are acting along the same action line and in the same direction the calculation is a simple case of the sum of the forces. Similarly if the forces are acting in opposite directions then the resultant force can be calculated by subtracting one from the other, with the greater of the two forces determining the resultant direction.

However, as stated earlier, forces are frequently multidirectional, and calculation of the resultant force by means of simple addition and subtraction is not always possible. In this case the calculation can be done graphically. If there are two forces involved then a *parallelogram of forces* can be drawn (Figure 1.21). For this you need to know the magnitude of the individual forces and the

Figure 1.21   Parallelogram of forces. Force A and Force B applied in the direction and quantity as indicated by the direction and length of the action lines. The resultant force will be Force C which also shows direction and quantity.

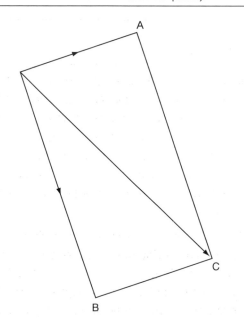

angle they make at their shared point of application. This is drawn to scale and then the two further sides are drawn in to complete the parallelogram. The diagonal from the point of application is measured and this will be the magnitude of the resultant force.

If there are many forces acting on a point then a polygon of forces can be drawn. Here, one vector is drawn to scale in the correct direction from the point of application. Then the next force is drawn, starting at the tip of the previous vector, again, drawn to scale and in the correct direction. This can be further added to in the same way — each additional vector line starting from the tip of the previous one. The final stage is the drawing of the resultant line, drawn from the tip of the final vector line to the original starting point. The direction and length of this 'resultant line' will represent the direction and magnitude of the resultant force.

Free Body Diagram

The free body diagram is a graphical method of calculating all the forces affecting an object / body in a particular position. When used for description of forces acting on the human body it usually involves drawing a 'stick man' and identifying the forces acting on the body. These are accurately represented by vectors showing both magnitude and direction, and must include body / body segment weight, ground reaction forces, forces produced by muscle contraction, force of friction and any other external forces such as resistance related to a specific activity.

It is beyond the scope of this book to describe how this and other methods are employed for the analysis of the complex force systems encountered in the study of biomechanics. The reader is advised to consult the recommended texts listed at the end of the chapter for further information.

Resolution of Forces

We have seen that the resultant force can be calculated using two or more forces. Similarly a force acting in a single direction can be considered as having more than one component, and so we can split the force into several separate components each with a different action line. This is often useful when considering the single force produced by a muscle which causes a rotary 'swing' of a bone around the joint axis. Splitting the force into two components can give a clearer picture of the differing effects the muscle's pull. For this the action line is identified as a line passing from one

Figure 1.22 Resolution of forces. The force of the contraction of the biceps brachii (A) can be resolved into two forces. Force B acts has an action line connecting the distal part of the moving segment to the axis of movement. In this diagram this will produce a compressive force across the joint. Force C is perpendicular to this and produces the 'swing' or rotary component of the movement.

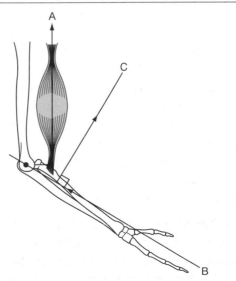

attachment to the other, usually longitudinally through the muscle belly, and the point of application of the force is the attachment of the tendon to the bone.

To illustrate this let us take the biceps brachii as an example. When the muscle shortens it produces flexion at the elbow joint and the bones of the forearm swing in a sagittal plane, turning around an axis passing through the elbow joint and lying in the frontal plane (Figure 1.22). This force A, from the contraction of the biceps muscle, can be resolved into two components. One, force B, acts along the shaft of the moving bone, passing through the axis. This will produce either compression or distraction between the joint surfaces. The second component, force C, is at right angles to this and produces the swing or rotary movement around the joint. Whether the joint is compressed or distracted will depend on the position of the elbow and will now be considered with reference to calculating the torque (or moment of force) of the 'swing' of a bone around a joint.

Levers

Definition: A lever is a rigid bar, or any rigid structure, that pivots about an axis, which is called a fulcrum. Two other forces are applied at some point along the length of the bar; these are called the effort and the weight or load. The effort tends to produce movement whereas the weight or load resists the movement of the lever around the fulcrum.

The body consists of many segments which can be considered as an interconnected system of anatomical levers. These levers are continually subject to internally and externally applied forces. To understand how these forces might affect movement it is necessary to apply the mechanical principles of levers in a little more detail. Each body segment can move around an axis or fulcrum provided by a joint. For the lever to move around the fulcrum, a force, *the effort*, is applied at any point along the lever. Provided this is sufficient to overcome the resistance, then the lever will move. In the body the effort is usually provided by the contracting muscles and the load is the weight of segment being moved, plus any additional weight/resistance to movement.

To calculate the effort and load, we also have to take into account the distance between each and the fulcrum. The distance from the load to the fulcrum is called the *load arm* and the distance from the applied effort to the fulcrum is called the *effort arm*.

The formulae used to calculate the magnitude of the forces are:

(Total) Effort = Effort × length of effort arm
(Total) Load = Load × length of load arm

When the Effort is equal to the Load the lever is said to be in balance or equilibrium, and the sum of the forces equals zero.

$$\Sigma F = 0$$

If the effort required to turn the lever is less than the load, then there is said to be a mechanical advantage.

Mechanical Advantage

Definition: The mechanical advantage (MA) is the ratio of the Load to the Effort.

$$\text{Mechanical Advantage} = \frac{\text{Load}}{\text{Effort}}$$

Therefore, expressed as a ratio, if the effort is equal to the load, the MA = 1

If the Effort required is greater than the Load it is said to have an MA < 1.
If the Effort required is less than the Load it is said to have an MA > 1.

The mechanical advantage of a lever depends on the relative positions of the fulcrum, and the applied effort and load. These can be in three different combinations and form the three orders of levers (Figure 1.23).

Orders of Levers

FIRST ORDER

In this type of lever the fulcrum always lies between the resistance and the effort. Simple mechanical examples are a seesaw and a set of balance scales. These may have an MA > 1 or an MA < 1, depending on the length of the load and effort arms.

Anatomical Example

An anatomical example of a lever of the first order is the articulation between the skull and the first cervical vertebra at the atlanto-occipital joint (Figure 1.23a). The joint is the fulcrum, the weight of the head is the load and the posterior muscles of the neck produce the effort. Remember that the weight of an object will act through its centre of mass and follow the line of gravity to the floor. In normal standing, the centre of mass of the head lies above the fulcrum and the head is 'balanced' on the cervical spine. However, if there is a small degree of flexion, this shifts the centre of mass (load) in front of the fulcrum and therefore the head tends to droop forwards. The effort to bring the head upright is applied by the cervical spine extensor muscle — lying behind the fulcrum. If the head is extended though, the centre of mass moves behind the fulcrum and the effort moves in front. However, the classification of the lever remains a first order one.

This order of lever can have an MA either greater or less than 1, depending on the distance of the effort from the fulcrum. If the effort arm is longer than the weight arm then it has an MA > 1, if the load arm is longer, then MA = < 1.

SECOND ORDER

In this type of lever the application of the load is always between the fulcrum and the effort (Figure 1.23b). Mechanical examples of this type of lever are the wheel barrow and a door with hinges on one side and a handle on the other. This order of lever always has a mechanical advantage greater than 1, as the effort arm is always longer. Therefore the effort required is always less than the load.

Anatomical Example

There are few good anatomical examples for the second order. One commonly used is the brachioradialis muscle when it is assisting with flexion at the elbow joint (Figure 1.23b). This muscle attaches to the humerus just proximal to the elbow and passes along the lateral border of the forearm to attach to the distal end of the radius. The fulcrum is the elbow, the load is the weight of forearm and hand — which, if you remember from earlier in the chap-

ter, will have its point of application through the centre of mass of the forearm. The effort is from the contraction of the muscle acting via its attachment to the distal end of the shaft of the radius. Therefore the position of each is as shown in the diagram.

Consider what would happen to the order of lever in this example if a heavy weight were placed in the hand. The weight would affect the position of the centre of mass — moving it distally. This would alter the relative positions of the load and effort. The effort would now lie between the load and the fulcrum turning it into a second order of lever with an MA < 1.

THIRD ORDER

In this type of lever the effort is always applied between the fulcrum and the load (Figure 1.23c). Mechanical examples of third order levers include a paper stapler. This type of lever always has a mechanical advantage less than 1, as the effort arm is always shorter. Therefore the effort required is always greater than the load.

Anatomical Example

The third order of lever is the type most frequently found in the body. The joint (fulcrum) is normally at the proximal end of the bone or segment, for example the elbow joint. The load is the weight of the forearm and hand, plus any additional resistance, for example a shopping bag. This additional load will shift the centre of mass of the segment, and thus the effective point of application of the load,

Figure I.23 The three orders of lever and anatomical examples. (a) First order, e.g. head balanced on the spine; (b) second order, e.g. brachioradialis as a flexor of the elbow; (c) third order, e.g. biceps brachii as a flexor of the elbow.

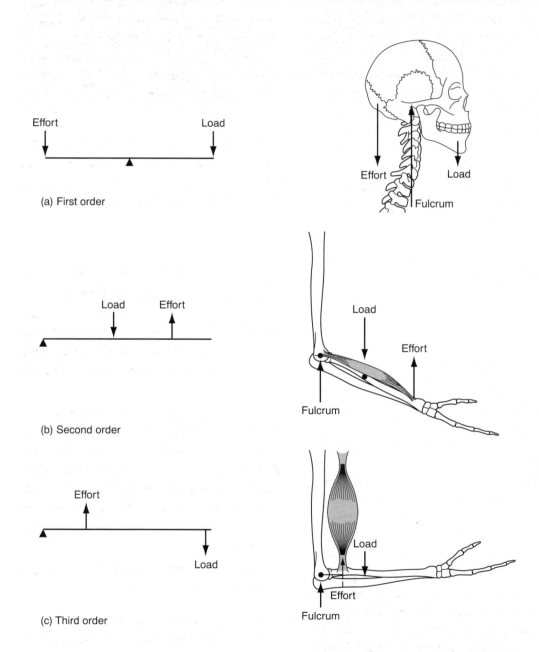

(a) First order

(b) Second order

(c) Third order

distally, increasing the length of the load arm. Finally, the effort required to move the load is produced by the contraction of muscles, for example, the biceps brachii working as flexors of the elbow (Figure 1.23c). This takes its attachment just distal to the elbow joint, and therefore has a relatively short effort arm.. This type of lever always has an MA < 1 and therefore the effort required will always exceed the weight of the load. Although it is not very efficient in terms of power, this arrangement is excellent for producing large movements of the distal end of the lever, which in our example is the hand, and keeping the muscle bulk crossing the joint to a minimum.

Practical Application

The body is comprised of a system of levers. These range from the long levers found in the lower limb to short levers formed by bony projections, such as the spinous and transverse processes of the vertebrae. Physiotherapists frequently use these anatomical levers to apply manual techniques, such as resisted exercise to a movement and passive joint mobilization techniques. Anteroposterior pressure on the spinous processes is used to produce movement and so mobilize the intervertebral apophyseal joints. However, there is considerable variation in the length and directions of these processes. There is also likely to be further variation in the force and direction of the applied pressure (both intertester and intratester differ-

ences) and finally there are many complex factors to be considered when calculating the resistance from the soft tissues in the area! We should be wary about being too dogmatic as to the mechanical effects of these techniques! For further discussion on this refer to Lee et al. (1996).

As seen in the example above, the order of the lever, and hence the effort required, can change when an external weight is applied; lengthening the lever may also have the same effect.

Torque or Moment of Force

Definition: Torque is the force that causes a turning movement of a lever around an axis. In the body this is usually the swing of a bone around a joint.

The SI unit for torque is newton-metres (Nm). Both force and length are included as the resulting number indicates not only force in newtons but also the length of the effort arm in metres. Torque can also be described as having direction, e.g. clockwise, or in the case of kinetic analysis we could use flexion/extension, abduction/adduction etc.

To calculate the effort required to resist the torque around the joint we need:

- The position of the axis of the joint;
- The point of application of the effort, and its line of action;
- The point of application of the load and its line of action;
- The load.

Figure 1.24 To illustrate the increase in torque around the hip joint with the knee extended. (a) Knee flexed: application of load is closer to axis; (b) Knee extended: application of load moves distally.

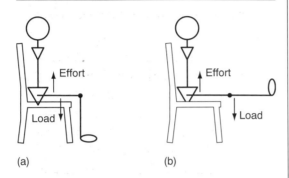

(a)   (b)

The equation to calculate the torque of a movement has the same principles as calculating leverage, and can therefore be expressed as:

$$\text{Load} \times \text{Load Arm} = \text{Effort} \times \text{Effort Arm}$$

The load is produced by the resistance to the movement, often from the weight of a limb.

The length of the load arm is the *horizontal* distance between a *vertical line* dropped from the axis and a *vertical line* dropped from the centre of mass of the moving part.

The effort is the force produced by the muscle contraction to maintain equilibrium (or greater if movement is required).

The length of the effort arm is the *horizontal* distance between a *vertical line* dropped from the axis and a *vertical line* dropped from the application of the effort — usually the tendon insertion.

Note the distances are horizontal measures between vertical lines transecting these specific points. We shall now see why this is important.

Let us take the example of hip flexion, first with the knee flexed and then with the knee straight

(see Figure 1.24). Before going into the calculations, sit down and try hip flexion both ways — making sure that you lift the back of the thigh clear of the seat. You should find that it is more difficult and requires more effort to do this with the knee extended. This is, in part, because the torque around the hip joint is greater with the knee extended. Why is this? We haven't increased the size of the leg. What we have done is *increased the length of the load arm*, by shifting the centre of mass distally.

For those interested in a hypothetical example of a calculation of this, see the text box.

Practical Example

If we use the formula and substitute some forces in kilograms (SI units are shown in brackets). First let us calculate the torque.

With knee flexed:
Load = weight of leg = 10 kgf (98.1 N)
Load arm = 50 cm (0.5 m), from axis of hip joint to centre of mass thigh with knee flexion
Effort = force from contraction of the hip flexors (unknown = E_1)
Effort arm = 10 cm (0.1 m), from axis of hip joint to tendon insertion

Therefore:

Load $\times$ load arm = effort $\times$ effort arm
Substituting numbers:
$10 \times 50 = E_1 \times 10 - (98.1 \times 0.5 = E_1 \times 0.1)$
$500 = E_1 \times 10 \ (49.05 \ Nm = E_1 \times 0.1)$
$E_1 = 50 \ kgf \ (490.5 \ N)$

Now:

With knee extended:
Load = 10 kg (98.1 N — unchanged)
Load arm = 75 cm (0.75m — increased

length of lever as extension of the knee shifts centre of mass distally)

Effort = Force of muscle contraction (unknown = E_2)

Effort arm = 10 cm (0.1 m − unchanged)

Therefore:

Load × load arm = effort × effort arm
Substituting numbers:
$10 \times 75 = E_2 \times 10 \; (98.1 \times 0.75 = E_2 \times 0.1)$
$750 = E_2 \times 10 \; (73.575 \, Nm = E_2 \times 0.1)$
$E_2 = 75 \, kg \; (735.75 \, N)$

The effort required to resist the torque or moment of force around the hip joint is greater when the knee is in extension; the 'load' moves distally so increasing the distance between the axis and the 'load'.

Practical Example

If applying manual resistance to a movement the position of your hands applying the 'load' or resistance is important. As the resistance increases so will the torque. This will affect the amount of effort required to resist the movement.

Take an obliging colleague and apply manual resistance to extension at the knee. First apply the resistance by placing your hands just distal to the knee joint. Then repeat the procedure with your hands placed just proximal to the ankle.

Can you detect a change in the amount of effort required to resist the movement? It should have been easier the second time, with your hands placed just proximal to the ankle. This is because you have increased the length of the 'load arm' and therefore increased the total load or resistance. Your colleague would have to work harder to overcome this increase in torque.

If a rotational force is applied to the distal port of a limb it will produce a twisting or torsional strain along the limb. This may result in ruptured ligaments or even fracture of the bone. Consider how this force would increase as the length of the lever increases. Skiing accidents often result in severe leg and knee injuries (the ankle tends to be supported by the ski boot), as the force of the torque is increased by the long lever provided by the ski.

On trying the practical task in the box, you may have noticed that the effort required also varied depending on the amount of flexion at the knee. This is due to a variety of factors, including:

- The position of the joint;
- The angle of pull of the tendon;
- The efficiency of muscle contraction in different ranges.

Another influencing factor may have been your own position/posture throughout the movement; a shift in your posture can influence the force of the resistance applied.

The three factors listed above all require some consideration in kinetic analysis of movement. We shall now take each and see how they influence the torque around a joint. To illustrate this we shall again use as an example flexion of the elbow produced by the contraction of the biceps brachii.

1. The *axis* of the movement is identified on the lateral side of the joint.

2. The *effort* is the force required to flex the elbow and, in this case, is produced by the contraction of the biceps brachii. The point of application of the effort is the attachment of the biceps tendon to the proximal shaft of the radius, just distal to the elbow joint. The line of application is a line passing upwards from this attachment, through the muscle belly, to its proximal insertion on the scapula.

3. The *load* is produced by the weight of the forearm and hand and, as described previously, its point of application is at the centre of mass. The centre of mass of the forearm is where the proximal $\frac{2}{5}$th meets the distal $\frac{3}{5}$th.

Position of the Joint

Remember, when calculating the torque, we use the horizontal length of the load arm from our vertical lines dropped from the axis and the centre of mass. It is a change in this that causes the variation of the length of the load arm and depends on the degree of flexion. For the same reason, there is also a slight variation in the length of the effort arm — although if the muscle is inserted close to the axis there is not usually such a significant change in length.

Look at the three positions in the diagrams, and compare the length of the load arm:

(Full extension = 0°)

1 With the elbow at 90°, the length of load arm (l^1) is at a maximum (Figure 1.25a).

2 With the elbow at 160°, the load arm (l^2) decreases (Figure 1.25b).

3 With the elbow at 40°, the load arm (l^3) also decreases (Figure 1.25c).

Therefore the effect of the load, i.e. the weight of the forearm, is at a maximum when the elbow is at a right angle, and the torque will be greatest in this position. As the elbow passes further into flexion, or further into extension, the length of the load arm decreases, thus decreasing the torque acting on the elbow joint.

However, even though the total load reduces, there is a loss of effort due to the angle of pull of the biceps.

The Angle of Pull of the Tendon

A force is most efficient in turning a lever when the line of application is perpendicular to the lever. In the body the torque produced by the muscle is most efficient when the angle between the tendon and the bone is at a right angle. Where there is a fixed axis of movement and fixed muscle attachments it is impossible to achieve this throughout the full range of movement. Consider our example.

1 With the elbow at 90°, the angle of pull (θ^1) is at a right angle, and therefore at its most efficient for producing the turning force around the joint (Figure 1.25a).

2 With the elbow at 160°, the angle of pull (θ^2) <90° (Figure 1.25b).

3 With the elbow at 40°, the angle of pull (θ^3) <90° (Figure 1.25c).

Why does either a decrease or increase from a right angle affect the force applied? For this we have to use the resolution of forces discussed previously.

When the elbow is nearing extension (Figure 1.25b) the angle of pull is less than 90°, and the effort can be resolved into two separate forces. Firstly there is the force with its action line drawn from the distal end of the bone and through the joint axis. This will produce a compressive force between the joint surfaces. Secondly, there is a force perpendicular to the first, which produces

Figure I.25   Showing the alteration in the load and the change in the angle of pull with varying degrees of elbow extension and the effect this has on the 'swing' and 'compression/distraction' of the joint. (a) At 90°, (b) At 160°, (c) At 40°.

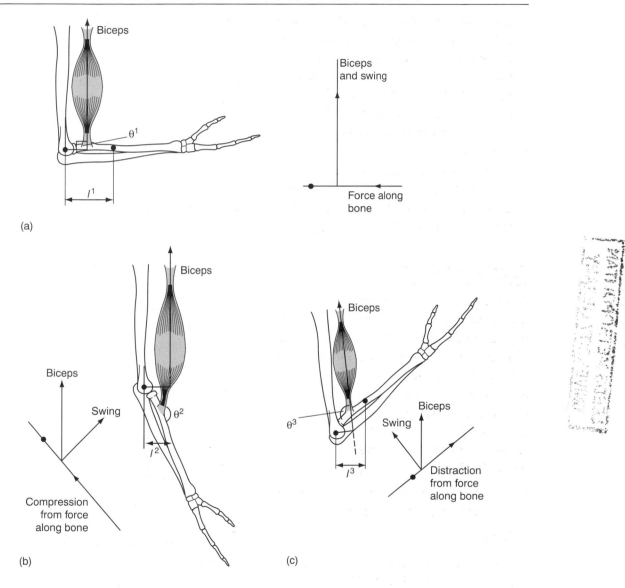

the turning force or 'swing' of the bone around the joint.

Compressive forces across joints may increase the friction between the surfaces, but their most important function is to increase the stability of the joint. Joints that require greater stability are overlaid with short, deeply situated muscles whose major role is to produce compression between the bones and so increase stability.

Consider the resultant forces when the elbow is nearing full flexion (Figure I.25c) and the angle of pull is greater than 90°. The effort produced can be resolved into two separate forces. That force acting through the joint axis will produce distraction between the articular surfaces. The force perpendicular to it will produce the swing of the bone.

From the above it can be seen that the turning effect of the muscle contraction will be reduced depending on the joint position. This does not automatically mean that the movement is always, proportionately, that much weaker. Frequently a joint has more than one muscle contributing to the turning effect. This means that if the tendon of one muscle is not at the optimum position for contributing to the swing (at right angles) of the bone around the axis, then another might be. For further discussion of this see Chapter 2.

Efficiency of Muscle Contraction

A muscle develops the most force or tension when it is acting in mid range, that is neither fully stretched nor fully shortened. There are many reasons for this and these will be covered when discussing the roles of muscle in Chapter 2.

Pulleys

To gain the optimum position for applying a force pulleys may be used.

Definition: A pulley is a grooved wheel with a rope passing in the groove; a load is attached to one end of the rope and the effort is applied to the other end.

The pulley wheel rotates around an axis. This allows the wheel to turn with minimal energy lost as heat due to friction. If the pulley is not in the form of a wheel then there will be friction between the wheel and the rope. This occurs when a pulley is in the form of a groove holding the rope in position. Although a pulley wheel is a low friction device, there is some loss of energy in the form of heat produced by friction between the wheel and its axle, but this is usually insignificant.

Mechanical pulleys are used to alter the angle of pull, for example when lifting a weight. The pulley wheel is attached above the weight. The rope passes from the weight, up around the wheel then back down to the point of application of the effort. This allows the force to be applied to the pulley rope in a downward, rather than upward, direction. This should be taken into consideration when moving a patient, where gravity assists the effort, rather than 'lifting' against gravity.

Anatomical pulley systems are found within the body. They may consist of a groove on the surface of a bone which is covered with smooth cartilage to reduce friction. A tendon passes in the groove, changing direction before its attachment to another area.

Practical Examples

Pulleys are frequently found in the clinical field and they are important components of hoists. Hoists are used to assist in the transfer of patients from bed to chair, wheelchair to bath etc. A pulley (or row of pulleys) is attached to an overhead frame and a rope passes from the canvas sling, supporting the patient, over the pulley wheel and then down again. The end of the rope is attached to a lever; this is at a height that enables the carer to apply the required effort in a downward direction. Although the effort required to lift the load is the same whether applied in an upward or downward direction, a downward force utilizes the effect of gravity and the carer's body weight to help muscular effort. Hoists, providing they are used correctly, reduce the risk of injury (particularly to the back). You may find that some hoists include numerous pulleys. Some of these may alter the direction of the force, whilst others may be positioned so that they actually reduce the amount of effort required to move the load. A block and tackle works on this principle.

Weight and pulley systems are found in 'multigym' apparatus used to apply resistance for strengthening muscles or muscle groups. By being able to vary the direction of the line of application, the patient can be positioned so that maximal force can be applied to a specific part of the range of movement.

Anatomical Examples

An example of an anatomical pulley is found where the tendon of obturator internus (a deep lateral rotator and stabilizer of the hip) passes across the posterior surface of the ischium. The tendon is formed within the pelvis and passes posteriorly around the ischium, just above the ischial tuberosity. This part of the bone is grooved, forming a pulley, for the tendon to pass through an acute angle to then cross the posterior surface of the hip joint and take its attachment on the femur.

Sesamoid bones, bones found within tendons, can also act as pulleys by distancing the tendon from the joint. This increases the length of the effort arm, thus increasing the torque, and can improve the efficiency of the angle of pull. The patella is an example of a sesamoid bone which improves the angle of pull of the quadriceps femoris muscles found on the anterior aspect of the thigh. The presence of the patella increases the angle of pull and also the length of the effort arm. Following surgical removal of the patella, the distance from the effort to the axis is reduced and the angle of pull is decreased. This affects the efficiency of the quadriceps muscle, requiring around 30% greater effort from the muscle to produce the same torque. (For further information see Nordin and Frankel (1989) and Peebles and Margo (1978).)

Stress and Strain

So far we have considered what constitutes a force and the effect forces may have on objects, especially relating to movement of the object. However, in addition to moving the object we must also consider the effect of forces internally, within the object. These are termed stress and strain.

Definition: Stress is the force *within* a material. The effect of stress is strain.

Definition: Strain is the resultant deformation or change in shape of an object which is subjected to stress. This deformation may be temporary or permanent and may occur immediately or over time, but it is always proportional to the stress applied.

Stress

Stress is measured as the force applied over an area, in newtons per square metre (N/m^2). There is a direct relationship between the force applied and the cross-sectional area of the object.

$$\text{Stress} = \frac{\text{Force}}{\text{Cross-sectional area}}$$

Anatomical Application

Think of the relative cross-sectional area of the bones of the skeleton — those with greater cross-sectional areas are the ones required for weight bearing. The femur in the thigh has a far greater cross-sectional area than the humerus in the arm. Conversely a bone's function can be determined from its structure. Consider the tibia and fibula in the leg; which bone do you think has a weight bearing role? It is obvious that the tibia is designed to take weight and the fibula, although important for maintaining stability of the ankle joint, is primarily useful for the attachment of muscles.

The effect of stress on an object depends not just on the cross-sectional area but also varies depending on the make-up of the object itself. Take a grape and a pebble between thumb and index finger, and pinch both equally hard. The force and stress is the same, but the resultant strain is very different, as the grape is squashed flat but the pebble remains intact. When comparing the grape and the pebble there are two factors to consider:

firstly the individual substance/s they are made of and, secondly, how these are arranged. These are known as the *material* and the *structure* of an object.

MATERIAL AND STRUCTURE

The ability of an object to withstand stress will depend on its mechanical properties. These are determined by both the mechanical properties of the materials and the mechanical properties of the arrangement of the materials, the structure, that gives the object its shape.

Definition: A material has the same molecular make-up throughout.

Definition: A structure is an arrangement of one or more materials in a way that is designed to sustain loads.

The type of stress occurring within an object will depend on the direction of the applied force (remember the 'force systems' discussed earlier?). Some of the different types of stress that are commonly encountered can be described as (Figure 1.26):

- Axial stress;
- Shear stress;
- Bending stress;
- Torsional stress.

Axial stress is a force acting on a body along its axis (e.g. colinear forces) which produces a stretch or compression strain within the object, causing either an increase or decrease in length. An increase in length is further defined as '*linear tensile stress*' whereas a decrease is '*compressive tensile stress*'.

Shear stress is produced when two opposing but parallel forces act on an object at different points (e.g. coplanar forces acting as a 'force couple'). The

Figure 1.26   The directions of applied forces.

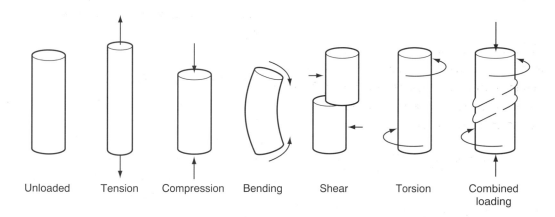

| Unloaded | Tension | Compression | Bending | Shear | Torsion | Combined loading |

resultant strain is an angular deformation within the object – imagine a square being 'stretched' into a rhomboid. Shear stresses are produced whenever any other of the stresses are applied.

Bending stress occurs as a result of forces causing a body to bend about an axis, that is one point of the object is relatively 'fixed'. If two coplanar forces are applied the axis will be between the forces, like bending a stick with both hands. However, there may be one or a combination of forces applied, causing many discreet areas of bending stress within the object. At each area or 'bend' there is a compressive stress on one side and a tensile stretch on the other, with some shear between.

Torsional stress is the stress generated by a force which causes a twist to occur in an object. This is a difficult type of stress to analyse as the strain produced will be a complex combination of bending, compression, shear and tensile stresses.

For further description and explanation on these different types of stress and strain, see Nordin and Frankel (1989).

Practical Application

The human body and its tissues need to withstand all of the above types of stress and when they fail to do this we see the results. Here are some examples of each.

Axial stress: Ligaments around joints are repeatedly subject to linear tensile stress. When the stress is excessive the result is rupture of the ligament. This is a common injury to the ligaments of the knee joint, especially during hard contact sports such as rugby and football. Weight-bearing bones, such as the calcaneus in the heel of the foot, must be able to withstand compressive tensile stress, for normal activity. However, jumping or falling from a height and landing on the heels can produce a crush fracture of the calcaneus *[heel bone] – in fact, if sufficiently great the force is transmitted through the lower limbs and to the spine, causing a* crush fracture of a vertebral body. *Check radiographs of the spine should be routine following a heavy fall landing on the feet.*

Shear stress: This occurs when there is a resisting frictional force between two surfaces. Think of a patient lying in a hospital bed. Perspiration may cause the skin and sheets to stick together. If he is 'dragged' up the bed — a shearing force occurs between the underlying tissues. The skin's delicate blood vessels may be stretched and torn with resultant bleeding just under the skin. A pressure sore may then develop.

Bending stress: The long bones of the lower limb are subject to this during walking and, in particular, running. The second metatarsal in the foot can sustain a fracture brought about by prolonged and frequent bending. This often occurs in soldiers and so is called a 'march fracture'.

Torsional stress: This twisting force along the bone can produce injuries such as fractures of the neck or femur, especially in elderly females. Torsional stress also causes fracture of the fibula just proximal to the ankle joint, where the mechanism of injury is twisting or turning on a soft muddy football pitch — the body and lower limbs turn but the studs of the boot, embedded in the soft mud, hold the foot securely in place.

As seen from the above rather simplified descriptions, stress analysis is a complex area of biomechanics. It is made particularly complex as the body consists of many different materials (i.e. the cells) grouped together to form structures such as bone, muscle, tendon etc. This means that any individual part of the body can be considered as a *structure* made up of different materials. Therefore, the ability of different areas of the body to withstand stress will depend on the specific mechanical properties of the cells of the area (i.e. the body's materials). In addition it will also depend on the relative positions and arrangement of all the materials to each other (i.e. the body's structure).

As this means that the body's response to stress will be varied, it is said to display *non-homogeneous* behaviour.

Definition: A homogeneous tissue is one that has uniform structure throughout and its mechanical properties will not vary from place to place within the material.

Strain

When stresses are applied some deformation, or strain, will occur. Obviously, as strain is a direct result of stress, it too will depend on:

- The force applied;
- The area of the cross-section of the bone/tendon.

$$\text{Stress} = \frac{\text{Force}}{\text{Cross-sectional area}}$$

However, it will also depend on:

- The mechanical properties of the material — that is, the elasticity and the yield point/point at which failure occurs.

Obviously the greater the force then the greater the stress and therefore strain. Similarly, the greater the cross-sectional area the lower the stress and the strain. To put it simply, a 'rope' made up one strand will easily snap, but another, made from many stands, will withstand a far greater stress before it snaps. But we must also consider what each strand is made from. Is it cotton, nylon or even wire? So we must consider the mechanical properties of the material and how they respond to applied stress.

STRESS–STRAIN CURVES

All objects when subject to stress will pass through the same stages before they break or rupture. However, the difference between them will be the magnitude of the stress required to produce rupture and the time it takes to pass through each stage. You can see this variation by taking a raw strand of spaghetti; if you apply a bending force it will soon snap. If you do the same to a cooked strand you will find that it will bend almost completely in half before it snaps or ruptures.

The stages through which the material or structure passes as stress is applied over time, can be shown graphically as a stress–strain curve (Figure 1.27). A stress–strain curve has the following stages or regions:

- Elastic;
- Plastic;
- Strain hardening;
- Necking;
- Rupture or failure point.

Let us describe these in further detail.

Figure 1.27 A typical stress–strain curve.

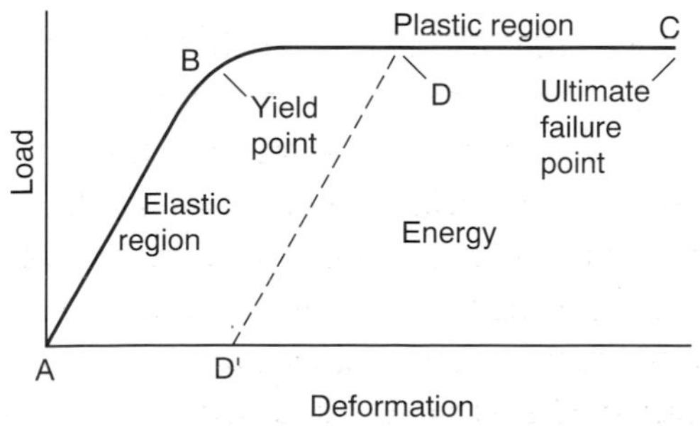

ELASTIC REGION

Definition: Elastic materials will deform in proportion to the load but will return to their prestressed state when the load is removed.

When the stress is first applied there will be some deformation of the material – however this is reversible due to the elastic properties of the material/s. Eventually, when the elastic limit is reached, continued stress will result in permanent deformation and the material will not regain its original state when the stress is removed.

This is an important concept for physiotherapists as muscle and ligamentous injuries (known as 'strains and sprains') are due to forces that exceed the elastic limit of the tissues, leading to stretching and rupture of the fibres.

The law that defines this is known as Hooke's law.

Hooke's law states that the strain produced is proportional to the applied stress, providing the elastic limit is not exceeded.

The amount of strain depends on the stiffness of the material and this relationship can be expressed as a ratio of stress to strain, and is known as *Young's modulus*, or the *modulus of elasticity*.

Definition: Young's modulus $= \dfrac{\text{stress}}{\text{strain}}$

As stated above, if the elastic limit is exceeded the next phase leads to permanent deformation of the material; this is called the plastic region.

PLASTIC REGION

In this region the material maintains or 'remembers' its new shape – this is plasticity. (You may also come across the term 'plasticity' with reference to the nervous system's ability to 'learn' and adopt new functions during the rehabilitation process.)

Definition: Plastic materials will deform in proportion to the load but the deformation is permanent and some or all of the new shape is retained when the load is removed.

Practical Example

Examples of materials that exhibit a high degree of plasticity are putty (including 'therapeutic putty' often used by physiotherapists when teaching hand exercises), wax (also used by physiotherapists), lead and many other soft metals. Tissues within the body tend to exhibit more elastic than plastic properties. It would not be desirable if our bones and tissues deformed when subject to normal degrees of stress and then remained that way! However it can and does happen — tissues may be overstretched due to disease or injury. When this occurs in ligaments, as in rheumatoid arthritis, it can lead to gross instability of the joint.

STRAIN-HARDENING REGION

During the later stages of the plastic region the material undergoes molecular changes — this is called strain hardening. It provides some resistance to further deformation, but eventually the material ruptures.

NECKING REGION

This occurs in linear tensile stresses. As the material is stretched the cross-sectional area decreases. If the cross-sectional area decreases then there is a decrease in the ability of the material to withstand the stress and *rupture or failure point* soon follows. We have all seen this when stretching Plasticine or chewing gum!

RUPTURE OR FAILURE POINT

This is when the material breaks. We see this when bones break and ligaments rupture. However, injuries to soft tissues may not produce a complete rupture with obvious discontinuity. There may only be a rupture of some of the fibres within the structure thereby weakening the tendon or ligament. This is common in 'overuse' injuries and may present as a chronic problem or may be asymptomatic until a force is applied, one that would normally be withstood, yet is sufficient to rupture the remaining intact fibres of the weakened tendon or ligament.

BRITTLE AND DUCTILE

A structure that easily breaks or ruptures is said to be *brittle*, whereas one that can deform considerably is said to be *ductile*. Most tissues within the body have a certain amount of ductility, although this decreases with age. (Refer to Le Veau (1992) for a more detailed discussion of the properties of biological materials and the effect of ageing.)

THE RESULT OF TIME ON STRAIN

If a steady stress is applied over time there may be a change in the shape of the material. This is in part due to the elastic properties already discussed but is also related to the material's *viscous properties*.

Definition: Viscous behaviour is a slow reaction to stress, the deformation is not immediate but occurs following a prolonged application of the stress. When the stress is removed the material does not return to the prestressed state.

In body tissue there is commonly a combination of elastic and viscous properties — this is called *viscoelastic behaviour* and the resulting deformation is called *creep*.

Definition: Creep is the gradual deformation that occurs within a material when a force is applied over a period of time.

Practical Example

Full range of movement at a joint may be prevented because of a fixed contracture (shortening) of the muscle, ligaments and/or joint capsule on one aspect of the joint. For example, shortening of the structures on the posterior aspect of the knee will prevent full extension. We can utilize the viscoelastic properties of these tissues, and by applying a sustained stretch to these shortened structures — for some minutes or even, in some cases, several hours — will encourage 'creep' or lengthening of the tissues. Provided this is done on a regular basis and the increase in length is maintained, then it is possible to regain full range of movement. As viscoelasticity is affected by temperature (becoming more viscous with increased temperature) heat may be applied to the tissues either before and/or during the stretch for maximum effect.

Summary

In this chapter we have reviewed some basic concepts concerned with the description and analysis of normal movement. After reading this and with some reinforcement from the practical application of these principles, it is hoped that you will be able to:

- Describe the body using appropriate terminology, e.g. anterior/superior, medial/lateral.
- Describe movement with reference to the anatomical position using the recognized terminology, e.g. flexion/extension.
- Describe a movement with reference to the axis and plane of the movement.
- Describe the difference between a slide, roll, spin and swing.
- Describe the magnitude of a movement using degrees or linear units.
- Using the above information, do a simple kinematic analysis of a movement at a major joint.
- Define mass, weight and force.
- Explain the significance of Newton's three laws of motion to normal movement.
- Define gravity, centre of mass, friction and pressure with reference to their relevance to movement.
- Explain the effect of force systems on an object, with reference to the magnitude of the force, its direction, the point of application and the resultant effect, and relate these to joint movement and muscle contraction.
- Explain how the order of lever affects the effort required to move a load.
- Define torque and explain how it varies depending on joint position.
- Explain how the efficiency of the muscle contraction varies with the angle of pull.
- Understand what is involved in a kinetic analysis of a movement.
- Define a pulley and describe how it affects the direction of an applied force.
- Understand the difference between stress and strain.

- Describe tensile, compression, bending, shear and torsional stress.
- Describe the difference between the material and the structure of an object.
- Define the regions of a stress–strain curve.
- Understand the difference between elasticity and viscosity.

References and Further Reading

Dvir, Z (1995) *Isokinetics: Muscle Testing, Interpretation and Clinical Application*. Churchill Livingstone, New York.

Galley, PM, Forster, AL (1987) *Human Movement: An Introductory Text for Physiotherapy Students*, 2nd edn. Churchill Livingstone, Edinburgh.

Kapanji, IA (1985) *The Physiology of the Joints: Volume Two Lower Limb*, 5th edn. Churchill Livingstone, Edinburgh.

Le Veau, BF (1992) *William's and Lissner's Biomechanics of Human Motion*, 3rd edn. WB Saunders, Philadelphia.

Lee, M, Steven, GP, Crosbie, J, Higgs, RJED (1996) Towards a theory of lumbar mobilisation — the relationship between applied manual force and movements of the spine. *Manual Therapy* 1: 67–75.

Low, J, Reed, A (1996) *Basic Biomechanics Explained*. Butterworth–Heinneman, Oxford.

McGuiness-Scott, J (1980) Benesh movement notation: An introduction to recording clinical data. Physiotherapy **66**, (8): 268–272.

Nordin, M and Frankel, VH (1989) *Basic Biomechanics of the Musculoskeletal System*, 2nd edn. Lea & Febiger, Philadelphia.

Norkin, CC and Levangie, PK (1992) *Joint Structure and Function: A Comprehensive Analysis*, 2nd edn. FA Davis, Philadelphia.

Peebles, RE and Margo, MK (1978) Function after patellectomy. *Clinical Orthopaedics* **132**: 180–186.

Roberts, SL and Falkenburg SA (1992) *Biomechanics – Problem Solving for Functional Activity*. Mosby Year Book, London.

Soderberg, G. (1997) *Kinesiology: Application to Pathological Motion*, 2nd edn. Williams and Wilkins, Baltimore.

Williams, PL and Warwick, R (1980) *Gray's Anatomy*, 36th edn. Churchill Livingstone, Edinburgh.

2

The Musculoskeletal Requirements for Normal Movement

JANE LOCKWOOD

Introduction
•
Chapter Objectives
•
The Skeletal System
•
The Articular System
•
The Muscular System
•
Summary

Introduction

Physiotherapists are concerned with the rehabilitation of normal movement and function. To assess this they might first examine the musculoskeletal system. However, as the body works as a complex whole, loss or impairment of any of the major systems will affect normal function. So, before reviewing in further detail the specifics required by the musculoskeletal system it is useful to look, in brief, at the major systems to identify their main roles:

- Skeletal system;
- Articular system;
- Muscular system;
- Nervous system;
- Cardiorespiratory system.

1 *The Skeletal System* The skeleton forms a framework giving the body shape. The bones also provide a firm site for the attachment of muscles and a mechanism for supporting and transmitting the weight of the body during normal movement. It is designed to withstand the external forces encountered during normal activity. The bones may also afford protection of the underlying organs, nerves and blood vessels. Finally, the bone marrow is also concerned with the production of blood cells.

2 *The Articular System* The bones are interconnected by articulations or 'joints' of the body. These provide simultaneous flexibility and

shock absorption during static and dynamic movement. A major purpose is to provide a means of altering the length of the limbs, for locomotion and prehensile (manual) tasks.

3 *The Muscular System* Muscles produce the controlled and coordinated movement required for normal activity. They are also important for supporting the joints during weight transference and shock absorption. In addition they help in the maintenance of the body temperature by producing the heat required to maintain the optimum temperature for normal cellular function.

4 *The Nervous System* This consists of the brain and the spinal cord (the central nervous system) and the nerves passing to and from the rest of the body (the peripheral nervous system). These are essential for normal movement and control of the other systems. The central and peripheral nervous systems provide a complex communication system for the initiation of movement and continuous sensory feedback required to control and modify static and dynamic posture.

5 *The Cardiorespiratory System* The heart, blood vessels, lymphatic vessels and the lungs are vital for the transfer of oxygen and nutrients to the tissues. They also remove the carbon dioxide and other waste products from the tissues. Working with internal organs such as the stomach, intestines, liver and kidneys, they maintain the energy requirements of the individual cells.

In this chapter we shall consider the roles of the skeletal, articular and muscular systems with reference to their contribution to the stability and mobility of the body. The roles of the nervous system will be considered in Chapter 3. Details of cell metabolism, renewal and repair are beyond the scope of this chapter and the reader is advised to consult a specialist text on human physiology.

In Chapter 1 we considered the major forces and some basic mechanical factors that affect normal movement. There was some reference to how the body adapts in response to these. This chapter will give an overview of the 'design' of the individual components of the musculoskeletal system, with particular reference to functional requirements. The mechanical properties of 'materials' (i.e. the tissues) and the 'structure' (i.e the specific arrangement of the tissues) will be considered.

In the body the difference between 'material' and 'structure' is not always clear cut. For example, tissue such as bone might be considered as an individual 'material'. Yet, because it consists of many different cells and intracellular matrix, it can also be seen as many different materials forming a 'structure'. This structure is an arrangement of bone cells, bone salts, collagen fibres, bone marrow and blood vessels. Each has its own mechanical properties, and forms a 'structure', such as an individual bone in the foot. This 'foot bone' is then just one component of the foot, which is a structure in its own right. For our purposes it is best to take the foot, or any discrete area of the body, as a 'structure' which is then made up from a specific arrangement of bones, ligaments, muscles, nerves and blood vessels etc.

Therefore, when considering the various parts of the musculoskeletal system, we shall use the terms 'material' and 'structure' rather loosely. The emphasis will be on how they fulfil the requirements for normal function.

Chapter Objectives

After reading this chapter the reader should be able to:

- Discuss the main histological features of the skeletal, articular and muscular systems with specific reference to normal function;
- Explain how the shape and arrangement of the bones, the joints and the muscles influence

their ability to fulfil their roles in normal movement.

The Skeletal System

Introduction

The skeleton is divided into the axial and appendicular skeleton (Figure 2.1).

Figure 2.1   The skeleton, showing the axial and appendicular (shaded) divisions. (Adapted from Clancy and McVicar, 1995, *Physiotherapy and Anatomy: A Homeostatic Approach*. Edward Arnold, London.)

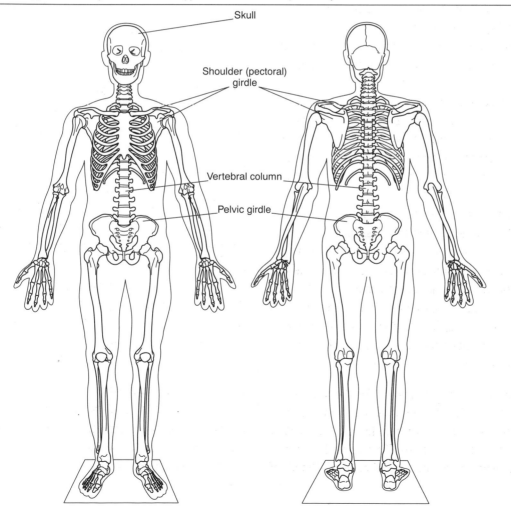

Skull

Shoulder (pectoral) girdle

Vertebral column

Pelvic girdle

The Axial Skeleton This is the trunk that comprises the skull, the vertebral column and the ribs. The axial skeleton is an important area for muscular attachment. Many of its bones also have a major role in the protection of the central nervous system and internal organs.

The Appendicular Skeleton This is formed by the bones of the upper and lower limbs and their girdles. The pectoral girdle connects the upper limbs to the trunk and the pelvic girdle connects the lower limbs to the trunk. The bones of the limbs form a system of levers, the fulcrum or axis at the joint allows the limbs to be shortened or lengthened. This means that there can be accurate positioning of the hand and foot for activities such as grasping an object or kicking a ball.

To fulfil the functional requirements of protection, mobility and weight transference we need a combination of rigidity and flexibility, often called *stability* and *mobility*. These are provided by the internal and external structure of the bone and by the articulations (joints) between individual bones and the surrounding soft tissues. Therefore we shall review:

- The histology of bone;
- The internal structure;
- The external shape.

We shall see how each fulfils these functional requirements. The contribution made by the joints and soft tissues will be discussed later in the chapter.

Histology of Bone

Bone consists of bone cells called osteocytes, which are important in producing the extracellular constituents. These lie in a matrix or ground substance consisting of collagen fibres, bone salts, and proteoglycan molecules. Collagen fibres are flexible but relatively inelastic. This means that they can withstand a certain amount of tensile stress. The fibres are arranged to follow the direction of these tensile forces. The bone salts provide rigidity and stiffness in the bone. Calcium, magnesium, sodium and fluoride, are the main bone salts. These are 'glued' together by proteins called osteonectins and hardened by hydroxyapatite crystals (Williams and Warwick, 1980). Bone is surprisingly flexible, and long bones can bend considerably before fracture occurs. This flexibility is provided by the proteoglycan gel, giving the bone elasticity so when stress is applied bending occurs, but not permanently. Without this elastic property bone would be extremely brittle and relatively low-impact activities, such as walking, might fracture weight-bearing bones. For further discussion on bone's ability to withstand tensile, compression and torsional forces refer to Nordin and Frankel (1980) and Frankel and Burstein (1964).

THE HAVERSIAN SYSTEM OR OSTEON

The arrangement of the cells and matrix is important. The cells and matrix are laid down in concentric layers called lamellae (Figure 2.2). These lamellae are fixed together by bundles of short collagen fibres that pierce adjacent layers and 'staple' them together. These are called *perforating fibres of Sharpey* and assist in the general ability of the bone to resist tensile stresses (Dempster and Coleman, 1960). Many concentric lamellae surround a central *Haversian canal* that contains the blood capillaries that are essential for the nutrition of the surrounding cells; they send off side branches, *perforating canals,* that link with adjacent Haversian canals. The Haversian canal and its 'own' surrounding lamellae is the *Haversian system* or *osteon.*

Figure 2.2   Structure of bone showing an osteon (Haversian system). (a) The arrangement of the osteons within the diaphysis of the bone. (b) An enlarged view of an osteon showing the osteocytes within lacan and the concentric lamellae. (Adapted from Van de Graaf, 1995, *Human Anatomy*, 4th edn., William Brown.)

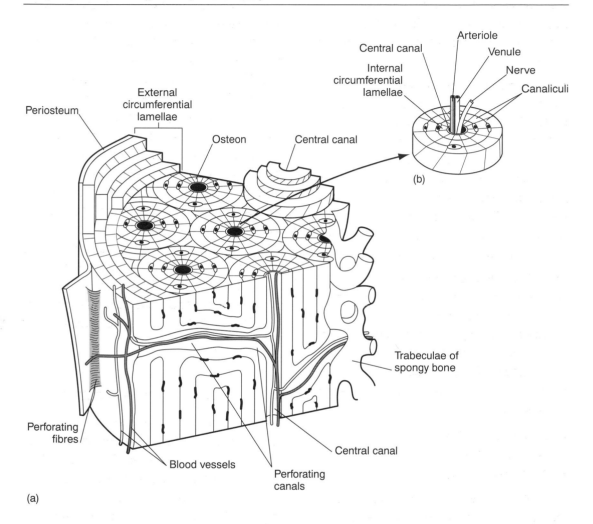

The collagen fibres in each lamella are generally parallel, but the fibres of adjacent lamellae are at an angle. This means that the directions of the fibres range from longitudinal to circumferential, with many running spirally around the shaft of the bone. This arrangement enables the bone to withstand tensile and torsional stresses from many directions. However, this arrangement varies considerably from bone to bone and even within the same osteon. There are also changes with increasing age, when the lamellae are less distinct and there are fewer circumferential fibres (Smith, 1960). This may lead to weakness of the bone, and so increase the risk of fractures.

A typical osteon is about 200 micrometres [μm)

in diameter (Nordin and Frankel, 1989). There are many Haversian systems within the substance of a bone, arranged like bundles of straws or tubes. Adjacent osteons do not have interconnecting collagen, but a layer of 'cement' glues the layers together. This is claimed to be a 'weak link' in the bone's strength (Dempster and Coleman, 1960), and tensile stresses in particular can pull osteons apart. It is the 'structural' arrangement of the layers and the bundles, together with the elasticity and stiffness (from the 'materials') that give bone the ability to withstand forces of many types and from varying directions.

Practical Application

When the organic matrix (proteoglycan) is removed the bone is extremely brittle. This is what we see when we inspect the skeletons found in the classroom. Note that the bone is lighter in weight but will easily break. Conversely if the inorganic salts (calcium etc) are removed, you are left with a 'bendy-toy' bone. This can be bent to a considerable angle without breaking and then return to its original shape.

For bone to withstand tension, compression and torsion forces, the constituents of bone have to be in the correct proportion laid down in appropriate directions. Too little calcium and the bone will bend leading to a permanent deformity. Years ago, this was frequently seen in children with rickets, a disease brought about by a deficiency of vitamin D. This is required for the intestines to absorb calcium. Besides poor nutrition, the lack of vitamin D in

these children was also possibly due to insufficient exposure to sunlight. This is because the formation of vitamin D is a complex reaction involving a precursor molecule found in the skin. This precursor molecule is modified in the presence of ultraviolet light and is finally converted to Vitamin D (calciferol) by the liver and kidneys.

Another vitamin deficiency affecting bone is scurvy. This is a condition caused by a lack of vitamin C. This leads to a decreased production of collagen and therefore the bones are weak. Here it is not due to insufficient calcium, but to a lack of collagen fibres. These are necessary to provide a scaffolding framework for the calcified matrix. Scurvy is generally caused by insufficient dietary intake of vitamin C and affects not just bone but all connective tissues that contain many collagen fibres. This can result in ulceration of the skin, haemorrhaging and poor wound healing.

The main source of vitamins is from the food we eat and its subsequent absorption through the membranes of the digestive system. If there is a problem with the absorption of the vitamin, this may result in 'soft' or 'crumbling' bones. Examples of this are from diseases such as cystic fibrosis or following surgical excision of part of the digestive system. Therefore it is important that the physiotherapist has information on the patient's past medical history and coexisting diseases. It may provide information which may contraindicate some passive techniques and the application of manual resistance.

Physiotherapists will frequently treat patients with osteoporosis, commonly found in elderly, postmenopausal females as it is caused, in part, by a decrease in the level of oestrogen but is also linked to lack of calcium in the diet and decrease in weight-bearing exercises (Putukian, 1994). This leads to an increase above normal in the absorption of bone matrix, leading to weakening and thinning, rarefaction, of the bone and thus an increase risk of fracture. Physiotherapists, by their involvement in rehabilitation and general health education and promotion (Preisinger et al., 1996), can contribute to the prevention of this process.

Now let us consider how the general internal and external structure of a bone is related to function.

Internal Structure

Where there are many osteons the bone is dense; this is *compact bone*. Compact bone is extremely strong, the arrangement of many pipes or tubes making a mechanically strong structure. However, a bone made entirely from compact bone would be extremely heavy and would require an enormous energy expenditure to produce movement. Therefore, to reduce the weight of bone, there are cavities, often filled with bone marrow. A large cavity forming the centre of the shaft of a long bone, is called a *medullary cavity*. This gives the long bone a tubular structure, which increases its mechanical strength, especially for resisting bending stress (Carter, 1985; Kummer, 1972).

All bones have an outer shell of compact bone. The ends of long bones and smaller bones have an internal structure that resembles a sponge or honeycomb. This is formed by many small cavities, separated by struts of bone and is called *cancellous bone* (also known as spongy or trabecular bone (Figure 2.3)). These struts of bone, called trabeculae, act as a 'scaffolding' framework. They are laid down in specific directions in response to external forces. These forces can be from the transmission of weight through the bone and from forces produced by the pull of muscle attachments. Trabeculae can show a complex arrangement, often forming 'Gothic arch' patterns, to resist multidirectional stresses. This is shown by their arrangement around the hip joint and pelvis arrangement of the trabeculae illustrated in Figure 2.4.

REMODELLING

The trabecular arrangement alters when the direction and/or amount of the applied stress changes. This is by a process called remodelling and occurs continually throughout life, albeit less efficiently as we get older. During this process the salts are absorbed by specialized cells called *osteoclasts* and the osteoblasts lay down new trabeculae aligned to withstand the altered line of force. There are many reasons why this internal structure of the bone may change. Examples are: (a) due to normal growth spurts in childhood and the associated gain in body weight, or (b) following repair of a fracture, especially when there is permanent change in the alignment of the shaft of the bone.

Figure 2.3   A long bone showing the central medullary canal surrounded by a layer of compact bone, with cancellous bone forming the trabeculae at the extremity. Key: SB = spongy bone; CB = compact bone; MC = medullary cavity. (Adapted from Moore, 1992, *Clinically Oriented Anatomy,* 3rd edn., Williams & Wilkins.)

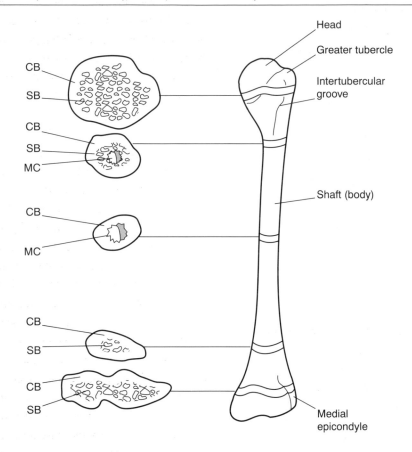

Clinical Application

To maintain strong trabeculae, bone must be subject to the same type of stress that occurs during normal function. Therefore an exercise programme that includes weight-bearing activities is ideal for maintaining the normal bone density (Preisinger et al., 1996). If a bone is deprived of normal stresses for a sustained period, then the number and size of the trabeculae decreases due to absorption of the bone salts. The general arrangement of the tra-beculae also undergoes some modification. This has been found in the astronauts who have spent weeks in weightless conditions (Arnaud et al., 1986; Tipton et al., 1996).

Of more relevance to the physiotherapist is the similar effect from periods of prolonged bed rest and therefore the importance of early mobilization and weight bearing. Long-term bed rest is avoided by the use of internal fixation of a fracture. This can be achieved by the insertion of an intramedullary nail or a metal plate

Figure 2.4   The 'Gothic arch' patterns of the trabeculae around the hip and pelvis (adapted from Kapanji, 1985 *The Physiology of the Joints: Volume Two, Lower Limb*, 5th edn. Churchill Livingstone, London.)

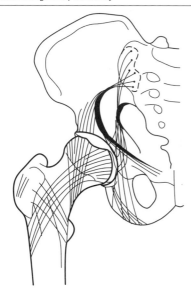

screwed to the shaft of the bone. However, a reduction in the bone density from loss of trabeculae can occur following the insertion of these implants. They absorb and redistribute the normal stresses encountered during normal function. This means that the fracture site won't regain its former strength until the implant is removed – usually within 24 months – and the limb resumes normal function, leading to the deposition of new trabeculae. (For further discussions on the internal fixation of fractures refer to Bunker et al., 1989)

External Structure

The external size and shape of the bone also decide its role for support, leverage and protection. Bones may be classified according to their external appearance (Figure 2.5).

LONG BONES

These provide excellent levers for movement and props for weight bearing. They consist of a shaft and two extremities called condyles. The shaft is a hollow tube of dense cortical bone surrounding a medullary cavity. The articular condyles are expanded to increase the surface area available for weight bearing through the joint. This will allow the force to be spread over a larger area and thus decrease the pressure and resulting strain at any one point. These condyles have a shell of compact bone surrounding trabecular bone. Besides long bones being a hollow tubular construction, they are usually slightly curved along their longitudinal axis. This curvature of bones about the long axis is important for withstanding compression and bending forces (Kummer, 1972). When stress is applied along this axis the curvature increases as the bone bends and will reform when the compressive load is removed, provided of course that the elastic limit is not exceeded. If you look at the skeleton, you will see many examples of this curved appearance. The shaft of the femur is slightly convex anteriorly, the metatarsals have a slight superior convexity and the radius and ulna both have a slight curvature.

The cross-sectional shape is also important in withstanding bending stresses along the length of a long bone. A round or cylindrical bone is good at withstanding torsional stress whereas a square cross-section can withstand bending stresses only in the planes of the parallel sides. However, a compromise is often required, which will withstand both torsion and bending in many directions. This is provided by a triangular cross-section. Examples of bones with a triangular cross-section are the tibia, the mid shaft of the femur and the proximal portion of

Figure 2.5   Classification of bones by shape: (a) long bone, e.g. femur; (b) short bone, e.g. tarsal bones; (c) flat bone, e.g. the scapula; (d) irregular bone, e.g. cervical vertebra.

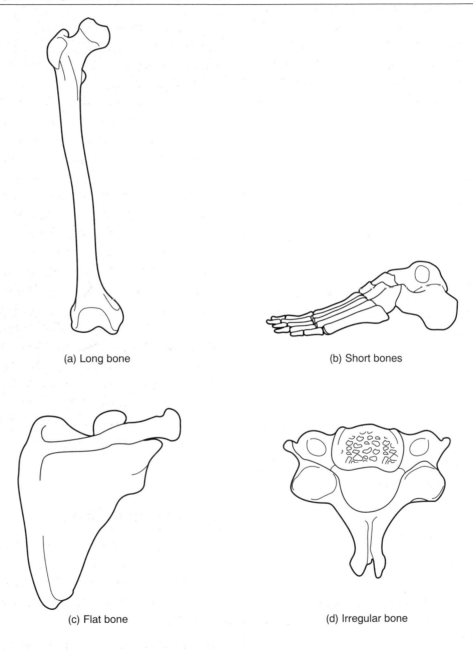

(a) Long bone

(b) Short bones

(c) Flat bone

(d) Irregular bone

the ulna. Many other smaller 'long bones' also display this feature. [For a discussion of the research relating to this refer to Frankel and Burstein (1965), Nordin and Frankel (1989), Kummer (1972).]

SHORT BONES

These are chunky or cuboid in appearance and are usually grouped together as in the tarsal bones of the foot and the vertebral bodies. They have an outer shell of cortical bone and an inner core of cancellous bone with the trabeculae arranged to transmit compressive forces occurring during weight bearing.

FLAT BONES

These consist of a shell of cortical bone (*diploe*) enclosing a thin layer of bone marrow with occasional supporting trabeculae. Flat bones form good bases for broad attachment of muscles, such as those attached to the scapulae. They also serve as a shell affording protection of internal organs and delicate structures, as seen in the bones of the skull. Due to their relatively delicate structure and few trabeculae they are not designed to withstand weight-bearing forces as the outer cortical layer will crack. However, some protection is afforded by the nature of the 'cancellous sandwich' which means that although the outer layer may crack, the 'filling' acts as a shock absorber and will compress so protecting the inner cortical layer intact.

IRREGULAR BONES

These do not fit into any of the above categories but may have features and therefore the properties of all three. The innominate bone of the pelvis, the vertebrae and the mandible are examples of irregular bones.

Anatomical Application

The mixture of features shown by an irregular bone is well illustrated by the innominate bone [Figure 2.4]. It has the broad 'flat bone' ilium superiorly, ideal for the attachment of the hip flexor muscle internally and the abductor and extensor muscles on its outer surface. The ischial tuberosity posteriorly, provides a short chunky bone ideal for weight bearing. If you sit on your hands, this is the bony protuberance you can feel. There are no obvious 'long bone' features, but pillars of bone are found to transmit the weight from the upper body and sacrum to the head of the femur. This bony pillar, with arched trabeculae, is the arcuate line and is part of the ilium. Other smaller pillars are found anteriorly. These are called the superior and inferior rami of the pubis and although not major factors in transmitting forces they are important in maintaining the arrangement of the bones of the pelvis as a ring [see below].

Arrangement of Bones

In addition to the above properties of bone, its roles will also be served by its position in relation to other bones and soft tissues. These make up an anatomical functional unit, such as the hand, the foot and the spine.

This arrangement of many smaller bones provides flexibility, allowing the unit to mould to the shape of the contact surface, for example the hand moulding to the shape of a cup or the foot to uneven ground. It also provides a relatively stable structure for support or weight transference and an ideal base for the attachment of muscles. This stability is conferred by the limited range of movement at the individual joints, so favouring stability at each joint. However, the sum of these small movements can produce a large range of movement. Think, for example, of the small range of movement available between individual vertebrae and yet the total range of movement in the spine.

We shall see later that joints are also important for preventing damage to the bone by providing flexible connections that 'give' rather than 'break' when stress is applied. These joints are an integral component of the arches and rings that form the structural arrangement of many areas of the body.

ARCHES

Examples of these are, again, found in the foot. The bones of the foot are arranged to form arches that run in anteroposterior (the medial and lateral longitudinal arches) and medial/lateral (transverse arches) directions (Figure 2.6). They are maintained by the specific shape of the bones, the

Figure 2.6   The bones of the foot arranged to form arches. The medial longitudinal arch has (a) a 'keystone' (the talus) and is supported from below by (b) short 'staples' (the short interosseous ligaments) and (c) long 'ties' (the long plantar ligaments and aponeurosis) and from above by (d) 'suspension ropes' (the tendons). (e) Bones of foot showing location of arches.

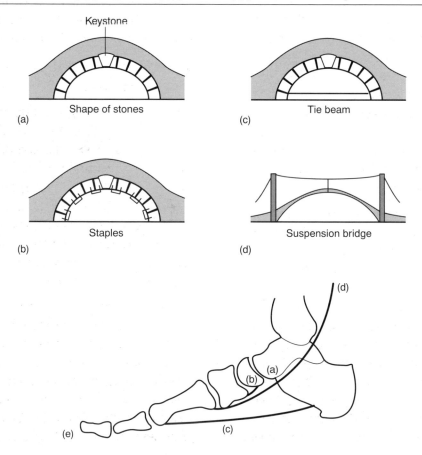

ligaments of the associated joints, active support provided by the muscles and the tendons which cross the joints.

Other arched structures, some fixed and some flexible, are found in the body. There are curves in the spine: both the cervical and lumbar *lordosis* have concavities directed posteriorly and the thoracic *kyphosis* has an anteriorly directed concavity. These provide flexibility, and when the spine is subjected to large longitudinal compressive forces the curvatures increase. This helps to dissipate the force that would otherwise be transmitted to the head, and risk injury to the brain.

Figure 2.7 If there is a severe discrepancy in leg length there is a compensatory scoliosis, the aim being to keep the head and, in particular the eyes, horizontal. (Posterior aspect.)

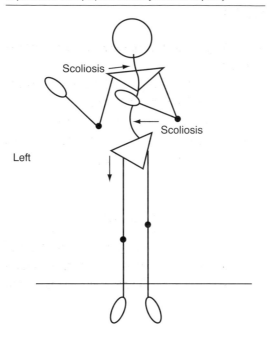

may be due to a difference in leg length. For example if the left leg is shorter than the right, this causes the pelvis to drop on the left (Figure 2.7). If the leg length discrepancy is severe, there is usually a scoliosis in the lumbar area (with the concavity to the right), and another further up the spine (the concavity to the left). These help to compensate for the difference in leg lengths and the aim is to keep the head in the normal horizontal and midline position.

RINGS

A ring is a particularly strong yet flexible arrangement. It allows some torsional stress, yet has inherent elasticity and regains its shape when the stress is removed. Examples where the arrangement of the bones forms a ring are found between the sacrum and the two innominate bones in the pelvis, the ribs and the bones of the skull. It is also the shape of the individual vertebrae encircling the spinal cord. If a ring loses discontinuity at only one point it tends to retain its basic shape (think of a broken hoop), and unless it is twisted the ends will tend to come together. However, if it is broken in two places the integrity of the ring is lost. This can occur in fractures of the rib. If the rib is broken in two places, the section between the fracture sites is unstable and known as a 'flail segment'.

Practical Application

Consider the torsional stresses applied to the pelvis during normal activity. Stand in front of a high step or stool – preferably 50 cm or more in height.

Place a hand on each iliac crest, with the index finger pointing to the anterior superior iliac spine and thumbs directed posteriorly. Compare the levels of your index fingers; these should be the same.

Now lift your left foot onto the step. What has happened to the relative levels of your index fingers? You should find that the left is now slightly higher than the right. This is from twisting or torsion of the pelvic ring. Most of this torsional stress produces a small range of rotation at the sacroiliac joints and the pubic symphysis, but the flexibility of the bones allows some twisting.

Similar torsional stresses are applied to the ribs that encircle the thoracic cavity when twisting and bending activities of the trunk occur.

The bones therefore play a major role in support, protection and movement. However, the flexibility which allows us to be so mobile and dexterous requires joints, between the adjacent bones.

The Articular System

Introduction

In all areas of the body there is a compromise between mobility and stability and frequently both are required. This depends on the functional role of the joint at a particular time. We shall now give an overview of the joints. The emphasis will be on how the requirements of stability and mobility are met by the histology of the tissues and by the arrangement of these tissues. These determine the type and shape of the joint.

We shall:

- Provide an acceptable method of classifying the joints;
- Relate the shape of the joint surfaces to the stability and mobility conferred;
- Consider the contribution made by the peri-articular and intra-articular structures to the stability and mobility of the joint.

Classification of Joints

Joints are classified by structure, or by range of available movement. There is obviously considerable overlap between the two methods as seen in Table 2.1.

Table 2.1
Classification of joints (adapted from Lindsay, 1996)

Classification by structure	Classification by range of movement		
	Immovable *Synarthrosis*	Slightly movable *Ampharthrosis*	Freely movable *Diarthrosis*
Fibrous	Sutures e.g. skull Gomphoses e.g. teeth in sockets in the mandible and maxilla	Syndesmoses e.g. the interosseous membranes connecting the shafts of the radius and ulna, and the tibia and fibula	
Cartilaginous	Synchondroses The cartilaginous plates between the epiphyses and shafts of long bones — allows for growth	Symphyses The bones are separated by a fibrocartilaginous disc e.g. between the pubic bones, the pubic symphysis	
Synovial			Synovial joints The bones are connected by a joint capsule, this is lined with synovial membrane and lubricated by synovial fluid e.g. hip, knee, shoulder

Immovable Joints

These are very stable joints and the two opposing bone surfaces are separated by either fibrous tissue or by cartilage (Figure 2.8).

SUTURES

These are found between the bones of the skull (Figure 2.8a). In childhood a layer of white fibrous tissue separated the bones. Growth of the bone is by gradual ossification of adjacent fibrous tissue. At the same time fibroblasts produce new fibrous tissue. When growth is complete the bones fuse and the layer of fibrous tissue becomes completely ossified. It is then called a *synostosis*.

Sutures are very stable joints as the joint surfaces fit closely together, so they are said to be highly *congruent*. The serrated edges lock together and prevent movement between the bones. In addition the fibrous layer is very thin but has a high proportion of collagen fibres that can withstand considerable amounts of compression and tension.

GOMPHOSES

These are unique to the articulation between the teeth and the jaw bones (Figure 2.8b). The roots of the tooth fit into a socket in the bone, and between the two is a thin layer of fibrous tissue. Fibrous tissue is compressible. This is important as it allows some flexibility and 'give' between the tooth and the jaw bone when chewing, acting as a shock absorber. Without this, forces repeatedly applied to the bone when eating might ultimately lead to a stress fracture.

SYNCHONDROSES

These form the growth zone found between two sections of a long bone (Figure 2.8c). The 'joint' is

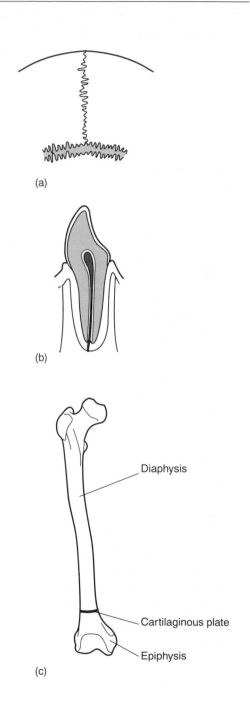

Figure 2.8 Immovable joints: (a) suture (in skull) (b) gomphosis (between tooth and jaw bone); (c) synchondrosis.

(a)

(b)

Diaphysis

Cartilaginous plate

Epiphysis

(c)

a layer of hyaline cartilage, a site of active cell replication to increase the length of the bone. The main shaft is the *diaphysis*, the cartilage layer the *epiphysial plate* and the end of the bone the *epiphysis*. When growth is complete, the epiphysial plate is ossified.

Anatomical Application

Immovable joints occasionally move and cause problems. Sutures can slip or lose contact through irregular growth of one bone; very occasionally they lose continuity due to trauma. The joint between the jaw and the teeth can become loose from gum disease or occasionally due to the reduction in collagen production as found in scurvy – a disease caused by a deficiency of vitamin C.

Synchondroses should be completely immovable and if movement does occur following abnormal stresses, it causes a 'slipped epiphysis'. This can have serious consequences on the longitudinal growth of the bone. A frequent site for this is the epiphyseal plate of the shaft of the femur. This condition usually affects adolescents, with boys having a slightly greater risk; 41% girls to 59% boys (Loder et al., 1996). It requires immediate medical attention and long-term immobilization. However, even after meticulous medical care there may be an alteration in the growth of the femur, leading to a discrepancy in leg length.

Slightly Movable Joints

The immovable joints described above are very stable, although some limited movement does occur between the bones. However, as there are no major ligaments connecting the bones they mainly rely on the shape of the joint surfaces, fibrous tissue and cartilage to connect the joint surfaces. There are two types of slightly movable joints, syndesmoses and symphyses (Figure 2.9).

Figure 2.9   Slightly movable joints: (a) syndesmosis, e.g. upper limb; (b) symphysis, e.g. spine.

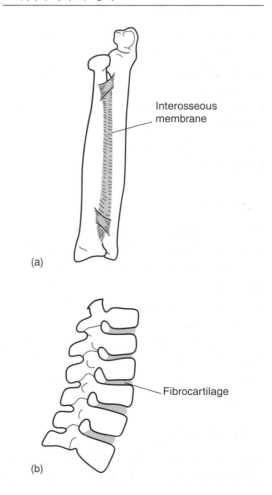

Interosseous membrane

(a)

Fibrocartilage

(b)

SYNDESMOSES

Here the articulating bones are separated by a considerable gap that is bridged by ligaments and/or a sheet of ligamentous tissue called an *interosseous membrane*. The radius and ulna in the forearm (Figure 2.9a) and the tibia and fibula in the leg are examples of syndesmoses, where an interosseous membrane serves to connect the bones. The ischium and the sacrum of the pelvis are connected by the extremely strong *sacrotuberous* and *sacrospinous ligaments*. The membranes and ligaments contain many collagen fibres laid down along the direction of the applied stress. These are important for maintaining the strong articulation and for absorbing some of the applied stresses. However collagen has visco-elastic properties. Too great a stress applied continually over a period of time can lead to permanent elongation and subsequent instability of the joint.

In addition to their supportive roles these membranes and ligaments also provide surfaces for the attachment of surrounding muscles, for example the attachment of the forearm and leg (crural) muscles.

SYMPHYSES

In a symphysis the bone ends are separated by a disc of white fibrocartilage attached to the joint surfaces. Examples are the joints between two vertebral bodies (Figure 2.9b) and the joint between the pubic bones. A symphysis forms a stable joint with only limited mobility as the disc attaches to each articular surface. In addition there are strong external ligaments connecting the bones. These pass across, often blending with, the surface of the disc, thus adding to the stability of the joint. The disc has an outer layer of collagen fibres and an inner nucleus of gel-like consistency. These contribute to its ability to withstand the compression forces, such as the ground reaction force transmitted from the lower limb when walking. The disc also allows some limited movement between the vertebrae.

The *nucleus pulposus* has hydrostatic properties which form a 'bearing' or fulcrum for the vertebra above and below. The nucleus compresses and deforms depending on the direction of movement. The outer *annulus fibrosus* can withstand tension and torsion due to the multidirectional arrangement of the collagen (and some elastic) fibres. For example, in flexion of the spine, the posterior region of the disc is stretched and the anterior compressed and the nucleus bulges posteriorly. The opposite occurs in extension. On rotation there is torsion of the disc between the vertebral bodies.

Although the movement available at each joint is small the total range is considerable. This means that there is stability between each. This is required for weight bearing and for the protection of the spinal cord, yet in total a reasonable degree of flexibility and movement is available in the spine for normal functional activity.

Freely Movable Joints

To enable a greater range of movement many joints of the body are lubricated by the production of synovial fluid. These are known collectively as *synovial joints* and form the only category in the freely movable group.

SYNOVIAL JOINTS

As we shall see these vary considerably in size and structure but the following features are present in a typical synovial joint (Figure 2.10):

Figure 2.10   A typical synovial joint.

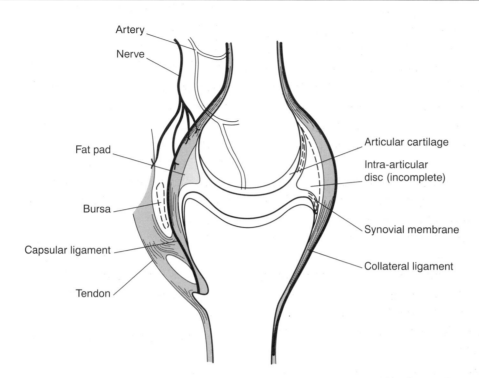

- Hyaline cartilage covering the freely movable articular surfaces;
- A fibrous capsule connecting the articulating bones;
- Ligaments around the joint providing additional support;
- Synovial membrane lining all the non-articular surfaces – this produces the lubricating synovial fluid;
- Intra-articular structures – these are found in some, but not all, synovial joints:
  Intra-articular ligaments and tendons assist in the stability of the joint;
  Intra-articular fibrocartilaginous discs and menisci increase stability and assist with shock absorption;
  Intra-articular pads of fat also assist with shock

absorption and prevent damage to the delicate synovial membrane.

The individual properties of these features, their arrangement and the shape of the joint surfaces all determine the mobility and stability of each synovial joint. These articular structures provide a static role in the mobility and stability at the joint. There is also a dynamic contribution from the activity of the surrounding musculature.

We shall consider how the properties and arrangement of these of the features listed above may contribute to the stability and mobility at the joint.

The Hyaline Cartilage
Hyaline cartilage covers the articular surfaces of most synovial joints, exceptions to this being the

temporomandibular joints of the jaw and the sacroiliac joints in the pelvis. These both have some fibrocartilage. Hyaline cartilage is smooth, shiny and has a high water content. This glassy smooth surface considerably reduces friction during movement and all surfaces of the joint that are in contact are covered by hyaline cartilage.

Anatomical Application

Hyaline cartilage appears to be a functional adaptation in response to movement between two bones. This means that the extent of the articular surface may vary between individuals. This depends on the range of movement frequently used. For example, people who habitually squat have an additional small articular facet on the distal surface of the tibia. These are called 'squatting facets'. They are generated in response to the increased range of dorsiflexion and articulate with reciprocal facets found on the upper surface of the neck of talus (Williams and Warwick, 1980).

The high water content makes it particularly well adapted to withstand compression. It reduces the pressure between the joint surfaces by distributing the forces evenly across the surface of the bones. This will be discussed further with the properties of the synovial fluid.

Hyaline cartilage is also found in other areas where friction occurs between two surfaces, such as lining the 'pulley wheel' grooves in bones. These serve to guide tendons to their point of attachment and prevent sideways movement when the muscle contracts.

Histology of Hyaline Cartilage Hyaline cartilage contains *chondroblasts,* specialized cartilage cells that secrete the ground substance consisting mainly of organic molecules called proteoglycans. The proteoglycans have viscoelastic properties which allow compression and subsequent reformation of the cartilage when subject to compression forces. *Fibroblasts* are also present and produce the many collagen fibres. Collagen fibres have the ability to resist tension along their length, and the fibres are laid down in a mesh-like arrangement within the cartilage. As such, they assist in the ability of the cartilage to withstand multidirectional shearing and compression forces. These are applied during movement when weight bearing. (For a discussion on this consult Hettinga, 1980.)

Hyaline cartilage has sponge-like properties with a high attraction for trapping water. It is this that gives cartilage its ability to be compressed on weight bearing yet able to regain its original thickness when the weight is removed. The thickness of the cartilage varies, from joint to joint and within the same joint. It is thicker in areas which are subject to greater pressure. For example, the cartilage covering the articular surfaces of the hip joint is thickest on the superomedial aspect of the head of the femur and the corresponding superior aspect of the acetabulum. These are the contact areas for transmitting the body weight in standing.

Clinical Application

Diseases such as osteoarthrosis and rheumatoid arthritis lead to a destruction of the articular cartilage, exposing areas of subchondral (deep to the cartilage) bone.

This loss of cartilage will increase the friction between the articular surfaces. This means that more energy will be required to do the movement as some of the energy will be lost as heat produced by the friction, instead of contributing to producing the movement. In addition to the loss of strength and range of movement there may also be the additional problem from pain.

The Joint Capsule and Ligaments

The bones of a typical synovial joint are connected by a capsule. This forms a flexible sleeve connecting the bones and it may be strengthened by additional bands of connective tissue called ligaments. Some ligaments, for example the *medial or tibial collateral ligament of the knee*, blend with, or are 'intimate' to the capsule. However others, such as the *lateral or fibular collateral ligament* are completely separate. Some are situated within the capsule, and these are then called *intra-articular ligaments*; examples of these are the *cruciate ligaments* of the knee joint.

The capsule and ligaments have a major role in limiting the range of movement available and thus make a vital contribution to the stability of the joint. Normal range of movement is limited when the capsule and/or ligaments are on a stretch and become taut. Capsular and ligamentous tissues consist of bundles of collagen and some elastic fibres. When these are not under tension the fibres have a slightly wavy appearance, but they straighten on the application of tensile forces.

The collagen fibres of the capsule and ligaments

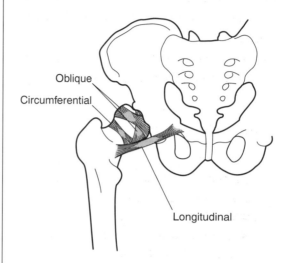

Figure 2.11 The multidirectional fibres of the capsule of the hip joint.

can withstand considerable tensile forces. The arrangement of the fibres in a ligament suggests the direction of the forces applied to that joint. For example the lateral collateral ligament of the knee joint has fibres that pass mainly vertically from the femur to the fibula. These prevent separation of the joint surfaces on the lateral side of the knee when an adduction (or *varus*) stress is applied during weight bearing.

A capsule or ligament that has to resist stress from many directions will have some fibres in a multidirectional arrangement. Consider the arrangement of the fibres of the hip joint capsule (Figure 2.11). The fibres are parallel, perpendicular (circumferential) and oblique to the neck of the femur, so they will restrict movement in most directions. (For further discussion on the role of ligaments in limiting movement refer to Evans (1988).)

Anatomical Application

The ability of a ligament to restrict movement depends on the fibres being taut. The range of movement allowed will depend on both the length of the ligament and direction of the fibres and the position of the joint. For example, the medial ligament of the knee has both vertical and oblique fibres. Their proximal femoral attachment is to a small area on the medial epicondyle of the femur. From this attachment the more posterior fibres pass vertically down to attach to the tibial condyle. The anterior fibres pass obliquely downwards and forward to attach more anteriorly to the upper part of the medial surface of the tibia. This obliquity, combined with an axis that alters throughout the range of movement, means that different fibres are taut in different positions (Figure 2.12).

[It may help your understanding if you draw the general direction of the posterior and anterior fibres on your own/a partner's knee, and do this practically. Although movement of the skin stops this being an accurate 'model', it might assist in visualizing the biomechanics of the movement.]

Now consider these three positions:

(a) In standing (Figure 2.12a): The knee is in extension and the distance between the ligament's attachments is at a maximum and most of the fibres are taut. Therefore, they are providing maximum support to the medial side of the joint and helping to compress the joint surfaces together. This is the position of greatest stability and is the position adopted when supporting the body weight in standing.

(b) In 20° knee flexion (Figure 2.12b): As the joint moves into the first stage of flexion there is a downward and backward movement of the femoral attachments. This causes the posterior fibres to become slack with tension maintained in the more

Figure 2.12   The triangular medial ligament of the knee joint. (a) In extension the posterior fibres are most taut. (b) In 20° flexion the posterior fibres lose tension yet the anterior fibres become taut. (c) In 90° flexion all the ligaments of the knee are slack and so allow the rotary movement (around a vertical axis) at the knee joint.

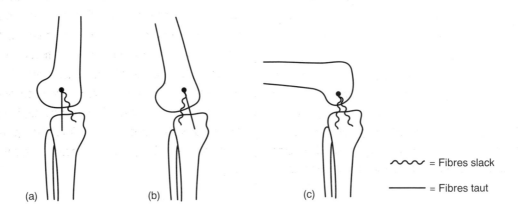

(a)   (b)   (c)

〰〰 = Fibres slack

—— = Fibres taut

oblique anterior fibres. Therefore some support is provided by the oblique fibres. The additional support required during any activity on a semi-flexed knee is provided by the active contribution of the surrounding musculature. In particular the quadriceps femoris and the postero-medial hamstrings, the semimembranosus and semitendinosis.

(c) In 90° flexion: The distance between the attachments of both parts of the ligament has decreased and they are now slack. Little stability is provided by the medial ligament; this then allows some rotation of the tibia on the femur, a movement not allowed when the ligaments are taut in extension.

Ligaments and tendons are commonly damaged from direct trauma or by the disease process. Obviously their ability to withstand stress will not only depend on their strength and position but also on the direction and speed of the applied stress.

The Normal Response of Ligamentous Tissue to Stress When ligaments are subject to stress, the first increase in length is from a straightening of the kinked fibres. As loading continues the elastic components will stretch. This is generally a linear relationship until the elastic limit is reached. The fibres will continue to stretch, passing into the plastic phase, and eventually rupture will occur. The exact length of the fibre when rupture occurs depends on the rate at which the force is applied. A sudden stress from a 'mistimed' football tackle may cause complete rupture of the medial ligament, whereas the same force applied slowly would not. This ability to withstand force applied over time is provided by the viscoelastic properties of the tissues, displaying the phenomenon known as 'creep'. Creep allows the application of a greater force over time before ultimate failure occurs. It is important to remember that the failure point will vary between the individual fibres. Care must be taken to avoid repeatedly overloading the ligament. This may cause rupture of a few fibres on each occasion leading to gradual, but cumulative, reduction in the overall strength of the ligament. Subsequent relatively low stress may cause a sudden and complete rupture of the remaining intact fibres and complete disruption of the ligament.

The rupture or stretching of ligaments around the joint will obviously lead to a reduction in its stability in certain directions. However, abnormal shortening of the ligament can lead to limitation of normal range of movement. If capsular and ligamentous tissues are immobilized in a shortened position then extensibility is lost, due to molecular changes and water loss (for further discussion on this refer to Donatelli (1981)). It is not only enforced immoblization that causes a loss of extensibility. If a ligament is not regularly stretched in the course of normal functional activity, it undergoes adaptive shortening, with a subsequent loss of movement. Therefore, to maintain full range of movement we should ensure that joints are regularly moved throughout full range. Ideally, this is done actively, but if a patient is paralysed or unconscious then passive movement of the joint may help to maintain range.

Clinical Application

Injury to ligamentous tissue is commonly presented to the physiotherapist, either as an acute sudden rupture or as a chronic 'overuse' injury. Both injuries lead to inflammation and repair of the damaged tissue. The laying down of new fibres is initially random and they must be encouraged to lie along the direction of the usual applied forces. This can be done by applying progressive tension to the area as healing takes place. This should be very gentle at first, increased gradually, until normal strength is resumed. There may be some scar tissue within the area of repair. This will contract and, unless stretched, there will be a resultant loss of the length of the ligament. Usually this is slight and has little effect on normal function, but it can be severe, and produce a fixed deformity.

These deformities can occur due to the joint being held in a flexed position, with the ligaments in a 'relaxed' position. Take, for example the knee joint. Usually in response to a painful inflammatory condition, for example rheumatoid arthritis, the knee is held in some flexion. The ligaments and soft tissues on the posterior aspect will shorten and those on the anterior aspect lengthen or 'creep' in response to the continuous stress. This process can be reversed and it is possible to gradually lengthen these shortened structures by applying traction or a splint. This takes considerable time and unless maintained in a stretched position the increase in length is 'lost'. (For a review of the effect of stretch on connective tissue with par-

ticular reference to physiotherapy see Smith (1995) and Threlkeld (1992).) The best solution is prevention of the deformity by the care team. This should include advice on optimum positioning and a regimen of specific exercises. These should help to prevent, or at the least reduce, any deformities.

Some ligaments have a greater proportion of elastic fibres than others. The ligamentum flavum of the vertebral column is highly elastic. During trunk flexion it is stretched and its elastic recoil contributes to the force required to regain the upright position. Although these ligaments, being highly elastic, lengthen fairly rapidly when loads are applied, once the elastic limit is reached they quickly rupture (Nachemson and Evans, 1968).

The Synovial Membrane and Synovial Fluid

Synovial membrane lines the internal surface of the capsule and covers all non-articular surfaces within the joint. It produces the lubricant *synovial fluid* and so is highly vascular. In appearance it is pink and shiny and is like slippery 'cling film'. It sometimes protrudes through a gap in the capsule to form a small pouch of synovial fluid called a *bursa(e)*. Bursae act by separating the capsule from an overlying muscle, tendon or ligament and form a lubricated cushion that reduces the friction between the structures. Folds of synovium may also project into the joint cavity and cover other intra-articular structures. Examples of this are the tendon of the long head of the biceps as it passes through the capsule of the shoulder joint (Figure 2.13), and the cruciate ligaments within the knee joint.

Figure 2.13   The long head of biceps brachii passing through the capsule of the glenohumeral joint enclosed by a synovial sheath.

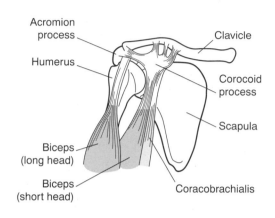

Acromion process
Clavicle
Humerus
Corocoid process
Scapula
Biceps (long head)
Biceps (short head)
Coracobrachialis

Clinical Application

These folds of synovial membrane can be 'nipped' between the joint surfaces, especially where the surfaces are roughened due to arthritis or trauma. This causes an inflammatory reaction resulting in hyperaemia, i.e. localized increase in the circulation. The membrane becomes swollen and there is an increase in the production of synovial fluid, called an effusion. This reaction to injury is visible in superficial joints such as the knee. On physical examination the joint will look red, shiny and swollen, the skin will feel hot and the patient will complain of pain. This reaction also occurs in more deeply positioned joints such as the hip, but the physical signs are not so easily detected. However, the patient will still complain of pain and there will possibly be a decrease in the range of movement. This may be from the protective 'guarding' spasm of the surrounding muscles.

The synovial membrane produces and absorbs the synovial fluid that looks and feels rather like egg white. Synovial fluid is important in the nutrition of the cartilage and lubricating the articular surfaces. It is similar to plasma found in the blood, with the addition of small amounts of protein and a substance called *hyaluronate*. This gives synovial fluid its viscoelastic and plastic properties (Williams and Warwick, 1980).

Methods of Lubrication   There are many theories of how synovial fluid lubricates the joint surfaces and so reduces intra-articular friction. Below is an overview of three of the more commonly accepted theories, which are weeping, hydrodynamic and boosted lubrication (Figure 2.14). All three theories are based on two fundamental principles of lubrication as described in the study of mechanical engineering. These are boundary and fluid-film lubrication:

- *Boundary lubrication* is produced by a single layer of molecules acting as a lubricant. The molecules behave as 'bearings' between the two surfaces.
- *Fluid-film lubrication* depends upon many layers of molecules that physically separate the two surfaces. In this case the movement occurs between the fluid molecules.

When the joint surfaces are not under compression the fluid is 'soaked up' by the hyaline cartilage. On compression, from the contraction of muscles crossing the joint and from weight bearing, the fluid is forced out. This is *'weeping'* or *'self'* or *'squeeze-film' lubrication* (Figure 2.14a), and forms a compressible film or layer separating the articular surfaces (fluid-film lubrication) which reduces friction. Additionally, when movement and sliding occur between the joint surfaces, a 'wedge' of fluid forms behind the leading

Figure 2.14   The tree main theories of synovial lubrication. (a) Weeping or self-lubrication: the pressure applied across the joint squeezes the synovial fluid out of the cartilage. (b) Hydrodynamic lubrication: a wedge of fluid is drawn into the gap, helping to keep the surfaces apart. (c) Boosted lubrication: the greater the pressure the more viscous is the synovial 'fluid'.

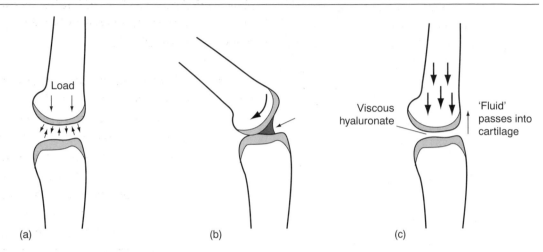

(a)   (b)   (c)

edges (Figure 2.14b). This wedge helps to separate the joint surfaces and so further reducing friction. This is *'hydrodynamic' lubrication* (Williams and Warwick, 1980).

However, these theories do not entirely account for what happens during a sustained pressure, which would have the effect of squeezing all the lubricating fluid from between the surfaces. Here it is thought that *'boosted' lubrication* comes into action (Figure 2.14c). The theory of boosted lubrication relies on the synovial fluid having an important property. This property is that the greater the pressure applied the more viscous is the synovial fluid. This is due to the 'fluid' component being forced into the cartilage, leaving the viscous hyaluronate in the joint space. This increased viscosity helps the fluid to 'stick' to the articular surfaces rather than being squeezed out by the pressure (Walker *et al.*, 1968, 1970, in Nordin and Frankel, 1989). In realitiy, it is more likely to be a complex integration of all of these

(and other) theories of lubrication, aided by the smooth, compressible and sponge-like properties of hyaline cartilage, that reduces the coefficient of friction in a synovial joint to around 0.02 (Armstrong and Mow, 1980, in Nordin and Frankel, 1989).

Intra-articular Structures

At the beginning of this section there was a reference to structures that lie within the joint capsule. We shall now consider how these may influence the functional role of a joint.

Intra–articular Fat Pads   These are found in most joints, to a varying degree. Their role is to assist in shock absorbency, reduce friction and act as protective cushions between the bone and the delicate folds of synovium. They also have a very minor role as a store of reserve 'fuel' for metabolism.

Intra–articular Ligaments and Tendons These are important for assisting in the stability of the joint. Examples of intra-articular ligaments are the cruciate ligaments of the knee joint. These pass from the femoral condyles, downwards to the superior surface of the tibia. A part of each is said to be taut in most of the range from full flexion to full extension. Thus they are important factors in providing stability throughout most functional activities (Norkin and Levangie, 1992). Tendons are also found within the joint capsule. An example of this is the long head of biceps brachii (Figure 2.13). This passes through the joint capsule of the shoulder joint, lying in the bony canal called the intertubercular sulcus or bicipital groove. This has an important role in stabilizing and controlling the head of the humerus in the glenoid fossa during movements of the shoulder joint, especially when lifting a heavy load (Kapandji, 1982).

Intra–articular Fibrocartilaginous Discs, Menisci and Labra These form additional plates of fibrocartilage that improve the contact area between the joint surfaces and so increase the stability of the joint. If we think back to Chapter 1, an increase in contact area reduces the pressure per unit area of cartilage. In addition these discs and menisci are made from fibrocartilage, which is compressible. They will therefore have an important role to play in increasing the congruency and shock-absorbing properties of the joint.

Examples of these are found as the menisci or semilunar cartilages of the knee joint. These crescent-shaped plates of fibrocartilage lie on the upper surface of the tibia (Figure 2.15). They deepen the concavity of the tibial articulating surface and therefore assist in the stability of the joint. They can however be damaged, especially during twisting movements of the knee when it is

Figure 2.15   The fibrocartilage menisci, deepening the concavity of the articular surfaces of the tibia.

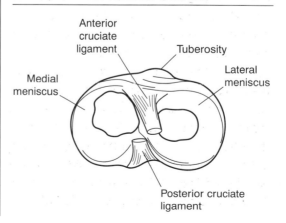

in flexion. This mechanism of injury is common in sports such as football and rugby football. When the ground is soft, the studs of the boot sink into the turf and fix the foot and leg. As the upper body and thigh turn a torsional stress is applied across the knee joint. If the knee is in extension and therefore 'locked' in a stable position there is usually little damage. However, frequently the knee is semi-flexed and relatively unstable. Then, the femoral condyle may trap part of the meniscus, tearing it, as the femur spins on the tibial plateau.

Intra-articular discs lie between the two articulating surfaces and can split the joint into two distinct cavities. An example is seen at the sternoclavicular joint, between the clavicle and the manubrium. Here the intra-articular disc is important for improving the congruency of the joint by increasing the surface area for the articulation of each bone.

Another example of an intra-articular disc is between the condyles of the mandible and the concave fossae of the temporal bones. These form the two temporomandibular joints of the jaw. The discs within these joints are thought to be extremely important in shock absorption and maintaining stability of the joint. The forces applied when biting and chewing can be considerable, although opinions on this vary (Williams and Warwick, 1980, p. 443). However there is complete agreement on its role in joint congruency and stability during movements (Hertling and Kessler, 1996).

Labra are lips of fibrocartilage attached to the rim of the joint socket, their other edge being free. They are found in the hip joint, as the *acetabular labrum* and in the shoulder joint, as *glenoid labrum* (Figure 2.16). Labra add depth to the socket, yet are more flexible than bone. This means that

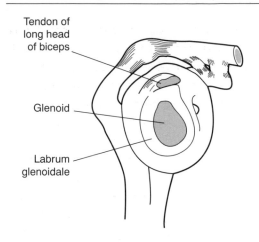

Figure 2.16 The fibrocartilaginous labrum forming a flexible extension so increasing the depth of the glenoid fossa.

Tendon of long head of biceps

Glenoid

Labrum glenoidale

they will increase the congruency and improve stability of the joint, yet will not severely limit movement. They are also thought have an additional role in assisting in the lubrication of the cartilage as they help to spread the synovial fluid over the cartilage during movement.

THE SHAPE OF THE JOINT SURFACES

The shape of the joint surfaces is important when accounting for the range and the direction of available movement. It also affects the inherent stability of the joint. Before we give examples, it is useful to review the three different types of movement that occur between joint surfaces. These are gliding, rolling and spinning and were first introduced in Chapter 1, when describing arthrokinematics.

The Movement Occurring between Joint Surfaces

The three types of movement are:

- Gliding or translation;

- Rolling;
- Spinning or rotation.

These all occur in various combinations during active movement and the proportions of each vary between individual joints, the range and direction of the movement occurring at the joint. Variation may also be from an increase in the resistance to the movement, for example, when kicking a football. It is important to remember that a loss, or change in the contribution, of these movements alters the biomechanics of the joint. This can lead to abnormal or limited movement. As such, a knowledge of these movements (which should include when they occur and the direction in which they take place) is required by the physiotherapist. This information is a vital 'ingredient' in the clinical reasoning process discussed in Chapter 6. When the lost or limited component of the movement is identified as a 'problem', then the patient management can be directed towards alleviating that particular problem. This may be by using techniques, such as passive mobilizations, which help to regain normal movement between the joint surfaces.

It is important to remember that when we describe these movements it is as if only one articulating surface is moving, the other being stationary or 'fixed'. Although this is sometimes the case, often *both* articulating surfaces move (but in opposite directions) and therefore contribute to the total movement.

1 *Gliding or sliding or translation* (Figure 2.17a) One joint surface moves across another. The contact point on the 'moving' surface remains the same as it slides across the 'fixed' surface. Imagine this as the blades of the skater sliding across the ice. The under surface of the blade is the moving contact point and the ice is the fixed surface. Another

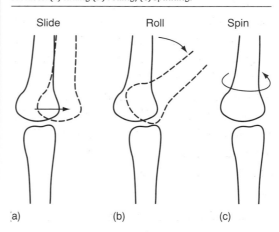

Figure 2.17   The three types of movement between two joint surfaces: (a) sliding (b) rolling; (c) spinning.

Slide   Roll   Spin

(a)   (b)   (c)

example is if the wheels of a car 'lock' and skid across a wet road.

Gliding usually occurs between relatively flat surfaces, like those of the cuneiform bones in the tarsus. It is also an important part of the movement between bones with reciprocally curved or 'concavoconvex' surfaces, where the convex 'ball' may skid over the concave 'socket'. This occurs as an important component in this type of joint such as the glenohumeral and knee joint.

2 *Rolling* (Figure 2.17b) Again one surface moves across the other. However, here the contact points of both the 'fixed' and the 'moving' surface continually shift as one bone rolls across the other. This is the movement that occurs between the wheels of a car and the tarmac as the car travels down the road.

Rolling occurs when a convex condyle rolls in a concave socket, as when the femoral condyle rolls forward on the tibial plateau during extension of the knee.

3 *Spinning or rotation* (Figure 2.17c) The moving bone spins on the surface of the stationary bone. In a pure spin the point of contact

remains the same for both the 'fixed' and the 'moving' surface. It is like spinning a plate or a coin on a flat surface. The analogy using the wheels of a car is turning the front wheels with the car stationary, as if trying to get out of a 'tight' parking space. Not a manoeuvre to be recommended as it subjects the tyre to considerable friction and increased wear and tear! Spinning occurs between the head of the humerus and the glenoid fossa during flexion of the humerus, especially when the movement is in the 'plane of the scapula'. When a pure spin occurs the axis of movement is fixed, and this is the essential difference between a spin and a roll. A fixed axis makes the joint like that of an articulated skeleton found in the classroom, where bolts connect the bones, forming fixed axes. However, our joints do not have fixed axes, so spins occurring at the joint are rarely 'pure' but usually in combination with some gliding and rolling.

In reality the gross movement at all joints can be accounted for in terms of translation, rolling and gliding. This 'gross' or 'combined' movement is often referred to as a *physiological movement*. If an individual component of the physiological movement can be performed actively and in isolation, it is said to be an *adjunct* movement. However, if the component cannot be performed in isolation actively it is said to be a *conjunct* or *accessory* movement.

To illustrate how these movements are combined we shall describe the movements occurring between the femoral and tibial condyles during extension of the knee joint when the foot is fixed by contact with the ground — that is, when it is acting as a 'closed kinetic chain'. (The principles of closed and open kinetic chains are described later in this chapter.)

First let us consider the position of the joint surfaces when the knee is moving from flexion to extension. In flexion, the posterior parts of the femoral condyles are in contact with the mid section of each tibial articulating surface. At the

Figure 2.18   (a) Fingers in extension. (b) Fingers in flexion and lateral rotation of phalanx. Note the deviation of the fingers towards the thenar eminence, caused by conjunct lateral rotation of the proximal phalanx on flexion of the metacarpal phalangeal joints.

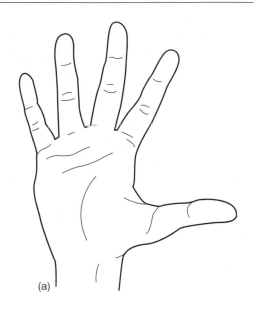

(a)

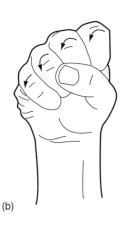

(b)

Practical Task

Although these accessory or conjunct (meaning = combined, joined together, associated; Fowler and Fowler, The Concise Oxford Dictionary, 1964) movements can't be performed in isolation actively, they can be reproduced passively.

Try the following:

Make a fist and note how the fingers deviate towards the lateral (thumb) side of the palm (Figure 2.18). This can, in part, be accounted for by conjunct lateral rotation occurring at the metacarpal phalangeal joint during flexion. Now try to reproduce this lateral rotation in isolation — it isn't possible! But if you firmly grasp a finger, you can passively rotate it.

Conjunct movements are essential components of normal movement and regaining them when limited or lost is the aim of most 'passive joint mobilization' treatments. The joint is passively manipulated to stretch the soft tissues and break down adhesions. This restores the normal range of the conjunct movement, and thus restores the range of the normal 'physiological' movement at the joint.

beginning of the movement, the femoral condyles *roll* forward on the tibia (Figure 2.19a). However, if this movement continues, they would 'fall off' the front of the tibia. So, to gain 'more' articular surface there is a backward *slide* of the femoral condyles on the tibia (Figure 2.19b). This *roll/slide/roll* sequence continues until the lateral side of the joint is in its 'close packed' position, and there is no further movement (MacConaill, 1964). However, the medial condyle of the femur continues to *slide* posteriorly until it becomes 'close packed' and fixed in full extension. This posterior translation, or glide, of the medial condyle is from a *rotation or spin* between the lateral condyles of the joint (Figure 2.19c). This occurs around a vertical axis through the lateral condyles, causing

Figure 2.19 Medial view of the knee joint. Full extension of the knee from flexion involves (a) rolling, (b) sliding and (c) rotation between the articular surfaces.

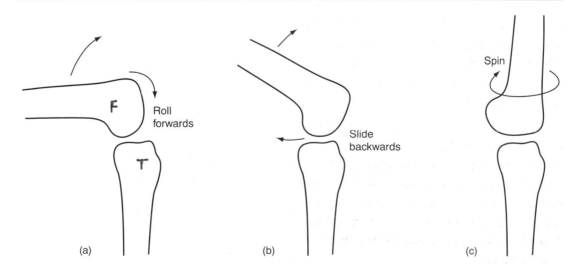

(a) Roll forwards F T

(b) Slide backwards

(c) Spin

the medial condyle to swing backwards (like a door on its hinges).

DEGREES OF FREEDOM

In Chapter I we looked at the terminology used to describe movements in various planes. A joint that allows movement in all three planes has *three degrees of freedom*. The hip and shoulder are examples of these, allowing flexion and extension in the sagittal plane, abduction and adduction in the frontal plane and rotation in the horizontal plane. Similarly, a joint that allows movement in only two planes has *two degrees of freedom*. Examples are the metatarsal phalangeal joints in the foot and the wrist joint, both allowing flexion/extension and abduction/adduction but no rotation. A joint with only *one degree of freedom* has more stability as movement in the other two planes is prevented. The elbow joint between the ulna and the humerus allows only flexion and extension and the ankle joint can only move through plantar and dorsiflexion.

Do remember that the movements and degrees of freedom above, only refer to the *physiological* movements occurring at the joint. During further arthrokinetic analysis of individual joint movement you will see how the contributions of *accessory* movements, occurring in the other planes, are also necessary for normal function.

Classification of Joints by Shape

Initially we classified joints by the range of movement available, e.g. slightly movable and freely movable joints. We shall now classify joints by the general shape of joint surfaces. We shall give some consideration as to how this influences the degrees of freedom and the available range of movement at the joint.

Articular surfaces are described as being either 'male' or 'female'. The male is a convex surface, and is usually the larger. This fits into a female, more concave surface. If the surfaces are flat or have both concave and convex features then the surface with the larger area is usually considered to be the 'male' surface.

There are seven categories for the classification of synovial joints by shape, which are as follows (Williams and Warwick, 1980):

- Plane joints;
- Hinge joints (ginglymi);
- Pivot joints (trochoid);
- Bi-condylar joints;
- Ellipsoid joints;
- Saddle joints (sellar);
- Ball-and-socket joints (spheroidal).

These are depicted in Figure 2.20 and described in Table 2.2.

Kinetic Chains

In biomechanical terms the movement occurring at a joint can be compared to those occurring between the links of a chain. If twisted at one end with the other end free to move, the chain will spin or rotate along its length, this is an *open chain*. However if the chain is twisted at one end and the other end is fixed, the links of the chain will twist and be subject to torsional stress and is said to be a *closed chain*.

Open Kinetic Chain When the chain is open, a twisting force at one end causes a rotation of the other. As it rotates it 'untwists' the chain and so no torsional stress occurs. Relate this to the upper limb when the hand is free to move. Rotation at the shoulder will produce a turning of the hand, as when reaching to take a cup off a shelf.

Figure 2.20 The seven main types of synovial joints and the movement available: (a) plane joint; (b) hinge joints (ginglymi); (c) pivot joints (trochoid); (d) bi-condylar joints; (e) ellipsoid joints; (f) saddle joints (sellar); (g) ball-and-socket joints (spheroidal).

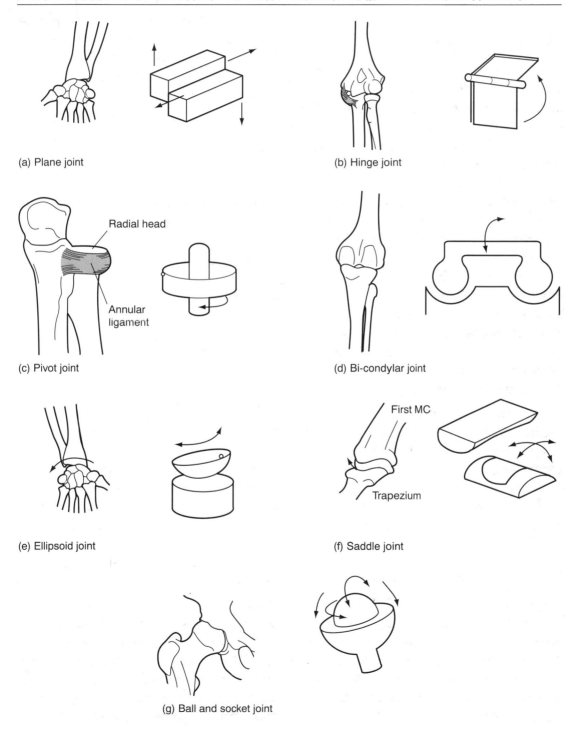

(a) Plane joint

(b) Hinge joint

Radial head

Annular ligament

(c) Pivot joint

(d) Bi-condylar joint

(e) Ellipsoid joint

First MC

Trapezium

(f) Saddle joint

(g) Ball and socket joint

Table 2.2
Classification of joints by shape (Reproduced, with permission, from Williams and Warwick, 1980, Cray's Anatomy, 36th edn. Churchill Livingstone, London.)

Classification	Description	Mobility and stability
Plane joints (Figure 2.20a) e.g. the intertarsal joints, the superior tibiofibular joint and the intervertebral facet joints	The joint surfaces are relatively flat.	Potentially these joints possess three degrees of movement. However the slight curvatures of the surfaces may restrict some movements and increase stability. Usually the mobility of these joints is restricted by strong, short ligaments passing from bone to bone. These can be ligaments on the surface of the joint and as interosseous ligaments that are situated deep between the bones. The range of movement in any direction is often small, and stability is favoured. Stability and mobility also depend on active contribution from surrounding muscles.
Hinge joints (Figure 2.20b) e.g. the elbow joint, ankle joint and the interphalangeal joint	A convex male surface fits into a concave female 'groove' or socket.	These allow only one degree of freedom of 'physiological' joint movement. Therefore, they are usually fairly stable. Movements in the plane at right angles to this are restricted by a combination of the shape of the joint surfaces and by strong collateral ligaments. These ligaments are often triangular, thus restricting side-to-side movement throughout most of the range. Stability and mobility will also depend on the active contribution from surrounding muscles.
Pivot joints (Figure 2.20c) e.g. the superior radioulnar joint and the atlanto-occipital joint	A round 'peg' of bone fits into a fibro-osseous 'ring'. Rotation of the peg within the ring is fairly free.	Movement is rotation around a vertical axis, therefore only one degree of freedom allowed. Stability in other planes is high, and rotatory movement is limited by ligaments and soft tissues, including the muscles.
Bi-condylar joints (Figure 2.20d) e.g. the knee joint and the temporomandibular joints (movement of one condyle always means movement of the 'partner')	Two convex 'male' condyles fit into two concave 'female' sockets.	Movement is mainly uniaxial, yet some rotation is allowed in the plane perpendicular to the first. The factors conferring stability are strong collateral ligaments – like those of the hinge joint. The congruency of the joint surfaces will affect the stability. The deeper the fossae, then the greater the congruency and the more stable the joint. The presence of two articulating condyles also aids stability. Stability and mobility will also depend on the active contribution from surrounding muscles.
Ellipsoid joints (Figure 2.20e) e.g. the metatarsal and metacarpal phalangeal joints	There is a curved egg-shaped male condyle with a reciprocally shaped concave fossa.	These joints allow considerable rolling and sliding, but minimal spinning. Therefore, flexion/extension and abduction/adduction are free, giving the joint two degrees of freedom. The stability is from the congruency of the surfaces and the position of the ligaments. Generally ellipsoid joints favour mobility at the expense of stability. Stability and mobility will also depend on the active contribution from surrounding muscles.
Saddle joints (Figure 2.20f) e.g. the carpometacarpal joint of the thumb, the ankle joint (although also considered to be a hinge joint) and the calcaneocuboid joint of the tarsus	As the name suggests each surface is convex in one direction and concave in the other.	This complex arrangement allows two degrees of movement, similar to an ellipsoid joint, yet the shape of the bones confers greater stability. There is also a small amount of conjunct rotation allowed – this is particularly important for opposition of the thumb. Stability and mobility will also depend on the active contribution from surrounding muscles.

Table 2.2 continued

Classification	Description	Mobility and stability
Spheroidal, 'ball-and-socket' joints (Figure 2.20g) e.g. the hip joint and the shoulder joint	As the name suggests these rely on an almost spherical (i.e. spheroid), male convex condyle articulating with a concave female 'socket'.	This is the most freely movable type of joint. It has three degrees of movement, but in reality it is multiaxial, so movement occurs in the many planes that lie between the three 'cardinal' planes of the body. Some stability is from the amount of congruency between the joint surfaces, but additional support is provided by the ligaments and soft tissues. Stability and mobility will also depend on the active contribution from surrounding muscles.

Here the upper limb is acting as an *open kinetic chain*.

Closed Kinetic Chain If the end of the chain is fixed, as, for example, when holding a stair bannister, the chain will not be able to 'untwist'. Any rotation at the shoulder produces a torsional stress across the joints (and bones) between the shoulder and the hand. The greater the rotation then the greater the torsional stress. In this instance the upper limb is acting as a *closed kinetic chain*.

The lower limb frequently acts as a 'closed kinetic chain' when the foot is 'fixed' to the ground by the body weight. However, if the foot is free, as it is during the 'swing' phase of walking, it becomes an 'open kinetic chain'. It is important to realize that either the distal or proximal end of a limb may be free to move and so 'open' the chain. We usually

Clinical Application

Whether the limb is acting as an open or closed kinetic chain is an important concept both for arthrokinematic analysis (analysis of movement between joint surfaces), and for kinetic analysis (analysis of forces). Closed kinetic chain activities produce greater torsional stress to the joints and soft tissues than open kinetic chain activities. Therefore, the muscles and joints of the area must withstand the additional demands that are imposed by 'closed chain' activities.

The stresses applied to the cruciate ligaments in the knee vary considerably. This depends on whether the foot is fixed or free. The cause of many injuries to these ligaments is a 'twisting' or turning of the body with the foot firmly 'fixed' in a muddy pitch. Here, as the upper body twists on a fixed foot the torsional stress causes a rupture of the ligaments in the knee. Following this type of injury rehabilitation should be directed to a functional approach. The re-education programme must include both open and closed kinetic chain activities. These should progressively stress, and therefore strengthen, the appropriate structures. (Refer to Irrgang (1993) for a review of the different approaches to the rehabilitation of the knee joint following injury to the anterior cruciate ligament.)

think of the lower limb acting as an open kinetic chain when the foot is free to move. However, the lower limb can act as an open kinetic chain when the foot is firmly fixed. In this instance, the torsion or rotatory force will move the proximal segment, the trunk and the rotation of the trunk will untwist the chain.

It is important, however, to remember that this is not always 'black and white'. There are occasions where resistance to movement tends to 'close' the chain. Consider what is happening when turning a stiff door knob. There is some 'opening' of the chain (i.e. untwisting) as the knob turns, yet the joints of the upper limb are subject to a moderate amount of torsion (the stiffer the door knob the greater the torsion).

The above section reviewed the mobility and stability of a joint with reference to the type of joint, the position and arrangement of the capsule and associated ligaments, and the shape of the joint surfaces. We have introduced the idea that muscles actively contribute to joint stability and mobility. We shall now expand on this by looking at the histology, shape and position of muscles, with particular reference to their roles in normal movement.

Muscular System

Introduction

Muscles are essential to normal function. Their role in producing and controlling movement is obvious, but their more subtle role in protecting joints is often overlooked. They serve to protect the joints by actively and passively limiting extremes of movement and by acting as shock absorbers. When muscles fatigue, they lose the ability to act as shock absorbers, and so more forces are transmitted to the cartilage and bone

(Markey, 1987). This may result in tissue damage and early degenerative changes. Therefore rehabilitation of muscle strength is required for restoring normal movement and for the protective role.

There are three major types of muscle:

- *Striated, voluntary or skeletal muscle.* This is concerned with stability and mobility of the skeleton and will be studied in some detail.
- *Non-striated, involuntary or smooth muscle* and *cardiac muscle*. Non-striated muscle has short fibres arranged as sheets of muscle. This type of muscle forms the walls of organs, blood vessels and respiratory passages.
- *Cardiac muscle.* This is only found in the heart. It forms the contractile tissue of the ventricles and atria.

The physiotherapist should understand the roles and the control of cardiac and involuntary muscle as they are vital for the maintenance of healthy tissues and homoeostasis.

Practical Application

When assessing patients, physiotherapists should be aware of possible problems linked to disease or malfunction of cardiac and involuntary muscle. Clinical problems such as a pain in the calf muscle may be due to poor circulation, leading to ischaemic pain, rather than local muscle injury. Similarly cardiac pain may be referred, and therefore felt by the patient in the shoulder and radiating down the arm. Of course there may be other causes of these symptoms. They might be pain from a 'trapped' nerve, which is compressed as it emerges from between the vertebrae of the spine.

This section will review the following:

- The histological make-up of skeletal muscle;
- Principles of muscle contraction;
- Group action of muscles and the individual role of the muscle within the group;
- Factors affecting the strength and range of movement.

The Histology of Skeletal Muscle

Muscle consists of specialized muscle cells, called *muscle fibres* or *myocytes*. A muscle fibre is between 10 and 100 µm in thickness and can be up to 30 cm in length, as seen in long muscles, such as the sartorius, a muscle in the anterior group of the thigh. Muscle fibres lie in parallel, separated by a thin layer of fibroelastic tissue called the *endomysium*. Fibres are grouped

Figure 2.21   A muscle, comprised of fibres grouped as fasciculi and then combined to form the muscle. (Adapted from Scott, 1996, in Kitchen and Bazin (eds) *Clayton's Electrotherapy*, 10th edn., WB Saunders.)

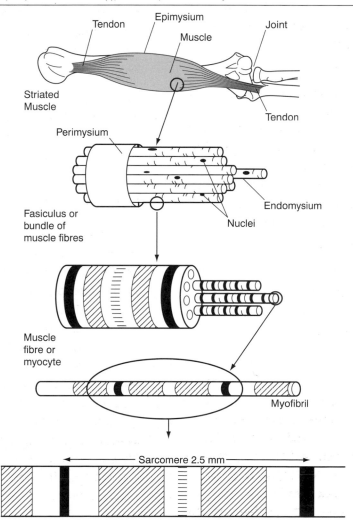

together to form a bundle, or *fasciculus*. Each fasciculus is held together by another fibroelastic sheath, the *perimysium*. The muscle is made from many fasciculi that are then enclosed in another sheath, the *epimysium,* alternatively known as *fascia* (Figure 2.21). Fascia serves to separate adjacent muscles by forming *intermuscular septa.* It also groups muscles together in anatomical compartments. These septa are important as they allow sliding between adjacent muscles and they also provide a surface for the attachment of muscle fibres. Many muscles fibres attach directly to the fascial sheath, and therefore do not extend from one bony attachment to the other.

The muscle fibre is the *contractile* element of the muscle and can actively shorten and lengthen. The connective tissues listed above, the vessels, nerves and tendons, form the *noncontractile elastic components* of the muscle. Those noncontractile tissues that lie between the muscle fibres are called *parallel elastic components*. Those that lie end-on to the muscles fibres are called *series elastic components*. Later in the chapter we shall discuss how the contractile and noncontractile components of muscle affect range of movement and force of muscle contraction.

THE SARCOMERE

The muscle's ability to shorten, lengthen and generate force is mainly provided by the contractile element of the muscle fibre. An individual muscle fibre has a cell membrane called a sarcolemma with many nuclei just beneath this membrane. Microscopically, it has a striped appearance, this is why skeletal muscle is called *striated muscle.* The stripes are from the different molecular constituents of the internal structure of the fibre (Figure 2.22).

The sarcomere forms the smallest individual contractile unit of the muscle fibre. They lie in series to make up the length of the fibre. It is the change in length of the individual sarcomeres that governs the total change in length of the muscle.

Each sarcomere contains microscopic fibres called myofibrils. There are two types of myofibril, each made from a different protein, called *actin* and *myosin*. The filaments of actin are thin and those of myosin are thick. They are arranged so as to produce the distinctive stripes of skeletal muscle. This pattern and its association with the mechanism of muscle contraction was first described by Huxley and Hanson (1954). These stripes form bands, lines and zones, shown in Figure 2.22.

The *Z line* is the boundary between adjacent

Figure 2.22   A sarcomere, showing the bands that give voluntary muscle a striated appearance.

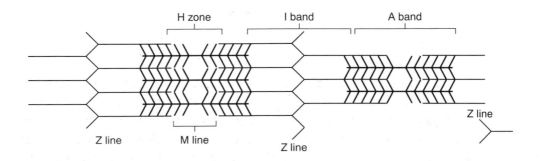

sarcomeres and is a disc of protein for the attachment of the actin myofilaments.

The *I band* lies either side of the Z line. It is a pale strip consisting of actin and strands of titin. Titin is an elastic fibre holding the thick myosin filaments in the centre when the sarcomere contracts. One titin molecule stretches from the M line to the Z line and loosely attaches to the surface of the myosin filament.

The *H zone* is the central section of the sarcomere and contains myosin myofilaments only.

The *M line* is the mid point of the sarcomere. It consists of fine protein filaments holding the myosin filaments in place.

The *A band* extends the length of the myosin and includes the H zone, the M line and the overlap between the actin and myosin myofilaments. This is the site for the 'cross-bridge' formation required for active muscle shortening and lengthening.

MUSCLE CONTRACTION: THE SLIDING FILAMENT THEORY

The physiology of muscle contraction can be found in detail in physiology texts: or refer to Billeter and Hoppeler (1992) for a more in-depth account related to muscle strength. However, at this point, a simplified account of this theory is important to understand and analyse muscle performance and injury.

When a muscle actively shortens the actin and myosin filaments overlap. It is the amount of overlap that governs the length of the sarcomere and therefore the total length of the muscle. Each actin fibre has on its surface molecules called tropomyosin and troponin molecules. There are 'active sites' found on the actin filament and when the muscle is not contracting these active sites are covered by tropomyosin.

The myosin myofibrils are made from bundles of myosin molecules. These have 'golf club' shaped heads that project from the myosin towards surrounding actin filaments. The head is attached to the filament by a hinge-like connection. This allows the myosin head to swing towards the centre of the sarcomere, the M line, and then back towards the Z line.

For a contraction to occur a nerve impulse passes to the muscle cells down the T tubules of the sarcoplasmic reticulum. As a result, calcium ions are released from the sarcoplasmic reticulum into the sarcoplasm. The calcium binds to the troponin which causes the tropomyosin to move deeper into the filament and expose 'active' sites on the actin. These active sites bind to the heads of the myosin. It is this binding of the actin to the myosin that forms the cross-bridge. The head swings on its hinge and pulls the Z lines together (Figure 2.23); this is the 'power stroke'. Following this, the myosin head detaches and swings back to its original position; this is the 'recovery stroke'. Provided calcium is still present, from the continued stimulation by nerve impulses, the head will attach to another active site, thus continuing to shorten the sarcomere. The calcium has to be actively removed from the area by *sarcoplasmic reticulum pumps* for relaxation to occur.

This whole process requires energy provided by adenosine triphosphate (ATP) stored within the myosin head. One molecule is required for the connection and one for the release of the head.

THRESHOLD STIMULUS

A muscle fibre will contract when the nerve stimulus is of sufficient intensity to release the calcium. This is a *threshold stimulus*. A nerve impulse weaker than threshold will fail to release the calcium and no contraction will occur.

Figure 2.23   Myosin heads attaching to the active sites on the actin filaments. This is followed by a swinging back of the heads drawing the Z lines together.

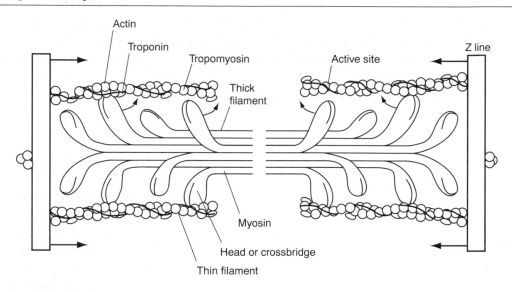

Furthermore a stronger stimulus will only produce the same force of muscle contraction, a *muscle twitch*. This is the 'all or none law of skeletal contraction'. If there are less than about 30 twitches per second, then the fibre will contract but the cross-bridges will detach before the next stimulus. This allows the muscle to 'relax' back to its former length. However, if the frequency of successive impulse is greater than 30 (range 30–100, depending on the type of muscle fibre; Williams and Warwick, 1980), each impulse will produce the twitch of the fibre before there is time for it to 'relax'. This means there is a progressive shortening of the fibre causing an increase in tension between the muscle attachments, so a stronger contraction is produced. This is a *tetanic contraction* (Figure 2.24).

A tetanic contraction is commonly reproduced experimentally, by applying an electric current over the nerve supplying the muscle. However, during a physiological contraction of muscle it is

Figure 2.24   A graph illustrating individual muscle twitches; when freqency increases they combine to form a tetanic contraction.

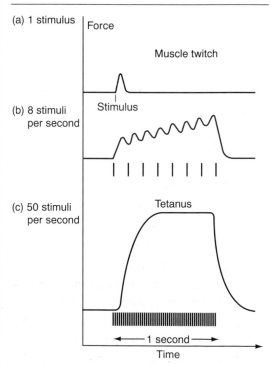

argued that a tetanic contraction seldom, if ever, occurs. Instead, some fibres will be contracting but others not. As one fibre stops contracting another will start, so it is the cumulative effect of many fibres contracting briefly, but in turn, that produces shortening of the muscle not just from a tetanic contraction of some (Williams and Warwick, 1980).

SUMMATION

Each muscle fibre is supplied by a nerve fibre. The nerve and the muscle fibres it supplies is a *motor unit*. When a nerve fibre transmits many subthreshold stimuli in quick succession, the transmitter substance produced at the *motor endplate* will 'summate'. This will then be sufficient to produce a muscle twitch; this is *temporal summation* (see Berne and Levy, 1996). Temporal summation also occurs at the synapse between two nerve fibres. However, nerve fibres are capable of another type of summation. This is called *spatial summation*.

It is important to remember that spatial summation *only* occurs at a *synapse*. It cannot occur at a motor endplate. It is beyond the scope of this chapter to give a detailed description of the transmission of a nerve impulse across a synapse, and the reader is recommended to consult a physiology text such as Berne and Levy (1996). However, this is an important physiological principle. It affects the number of motor units active at any time, and therefore the force of a muscle contraction, so it is worth a brief mention at this point.

Spatial summation occurs when *two or more nerves* both fire at the same synapse and *simultaneously* produce a subthreshold stimulus. Individually, each stimulus produces only a small amount of transmitter substance. This is insufficient to produce an effect at the post-synaptic membrane, and so no impulse is transmitted across the

synapse. However, the *total* amount of transmitter substance is sufficient to produce an effect. This effect is to stimulate the production of an impulse along the post-synaptic nerve. This might be a motor nerve supplying its muscle fibres and so increase the number of contracting fibres.

Practical Application

Physiotherapists frequently utilize temporal and spatial summation to improve a patient's performance, particularly when using facilitatory techniques such as proprioceptive neuromuscular facilitation (PNF). Manual resistance to a movement, combined with verbal encouragement will facilitate an increase in the number of impulses passing to the muscle. This is from an increase in stimulation of motor neurones at the anterior horn. The anterior horn is within the spinal cord. There will be both temporal and spatial summation, increasing the number of muscle fibres stimulated and thus the force generated by the muscle contraction. The exact mechanisms behind the facilitation are complex, but you may personally have experienced the 'boost' to performance that can come from verbal encouragement alone.

As mentioned earlier, each muscle fibre obeys the 'all or none rule'. Force is generated only when the frequency of the 'twitches' is sufficient to produce shortening or tension within the muscle. Before discussing other factors that can affect muscle tension and force of contraction, we shall review the different types of muscle activity and roles of muscle.

Types of Muscle Activity

As seen from the above, when a muscle contracts, cross-bridges form and *muscle tensions* is generated. This tension may lead to shortening of the muscle and so draw the attachments closer together. However, tension is also generated when a muscle is actively lengthening or even just maintaining the same length. These three different types of muscle work are all required for normal movement and the mechanism for each is described below.

CONCENTRIC SHORTENING

When a muscle shortens the muscle is said to be working *concentrically*. This is the action that is normally associated with a muscle contraction. For example, when abducting the arm against gravity, the deltoid (on the superior aspect of the shoulder joint) will work concentrically

Figure 2.25   The deltoid of the shoulder: shortening (concentric muscle work) produces abduction against gravity; a controlled lengthening (eccentric muscle work) produces adduction; and when working isometrically the limb is held in abduction.

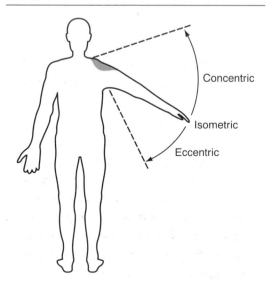

(Figure 2.25). Cross-bridges form and the myosin head swings towards the M line. This pulls the Z lines together and the overlap between the actin and myosin filaments increases as the sarcomere shortens.

Initially, the tension generated between the two attachments does not produce movement. This is because at first it has to 'take up the slack' in the series elastic components, such as the tendons. Only when these are stretched tautly can the continued shortening of the fibres generate a force sufficient to produce movement of the bone. Interestingly, the initiation of a movement will require a greater force than that required to continue the same movement. This is because inertia has to be overcome at the start of the movement.

ECCENTRIC LENGTHENING

A muscle might be active yet increase in length. Here it is said to be working *eccentrically*. Eccentric muscle work controls movement that would otherwise occur by gravity alone. For example, after abducting the arm, to slowly lower it back down to the side requires eccentric work of the deltoid (Figure 2.25). During eccentric muscle work, the cross-bridges form and the myosin heads swing towards the Z line (i.e. in the opposite direction to concentric muscle work). The overlap between the actin and myosin decreases and the sarcomere increases in length. In this lengthened position new cross-bridges immediately form and the process is repeated. This results in the muscle doing a controlled lengthening.

Concentric and eccentric muscle work are sometimes called *isotonic shortening* and *isotonic lengthening* respectively (iso = same, tonic = tension). Although this is accepted terminology, it is not strictly accurate as the tension generated within the muscle is not the same throughout the range of movement. It will vary as the muscle alters in length and the position of the joint influences the torque around the joint. This will be overviewed later, but for a more detailed explanation of this consult Pitman and Peterson (1980).

ISOMETRIC MAINTENANCE OF A CONSTANT LENGTH

Muscles are often required to hold the joint in a static position. The muscle is working actively and tension is generated within the muscle. However, the distance between the muscle attachments remains the same. This is a *static* or *isometric* muscle contraction. As when holding the arm out in abduction, although not moving the deltoid will still be working (Figure 2.25). In an isometric contraction the cross-bridges form, disengage and reform. Each time the myosin head attaches to the same active site on the actin filament. Think of them 'running on the spot', maintaining just enough tension to prevent movement, but not too much, as this would produce movement. Again, although we call this an *isometric contraction* (iso = same, metric = length) it can be argued that minimal shortening will initially take place. This will again act to 'take up the slack' in the series elastic components. (For further details refer to Pitman and Petersen (1980).)

RECIPROCAL LENGTHENING AND SHORTENING

When one set of muscles (the *agonists*) work concentrically so shortening the muscle to produce movement, for example deltoid producing abduction of the shoulder, there must be a reciprocal lengthening of the opposing group, the *antagonists*. In our example these are the adductors. Similarly, if the agonists are working eccentrically, that is, actively lengthening, there must be a simultaneous 'gathering up' or shortening of the antagonistic muscle fibres. In our example, when lowering the arm back down to the side, the adductors will reciprocally shorten. Both reciprocal lengthening (also called 'reciprocal relaxation') and shortening are involuntary processes. Even though they require the formation and breaking of cross-bridges, the connections between the myosin and actin are weak and the energy required minimal. Therefore this reciprocal activity is not usually classed as *active* muscle work.

Loss of reciprocal lengthening or relaxation may be seen in patients with dysfunction of the central nervous system. This can lead to increased tension in certain groups of muscles and an inability to relax when the opposing group is working concentrically. This is known as *spasticity* and it can be reduced by some therapeutic techniques and careful positioning of the patient. For further information on this consult a clinical neurology text, such as Fredericks and Saladin (1996).

Practical Task

The best way to ensure that you understand these different types of muscle work is to experience them. Try this:

Stand up and then slowly crouch down into a squatting position. During this movement the knees start in extension and finish in flexion. What actually causes this to happen? The answer is gravity. However, if it was gravity alone, once your knees started bending they would 'jackknife' into full flexion and you would collapse in a heap on the floor!

Now do it again, feeling which muscles are working in the thigh. You should feel activity in the quadriceps femoris, on the anterior aspect of the thigh. They are actively lengthening, i.e. working eccentrically. They are controlling the effect of gravity on the body, and so allowing knee flexion to occur slowly, and preventing the knees from jackknifing.

If you now stand up from the squatting position, you should feel the same group of muscles working. This time they are working to produce extension of the knees – not to control flexion. In this case they are actively shortening and so are working concentrically. Finally, try going down into a squat, stopping after about 30° of knee flexion. Hold it there for a few seconds – you should start to feel the effects of this very soon and the quadriceps femoris muscles will soon start to hurt! This time they are neither controlling flexion nor are they producing extension. They are working to support the weight of the body and hold the knees in flexion. They are maintaining a constant length and are working statically or isometrically.

Try making other muscles work in these three ways. Start with the biceps brachii, which is the muscle on the anterior aspect of the arm that produces flexion of the elbow joint. Then the calf muscles, which produce plantarflexion and finally the anterior abdominal muscles, rectus abdominus, which produce flexion of the trunk. All muscles can work in these three ways and it is important to include exercises that require all three when planning a rehabilitation programme.

Group Action of Muscles

Muscles do not work in isolation but must work together, in a controlled and coordinated manner. This is *group action* of muscles. We shall now consider the various roles that a muscle may adopt during movement. However, during a complex activity one specific muscle, or group of muscles, may take on all these roles at different stages of the movement.

Muscle fibres passing from one attachment to another may cross one or more joints. These attachments are sometimes referred to as a proximal 'origin' and a distal 'insertion'. However, this can be misleading terminology. It implies that the 'origin' is fixed and contraction of the muscle produces movement of the insertion only – drawing it towards the origin as the muscle shortens. This is not so – when muscle contracts the tension has an effect on all the attachments, pulling them together. Therefore, we usually refer to these in general as *muscle attachments*. Further description may be provided by terms such as proximal, distal, medial etc.

In normal activity there is usually more movement at one attachment than at the other. This means that the 'less mobile' attachment has to be 'fixed' so that shortening of the muscle will produce movement of the 'mobile' attachment. To ensure that this is coordinated and smoothly executed, the muscles work in different roles, acting as:

- Prime movers or agonists;
- Antagonists;
- Fixators;
- Synergists.

To illustrate this, we shall take the example of flexion of the elbow, as if lifting a book off the table, and consider the roles of the major muscles involved in this movement.

The Prime Mover or Agonist

This is the term given to the muscle (or muscle group) producing the major movement. In our example the prime mover is the biceps brachii. The proximal attachments of the biceps are to the coracoid process and the supraglenoid tubercle, both of which are on the scapula. Its main distal attachment is to the tuberosity of the radius, just distal to the elbow joint (Figure 2.26a). The biceps muscle crosses three joints, namely the gleno-humeral joint, the elbow joint and the superior radioulnar joint. Therefore, shortening of the muscle will tend to produce flexion at the gleno-humeral joint, flexion at the elbow joint and, as it winds around the shaft of the radius, also rotation of the radius to produce supination of the fore-arm.

The Antagonist

This is the muscle that produces the opposite movement to the agonist, in our example the antagonist is the triceps berated (Figure 2.26b). Triceps, acting as a prime mover extends the

Figure 2.26   To pick a book off a table various muscles work in different roles. The biceps brachii is the prime mover (a) with the triceps brachii the antagonist (b). The muscles connecting the scapula to the vertebral column act as fixators to stabilize the scapula (c), and finally the quality of the movement is provided by the pronators, preventing unwanted supination (d).

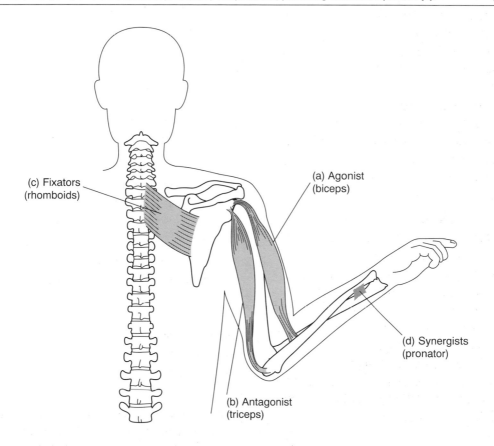

(c) Fixators (rhomboids)

(a) Agonist (biceps)

(d) Synergists (pronator)

(b) Antagonist (triceps)

elbow. As an antagonist to flexion of the elbow, it must relax or lengthen (i.e. the reciprocal lengthening we discussed earlier), as the agonist contracts and shortens, so allowing elbow flexion to occur.

Fixators

Fixators act to fix or stabilize a bone and so provide a firm base for the attachment of another muscle (usually the prime mover). In our example, the proximal attachments of the biceps are to the scapula and the distal attachment to the radius. When the biceps contracts, the muscle shortens and there is a force pulling both the radius and the scapula closer together. As the movement required is flexion of the elbow, we must prevent movement of the scapula. This is provided by other muscles, working as fixators, which stabilize the scapula. These are the muscles that connect the scapula to the vertebral column, for example the rhomboids and the trapezius (Figure 2.26c). Generally, fixator muscles are the more proximal, sheet-like muscles, such as those found in the trunk. However, this is only a generality, and other smaller muscles within the limbs can also work as fixators.

Synergists

Synergists are muscles that work together ('synergy' means working together) with the prime movers. They improve the fine control and quality of the movement and prevent any unwanted movement produced by the unopposed action of the prime mover. In our example, we have already said that the biceps not only produces flexion but also supination of the forearm. To prevent supination, synergistic muscle work is needed. This is from the muscles that pronate the forearm, in particularly pronator

quadratus, which will work to prevent supination at the radioulnar joints (Figure 2.26d).

Practical Examples

Students frequently have difficulty in distinguishing between the role of a fixator and that of a synergist. Remember, the former is stabilizing or fixing a bone to provide a stable base for the attachment of the prime mover. The latter are concerned with the general quality of the movement produced by the prime mover. Difficulty in distinguishing between them is not surprising, as the difference in the roles of a muscle is sometimes a 'grey' area. This is especially true when they are involved in a complex movement because then they may act as both fixators and synergists. Let us think about our example of elbow flexion. Here we said that the muscles connecting the scapula to the vertebral column were acting as fixators. Consider their role if the scapula was required to retract at the same time as elbow flexion. For example, as when pulling a door open. In this case they may be working as synergists (working with the prime mover for retraction, i.e. the trapezius) and fixators (for the biceps brachii) simultaneously.

Synergistic activity is often required when muscles cross, and therefore act on, more than one joint. In this case they might limit the movement to one specific joint. This is often required to put a joint in the optimum position for function and so to allow the prime movers to work most efficiently. In our example we were picking up a book. Let us take this one step further and consider the muscle activity in the forearm, wrist and hand. To pick up the book we require flexion of the fingers. However, the finger flexors also flex the wrist, to prevent this, the wrist extensors will work synergistically and hold the wrist in extension. This puts the flexors at an optimum length for powerful flexion of the fingers. To illustrate the point, try it yourself, and make a fist. What position does your wrist automatically assume? You will find that it is extension, to allow the flexors to produce a powerful grip.

In addition to the main roles muscles may adopt when working together, muscles may also be described as working as a *shunt* or a *spurt* muscle.

The muscle is working as a *spurt* muscle when it is producing the swing of the mobile bone, that is, producing the angulation at the joint. A *shunt* action is seen when the muscle provides a compressive force across the joint. This prevents any distraction of the bones, as this may decrease the stability of the joint. A particular muscle may work as either a shunt or a spurt muscle during the full range of movement at a joint. This will depend on both the position of the joint and whether it is the distal or proximal attachment that is free to move

Practical Example

Think about hammering a nail into a piece of wood. This involves, fast repetitive elbow flexion and extension. The weight of the hammer in the hand increases the centrifugal force produced by the 'swing' of the movement. The centrifugal force distracts the joint surfaces at the elbow

joint. This distraction force would put an unwanted stress on the capsule and ligaments of the joint. To prevent, this another muscle, the brachioradialis acts, as a shunt muscle and pushes the joint surfaces together. The brachioradialis is attached proximally to the shaft of the humerus, just superior to the lateral epicondyle. Its distal attachment is to the distal end of the radius, just proximal to the radial styloid. The position of these attachments provide a compressive force across the joint when the muscle contracts and shortens.

Distraction is not only produced by centrifugal force. The angle of pull of the tendon can produce the same effect. For example, when the biceps is producing flexion of the elbow in a range greater than 90°, the force can be resolved into two. One produces the swing of the forearm flexion, the other a force along the forearm, which acts to distract the joint surfaces. Here, the brachioradialis will act as a shunt muscle to provide the compressive force needed to counterbalance the distraction (Figure 2.27).

Factors Affecting Strength and Range of Normal Movement

These can be summarized as:

- The force or tension developed by the contractile components;
- The assistance and resistance from the noncontractile viscoelastic components;
- The length and position of the muscle;

Figure 2.27 During flexion of the elbow, when it is greater than 90° the biceps brachii will act as a 'spurt' muscle, producing the swing of the bone with some distraction of the joint surfaces. The brachioradialis acts as a 'shunt' muscle, adding a compressive force to stabilize the joint.

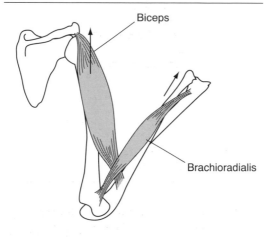

- The range of muscle work (length–tension relationship), the angle of pull and torque.

The Contractile Components

This depends on:

- Fibre type;
- Fibre diameter;
- Number of fibres;
- Neural control;
- Arrangement of the fibres/the shape of the muscle.

FIBRE TYPE

Muscle fibres may be classified according to their metabolism. They are then called either 'fast twitch' or 'slow twitch' fibres, fast fibres having a larger diameter than slow fibres.

Slow–Twitch or Type I Fibres

Slow-twitch oxidative (SO) fibres are also known as Type I fibres. They have a slow contraction time.

This is governed by the time taken for the myosin to 'attach' to the actin in cross-bridge formation. These slow fibres take 90–140 ms. Their metabolism is mainly dependent on aerobic (oxidative) respiration. As such they require an abundant blood supply (which gives them an alternate name, which is 'red' fibres), to provide the oxygen required for metabolism. Slow fibres do not fatigue easily, which means that they can work for a long time, but they sacrifice strength for endurance. These fibres predominate in muscles concerned with posture and repetitive activities that require less muscle strength but more 'lasting power'. An example of a 'slow' muscle is the soleus in the calf. Even when standing still there is some activity in this muscle, helping to keep the body balanced over the feet.

Fast–Twitch or Type II Fibres

Fast muscle fibres can be divided into two main types:

Type IIA are fast-twitch oxidative-glycolytic (FOG) fibres, which can perform both aerobic and anaerobic (glycolytic) activity. They are therefore an intermediate group between the Type I slow-twitch and the fast-twitch Type IIB. This means that they must have a reasonably good blood supply, and are relatively resistant to fatigue.

Type IIB are fast-twitch glycolytic (FG) fibres. As expected they will be capable of anaerobic activity for short periods. The blood supply is generally less abundant than that to the slow fibres (which leads to their alternative name of 'white' fibres). They have a relatively large fibre diameter and can develop considerable amounts of tension during muscle contraction. However, this increase in tension is partly due to the speed at which the myosin can generate new cross-bridges and 'pull' the Z lines together. This takes 40–90 ms, considerably

Table 2.3
Major differences between fast and slow fibres

Characteristic	Type I: slow fibre	Type IIB: fast fibre
Metabolism	Aerobic	Anaerobic
Blood supply	Abundant	Less abundant
Fibre diameter / appearance	Small diameter / red	Large diameter / white
Resistance to fatigue	High	Low
Cross-bridge formation	Slow (90–140 ms)	Fast (40–90 ms)
Cross-bridge duration	Longer	Shorter
Energy consumption	Low	High
Force generated / fibre	Low	High
Function	Postural control, high endurance activities (the marathon runner)	Explosive, high intensity activities (the sprinter)
Example of skeletal muscle	Soleus	Gastrocnemius

faster than the 90–140 ms of the slow fibres. Unfortunately they are not as efficient in terms of energy consumption. Although the cross-bridges attach readily they also detach more quickly than those of slow fibres. This means, to maintain a contraction of each type for the same time-span, the fast fibres will make / break and remake more cross-bridges than the slow fibres. As we have seen, making cross-bridges requires energy from the ATP. Therefore the fast fibres will use more energy than fast fibres. Gastrocnemius, again in the calf and just superficial to the soleus, is an example of a 'fast' muscle. This, unlike soleus, is not active in quiet standing, but comes into action during more strenuous activities, such as jumping and running.

In summary, we can generalize the major differences between fast and slow fibres as shown in Table 2.3.

Practical Application

It has been found that the proportion of fast and slow fibres decides the exercise capabilities of the muscle. Marathon runners have a greater proportion of slow fibres, whereas sprinters will have more fast fibres. This is thought to be largely genetically predetermined. However, there is some evidence that an athlete can be 'trained' to induce fibre type conversions from Type IIB to IIA and, less frequently, IIA to type I (Billeter and Hoppeler, 1992). Following immobilization, muscle fibres atrophy. The slow fibres are the first to atrophy (Appell, 1990). However, they have been found to have a better recovery rate than the fast fibres, but more important is to prevent immobilzation atrophy. It is preventable with good management and patient education, an important role of the physiotherapist (Kannus et al., 1992).

All skeletal muscles consist of a mixture of both types of fibre. Larger, flatter muscles are often found to have more slow fibres and are mainly concerned with posture. Muscles that contain a majority of fast fibres are quiet for most normal activities, being usually brought into action for fast or powerful movements. The type of fibre is determined by the frequency of the nerve impulses it receives from its motor supply. This was shown experimentally by transposing 'fast' and 'slow' muscle nerve supplies (Butler *et al.*, 1960). Over time the muscle fibre changed to 'match' the nerve impulses. There is also evidence to show that as we get older fast fibres are replaced by slow fibres. This may be attributable to disuse of the fast fibres as physical activity decreases, rather than age alone (Kovanen *et al.*, 1989).

FIBRE DIAMETER

So far we have seen that muscle fibres differ in their ability to resist fatigue according to their means of metabolism. Slow oxidative (SO) fibres are more resistant to fatigue than fast glycolytic (FG) fibres, with the fast glycolytic-oxidative (FOG) lying somewhere between. However, just because a muscle is resistant to fatigue does not automatically mean that it will generate less force. The factors that govern the relationship between force generated and fibre type is complex. However, fibres with a large diameter generate more force than those with a smaller diameter. Therefore 'fast' fibres can generate a more forceful single twitch than slow fibres (Billeter and Hoppeler, 1992).

NUMBER OF FIBRES

A muscle with more fibres will produce a more forceful contraction. Obviously if those fibres are the thicker fast-type IIB, then the muscle bulk will be greater still. Muscle fibres usually lie parallel to each other. Therefore, the force produced by a muscle will be related to the total cross-sectional area of the muscle. We say 'total' deliberately as

this varies enormously, depending on the arrangement of the fibres within the muscle. This means that the total cross-sectional area of a muscles fibres might not be apparent from its gross shape. This will be referred to again when we consider differing arrangements of muscle fibres.

NEURAL CONTROL

We have seen that to generate muscle tension there must be to be a continuous flow of nerve impulses. When nerve impulses are infrequent, the cross-bridges can disengage between each impulse, allowing the sarcomere to lengthen as the actin and myosin slide apart. When this occurs tension decreases or is lost completely. However, when the impulses are frequent there is the continuous formation of new cross-bridges, producing a progressive shortening of the sarcomere and increase in muscle tension. For most activities not all motor units are brought into action. It is only when an exceptionally powerful contraction is required that all the muscle fibres will be recruited, and maximum tension can develop.

ARRANGEMENT OF THE FIBRES/MUSCLE SHAPE

The arrangement of the muscle fibres within the muscle affects the shape of the muscle. Remember, the amount of tension generated by a muscle is that from all the individual muscle fibres. Similarly, the direction of the force produced by the muscle is determined by the direction/s of the forces produced by the individual fibres. We do this by applying the principles of resolution of forces, outlined in Chapter 1. For example, if the fibres of a muscle lie parallel to each other, then the force of each will summate. They will be a colinear force system and their lines of force will all be in the same direction. If, however, some are arranged obliquely, as in 'pennate' muscles, then it is not a question of simply summating the forces. Here, the forces must be resolved into different components and the resultant force calculated. Examples of these will be seen later when we classify muscles by general shape.

Attachments of Muscle to Bone

The shape of a muscle depends in part on its attachments. Obviously a triangular muscle will have one broad and one narrow attachment. Muscle fibres may attach to the bone or other tissues directly, but commonly the muscle fibres attach to a tendon and the tendon attaches to the bone. A tendon can be a round cord or a broad flat sheet, an *aponeurosis*. Frequently, they are somewhere between the two, and a muscle may have a rounded tendon at one attachment and a broad aponeurosis at the other, for example the adductor longus in the thigh. Tendons are histologically similar to joint capsules and ligaments, but are generally slightly more elastic. They consist of parallel bundles of collagen and some elastic fibres grouped together by a layer of connective tissue, the *epitenon*. These form yet more bundles that are finally bound together by a smooth sheath of connective tissue, the *paratenon*. The fibres of the tendon and tendon sheath blend with muscle tissues at one end and the periosteum and bone at the other. The fibres connecting the tendon to the bone are called *fibres of Sharpey*. Although the primary function of a tendon is to transmit the force of the muscle contraction to the bone, as stated above, they do have some viscoelastic properties. These are important both in preventing rupture of the tendon and in the control of muscle length. When the muscle contracts, the tendon 'gives' and there is a slight increase in length. Initially this is from a straightening out of the wavy collagen fibres, then from the immediate lengthening of the elastic tissue. Following this any increase in muscle tension will move the bone. However, consider what might happen if the bone was fixed and no movement occurred, as in an isometric contraction against resistance. Here, continuing stress will cause the tendon to stretch some more. This is due to 'creep', the lengthening of the fibres viscous properties, which occurs when tension is applied over time.

Practical Application

The viscoelastic properties of soft tissues are extremely important and must be considered when assessing patients who have increased or decreased range of movement. For example, if a patient presents with limited extension at the knee joint, this might be from an adaptive shortening of the tissues on the posterior aspect of the joint. To correct this the physiotherapist may use passive manual techniques, producing 'creep' and lengthening of the tissues by applying a long slow stretch. In some cases it may be necessary to splint the limb, holding the knee in extension to maintain this increase in tissue length or the increase may be maintained by exercise alone.

When muscle is held in a lengthened position, in addition to 'creep' of the noncontractile components, there is also some actual lengthening of the muscle fibres. This is from the addition of sarcomeres at the ends of the muscle fibre. This is serial addition of sarcomeres (Williams and Goldspink, 1971).

Tendons need to withstand high tensile forces, but they also need to be flexible, to bend through angles of 90° or more. The tibialis posterior tendon has to bend as it passes behind the medial malleolus at the ankle and again as it enters the sole of the foot. As it passes round the malleolus it lies in a bony groove. This acts as a pulley and alters the direction of the line of pull. It does increase the friction between the tendon and underlying bone, which over time would lead to fraying and possible rupture of the tendon. To decrease this friction a synovial sheath surrounds the tendon (see earlier section). This consists of two layers of synovium, and between them is a film of synovial fluid. This acts as a lubricant, allowing sliding between the tendon and its sheath and least friction.

Practical Application

Tendons with surrounding synovial sheaths are common. They are sometimes damaged and inflammation of the sheath occurs. This is a painful condition called tenosynovitis. *The inflammatory process produces an* inflammatory exudate *which causes localized swelling and then fibrin is deposited on the inner surfaces of the sheath. The fibrin makes the surface of the sheath rough, and 'grating' occurs; sometimes this is felt on palpational over the area, as the two layers try to slide against each other.*

One example is found at the wrist joint and affects the extensor tendons. It is a symptom of repetitive strain injury. *This is one of a group of conditions, known collectively as 'cumulative trauma disorders'. It frequently affects typists and computer operators, but can occur in any worker involved in tasks requiring small range, repetitive movements with insufficient rest periods (English et al., 1995). The management of this condition is primarily rest, often requiring a splint. This may be used together with other manual and/or electrothermal techniques that might encourage a decrease in the inflammation and speed up healing and the restoration of normal function. Of course, prevention is better than cure, so education of the worker and the employer is essential (see Chapter 13).*

Classification of Muscles by Shape

The two important factors to consider are:

- Length and position of the muscle/muscle fibres;
- Number of fibres.

Fibre length: As said earlier, muscle fibres consist of sarcomeres in series. When a fibre contracts all of its sarcomeres shorten. So how does this alter the range of movement? Let us consider the effect of the contraction of a 'short' fibre, with relatively few sarcomeres, compared to that of a 'long' fibre with many sarcomeres. It has been found that a sarcomere, when fully contracted, will be reduced in length by about a third of its original or *resting* length. If the muscle has a resting length of 6 cm, it follows that at the end of a maximum contraction it will decrease in length to 4 cm. This is a reduction of 2 cm. However a long muscle, with a resting length of 60 cm, after a maximal contraction will be 40 cm. Think of the effect this has on the muscle attachment. A longer muscle will pull its attachment though a greater distance than the shorter muscle, so we can generalize that a longer muscle has the potential to produce a large range of movement. Besides shortening over a considerable distance, usually they are more superficial. This may give a better angle of pull between the bone and the mobile segment, so increasing their efficiency. On the other hand, shorter, more deeply situated muscles are important stabilizers of joints. They act as 'adjustable ligaments' often lying parallel to the axis of movement as they pass across the joint. However, this deeply situated position and lack of length mean that they are less efficient in producing large 'swings' of movement around the joint.

Number of fibres: A muscle with more fibres has a greater total cross-sectional area and so is capable of generating more force.

These two principles of muscle length and cross-section can be related to the gross shapes described when classifying skeletal muscle. In addition, the muscle attachments and the direction of its fibres will influence the direction, the force and the range of the movement.

Muscles categorized according to shape are said to have one of the following arrangements (see Figure 2.28):

- Quadrilateral;
- Strap;
- Fusiform;
- Triangular;
- Pennate;
- Spiral.

QUADRILATERAL MUSCLE

The overall shape of the muscle is flat and square (Figure 2.28a). The muscle fibres are parallel, extend the length of the muscle and are attached to the bone by short flat tendons. If the fibres are short then the range of movement produced is small. Quadrilateral muscles are often found in situations where support is required to stabilize two adjacent bones. For example, the pronator quadratus in the forearm is important in providing stability between the distal radius and ulna, so preventing separation (*diastasis*) at the inferior radioulnar joint. Larger muscles, such as the gluteus maximus, may also be quadrilateral in shape. As well as being an important hip extensor and lateral rotator, it can also assist in the stability of the hip joint. Some fibres run parallel to the neck of the femur, so when they contract they compress the head into the acetabulum. However, the more deeply situated quadratus femoris is better positioned for this stabilizing role.

STRAP MUSCLE

In this type of muscle the fibres are parallel and may extend the whole length of the muscle (Figure 2.28b). For example the sartorius in the thigh. The fibres of strap muscles may be intersected along their length by tendinous bands, as seen in the rectus abdominous on the anterior aspect of the trunk. These muscles have longer fibres and so are capable of producing a greater range of movement.

FUSIFORM MUSCLE

This type of muscle belly is spindle shaped (Figure 2.28c). Most fibres attach to a cord-like tendon at each end. A variation of the fusiform arrangement is when two or three muscle bellies converge on one tendon. These are called *bicipital* and *tricipital* muscles. In all of these, the fibres are approximately parallel to the line of pull of the muscle. This arrangement gives optimum range and as there are many fibres, a substantial force is produced on contraction of the muscle.

Figure 2.28   Classification of muscle by shape: (a) quadrilateral; (b) strap; (c) fusiform; (d) triangular; (e) pennate; (f) spiral.

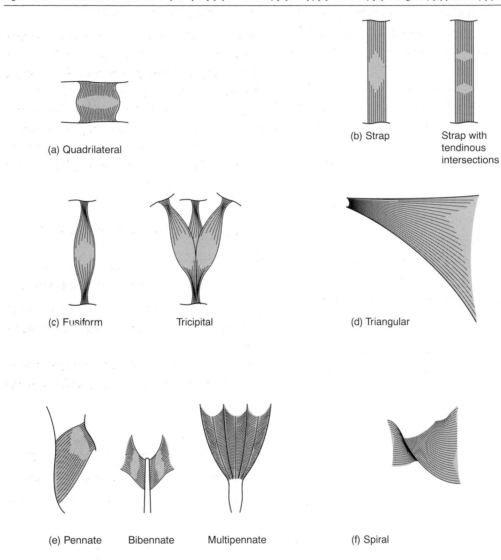

(a) Quadrilateral

(b) Strap

Strap with tendinous intersections

(c) Fusiform

Tricipital

(d) Triangular

(e) Pennate   Bibennate   Multipennate

(f) Spiral

TRIANGULAR MUSCLE

This muscle has a broad flat tendon or aponeurosis at one attachment and at the other it converges to a cord-like tendon (Figure 2.28d). An example of a triangular muscle is the gluteus medius, an abductor of the hip joint. This arrangement means that some fibres insert into the tendon at an angle. They are therefore oblique to the resultant line of pull of the tendon. However, this arrangement has a major advantage in that the force applied to the broad attachment, or 'base', of a triangular muscle is evenly spread over a greater area.

PENNATE MUSCLE

The fibres in this type of muscle are arranged like the barbs of a feather (Figure 2.28e). They arise from a broad attachment and pass obliquely to a central shaft of tendon which continues as the 'quill' of the feather and attaches to the bone. Pennate muscles can be *unipennate, bipennate* and *multipennate* depending on the number of 'barbs' or sets of fibres present. Where the fibres converge from all sides to a central tendon, they are called *circumpennate*. Examples of each are: unipennate, the flexor pollicis longus; bipennate, the dorsal interossei in the hand; multipennate, the middle fibres of deltoid; and circumpennate, the tibialis anterior.

Pennate and triangular muscles all have fibres with an oblique line of pull. The resultant force of the fibres decides the direction of the force applied by the main tendon. The force of each fibre can be resolved into two, one passing in the same direction, and the other perpendicular to, the central tendon. The advantage of this arrangement is that many fibres converge on the central tendon. This gives, in total, a large cross-sectional area of muscle fibres and so produces a powerful contraction. Triangular and pennate muscles are usually found where force or precision is required at the expense of a large range of movement.

SPIRAL MUSCLE

Here, the fasculi twist as they pass from one attachment to the other (Figure 2.28f). For example, the latissimus dorsi muscle, as it passes from the lower thoracic and lumbar vertebrae to the humerus, twists through 180°. Spiralized fibres tend to despiralize as the muscle contracts. This can produce rotation of the moving bone. For example, in addition to producing adduction and extension of the humerus, the latissimus dorsi is also an efficient medial rotator of the humerus. (However, note that muscles do not have to be spiral in arrangement to produce a kinematic rotation at a joint and the attachment of the latissimus dorsi on the anterior aspect of the humerus, so anterior to the rotational axis, also favours medial rotation.)

Some muscles fibres are arranged in combinations of the above. Here, different parts of the muscle often perform different functions. For example the deltoid is an abductor of the humerus. Its fibres are in three distinct groups. The middle group are multipennate, for strength, flanked by triangular posterior and anterior section groups. These produce the larger range of movement required at the shoulder.

The Series and Parallel Elastic Components

The elastic components of muscles are either:

- In series – mainly consist of tendons and other elastic components lying end-on to the muscle fibres;
- In parallel – consist of septa, tendons, nerves and blood vessels that lie in parallel with the muscle fibres.

See Figure 2.29.

Figure 2.29   Diagrammatic illustration of the contractile components with relation to the viscoelastic components in parallel and in series.

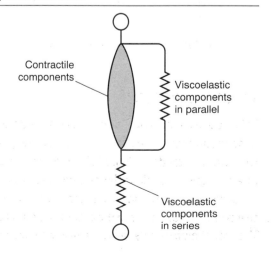

Contractile components

Viscoelastic components in parallel

Viscoelastic components in series

Active muscles, whether working concentrically, eccentrically or isometrically, develop a force within the muscle that we call muscle tension. This tension has to have force great enough to overcome the forces resisting the movement. These 'resistances' are both from external and internal forces. External resistance is from the weight of the limb and any additional load, for example a bag of shopping or a football when kicked. Internal resistance is from the noncontractile tissues in and around the muscle and any frictional force between the joint surfaces. As discussed earlier, friction between joint surfaces varies, depending on factors such as the type of joint and the shape of the joint surfaces. However, the internal resistance from the viscoelastic elements need considering in some more depth.

In the section on muscle histology we saw that, in addition to the contractile sarcomeres, there is also an abundance of connective tissue. This forms sheaths around the muscle fibres, intermuscular septa between the muscles, and tendons and aponeuroses for muscle attachment. It is also found in the walls of blood vessels and around nerve fibres. All these make up the noncontractile elements of muscle, and they demonstrate some viscoelastic behaviour. Therefore these tissues can act as a resistance and even, in some situations, can assist the muscle contraction. This depends on whether they lie in series or parallel to the muscle fibres, therefore they are usually called the 'series elastic components' and the 'parallel elastic components' of skeletal muscle

Those in series are usually concerned with connecting the muscle to bone. Those in parallel are frequently the connective tissue surrounding the muscle fibres, fasciculi and the muscle (the endomysium, epimysium and perimysium). They also include tendinous tissue that lays internal to or on the surface of the muscle, and blood vessels and nerves running between the muscle fibres. Besides these, which are all outside the muscle fibre, there is also a certain amount of viscoelastic behaviour from the cross-bridges within the sarcomere (Figure 2.29).

All these tissues have both elastic and viscous properties; the degree of lengthening (strain) will vary with both the forces (stress) applied and the time for which it is applied. We shall review some basic points relating to this. However, for further discussion on this topic, see Magnusson et al. (1996), Safran et al. (1988), Purslow (1989), Borg and Caulfield (1980) and Kovanen et al. (1984).

THE ELASTIC COMPONENTS OF THE PRIME MOVER

Consider what happens when the prime mover undergoes a concentric contraction. The initial tension and shortening will stretch the series elastic components, but reduce the tension on those in parallel. Once those in series are taut the continuing tension is transmitted to the bone and movement occurs. This tension in the series elastic component is stored as potential energy. This potential energy is released when the muscle relaxes, allowing the tendon to 'recoil', and regain its original length. Therefore, recoil plays an important part in returning the muscle to its 'resting length' following a concentric contraction, so the elastic components are important in determining the resting length of the muscle. Most muscles resume their 'resting length' when a relaxed position is adopted; however, the true resting length is the length of the muscle when all of its attachments are cut free.

This recoil, besides returning the muscle to its resting length, also adds to the force of a muscle contraction. For this, the muscle and its connective tissues (both in series and in parallel) are stretched passively, immediately prior to a muscle contraction. This principle is employed by physiotherapists when applying manual therapeutic techniques such as proprioceptive neuromuscular facilitation. Here, a passive stretch of the muscles is part of the technique for improving muscle function. It can also be deliberately employed in athletic training, where this type of exercise is called 'plyometrics'.

If no movement occurs from the increase in muscle tension, for example if attachments are fixed, then the tension continues to increase within the muscle as it performs an isometric contraction. This tension is transferred to the series elastic components. If this is prolonged, they will continue to lengthen (creep) due to the viscous properties of the tissues until the force generated exceeds the elastic limit or yield point. When this is reached, the tissues will either irreversibly lengthen or even rupture. Rupture often occurs when the tendon has been previously damaged, resulting in the loss of overall strength of the tissues.

If the muscle is working eccentrically (actively lengthening), the series components will be on a stretch throughout the contraction. However, the parallel components will only start to elongate when the muscle length exceeds the 'resting length' of the muscle. As the muscle eccentrically extends the parallel components will become progressively longer. It is the tension from these that assists in preventing over-stretching of the muscle and damage to the fibres and sarcomeres.

Practical Application

An example of a plyometric manoeuvre is contraction of the calf muscle immediately after jumping from a moderate height of 110 cm (these are 'depth jumps'). On landing, the foot and ankle are forced into dorsiflexion, stretching the series and parallel elastic tissues. If this is followed by an immediate contraction of the stretched muscles (as by instructing to 'jump as high as possible'), the force of the contraction increases (Hakkinen et al., 1985). Part of this increase in power can be attributed to the release of the stored potential energy, the elastic recoil of the noncontractile elements. There are also complex neural mechanisms involved in this increase in force, which are also affected by attitude and motivation. A third major factor in this increase in muscle tension, is that this recoil restores the muscle fibre to an optimum length for an efficient contraction. This is explained later, in more detail, in the section on muscle length–tension curves.

THE ELASTIC COMPONENTS OF THE ANTAGONISTS

We have seen that when the prime mover shortens there must be a passive lengthening of the agonists. This depends on the extensibility of the series and parallel elastic components. If the antagonists lose extensibility and therefore length, they will limit movement. This limitation of movement is said to be caused by *passive insufficiency* of the antagonists.

Clinical Application

*Both series and parallel viscoelastic com-
ponents should be stretched before exercise to prevent damaging the tissues. This
should be a slow prolonged stretch — the
stretch must be held for long enough to
allow elongation of the more viscous collagenous sheaths (Malachy et al., 1992).
These viscoelastic properties of tissue
may also be increased by heat (Strickler
et al., 1990). This is a principle used by
physiotherapists when using treatments
that heat the tissues. This is followed by a
sustained stretch in order to increase the
length of the shortened ligaments and/or
scar tissue.*

*Do remember that muscles immobilized in
a shortened position, lose elasticity of the
noncontractile elements. In addition,
there is a reduction in the number of
sarcomeres, so reducing the length of
the muscle fibres. It has been found that
an intermittent stretch, even as little as half
an hour per day, is sufficient to prevent
sarcomere loss; it may even be sufficient to
increase in the number of sarcomeres in
series (Williams, 1990). This is particularly
relevant to the physiotherapist when
treating patients who may be unable or
reluctant to stretch the muscles and soft
tissues.*

PASSIVE INSUFFICIENCY

A certain amount of passive insufficiency is normal, and all muscles have a desired maximum
length. This is important for limiting excessive
movements at a joint. Excessive movement would
lead to an unstable joint, even damaging the joint
surfaces and ligaments. However, excessive passive insufficiency is abnormal and limits normal
range of movement. So, the extensibility of the
opposing tissues should be considered when
assessing joint range. For example, the hamstrings
produce movement at both the hip and the knee
joint, so they are called 'two-joint muscles'. They
cause active knee flexion and hip extension. This
means that they are fully stretched when the hip is
flexed and the knee extended. Muscles that pass
over two joints normally restrict some of the
movement at one or both of the joints. This is
because they have insufficient extensibility/
length, to allow both joints to move through
full range simultaneously. Therefore, when assessing the range of hip flexion, you must ensure that
you eliminate any passive insufficiency from the
hamstrings. This is by ensuring that hip flexion is
measured with the knee in flexion. If the knee was
in extension the hamstrings would restrict full hip
flexion, limiting the movement by passive insufficiency. The degree of restriction to movement
from passive insufficiency depends on the extensibility of the muscles. This varies between individuals: some, such as trained athletes and gymnasts
have very extensible muscles, whilst others,
'couch potatoes!' have normal limited range of
movement due to soft tissue shortening.

Practical Application

*Even though variation in muscle length is
normal, muscles may become abnormally
short for a variety of reasons. These
include habitual poor posture and/or
inactivity, which prevents certain muscle
groups from being fully stretched. This
can lead to adaptive shortening of both*

the contractile and noncontractile components of the muscle and is frequently found in muscles which cross more than one joint. In severe cases this shortening produces fixed deformities, gross limitation of normal movement and function, and even overstretching and subsequent damage to opposing structures. This is one of the problems that must be addressed in the treatment of muscle imbalance.

Some of this lack of extensibility of a muscle will be from permanent shortening of the series and parallel elastic components; however, it may also be from loss of length of the muscle fibres. It has been found that muscle fibres that are held in a shortened position, or are not regularly stretched through full range, lose sarcomeres and so the length of the contractile component physically decreases (Williams, 1990). The physiotherapists motto and advice to all should be 'if you don't want to lose it, use it!'

The Range of Muscle Contraction (Length–Tension Relationship) and Angle of Pull

These affect the force and amount of movement and depend on:

- The range, described as either inner, middle or outer range and the effect this has on the efficiency of the sarcomere;
- The angle of pull of the muscle attachment and the effect this has on the movement.

THE RANGE OF THE MUSCLE WORK

The length of the muscle is an important factor in governing the force/tension it can generate. When a muscle starts from fully stretched and contracts to its shortest length, it has worked through *full range*. For ease of description we can split this range into equal thirds, named *outer, middle and inner range*. Outer range starts from when the muscle is fully stretched and inner range is the final phase of shortening. Obviously the phase between these two is middle range. These ranges are not particularly precise but are useful descriptors of muscle activity (Figure 2.30).

The tension produced by a muscle varies depending on the range. This is, in part, due to the number of cross-bridges formed and in part, from the viscoelastic components. Let us consider these in relation to range of muscle work.

Outer Range
When the muscle is contracting in its outer range, and it starts from a lengthened position, the actin and myosin have least overlap, fewer cross-bridges can bind and so less tension is produced (Figure 2.30a). We have seen that in normal muscle, the length of the muscle will be self limiting. This is from the passive tension developed by the resistance of the series and parallel elastic components. Under normal circumstances, this prevents complete disruption to the overlap of the actin and myosin filaments. In addition, when the muscle is contracting from a lengthened position, the recoil of the stretched elastic components (series and parallel) contributes to the developing muscle tension. This helps the muscle to shorten into middle range, which is the optimum length for the actin and myosin overlap.

Figure 2.30   The quadriceps femoris, working as knee extensors throughout full range. (a) outer range, (b) middle range, (c) inner range with the associated actin/myosin overlap within the sarcomere.

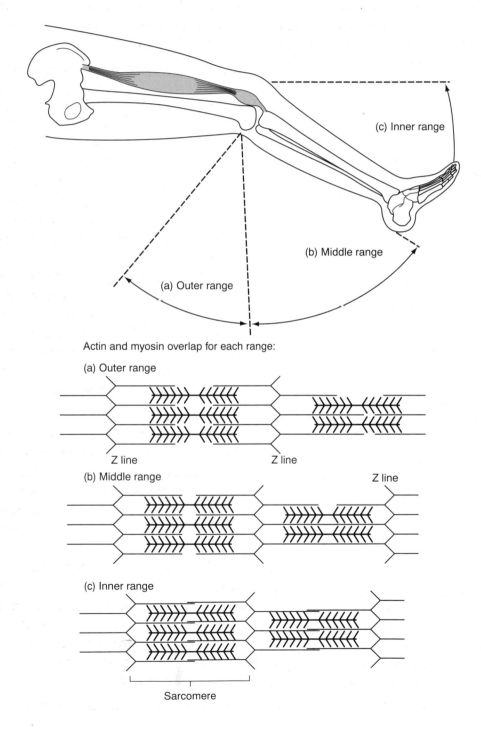

Middle Range

Maximum tension is generated in this range as the overlap between the actin and myosin filaments provides the optimum number of sites for cross-bridge formation (Figure 2.30b). As discussed earlier, the more cross-bridges formed then the greater the force generated by the muscle fibre.

Inner Range

If the muscle is contracting in inner range it is in a shortened position (Figure 2.30c). The actin and myosin filaments overlap each other. This decreases the number of sites available for cross-bridge formation and therefore less force is generated. There is no contribution from the recoil of the parallel elastic components (they are under no tension in this position), and in addition, the series elastic components of the prime mover, and the series *and* parallel components of the antagonists are stretched. These all form additional internal resistance to the muscle contraction, so reducing its efficiency.

Active Insufficiency

Movement when limited by the inability of the agonist to actively shorten is called *active insufficiency.* This occurs when the muscle is working in inner range. Muscles working in this range may be unable to shorten sufficiently to produce the full range of movement available at the joint. For example, consider the range of knee flexion, both actively and passively. Stand in the anatomical position. Now do active flexion of one knee, so bringing the heel towards the back of the thigh. You will find that the heel does not touch the thigh, but this is not due to lack of movement at the joint. Prove this to yourself, by reaching down and taking hold of the foot and passively pull your heel up, bringing the knee into further flexion. Now, the movement is limited by contact of the soft tissues of the calf and thigh. So, in this case, the inability of the hamstrings to produce full range of active knee flexion is caused by active insufficiency. They are physically unable to shorten any further.

To relate this to the activity within the sarcomere; as the sarcomere is fully contracted there is a great deal of overlap between the actin and myosin, which means that there are no free active sites on the actin for cross-bridge formation. However, if you bring your hip joint further into flexion, you may find that you can get more knee flexion. This is because flexion of the hip has stretched the hamstrings and so lengthened the sarcomere, resulting in an increase in available active sites. Abnormal active insufficiency of a muscle may be due to permanent lengthening of the muscle, which is usually from overstretching of the elastic components — beyond the elastic limit. This means that the recoil of the elastic tissues is lost and there is a resultant increase in the resting length of the muscle. The body's natural response to this is to increase the number of sarcomeres, by adding sarcomeres in series.

This is one of the reasons given for the occurrence of stress incontinence following childbirth. In the later stages of pregnancy and during the birth, the tissues of the pelvic floor may be stretched beyond their elastic limit. This can result in permanent lengthening of the tissues, so sarcomeres are added in series. This increase in length of the pelvic floor muscles means that even on a maximal contraction, the muscle is unable to shorten enough to shut the external sphincter. This means that there may be an involuntary loss of urine, particularly during strenuous activity or when laughing and coughing. All of which may increase the intra-abdominal pressure.

To avoid serial addition or loss of sarcomeres, it is

best to immobilize muscles in their middle or resting length. However, ligaments should be near full stretch, to prevent adaptive shortening. Sometimes there has to be some compromise, as optimum position for both is not possible. For example, generally when the knee is in extension, the major ligaments are taut. However, the quadriceps are in inner range, so risking a decrease in muscle length. The hamstrings are in outer range (especially if sitting with extended knees and flexion at the hip joints), so risking an increase in muscle length. This is the position often adopted for immobilization of the lower limb, but usually active knee flexion starts at the earliest opportunity.

The Overall Effect of Muscle Contraction and Noncontractile Elements on Intramuscular Tension Throughout Full Range

The graph (Figure 2.31) summarizes the above and shows the actual tension developed by a muscle throughout range (solid line) and the resulting tension, after the contribution from the passive elements (dotted line). You can see from this that a muscle will normally produce its maximum tension when it is working in middle range. This is usually its 'resting length' (remember, this is the length that a muscle adopts if both attachments were cut free and the muscle detached). At the two extremes of muscle length/range the force generated decreases, so outer and inner ranges

Figure 2.31   A graph showing the tension developed by a muscle contraction throughout range (solid line) and the resultant tension following the effect of the visoelastic passive components of the agonist (dotted line).

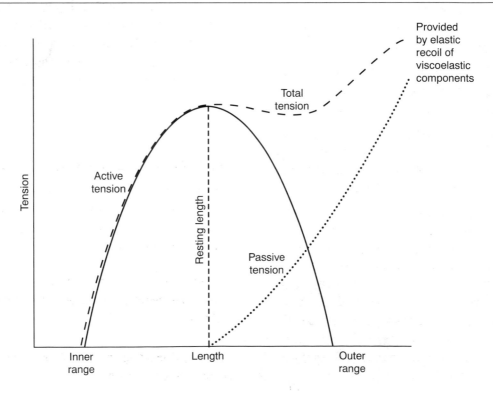

are usually less efficient at generating increased muscle tension. However, outer range is assisted by recoil of agonist elastic components, and inner range is resisted by the stretching of the antagonist elastic components.

Practical Task

All muscles have some passive and active insufficiency, and it is the combined group action of muscles that prevents this from interfering with normal function.

Earlier in this chapter you were asked to make a fist and observe the position of the wrist joint. If you remember correctly the wrist was in extension. This is by the synergistic activity of the wrist extensor muscles.

But why?

Now try making a fist again, but this time allow the wrist to flex (from the unopposed action of the finger flexors).

You should now find that you are unable to make such a powerful clenched fist, as the fingers are unable to flex fully.

This can be explained: in part it is from passive insufficiency and in part from some active insufficiency. We shall first of all explain the passive insufficiency.

Remember, this is from lack of length of the antagonists. Here, the antagonists are the muscles and tendons on the dorsum of the wrist and hand, the extensor muscles. When the wrist and fingers flex they become fully stretched over the dorsal surface. They are unable to lengthen any further, so preventing full flexion of the fingers. This means that you cannot make a tightly clenched fist.

The active insufficiency is from the long muscles that flex the fingers. If the wrist is in flexion, the finger flexors are in a shortened position and working in inner range. As discussed earlier, in inner range the sarcomeres are unable to shorten further. This means that muscle cannot actively pull the fingers into full range of flexion. A tight fist requires full flexion of the fingers.

The brain is able to produce functional movement by coordinating muscle activity, that is 'group action' of muscles. If the neural control of this is lost then muscles may still 'work' but coordination and function may be lost. This is seen in patients who have lost the nerve supply (the radial nerve) to the wrist extensors. On attempting to make a fist, the hand and wrist 'claw' into flexion. Function can be improved by applying a 'cock-up' splint, this permanently holds the wrist in slight extension, putting the flexors in an optimum functional position.

THE TORQUE AND THE ANGLE OF PULL

We have seen that muscle tension is related to the muscle range and so the force produced by the muscle varies with movement at the joint. This force is also affected by:

- The length of the moment arm;
- The angle between the muscle attachment and the bone.

Both vary depending on the position of the joint. Let us take each in turn.

The Moment Arm

In Chapter 1 we discussed levers and saw that by altering the distance between the application of the load and the axis of movement we change the torque, which is the turning force around a joint. Let us consider how this can also affect the effort required to produce movement of the bone or limb.

The effort arm is the perpendicular distance from the point of application of effort to the joint axis. As we have seen, axes of joints are rarely fixed and they shift during movement, every position having its own *instantaneous centre of rotation*. However, we usually identify a specific point by taking a 'good approximation' of all these; this is then the axis of movement.

The point of application of the effort is identified as the mid point of the muscle's attachment to the bone. It is important to remember that the *effective length* of the load arm varies depending on the position of the joint. This means that the force required to overcome the load varies accordingly. To remind you, the point of application of the load is the centre of mass of the segment. The perpendicular distance between the centre of mass and the axis alters as the bone swings around the joint.

Let us take as an example the biceps brachii working as a flexor of the elbow joint. This is shown in Figure 2.32, in full extension, 90° flexion and full flexion. You can see that the distance between the axis and the load is greatest when the elbow is at a right angle. Therefore, in this position, the muscle must generate greatest force to produce movement. However, the body is adapted for this, so in this position the muscle is working in middle range, which, as said earlier, is the optimum range for generating muscle tension. Generally, but not always, this is the case, and muscles acting on the joints work in their middle range when maximum force is required. In addition to torque there is also a change in the tendon's angle of pull; this too will have an effect on the resultant effort.

THE ANGLE OF PULL

You should remember from Chapter 1 that a force will have maximum effect when applied in the same direction as the intended movement. We have seen that most movement in the body comprises of a bone turning around a joint axis. When the effort is applied via a muscle attachment, usually a tendon, it produces a maximum effect when the angle pull is 90°. In our example in Figure 2.32, this is when the joint is also approximately at a right angle.

If you look at Figure 2.32a, you can see that as the elbow moves further into extension, the angle of pull decreases. Here the muscle force can be resolved into two components, one producing the swing of the bone, and the other passing through the shaft of the radius producing compression between the articular surfaces (acting more in the role of a 'shunt' muscle).

At the other extreme (Figure 2.32c), in full flexion, the angle of pull is greater than 90°. Here the force can again be resolved into two components, one producing the swing (acting as a 'spurt' muscle) and the other producing a distraction force across the joint.

Therefore we can generally accept that a muscle will produce its most efficient movement of a load when the applied effort is at its greatest distance from the axis of movement and the angle of pull of the applied effort is 90°.

Figure 2.32   Showing biceps brachii and how the angle of pull and the length of the load and effort arm change throughout the range of movement: (a) full extension, (b) 90° flexion and (c) full flexion.

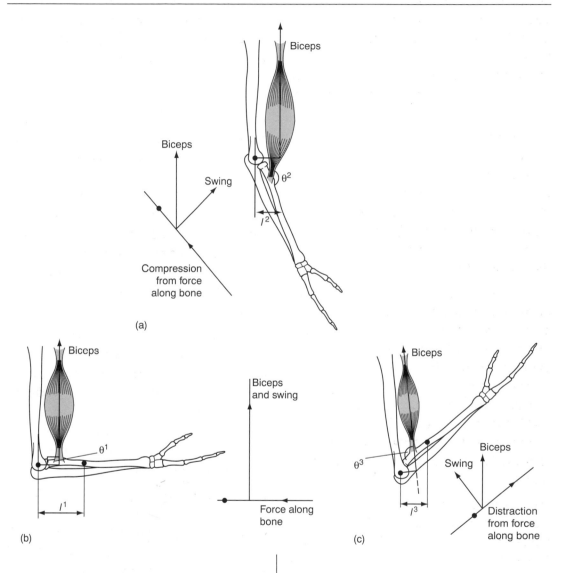

Summary

This chapter has covered the major roles of the musculoskeletal components and how they contribute to normal movement. At the start we said that these roles could be generalized as being concerned with either 'stability' or 'mobility'.

Looking at these might provide us with a suitable means of summarizing the main points discussed (see Table 2.4). However, do remember that these are the two functional roles at each extreme and most areas of the body require a compromise. This will allow some mobility alongside a certain amount of stability.

Table 2.4
Summary of the components of the skeletal, articular and muscular systems

Support/stability/small range of movement	Mobility/large range of movement
Skeletal system	**Skeletal system**
Histology Rigidity provided by the minerals in matrix Tensile strength by the collagen fibres and absolute strength by the 'tubes' formed by ostoen arrangement	*Histology* Some flexibility provided by proteoglycan gel matrix Rigidity required for muscle attachment provided by collagen and minerals
Internal structure Outer layer of compact bone provides protection and rigidity Inner arrangement of trabeculae contributes to strength of bone	
External shape Short or irregular bone with large surface area for support/weight bearing	*External shape* Long bones form levers for movement, triangular cross-section gives flexibility yet strength
General arrangement Bones arranged to form arches/rings for added strength	*General arrangement* Bones arranged to form arches and curves for some flexibility Grooved surfaces and sesamoid bones act as pulleys to improve angle of pull
Articular system	**Articular system**
Type of joint Fibrous joints' (immovable or slightly movable) increased friction between joint surfaces aids stability and congruency Uniaxial joints for stability Larger articular surface area decreases pressure yet increases friction Often have large surface area to increase contact/congruency between joint surfaces, also increased by the slightly compressible nature of the cartilage	*Type of joint* Synovial joints have less friction so mobility is favoured Methods of synovial lubrication decrease friction Multiaxial joints for increased mobility Smaller articular surface area decreases friction, yet pressure will increase Decrease in contact/congruency between joint surfaces increases mobility
Ligaments Collagen fibres often have a multidirectional arrangement to resist tensile stress in many directions Short ligaments reduce movement between bones	*Ligaments* Collagen fibres more parallel Long ligaments allow greater range of movement May contain elastic fibres which recoil following a stretch thereby assisting active movement

Table 2.4 continued

General arrangement
Many smaller joints acting will allow greater movement overall yet maintain optimum stability between individual bones

Muscular system

Fibre type
Slow Type I fibres resist fatigue so can provide long-term postural support required for stabilizing joints

Fibre arrangement
Short fibres, often oblique to tendon, so forming pennate muscles which sacrifice large movement for increased strength

Muscle position
Frequently deep, shorter and attached near to the joint to provide 'adjustable ligaments'
Positioned to apply transarticular compression ('shunt' action) to increase stability
May have many fibres so increasing the total cross-sectional area to increase force/stability

Muscle action
Muscles concerned with stability frequently are primarily postural muscles and their major role may be as fixators for the prime movers

General arrangement
Individual joints may possess a large range of multiaxial movement; this increases mobility with loss of inherent joint stability

Muscular system

Fibre type
Fast Type II fibres are ideal for sudden high speed movement required for mobility yet rapidly fatigue

Fibre arrangement
Longer fibres forming strap, triangular, bicipital muscles to produce large range of movement

Muscle position
Often more superficial with distal attachments
Positioned to provide the optimum mechanical advantage for producing the 'swing' around the joint ('spurt' action)
May sacrifice power for less bulk and there may be fewer fibres so decreasing the total cross-sectional area with a resultant loss of force
Noncontractile viscoelastic components may increase (agonists) or decrease (antagonists) range of movement

Muscle action
Muscles concerned with mobility usually have a major role as prime movers

References and Further Reading

Appell, HJ (1990) Muscular atrophy following immobilisation: A review. *Sports Medicine* 10 (1): 42–48.

Arnaud, SB, Schneider, VS, Morey-Holton, E (1986). Effects of inactivity on bone and calcium metabolism, in Sandler H, Vernikos, J (eds) *Inactivity Physiological Effects*. pp. 49–76, Academic Press, New York.

Bear, M, Connors, B, Paradiso, M (1996) *Neuroscience: Exploring the Mind*. Williams & Wilkins, London.

Berne, RM Levy, MN (1996) *Principles of Physiology*, 2nd edition. Mosby-Year Book Inc., St Louis, USA.

Billeter, R, Hoppeler, H (1992). Muscular basis of strength, in Komi, PV (ed) *Strength and Power in Sport*. Blackwell Scientific Publications, London.

Borg, TK, Caulfield, JB (1980) Morphology of connective tissue in skeletal muscle. *Tissue and Cell* 12 (1): 197–207.

Bunker, TD, Colton, CL, Webb, JK (eds) (1989). *Frontiers in Fracture Management*. Martin Dunitz, London.

Butler, AJ, Eccles, JC, Eccles, RW (1960) Intersections between motoneurons and muscle in respect of the characteristic speeds of their responses. *Journal of Physiology* 150: 417–439.

Carter, DR (1985). Biomechanic of bone, in Nahum, AM, Melvin, J (eds) *The Biomechanic of Trauma*, pp 135–165. Appleton-Century-Crofts, Norwalk, CT.

Clancy, J, McVicar, AJ (1995) *Physiotherapy and Anatomy: A Homeostatic Approach*. Edward Arnold, London.

Dempster, WT, Coleman, RF (1960). Tensile strength of bone along and across the grain. *Journal of Applied Physiology* 16: 355–360.

Donatelli, R (1981). Effects of immobilization on the extensibility of periarticular connective tissue. *Journal of Orthopaedic and Sports Physical Therapy.* **3** (2): 67–72.

English, CJ, Maclaren, WM, Courtbrown, C, Hughes, SPF, Porter, RW, Wallace, WA, Graves, RJ, Pethick, AJ, Soutar, CA (1995). Relations between upper limb soft tissue disorders and repetitive movements at work. *American Journal of Industrial Medicine.* **27** (1): 75–90.

Evans, P (1988). Ligaments, joint surfaces, conjunct rotation and close pack. *Physiotherapy* **74** (3): 105–114.

Fowler, HW, Fowler, FG (1964). *The Concise Oxford Dictionary,* 5th edn. Oxford University Press, Oxford.

Frankel, VH, Burstein, AH (1965) Loading capacity of tubular bone Kenedi, RM, (ed.). In *Biomechanics and Related Bio-engineering Topics,* Proceedings of a Symposium. Pergamon Press, Oxford.

Fredericks, C, Saladin, L (1996). *Pathophysiology of the motor systems: Principles and clinical presentations.* FA Davis Company, Philadelphia.

Hertling, D, Kessler, RM (1996) *Management of Common Musculo-skeletal Disorders,* 3rd edn. Lippincott, New York.

Hettinga, DL (1980) III. Normal joint structures and their reactions to injury. *Journal of Orthopaedic and Sports Physical Therapy* 1 (3): 178–184.

Huxley, HE, Hanson, J (1954) Changes in the cross striations of muscle during contraction and stretch and their interpretation. *Nature* **173**: 973–976.

Irrgang, JJ (1993) Modern trends in anterior cruciate ligament rehabilitation: nonpostoperative and postoperative management. *Clinics in Sports Medicine* **12** (4): 797–811.

Kannus, P, Jozsa, L, Renstrom, P, Jarvinen, M, Kvist, M, Lehto, M, Oja, P, Vuori, I (1992) The effects of training, immobilisation and remobilisation on musculoskeletal ti. 2. Remobilisation and prevention of immobilisation atrophy. *Scandinavian Journal of Medicine and Science in Sport* **2** (4): 164–176.

Kapanji, IA (1982) *The Physiology of the Joints: Volume One, Upper Limb,* 5th edn. Churchill Livingstone, London.

Kapanji, IA (1985) *The Physiology of the Joints: Volume Two, Lower Limb,* 5th edn. Churchill Livingstone, London.

Kovanen, V (1989) Effects of aging and physical training on rat skeletal muscle. *Acta Physiologica Scandinavica* 135 (Suppl): 577.

Kovanen, V, Suominen, H, Heikkinen, E (1984) Mechanical properties of fast and slow skeletal muscle with special reference to collagen and endurance training. *Journal of Biomechanics* **17** (10): 725–735.

Kummer, BKF (1972) Biomechanics of bone: Mechanical properties, functional structure, functional adaptation. In Fung, Y C, Perrone, N and Anliker, M (eds), *Proceedings of the Symposium on Biomechanics: its foundations and objectives.* Prentice-Hall, Inc., New Jersey.

Lindsay, D (1996) *Functional Human Anatomy.* Mosby-Year Book Inc., St Louis.

Loder, RT *et al.* (1996) The demographics of slipped capital femoral epiphysis: An international multicentre study. *Clinical Orthopaedics and Related Research.* Jan, Number 322, pp. 8–27. Lippincott-Raven, New York.

MacConaill, MA (1964) Joint movement. *Physiotherapy* **50** (11): 359–367.

Magnusson, SP, Simonsen, EB, Aagaard, MS, Kjaer, M (1996) Biomechanical responses to repeated stretches in human hamstring muscle in vivo. *American Journal of Sports Medicine* **24** (5): 622–628.

Markey, KL (1987) Stress fractures. *Clinics in Sports Medicine* **6**: 405–425.

Moore, KL (1992) *Clinically Oriented Anatomy,* 3rd edn. Williams & Wilkins, USA.

Mow, VC, Proctor, CS, Kelly, MA (1980). In Nordin, M and Frankel, VH (eds) *Basic Biomechanics of the Musculoskeletal System,* Chapter 2, 2nd edn, Lea and Febiger. Philadelphia.

Nachemson, AI, Evans, JH (1968) Some mechanical properties of the third human interlaminar ligament (ligamentum flavum). *Journal of Biomechanics* I: 211–220

Nordin, M, Frankel, VH (1989) *Basic Biomechanics of the Musculoskeletal System,* 2nd edn. Lea and Febiger, Philadelphia.

Norkin, CC, Levangie, PK (1992) *Joint Structure and Function: A Comprehensive Analysis.* 2nd edn. F A Davis Company, USA.

Pitman, MI, Peterson, L (1980) in: Nordin, M, Frankel, VH (1980). *Basic Biomechanics of the Musculoskeletal System,* Chapter 5, 2nd edn. Lea and Febiger, Philadelphia.

Preisinger, E, Alacamlioglu, Y, Pils, K, Bosina, E, Metka, M, Schneider, B Ernst, E (1996) Exercise therapy for osteoporosis: results of a randomised control trial. *British Journal of Sports Medicine* 30: 209–212.

Purslow, PP (1909) Strain induced reorientation of an intramuscular connective tissue network: implications for passive muscle elasticity. *Journal of Biomechanics* 22 (1): 21–31.

Putukian, M (1994) The female triad: Eating disorders, amenorrhea and osteoporosis. *Medical Clinics in North America* **78** (2): 345–356.

Safran, M, Garret, JR, Seaber, AV, Glisson, RR, Ribbeck, BN (1988) The role of warm up in muscular injury prevention. *American Journal of Sports Medicine* **16** (2): 123–129.

Scott, O (1996) Sensory and motor nerve activation. In Kitchen, S and Bazin, S (eds) Clayton's Electrotherapy, 10th edn. p. 73. WB Saunders, London.

Smith, N (1995) Connective tissue: its molecular structure and responses to movement and manual therapy. *British Journal of Therapy and Rehabilitation.* Vol 2, number 12, pp 659–662.

Threlkeld, AJ (1992) The effects of manual therapy on connective tissue. *Physical Therapy* **72** (12): 893–902.

Tipton, CM, Greenleaf, JE and Jackson, CGR (1996) Neuroendocrine and immune system responses with spaceflghts. *Medicine and Science in Sports and Exercise* **28**: 988–995.

Van de Graaf, KM (1995) *Human Anatomy,* 4th edn. William Brown.

Williams, PE (1990) Use of intermittent stretch in the prevention of serial sarcomere loss in immobilised muscle. *Annals of Rheumatic Diseases* **49**: 316–317.

Williams, PE, Goldspine, G (1971) Longitudinal growth of striated muscle fibres. *Journal of Cell Science* **9**: 751–757.

Williams, PL and Warwick, R (1980) *Gray's Anatomy,* 36th edn. Churchill Livingstone, London.

3

Physiology of Motor Control

SIMON MOCKETT

Introduction

This chapter will deal with the physiology of motor control. It is not intended to be a detailed description of the neuroanatomy or of the finer details of neurophysiology, both of which are available separately in specialist texts. The intention is to provide sufficient information to enable you to understand the principles involved in the control of human movement and to promote interest in the topic so that further reading may be encouraged.

Chapter Objectives

After reading this chapter you should be able to:

- describe the general arrangement of the central nervous system;
- describe the innervation of the muscle spindle and Golgi tendon organ;
- explain the function of the muscle spindle and Golgi tendon organ;
- discuss the interaction between sensory systems;
- describe the function of the cerebral cortex, cerebellum and basal ganglia;
- explain the mechanisms by which motor plans are executed;
- discuss the consequences of error, injury or disease;
- describe the differences between high and low muscle tone;
- appreciate the importance of understanding the motor control of human movement as a basis for the therapeutic management of patients.

The Central Nervous System

Without the central nervous system (CNS) our bodies would be elegantly constructed but would not function. Indeed when the CNS is injured or develops disease, function is very quickly reduced, e.g. brachial plexus lesions, stroke, paraplegia or multiple sclerosis.

The CNS can be regarded as having:

1 An input system (sensation);
2 An interpreting and integrative system coupled with central processing (higher centres);
3 An output system (motor).

In order that movement is smooth, coordinated and as we intend, all three must work efficiently. If the sensory system is faulty we do not know where we are or what is happening to us. If the motor system is faulty then the commands will not be executed as intended. If the central processing systems are at fault then the possibilities for abnormality are numerous.

Before carrying on in too much detail a general overview of the central systems will help. Figure 3.1 is a schematic of the CNS which contains the major anatomical features referred to.

The sensory system consists of sensory receptors throughout our body which respond to stimulation. As a result nervous impulses are transmitted along neurones (nerve cells) to the CNS (most commonly the spinal cord). Here they either pass directly up the spinal cord or they synapse with other neurones which then pass up the spinal cord. Some neurones will synapse with motor neurones to effect an immediate motor response (the withdrawal reflex is an example of this type of arrangement), others will synapse with many other neurones to disseminate the information throughout various areas of the CNS, e.g. higher centres, cerebellum, so that complex functions such as balance and coordination can be carried out.

Figure 3.1 Schematic of central nervous system. Each major area is named and a synopsis of its function is given in italics. The sensory pathway is shown as a dashed line; the motor pathway is shown as a dotted line.

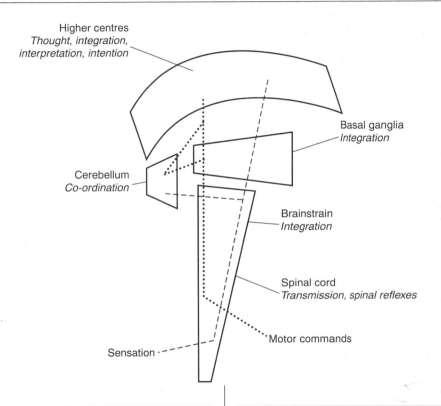

Higher centres
Thought, integration, interpretation, intention

Basal ganglia
Integration

Cerebellum
Co-ordination

Brainstrain
Integration

Spinal cord
Transmission, spinal reflexes

Motor commands

Sensation

Physiological Examples

1 You reach out to pick up a saucepan off the cooker. The handle is hot and burns. The immediate response is to let go.
So what has happened?
The sensory neurones in your hand are stimulated by the noxious stimulation of the hot saucepan. The impulse is received at the spinal cord. Here there is a synapse with the motor neurones that will move your hand away. Also there are other synapses which will send messages to your CNS to inform you what is going on. Your hand will hurt later! It is more important to remove it

from the source of the damage than to wait and have a bit of a think about how hot the saucepan might be!
2 As you move around you don't normally trip up or bump into things.
Why not?
As you move around your CNS is planning movements against a background of 'knowledge' of where you are in time and space. This information comes from the interpretation of information from your sensory systems. Neurones are firing all the time to tell your nonconscious mind about the length and tension of your muscles, the position of your joints, the movement of your

body and the relationship of centre of gravity and base of support, etc. So, if you know where you are, where you are going and you can see what is in the way then you don't bump into it.

Clearly if we don't pay attention or are ill or if the systems are damaged then the situation changes.

Once information is passed up the spinal cord it will be received by a number of different centres in which it will be integrated with information from other sources before being interpreted or used. The brainstem (which is at the base of the brain, see Figure 3.1) has within it a number of nuclei which will either add or separate information from the original message before it is passed to higher centres such as the cerebellum (whose function is coordination) or the basal ganglia (whose function is in movement control). The package of information may then be passed either directly or as an interpreted message to the sensory cortex. Once this reaches the cortex we will 'know' it. That conscious sensation is the province of the sensory cortex.

Key Point

Not all sensory information comes to consciousness. The only conscious appreciation of sensation is that which reaches the sensory cortex. Other information which is invaluable may be used by nonconscious elements of the CNS, e.g. cerebellum.

To activate a movement there needs to be the desire to move, followed by a plan and a pro-gramme to be executed. Thus the motor cortex will inform the basal ganglia and the cerebellum of the plan for a movement before the nervous impulses are sent to the spinal cord to stimulate the neurones which will cause the muscles to contract. Once this is happening there will be a change in the level and nature of stimulation on the sensory receptors and a different set of sensory stimuli will arrive at the CNS.

Key Point

It is apparent therefore that the sensory and motor systems are intimately linked and the performance of smooth movement relies heavily on all elements of the system.

Sensation

Sensation relies on stimulation of receptors which will then pass information to the CNS to effect a response or to be interpreted. There are many different types of receptor and the means by which they are classified varies. The main classes are:

1 *Exteroceptors* which respond to stimulation of the body's surface, for instance touch or temperature;
2 *Interoceptors* which respond to stimulation of the viscera for instance baroreceptors and those in the mesentery;
3 *Proprioceptors* which respond to stimulation within muscles or around joints; for instance muscle spindles or Golgi tendon organs.

Within each of these receptors there are gradations of sensitivity and speed and nature of

Table 3.1
Classification of nerves by type, diameter and velocity

Fibre type	Conduction velocity (m/s)	Diameter (μm)	Function
Sensory			
Ia (Aα)	70–120	12–20	Sensory from muscle spindle
Ib (Aα)	70–120	12–20	Sensory from Golgi tendon organs
II (Aβ or γ)	15–70	3–12	Sensory from muscle spindle, pressure receptors, touch
III (Aδ)	12–30	2–5	Sensory from pain receptors (fast pain), temperature and touch
IV (C)	0.5–2.0	0.2–2.0	Pain (slow), crude touch
Motor			
Aα	70–120	12–20	Motor to extrafusal fibres
Aγ	15–30	3–6	Motor to intrafusal fibres

Note that the naming of sensory nerves is not consistent among authors. Therefore for sensory nerves both of the common names are given. It is also not uncommon for both sets of names to be used concurrently within texts so watch out for that.

response. Some classifications are based on this difference and sensory neurones are classified and termed by their diameter and conduction velocity. These qualities reflect their function, see Table 3.1. The following sections will explore the functions of proprioceptors and exteroceptors in the context of movement.

Proprioceptors

With your eyes shut you can tell whether you are standing up or sitting down, you know where your limbs are and whether they are moving. If they are moving you can tell how fast or slow. You can brush your hair without looking, and touch your face.

To do all these types of things you need to know the position of your body and all of its component parts in space, but not necessarily at a conscious level. This is *proprioception*.

Proprioceptors are receptors which inform the CNS about the state of our joints and muscles.

They respond to muscle length and tension during static and moving conditions. Also there are joint receptors that respond to the deforming of structures around and within joints to inform the CNS about movement – either planned or unplanned.

The Muscle Spindle

The muscle spindle is the most important intramuscular proprioceptor. It is shown diagrammatically in Figure 3.2. Its function is to detect and respond to change and rate of change, in muscle length. Remember this as you read the following section. Also refer to Table 3.1 for details of characteristics of the neurones involved if you need to.

Muscle spindles are organelles within the muscles. They are arranged in parallel with the fibres of the muscle (extrafusal fibres). They are several millimetres long but only a few micrometres in diameter. Each muscle spindle has a connective tissue sheath which encloses 2–12 intrafusal fibres. The

Figure 3.2   Muscle spindle.

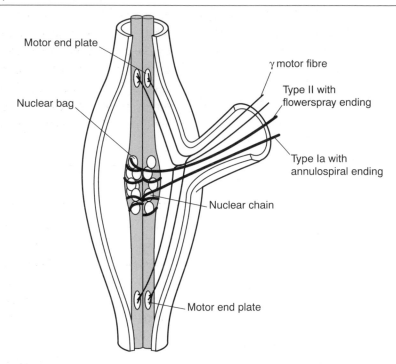

- Motor end plate
- Nuclear bag
- γ motor fibre
- Type II with flowerspray ending
- Type Ia with annulospiral ending
- Nuclear chain
- Motor end plate

basic arrangement of the intrafusal fibre is that of a central area or equator which is densely populated with nuclei. At the outer edges or poles, beyond the equatorial regions, are contractile elements. There are different types of intrafusal fibres. Nuclear bag fibres are so called because the equatorial region is expanded. This is in contrast to nuclear chain fibres which are smaller and have fewer nuclei.

Each muscle spindle has its own sensory and motor supply. Its sensory supply is so that it can respond to changes in the length of the extrafusal muscle fibres. Its motor supply is so that it can change its own length in response to changes in the length of the extrafusal muscle fibres and thus have a greater dynamic range.

The sensory supply is via a single Type Ia and a single Type II neurone irrespective of the number of intrafusal fibres. These are arranged so that the Type Ia neurone receives input from the nerve endings which wrap around the equatorial region. These are called *annulospiral nerve endings*. The Type II are arranged at the edges of the equatorial regions and invest but do not enwrap the intrafusal fibres. These are called *flowerspray nerve endings*.

The motor supply is via Aγ motor neurones which are also called fusimotor neurones. They originate in the anterior horn of the spinal cord, where they are intermingled among the Aα motor neurones which supply the extrafusal fibres. This is functionally relevant as will be seen later. There are two classes of Aγ motor neurones to the spindle.

1 *Plate endings* which have discrete motor end-plates on the contractile poles of the nuclear bag fibres;

2 *Trail endings* which have extensive network of endings and are mainly attached to nuclear chain fibres. If you want to read more about this, it is dealt with well in *Gray's Anatomy* (Williams *et al.*, 1989).

There is a constant flow of impulses being discharged via the sensory neurones informing the CNS about the relative length of the muscle spindle to the extrafusal fibres. As the muscle spindle is lengthened then the equatorial region is deformed. The rate of discharge of impulses is a function of the *length* of the muscle spindle. However, there are differences in function between the types of sensory fibre. At any given length there is a sustained or static rate of discharge, but if the muscle is stretched *(lengthened)* then the rate of discharge changes. The rate of discharge from Type Ia fibres changes as a function of the velocity of the change in length whereas the Type II fibres are a function of the absolute length. During shortening the same situation applies only the direction changes, i.e. it is the reverse of lengthening.

The muscle spindle also has a motor supply of its own via the γ system. If the γ motor neurone is stimulated and causes the contraction of the poles of a muscle spindle which were held at a fixed length then the equatorial region would be deformed and its rate of discharge would increase. Similarly if the stimulation of the γ motor neurone was reduced, then the amount of deformation of the equatorial region would decrease, as would its consequent discharge of impulses. Thus alteration of the amount of γ motor neurone activity can affect the sensitivity of the central equatorial region to changes in length not mediated by the γ system. Thus individual muscle spindles can have a wide dynamic range.

It is important to note that muscle spindle receptors do not signal absolute extrafusal muscle fibre length. Rather they give information about relative length and change of length. Because of their dynamic nature any given rate of discharge can correspond to a variety of extrafusal muscle lengths. For interpretation of the absolute length then the CNS needs to integrate both the afferent impulses and the efferent γ motor impulses.

It has been suggested that static information arises from the chain fibres which are served by the trail endings, and that dynamic information arises from the plate endings (Berne and Levy, 1988). Since the trail endings are more prevalent in the nuclear chain fibres it is speculated that these monitor static states; conversely nuclear bag fibres contain more plate fibres and that these respond to dynamic velocity related change. However, the situation may not be quite as clear cut as this.

It can be seen that the muscle spindle is a very complex receptor organ. The receptors respond to relative length and rate of change of length. Their sensitivity can be adjusted and differentially controlled via the γ motor system. Because of the complexity of the situation it is important that the activation of the intrafusal fibres is closely coordinated with the Aα motor neurone recruitment of the extrafusal fibres. Indeed this coactivation allows precise and sensitive control of movement.

Practical Example

Imagine you are bending your elbow against a slight resistance.

Before you begin: Muscle spindles will be sending impulses at their 'normal' rate.

As you start to move: The Type Ia and Type II fibres will be stimulated and will 'fire' at a different rate. You are able to interpret this as movement.

If you move faster: The rate of firing of Type Ia fibres will increase to a greater extent than Type II.

Look back over the previous section to make sure you can explain why.

However, the muscle spindle is a length detector. It infers but does not respond to the force being generated by the contraction of the extrafusal fibres. That is the domain of the Golgi tendon organs.

Golgi Tendon Organs

Since the muscle spindle only gives, at best, inferred information regarding the force being generated by the contractile extrafusal units, it is necessary to have sensory organs that can provide such information. This is the role of the Golgi tendon organ (GTO). If force is to be registered then the receptor needs to be in series with the contractile elements. They are found at, or near the junction between muscle fibres and tendons. They are 500 µm long and 100 µm in diameter at rest. They consist of a small bundle of tendon fibres (intrafusal fasciculi) wrapped in a capsule. This capsule is thin and is pierced by at least one thickly myelinated Ib fibre. Inside the capsule the Ib fibre(s) divide and disperse between the intrafusal fasciculi. Figure 3.3 gives a diagrammatic representation of the Golgi tendon organ.

The GTOs are very sensitive and highly active when the tendon is stretched, whether that stretch be passive or active. The deformation of the GTO probably occurs because as force is generated by the contractile unit the collagen

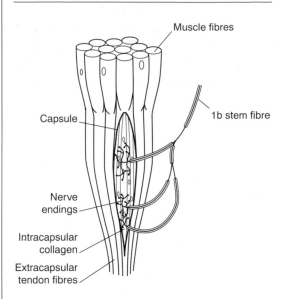

Figure 3.3   Golgi tendon organ.

fibres within the tendons tend to lie parallel and closer together. So, as more force is generated the GTO is deformed more. The Ib fibres are stimulated more and there is a greater firing of impulses. According to Berne and Levy (1988), the threshold for stimulation of a GTO may be for forces as low as 0.1 gram. Also they are slowly adapting so they are able to continue to provide information about the force being generated.

This is particularly important given the proportion of static muscle work which occurs in functional activity.

It would be worth thinking for a moment about what you know about isometric muscle work and functional considerations such as fixator and synergistic activity. What might the role of the role of the Golgi tendon organs be? Also bear this in mind when you read Chapter 10 on Neuromuscular Therapeutic Techniques.

It is also important to be aware that GTOs give information about the specific musculotendinous unit in which they reside and not an average for the whole muscle. In this way very accurate information is received regarding generated force or tension. Also of note is the fact that active contraction of the muscle fibres will cause a greater firing rate than a passive stretch because active contraction is more effective in elongating the tendon and thereby deforming the GTOs.

Function of Muscle Spindles and Golgi Tendon Organs

It has already been shown that the muscle spindles respond to changes in length of muscle fibres and that GTOs respond to the tension (force) being developed. This information can be used in a number of ways, each interacting and complementary.

At the most basic level information from these receptors can be involved in protective reflexes. By consideration of these reflexes it is possible to demonstrate pathways along which information travels and the principal synaptic connections along the way (see later). However, without seeking to devalue these reflexes, if this was the only function for these organelles then such an elaborate and elegant system would not be required. Therefore, it must be that the role extends to one of proprioception. That is the constant feedback of the state of the muscles in response to changes in the external environment, the motor system stimulation and the interaction between them all. In this way the individual is able to initiate appropriate motor plans from a position of 'knowledge' of their current position and then to control the movement of their body in a smooth and coordinated way.

How is this achieved?

In order to answer such a question it is necessary to consider the reflex actions in which the muscle spindle and GTO are involved and how this might be used in an integrative way as well as for protection.

REFLEX ACTIONS INVOLVING THE MUSCLE SPINDLES.

The reflexes in which the *muscle spindles* are active are the *spinal stretch reflexes.*

The most obvious example of this type of reflex is the stretch reflex typified by the knee jerk, which will be used as the example (see Figure 3.4). From the diagram it can be seen that the sensory nerve travels from the muscle spindle towards the spinal cord, enters the spinal cord via the dorsal horn and forms an *excitatory* synapse with the Aα motor neurone to the same muscle.

When the tendon hammer hits the patellar tendon it causes a sudden and unexpected stretching of the quadriceps muscle fibres. This results in a sudden increase in length on the intrafusal muscle fibres (muscle spindles). As a result there is an increased firing of the sensory fibres (Type Ia probably). Impulses will travel along the sensory nerve causing excitation of the Aα motor neurone to the quadriceps, which then contract. This is seen as the knee joint extending slightly before returning to the resting position.

The function of the circuit was to return the muscle spindle to its previous position by reducing the lengthening effect of the extrafusal fibres by making them contract, i.e. shorten, and in this way return the firing rate of the intrafusal fibres to their previous level.

The function of the reflex may be twofold. The most apparent is protective. Sudden changes in length are potentially damaging. Therefore a mechanism which restores the status quo will

Figure 3.4 Patellar reflex including reciprocal inhibition. Arrows indicate nerve impulses. (a) A tap to the patellar ligament stretches the spindles in quadriceps femoris. (2) Spindles discharge excitatory impulses to the spinal cord. (3) Motor neurones respond by eliciting a twitch in quadriceps, with extension of the knee. (4) Ia inhibitory internuncials respond by suppressing any activity in the hamstrings. (Adapted from Fitzgerald, 1996, *Neuroanatomy: Basic and Clinical*, WB Saunders, London.)

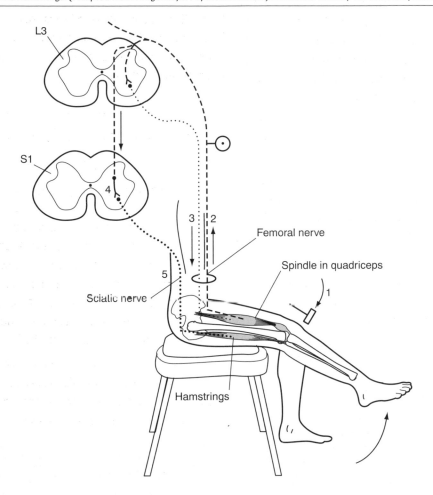

lessen the potential for harm. Secondly the reflex may actually be used to initiate movement. If the degree of contraction of the muscle spindle's contractile elements were deliberately altered then an extrafusal muscle fibre would contract. If there was a phased and coincident stimulation of the extrafusal fibre by impulses descending from the brain then the degree of recruitment would be increased. This is particularly so when counteracting the effect of gravity. The later example of standing might help you to understand this better.

Remember also that the γ motor neurones are able to alter the length of the muscle spindle so that it is sensitive over the whole range of the muscles length (see above).

REFLEXES INVOLVING THE GOLGI TENDON ORGANS

Unlike the muscle spindles, GTOs respond to tension. The pathway for the Type Ib neurones which supply them is slightly different to the muscle spindle and is shown in Figure 3.5. The Type Ib neurones enter the spinal cord via the dorsal horn and forms an excitatory synapse with an interneurone. This interneurone forms an *inhibitory* synapse with the Aα motor neurone.

Therefore if there is an excessive rise in stimulation of the GTO then they will inhibit the contraction of the muscle fibres supplied and thus reduce the level of contraction. The function is clearly protective.

With both of these reflexes it is important to note that they do not happen in isolation. When an agonistic muscle is caused to contract then the antagonistic muscle is caused to relax, and vice versa. This is also known as the principle of reci-

procal innervation/relaxation and may be used therapeutically. Other chapters will deal with the therapeutic techniques which apply this principle.

Details of the variety of reflexes are available elsewhere and will not be dealt with here. Davies (1994) explains them well and in the context of therapeutic intervention.

The Role of Muscle Spindles and Golgi Tendon Organs in Voluntary Motor Actions

It is important to note that the information being transmitted from the muscle spindle and GTOs does not only feature in reflex pathways. This information is important in the planning and execution of motor actions. As a consequence collateral pathways transmit information up the spinal cord to higher centres in the brain.

There also has to be integration with other types and sources of sensory information. In order to focus on what this might be and the organization involved consider the following example.

Figure 3.5   Golgi tendon organ reflexes. Sensory nerve fibres from Golgi tendon organs form synaptic contacts with interneurones in the spinal cord. These interneurones inhibit motor neurones supplying the muscle to which that Golgi tendon organ is attached. (Reprinted with permission from Lamb *et al.*, 1991, *Essentials of Physiology,* Blackwell Scientific Publications, London.)

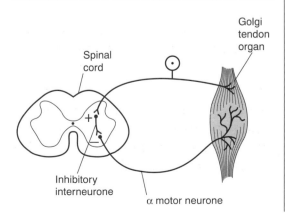

Practical Task

When holding a pen how do you know where it is and what shape it is, without looking at it?

Initially there will be a stimulation of the sensory receptors (transducer) in the fingers. This information will be transmitted to the spinal cord and from there to the brain. However this information will need to be quite detailed.

Which areas of the skin on the fingers are being stimulated? What position are the joints in? How much are the muscles changing in length and tension?

In order to investigate shape then there needs to be an exploration of the pen. This requires action of the receptors that respond to change (the phasic type of receptors) since those that fire as long as a stimulus is provided (the tonic type of receptors) are already being stimulated by the pressure of pen in the hand. Therefore the pen is rolled in the finger tips. This stimulates a variety of phasic receptors each of which will fire when stimulation starts and again when it stops. As the fingers are moved then there will be a change in either the length, or tension, or more likely both, of the muscles involved. This will cause firing patterns from the muscle spindles and Golgi tendon organs to change. With this information the CNS can interpret the impulses to recognize the afferent impulses from finger tips in conjunction with information about joint position and muscle length and tension as being a pen.

From this description it is clear that the area supplied by each transducer is discrete as is the supply to each afferent neurone. This allows and facilitates the interpretive function. The discrete area is known as the receptor field. Also, because neurones are linked to specific transducers then when they are stimulated the sensory system interprets that as a specific sensation even if the stimulation of the transducer is by another means. Fredericks and Saladin (1996) give some interesting examples of this.

Exteroceptors

The example above has brought up the issue of exteroceptors and their function. It is easiest to consider them in two types: those that respond to change (phasic type receptors); and those that respond continuously as long as the stimulus persists (tonic type receptors). The primary function of the sensory system (in the context of this chapter) is to inform the CNS at either a conscious or nonconscious level of the position of the body both spatially and temporally. In order to achieve this there needs to be an integration of the afferent sensations. Those from the skin or surface is termed exteroception, whereas that from within or due to muscle action is proprioception.

The sources of the stimuli are many and varied. In essence there are transducers which cause an effect on neurones which, if a critical threshold is reached, fire and send impulses to the spinal cord. There is a large variety of sensory transducers, and definition of the exact sensations to which they respond is not without dispute (Berne and Levy, 1988). However, they tend to fall into two types and the principles are quite clear.

Phasic Receptors

Phasic systems only generate action potentials when changes in stimulation occur. However, they are often poor at distinguishing between increases or decreases in intensity, and can only detect that it has changed.

Pacinian corpuscles are sensitive to pressure or vibration and are therefore phasic receptors, i.e. are stimulated by change in the sensation. As the pressure on the corpuscle rises a generator potential is initiated. If this is sufficient then it can lead to the initiation of an action potential. If not then the *generator potential* will quickly decay and cause no functional effect. If the critical level is breached then a regenerative action potential (saltatory conduction) will be transmitted to the spinal cord. The importance of the structure of the corpuscle is that due to its viscoelastic properties it acts as a temporal filter for mechanical stimuli so that only transient pressure changes reach the central element which is where the sensory nerve ending is located. What this means is that if you squash it it responds to the change and causes the nerve inside to be stimulated. However, if you maintain the 'squashing force' then the elastic nature of the corpuscle means that it will absorb the force and not transmit it to the nerve ending and so there will be no new stimulation. When you then remove the 'squashing force' the elastic recoil will cause a pressure change on the underlying nerve which will then transmit another impulse.

It is interesting to note that if the nerve ending is stripped of the corpuscle it is tonic.

The important point is that in the complete system the neurone will fire only in response to *changes* off pressure, when that change in stimuli is sufficient to cause a change in stimulation beyond a critical threshold.

Tonic Receptors

Tonic systems on the other hand increase or decrease monotonically with stimulus strength. That is if the stimulus (above a critical threshold) persists then the neurone will continue to fire impulses. This, however, makes small changes in stimulus difficult to detect.

Tonic receptors, unlike phasic receptors, maintain a generator potential with very little decay, or loss of potential, throughout the duration of the stimulation. Also once the generator potential exceeds the critical threshold for action potentials, then the sooner it can fire again. Thus the greater the degree to which the stimulus exceeds the critical threshold the greater will be the frequency of firing of the sensory neurone. That is, the firing frequency is monotonically related to the intensity of stimulation.

There is a great variety of transducers which are found attached to or in the vicinity of sensory nerve endings and there is supposition as to their effects and the sensation to which they respond.

Table 3.2
Sensory transducers by type, nerve fibre and function

Type of transducer	Type of nerve fibre	Type of function
Meissner	Aα	Rapidly adapting mechanoreceptor, very sensitive to touch
Pacinian corpuscle	Aα	Rapidly adapting mechanoreceptor, very sensitive to touch
Ruffini end organ	Aα	Slowly adapting mechanoreceptor information on proprioceptive states
Merkels disc	Aα	Rapidly adapting mechanoreceptor
Thermoreceptors	A δ or C	Respond to change in temperature
Nocioceptors	A δ or C	Respond to nocioceptive (painful) stimuli
Free nerve endings	A δ or C	Respond directly to stimulation, conduction rate determined by diameter. Sensitive to touch and pain

This was thought to be unclear though more recently the situation has clarified and is shown in Table 3.2. However, the precise consideration of the nature and function of individual transducers is not required. Suffice to know that the neuronal characteristics will affect conduction speed and that will be an influence on function.

Possible Functions of Exteroceptors by Type

$A\alpha$ fibres originate in muscle spindles and Golgi tendon organs (see above). Their action is to subserve spinal reflex reactions though their function is more likely kinaesthetic. $A\beta$ and $A\gamma$ transmit information about touch and kinaesthesia. $A\delta$ convey information about cruder forms of touch, temperature and pain. C fibres convey information about touch and pain. It is immediately apparent that there is some overlap and also that there is a discrepancy in the speed of conduction. This is all functionally relevant.

Fibres which transmit information which require rapid integration will obviously transmit faster. Such neurones would be those involved in proprioception, for example. Others which have protective functions will also be fast but it is not necessary to experience qualitative differences until later, therefore some sensations can transmit more slowly.

Practical Task

Think for a moment how this fits in with the example of the pen.

What might be happening to allow you to appreciate that the pen is in your hand?

Look back over the functions of the proprioceptors and exteroceptors and speculate.

Also ponder on your own experience of other sensations such as pain. You know that some sensations travel faster than others. How many of us have felt the pressure of stubbing our toe and then moments later felt the pain? The same happens if you hit your thumb with a hammer or cut yourself on an envelope.

Refer back to Table 3.2 and consider the functions more closely.

The Spinal Cord

We have seen already that neurones reach the spinal cord and enter it and also that synapses occur with other neurones that exist there. It is necessary to have an appreciation of the internal arrangements of these systems though not necessary to embark upon a detailed examination of the anatomy which is widely available in neuro-anatomy texts.

The spinal cord extends from the foramen magnum to the first or second lumbar spine. It is covered by the meninges some of which extend to the vertebral foramen. Meninges are innervated so any impingement upon them is exquisitely painful. Think of this when you see people with neck or back pain.

There are nerves which pass up the spinal cord, others which pass down and yet more that connect within it. Those passing up or down tend to go to or arise from centres within the brain. These are then known as the ascending or descending tracts respectively. Like everything else in the CNS they are arranged together in functional bundles.

Figure 3.6   Major tracts of the spinal white matter at midcervical level. Ascending tracts are on the left; descending tracts are on the right. (Reproduced, with permission, from Barr and Kiernan, 1993, *The Human Nervous System*, 6th edn. Lippincott, London.)

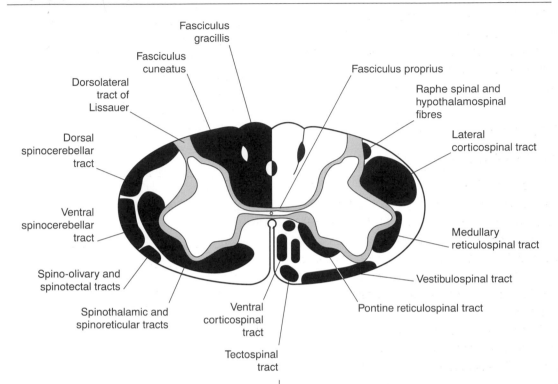

They are easily seen in cross-sections of the spinal cord as in Figure 3.6.

Ascending Tracts

Sensation from the periphery can be regarded as having three conceptual elements which all impact into the CNS: namely, what the environment is like, what the environment is doing to the person and how the person might react to the sensation. In essence these three elements fall into three integrated systems:

1 The dorsal column–lemniscal system;
2 The spinothalamic system;
3 The reticulospinal system, respectively.

The dorsal column–lemniscal system deals with inputs which are served by neurones which are large in diameter and fast conducting. These are serving organelles which are sensitive to change (for the most part) and thus rapidly adapting. This is ideal for functions that require precise discrimination such as proprioception and discriminative tactile exploration. Thus, it is these pathways which transmit information that will eventually be used to interpret position in time and three-dimensional space.

Dorsal column–lemniscal pathway destinations are the nuclei of the medulla. From there, second order neurones project up to the thalamus. In addition there is an important projection to the cerebellum. The nature of the sensations is essentially proprioceptive and fine and discriminative touch.

Related to this tract, though not within it, is the spinocerebellar tract. The nature of the sensory information passing in this tract is essentially proprioceptive so that interpretation of body position can be assessed in collaboration with precision sensations.

An important difference between these two pathways is that information transmitted in the dorsal column—lemniscal system is potentially conscious in that there are connections to the sensory cortex for some neurones whereas the information in the spinocerebellar pathways is not conscious.

The spinothalamic system deals with inputs from slower conducting neurones. These neurones are either serving organelles, or they are free, and they respond to cruder types of sensation such as temperature, pain or coarse touch. There are two substantial divisions: Aδ and C fibres. The former is faster conducting and has the function that alerts the CNS to imminent danger of, or virtually instantly to, damage. The C fibres warn of past injury and have a protective function to prevent further damage.

The spinothalamic pathway destination is the thalamus, with projections from there to the sensorimotor cortex. The nature of the sensations is essentially other skin sensations such as temperature, coarse touch and so on.

The reticulospinal system is very much less well defined though is very extensive. It would seem that its function is to allow us to receive qualitative inputs about the degree or nature of the sensation being received from which to make a response.

The reticulospinal pathway destination is rather diffuse through the reticular formation of the brain. The nature of the sensations is of a general level. This pathway is served by less spatially or type specific neurones and organelles than the other pathways. It appears that they respond to overall levels of sensory input upon which to make a response. This is best understood in terms of a general response; for example, when the room a person is in gets warmer they will react. They might take off their coat, fan their face, open a window etc. But which particular part of them got too hot? Probably all of them. Which organelles responded in the sort of way described in the spinothalamic tracts or as protective reflexes? Probably not many. So how did they know to react? Apart from a more complex investigation of core temperature and the like the simple answer is the general level of increased reticulospinal activity.

When considering precision movements then the effect of visual guidance systems and optical reflexes are vital. The physiology of vision is beyond the remit of this chapter. (The chapter by Stein in Cody (1995) is particularly good.) However, it is clear that what we can see will help us to interpret our environment and our place within it. We tend to look at and remember our position and then, if we are to move, predict our new position. Usually this works well. But if we are unable to see clearly, unable to process or interpret the information, problems arise. This is often the case in stroke patients who have perceptual difficulties.

Practical Example

This is evident to anyone who tries to move around even a familiar room wearing a blindfold or even just in the dark. The consequences of lost or impaired vision are obvious. However, it is worth considering the plight of those people who have an impairment of the ability to correctly interpret what they see. An example of this might be the stroke patient who has a depth perceptual dysfunction. A line on the floor (such as where the colour changes between carpets) may appear to them to be a step. Likewise a step may be just another colour change. If they are already not in complete control of their movement then difficulties like these may lead to either accidents or a fear of accidents sufficient to disable them further.

balance (most of the time!). But it is possible to overload the system. If we turn too quickly then we do become disorientated and may stagger. Try standing up and turning around several times quickly and you may become dizzy. But the sensation should soon pass.

Anyone who has ridden a fairground Waltzer or similar ride will know the disorientation is temporary (and to some enjoyable). But if that disorientation were permanent then the situation would be very different. Such is the situation which affects people with vestibular disease.

Similarly, in large-scale movements balance reactions which are modulated by the vestibular system are crucial. Again details of the vestibular system are beyond the remit of this chapter but it is important to note that information from the vestibule and semicircular canals in the ear is relayed to the vestibular nucleus in the brain. This information is vital to the interpretation of three-dimensional movement of the head. Therefore it allows interpretation of movement in three planes. Details of this system can be found in most physiology textbooks. The importance here is that the information regarding the upright posture and positions of balance are immediately interpretable and responses to restore any perceived loss of balance can be instigated immediately.

Practical Example

We know this works. If you turn quickly round a corner you don't fall over. We can play games that require many quick changes of posture and yet still keep our

The Brain

So far we have seen that stimuli cause an impulse to be propagated in neurones which then pass into the spinal cord where they either cause a motor efferent to be stimulated or they are passed to the brain. But whereabouts?

The brain itself is a structure of enormous complexity so we will restrict ourselves to the nuclei of principal interest. The sensory information passes to the thalamus, sensorimotor cortex and to the cerebellum (either directly or indirectly). It is these areas that will be considered next.

The general topography and principal function are shown in Figure 3.7.

It is clear that the input from the periphery to the principal destinations shown in Figure 3.7 are not the sole destination of the inputs and that there is considerable distribution of input through the brain.

Figure 3.7 The general topography of the brain.

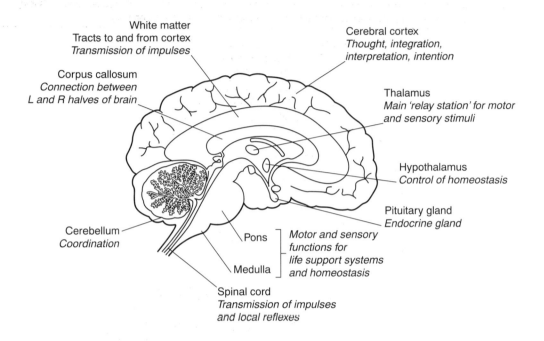

White matter
Tracts to and from cortex
Transmission of impulses

Cerebral cortex
*Thought, integration,
interpretation, intention*

Corpus callosum
*Connection between
L and R halves of brain*

Thalamus
*Main 'relay station' for motor
and sensory stimuli*

Hypothalamus
Control of homeostasis

Pituitary gland
Endocrine gland

Cerebellum
Coordination

Pons

*Motor and sensory
functions for
life support systems
and homeostasis*

Medulla

Spinal cord
*Transmission of impulses
and local reflexes*

At a conscious level there is a sensory 'map' on the somatic sensory area, sometimes called the sensorimotor cortex (see Figure 3.8). There is a general level of overlap amongst these neurones with specificity of individual cells being precise in terms of interpretation of sensations at specific body parts. As a result it is possible to plot the areas of the body represented on the area of cells – this is the so-called sensory homonculus. Figure 3.8b shows the homonculus.

The area of cortical tissue given over to each area of the body indicates the level of complexity of sensory information and processing which occurs for that part. So our hands are given a lot of space and our thumbs are given disproportionately more. So our hands are important sensory organs. Imagine then the consequence of poor sensation in the hands of a person with multiple sclerosis or with a nerve lesion in the arm.

Practical Task

Look at the homonculus and rationalize the distribution for other areas and think of why it might be as it is.

As well as interpreting the sensory information at a conscious level there are a number of centres within the brain which are essential to normal function but are not conscious. This level of information is received by the cerebellum and the thalamus. The cerebellum also has a homonculus but it is less well defined than on the cerebral cortex. The main function of the cerebellum is coordination. The constant reception of sensory stimuli regarding the position of the body and body parts is essential.

The thalamus is the major 'relay station' for

Figure 3.8   Somatic sensory area of the cerbral cortex. (a) The somatic sensory cortex is situated just behind the central sulcus on a ridge known as the postcentral gyrus. (b) Signals from different parts of the body are sent to different regions of the somatic sensory cortex: body regions with the highest tactile discrimination have the largest areas of cortical representation. (Adapted, with permission, from Lamb et al., 1991, *Essentials of Physiology*, Blackwell Scientific Publications, London.)

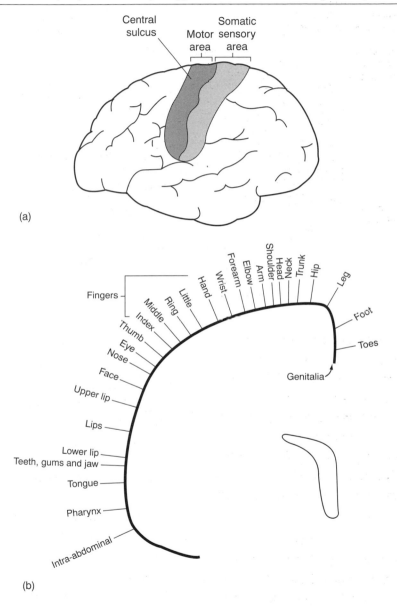

(a)

(b)

sensory information. The thalamus receives information from the sensory receptors either directly or indirectly. Then the information is 'sorted' by site and type before being moved on to other centres. Thus the sensations from the same body parts are gathered together before being given to the sensory cortex to deal with. The same principle applies to types of sensation.

Functioning of the Sensory System

When movement is being planned or executed it is important that the brain is aware of position of body parts in time and space. Once movement is occurring then it needs to be continuously updated on the situation. As a result there is a map or plan of expected events laid down. In this way early interpretation of deviation from the plan can be highlighted. In effect the brain tells itself 'this is what I am expecting to happen' and inhibits incoming information in such a way that it can monitor that and 'listen' for answers to the question 'is anything different happening?' Whilst this is a somewhat crude representation of rather complicated physiology it does account for the ability to concentrate on specific areas of the body and on specific tasks to the exclusion of others. Incidentally this may also be a function of the limbic system inputs to the basal ganglia (see below).

It is clear that the pathways allow interpretation of sensations. It is also clear that this can be refined. This can happen in a number of places but the principle remains the same. That is, the ratio of important and relevant signal to irrelevant and unimportant ones (the signal:noise ratio) must be modified to best advantage so that we can attend to what is important rather than have to attend to all the sensations that enter the sensory system. To that end a number of features are built into the system. Some neurones and their organelles only respond to change (i.e. are phasic), therefore in the absence of change they do not exceed the critical threshold for an action potential to be generated. However, others respond to specific stimuli all the time (i.e. are tonic) and can sustain action potential discharges. When we do not want or need to attend to these inputs they can be inhibited by either pre- or post-synaptic inhibition. The purpose here is to differentiate between extraneous and important elements. This is crucial in movement so that as we move we can concentrate on what is important so that we get it right, and other sensations are ignored temporarily.

Key Points

Summary of sensory inputs by function

Appreciation of the environment (hot, cold etc.)

- *where am I in it (proprioception)*
- *interpretation of effect of environment (pain)*
- *planning of a response (comfort)*
- *planning of movement*

Monitoring of movement

Sensation by pathways
Spinothalamic

- *spinocerebellar*
- *spinoreticular*

Other pathways are involved (see specialized texts for details)

Involvement
Spinal reflexes

- *conscious perception*

Motor function

Practical Task

Look now at Figure 3.15. The shaded boxes are the principal sensory elements which have been referred to in the previous

Motor Activation Systems

Movement can be thought of as having three basic elements: a plan, a programme and an execution. It is convenient to think of these as a series of events (and descriptively that is how it will be done initially); however it is now evident that they occur to a greater extent in parallel (Shumway-Cook and Woollacott, 1995). It is worth noting at the moment that the CNS is active much longer before a movement occurs than would be necessary if a linear series was all that was required (Fitzgerald, 1996; Lemon, 1995). It appears that information passes several times between various brain centres before being transmitted to the spinal cord.

Motor neurones project from the brain to the spinal cord to activate the motor neurones (both α and γ) to instigate events which will lead to contraction of muscles and alteration of the sensitivity of the muscle spindles within them. Several areas of the brain have been identified as having motor functions, most importantly the primary motor cortex, premotor cortex, basal ganglia and cerebellum.

Other areas contribute to this outflow especially areas of the sensorimotor cortex (see above) and other motor activating areas.

The function of the various areas has been the cause of considerable study. In humans, fibres which project *directly* from the motor cortex to the spinal cord seem to control skilled movements of the hands (and to a lesser extent feet). Lemon (1995) claims that they may also control some elbow and shoulder functions. This is presumably due to the complexity of human hand movements. In lower order animals these pathways are either less extensive or do not exist. However, it would be a mistake to overemphasize the contribution of the direct corticospinal pathways since other pathways are also important as evidenced by the effects of lesions of the brain. So how is the motor command organized?

Organization of Motor Commands

Figure 3.8 shows the main cerebral area involved. It should be recognized that there are others. To make sense of the system we need first to establish what might be happening at a spinal cord level since that is the 'final staging post' for commands to leave the CNS. Once that is done we can consider the nature of the commands that are presented to the spinal cord.

Spinal Cord

Look again at Figure 3.6 which shows the cross-section of the spinal cord to orientate yourself.

It is in the anterior horn of the grey matter that the cell bodies of motor nerves are found. They are both alpha and gamma types. Remember that α motor neurones supply the extrafusal fibres and motor neurones supply the intrafusal motor fibres. If you are unsure about this it is worth looking back at the muscle spindle. The axons

Figure 3.9 (a) Cell columns in the anterior grey horn of the spinal cord: somatotopic organization. (Adapted, with permission, from Fitzgerald, 1996, *Neuroanatomy: Basic and Clinical*, WB Saunders, London.) (b) Cross-section of a cervical segment of the spinal cord showing functional arrangement of spinal motor neurones. (The arms are innervated by motor neurones located in the cervical segments of the spinal cord.) Motor neurones supplying the arm extremities are located at the lateral margin of the ventral horn: motor neurones innervating the upper arm are at the medial margin of the ventral horn. Extensor motor neurones are found ventral to flexor motor neurones. (Adapted from Netter SH (1972) *CIBA Collection of Medical Illustrations: Nervous System*, vol. 1, CIBA, New Jersey.)

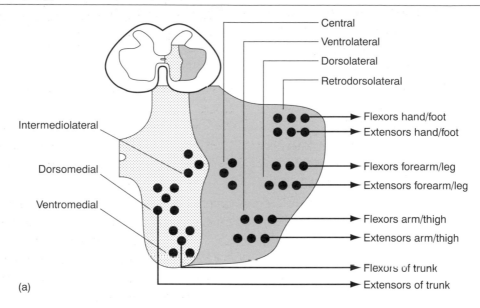

(a)

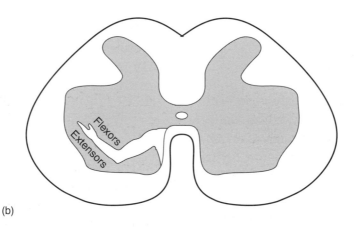

(b)

from these cell bodies exit through the anterior roots and pass, as a peripheral nerve, to the specific muscles they supply. There is a consistent organization to them in the anterior horn, with cell bodies from flexor muscles being more central than extensors and the upper limbs being more lateral than the lower limb, with the trunk being medial to both, as seen in Figure 3.9.

These anterior horn cells receive information from higher centres which is either excitatory or inhibitory which will then affect the level of stimulation received by individual muscles depending upon the action required. For example, if the muscle is an agonist then there will be a gradual increase in excitation of both alpha and gamma systems, if it is an antagonist then there will be a gradual decrease in stimulation. If it is a synergist or fixator then the level of stimulation will be adjusted so that isometric contraction of extrafusal fibres is allowed and there is appropriate stimulation of the gamma system. Remember also here that the effects of stimulation of the muscle spindles and Golgi tendon organs are vital since these inputs allow control but will also tend to stimulate the anterior horn cell.

If these adjustments do not happen sequentially and to the correct level then the muscle spindles may respond too quickly or too slowly. Therefore the feedback to the brain is not correct and the movement will not be coordinated. This compromised movement control is often seen in patients with damage to their central nervous system.

Clinical Example

Think for a moment about the plight of the patient with a complete lesion of the spinal cord. Not only will there be no means of sending motor commands down past the site of the lesion there will be no means of receiving sensory information from any level below. More than that, if the cord below the level of the lesion survives and does not die then local spinal reflexes can be set off. This is known as isolated cord syndrome and can be the source of considerable difficulty for the patient and their carers. For example, moving the limb too fast can cause reflex contraction of the muscles over which the patient has no control. Similarly such movements as the patient can make may affect other parts they cannot control and set off reflex actions.

Some conditions manifest themselves with destruction of specific areas of spinal cord tissue. Poliomyelitis for instance destroys the anterior horn cells. There is no possibility of the dead cells being replaced with other neurones so the patient loses the ability to stimulate the muscle fibres supplied by that nerve. So when you see these patients often the muscles are wasted. This can lead to considerable problems or even death if the respiratory muscles are affected. Fortunately as a result of vaccination programmes poliomyelitis is much less common than it once was.

How are the neurones in the spinal cord controlled? The simple answer is by higher centres. But which and how is the source of much research.

Roles of Higher Centres

The higher centres which will have an effect on movement and the pathways by which they affect the anterior horn cells or each other are shown in Figure 3.6. It is important to appreciate that the centres communicate with each other to a huge extent. In fact there are probably more neurones that have connections entirely within the CNS than there are ones that have connections outside it.

Table 3.3 shows each centre, the means by which it connects with the spinal cord, its function and the likely problem if the centre fails or becomes

Table 3.3
Each major centre and its connections with spinal cord. Effect of dysfunction also shown

Centre	Function	Connection to or from periphery	Consequence of dysfunction or failure
Cerebral cortex	Precise motor control	Corticospinal tract	Loss of precise movement especially of hands
	Interpretation of sensory information	As third order neurones from thalamus	Loss or alteration of sensation or perception (interpretation)
Basal ganglia	Integration of motor control	Striatocortical tracts Striatocerebellar tracts	Loss of automatic or learned movement Alteration in muscle tone Unintentional movement occurs
	Intepretation of sensation	Spinothalamic tracts	Loss or alteration of sensation or perception (interpretation)
Subcortical nuclei (red nucleus, olivary nucleus, reticular formation etc.)	Nonconscious parts of movement, such as fixation, synergy and tone adjustments	Rubrospinal tract Reticulospinal tract	Abnormal sequencing of movement
Vestibular nucleus	Postural adjustment	Vestibulospinal tract	Loss of balance reactions
Cerebellum	Coordination	Cerebellocortical pathways	Loss of coordination Altered muscle tone

dysfunctional. Some of these will then be described in a bit more detail.

Cerebral Cortex

The cerebral cortex receives information from many centres which it is able to interpret. In motor terms it sends commands to the spinal cord either directly or indirectly. The pathways are called corticospinal tracts or pathways.

The corticospinal pathways that pass directly onto motor neurone pools in the spinal cord are attributed by most authors as having the function of dexterity of the distal parts of limbs and are vastly more extensive for the hand. There is good evidence for this from patients who have damaged these tracts and lost precision in hand movements but retained gross control of the limb. For instance gripping and holding may well be possible but threading needles or playing the violin would not. Most connections would have an effect on the hand (see above). This is seen across species with different levels of manual dexterity. Thus they are most extensive in man and other high primates, less so in other apes and hardly at all in lower mammals and absent in other species (Lemon, 1995). During development there is a parallel maturation of distal dexterity and the connections of these pathways.

The pathways terminate in the interneuronal pools of the spinal cord. As well as allowing the activation of intended motor neurones this also allows the suppression of stretch reflex activity and the coactivation of α and γ motor neurones. Similarly there can be co-contraction of synergists and fixator muscles together with inhibition of antagonists.

From this it appears that nerve fibres which project directly from the cortex are related to function rather than to the recruitment of specific anatomical groups of muscles.

It is known that individual fibres can cause effects on the anterior horn cells of several muscles because they have collateral branches (Lemon, 1995). They therefore facilitate function since the small groups of muscle fibres supplied in common will tend to act synergistically. Therefore by recruiting the specific groupings of projection fibres, groups of muscle fibres in various muscles will be recruited at the same time. This will tend to raise the potential towards threshold in a greater number of muscle fibres. Since the groups of muscle fibres are the ones which will act together most frequently this will facilitate recruitment and therefore function. In this way the vast array of movements possible in the body can be coordinated without the need for enormous individual specificity for the recruitment on individual motor units centrally. That is by recruiting different projection fibres there will be a different recruitment of motor neurones and therefore a different motor event.

This also indicates that different projection fibres can converge on each α motor neurone.

In order to control these processes the motor cortex has a 'map' of the body parts in much the same way as the sensory cortex has a map for interpreting sensation, see Figure 3.10. Those requiring greater degrees of coordinated activation are represented most extensively. There is considerable overlap of body parts to specific cells thus facilitating the coordinative group action of the projection fibres without compromising their precision function. As with the sensory homunculus which was considered earlier, the motor homunculus is not a uniform representation of the body on the cortex. Instead those areas requiring greatest precision dominate the cortical tissue.

Practical Task

Consider for a moment those areas with the largest representation and the complexity of their functions and then compare them with those areas that are less well represented. Then compare the motor homunculus with the sensory homunculus. What does it mean?

The motor cortex receives input from the sensory systems. The majority seems to be from the muscle receptors though those from the skin, especially for skilled movement of the hand, are also important. Thus the motor cortex is able to interpret both sensory and motor 'maps'. Output is in terms of movements rather than specific muscles and is selected with reference to the sensory input. The cortical control of movement allows the recruitment of functionally relevant groups of cells to produce the desired outcome even if that requires activity in agonists, antagonists, fixators and synergists.

Figure 3.10   Motor cortex. (a) This area occupies a strip of cortex just in front of the somatic sensory cortex. (b) Different parts of the body are controlled by different regions of the motor cortex: those muscles which may be controlled most precisely have the greatest area of cortical representation. [Adapted from Penfield WG and Rasmussen T (1950) *The Cerebral Cortex of Man*, MacMillan, London.]

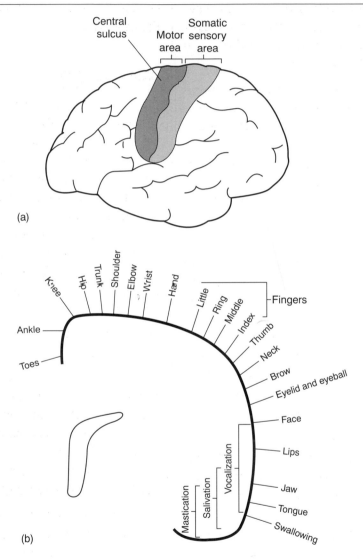

(a)

(b)

The cortical cells that are activated will cause effects on the neurones of the spinal cord. Because the projection cells can connect with motor neurones to several muscles, the reverse is also true that there is representation of an individual muscle on several projection fibres. This means that just as one projection fibre can serve many muscles so can a muscle be served by many projection fibres.

Lemon (1995) has described fast- and slow-conducting direct corticospinal neurones. He suggests that the fast fibres 'shape' the pattern of muscle activity and the slow ones provide the ongoing drive to control the posture and force of the movement. This is entirely plausible given that the ratio of fast to slow fibres is 1:10. He was restricting his explanations to hand function but there is no reason to suppose that other areas of the body are treated remarkably differently in function even if they are in degree.

For the critical threshold to be reached which generates an action potential in a neurone a number of impulses from other neurones may need to be received. This is called summation. Summation can either be many impulses received from one neurone onto the 'target' neurone (temporal summation) or sufficient impulses received from a number of different neurones.

In the arrangement described above it is clear that summation must occur before an action potential will be transmitted by the α motor neurone. This facilitates the coordinated function of the brain and spinal cord arrangements. This is essential, because the α motor neurones will be served by many fibres. If they responded in a simple 1:1 ratio then the level of coordination possible would be reduced and the need for brain to spinal cord neurones would increase dramatically.

An important feature of this system is that it is dynamic and adaptive. Following lesions the system has shown itself to be able to reorganize to a functional extent. The recovery seen in stroke patients is evidence of the reorganizing potential. This is the principle of neuroplasticity (the ability of the CNS to develop new synapses and therefore functions) which can be used to explain such reorganization and also be extended to explain how learning occurs. Detailed explanation is not relevant here but readers are encouraged to explore texts dealing with such phenomena (such as Kidd et al., 1992).

The precision of movement can be accounted for by corticospinal pathways but other elements, such as postural control, synergy and fixator function need to be taken into consideration. This is the role of the basal ganglia and the cerebellum.

Basal Ganglia

The basal ganglia consist of five nuclei: globus pallidus, putamen, caudate nucleus, substantia nigra and the subthalamic nuclei. They are present in both halves of the brain and are arranged as shown in Figure 3.11. Their function is the control of posture and 'background' adjustments which are necessary when moving. Also they seem to prepare the cortex for movement since they are active some 800 ms before the cells of the motor cortex (Lemon, 1995). Therefore it is likely that they modify the motor output before the output is transmitted elsewhere.

The major input to the basal ganglia is from the motor cortex.

The major output from the basal ganglia is to the motor cortex via the thalamus. Other areas receiving output are the superior colliculus (to guide eye movements), the reticular formation (for general levels of attention, activation and so on) and the pedunculo-pontine nucleus (to provide input to the cerebellum).

The main receiving nuclei are the caudate and putamen (together known as the striatum) and the main output is from the globus pallidus and the substantia nigra.

Cortical input to the striatum is excitatory and originates from the premotor, supplementary and motor areas. Output towards the thalamus can be via either of two routes: a relatively direct loop which is excitatory, and a relatively indirect loop which is inhibitory.

Figure 3.11   A coronal section showing the main cell masses (shaded) of the basal ganglia. VA, ventral anterior thalamic nucleus; VL, ventral lateral thalamic nucleus. (Reprinted with permission from Brodal, 1981, *Neurological Anatomy*, 3rd edn, Oxford University Press.)

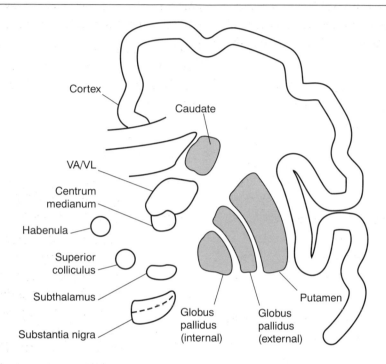

The detailed organization of the loops is not yet clear but that will not matter for the moment. What is clear is that either all motor inputs from all cortical motor areas converge on the same area of the striatum or that some areas contribute substantially more importantly. Either way the major output is to the premotor and motor cortices via the thalamus. The arrangement is shown schematically in Figure 3.12.

There are some important features of the output. The majority of the output to the thalamus from the basal ganglia is inhibitory (the thalamic output to the sensorimotor cortex is excitatory). Also, at rest their cells fire at high frequency. These two factors have led to the suppositions of basal ganglial function.

There now appears to be a consensus that removal

Figure 3.12   Summary of connections between major nucleii of the basal ganglia.

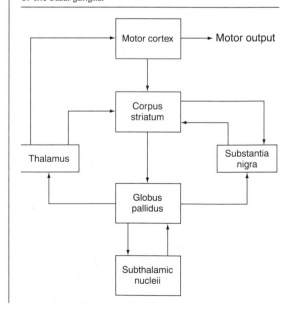

or lessening of the firing of the inhibitory output 'allows' movement to occur, whilst simultaneous increase in other elements will inhibit unwanted movement. Thus for a given pattern of movement the desired elements will be facilitated and the undesired inhibited.

It seems more likely that basal ganglia are related to postural and 'background' functions since subsequent to lesions within the basal ganglia movement can still be performed, albeit poorly. However, there is debate as to whether there are parallel or series events in the loops. The argument for parallel is that the range of firing patterns implies many functions occurring simultaneously. These involve *preparation* for movement as well as ongoing movement situations. However, series events are more easily rationalized.

There is also a notion that the basal ganglia function in automatic or sequential events. The evidence for this is that when actions which have a regular pattern have been learned, there is increased activity just *prior* to switching to the next element. In this situation it is presumed that the control has been handed over from the cortex to the basal ganglia (Lemon, 1995).

Interestingly the limbic system (which comprises the limbic lobe and subcortical nuclei and is the area which is thought to influence emotional responses) also has good connections into the striatum. The implication from this is that emotions, attitudes and concentration factors will have an effect on motor processes. This compares well with common experience and seems a logical reasoning for these inputs. For example, how many athletes achieve a higher level of performance in the heightened states of tension during important competitions? How many 'freeze' or 'tie up' because of fear? How many people perform a practical skill less well when they are being watched especially if this is in an examination?

Similarly other somatosensory inputs are received, mainly from the deep receptors rather than from skin. This input helps the processing of information.

Clinical Examples

It is worth thinking for a moment of some clinical situations that might be relevant applications of these processes.

When learning a new skill, whether it is walking in a child or sport in an adult or a clinical skill as a professional, there needs to be a learning phase. During this phase the individual knows what they want to do. So they stimulate the neurones to achieve the movement as best they can. The feedback from the sensory system then allows a computation of how close the actual movement was to the intended. (This is actually the function of the cerebellum.) Gradually with practice refinements take place until the movement is performed to the maximum ability of that person. With a new skill the person has to attend to what they are doing. Eventually it is learned and can become automatic. At this point the cerebral cortex is needed less and less and the activation can be 'devolved' to the basal ganglia.

Physiotherapists use this when treating patients who have injured themselves and need to relearn how to move. This need not necessarily be a neurological injury. A sportsman who has broken his leg will need to regain strength and range of movement but will also need to relearn control and timing.

Concentration is needed so that the 'interference' of information not relevant to the performance of the movement (noise) can be reduced, thereby improving the signal: noise ratio.

Eventually the movement becomes 'second nature'; perhaps it is now learned by the basal ganglia and the cerebellum (see later).

So overall the basal ganglia appear to act mainly for postural guidance or in automated patterns of movement. They act to prevent motor activation (i.e. as a braking system), so that they can both facilitate desired and inhibit undesired actions.

Clinical Example

This fits well with what is observed in basal ganglial disease for example. Movements are of poor quality, depending upon whether the indirect or direct pathways have been affected. This can lead to either an excessive output which would result in reduced spontaneous movement (hypokinesia) or a reduced input which could result in excess spontaneous movement (hyperkinesia). There is also the possibility of involuntary movement occurring without the patient willing them to, as in conditions exhibiting chorea (involuntary contraction of some muscles in short bursts), athetosis (slow sinuous writhing movements of parts or all of the body) or tremor (fairly fast rhythmical movements of body parts).

So when a movement is planned the frontal cortex sends the intention to the motor activating areas. There are then a number of possibilities. Firstly there appears to be a processing of information between the cortex and the basal ganglia and back to the cortex prior to any information being transmitted to the spinal cord. Once it does leave the brain there has already been a considerable amount of processing. Precision actions will be coordinated via the direct cortico-spinal pathways and automatic and postural effects will result from outputs from the corticobasal ganglial-cortical loop as well as from other motor nuclei such as red nucleus (whose method of function in humans is unclear), reticular formation and vestibular system.

The reticular formation is a very complex arrangement of nuclei. It has both sensory and motor elements to it. Whilst there really is no easy explanation of its function it is true to say that it has responsibility for the degree of excitation that is imposed upon the nervous system either as a whole or to specific areas.

The vestibular system is allied to the control of balance and the detection and interpretation of movement of the head. It is vital in the provision of sensory feedback of movement and feeds directly into the basal ganglia. There are also pathways to the spinal cord that allow for adjustments that can reflexly adjust in response to sudden movements.

However, whilst all this will lead to a movement of considerable complexity there is no means within this set-up for determining whether it will be the exact movement that was desired. Matching intended to actual is the role of the cerebellum.

Cerebellum

The cerebellum is essential for good function. Lesions of the cerebellum are devastating to motor events. However, as can be seen from the previous section the cerebellum does not feature in the main pathways for motor output. Instead it resides as a parallel system.

The cerebellum is often referred to as a computer–comparator system. What this means is that it seems to be able to compute the likely outcome of an intended or programmed set of motor impulses and compare them to the intended outcome. If the match is good then it allows the motor pattern to persist or continue. On the other hand, if there is a discrepancy then the cerebellum acts to correct the mismatch by stimulation of the motor activating nuclei. Clearly for such an elegant system to work the cerebellum must be constantly informed about the position of the body in time and three-dimensional space. Similarly it will require accurate details of the intended motor plan and the precise details of how that will be activated.

The following sections deal with the input to the cerebellum, followed by the output system.

CEREBELLAR AFFERENTS

Input to the cerebellum is via a number of important pathways and is very complex. A summary is shown in Figure 3.13. For the sake of understanding only a summary will be given here but if you are interested then the majority of neuroanatomy texts deal with it in detail. The major areas from which information is received is from the motor, visual and auditory cortices, other central

Figure 3.13   A schematic representation of tracts into and out from the cerebellum.

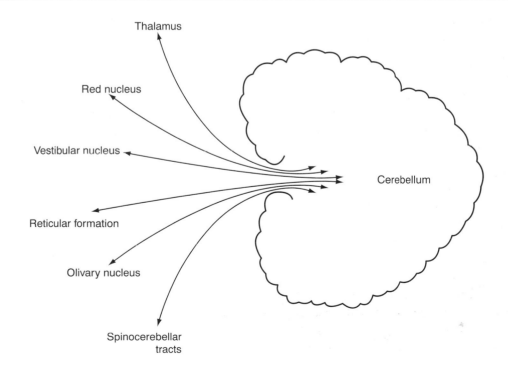

Thalamus

Red nucleus

Vestibular nucleus

Reticular formation

Olivary nucleus

Spinocerebellar
tracts

Cerebellum

nervous system nuclei (e.g. pontine nuclei and vestibular nuclei), and either directly or indirectly from the spinal cord.

Sensory information from the spinal cord is mapped onto the cerebellum in much the same fashion as on the cerebral cortex, though the cerebellum has two maps — one on its anterior lobe and another on the posterior lobe. Why this might be is not clear.

Input from the auditory and visual cortices is situated in the area of the cerebellum between the two sensory maps just described. This may be relevant since head control is vital in most movements. Ask any golfer for example!

Input from the spinal cord is via a number of pathways. The spinocerebellar pathways themselves are divided in terms of the areas from which the sensations they carry originate. According to Berne and Levy (1988) the dorsal and ventral spinocerebellar relay information from the thoracic and upper lumbar regions whereas the cuneocerebellar (which carries information from the dorsal column–lemniscal pathways) and rostral spinocerebellar relay from the cervical regions. Clearly this is the spinal area rather than the area of the body. So the whole of the body is represented on the cerebellar cortex. In addition it should be noted that the upper limb has a greater distribution than the lower limb reflecting the greater degree of coordination required for precision movements.

Other important areas of input are from the reticular formation.

Clinical Example

It is obvious at this stage, leaving aside detail of how this information is to be processed, that any interference with these afferent fibres will deprive the cerebellum of essential information.

Given its role as a computer–comparator if it doesn't 'know' where you are then its chances of computing your position accurately are dramatically reduced.

The type of incoordination can be either:

sensory: where the sensory information is either not received or is faulty; or

cerebellar: in which the sensory information is processed incorrectly.

This is often differentiated using Rhomberg's test. Get a patient to stand up and stay as still as they can. Close their eyes. Normally people wobble slightly. If they wobble a lot more then they have sensory ataxia. If they wobble excessively with their eyes open and with their eyes closed and the wobbling is unchanged between having eyes open and eyes shut then they have cerebellar ataxia.

Motor pathways are also important principal origins for inputs. Clearly if the purpose of the cerebellum is to compute intended against actual movement then it has to 'know' what was intended. These inputs are shown in Figure 3.13.

CEREBELLAR EFFERENTS

The output from the cerebellum is organized in a logical and predictable manner. The manner of the effect they have is the subject of later sections but they can be summarized to give a good appreciation of their function.

1 Cells of the vermis (medial cortical zone) influence the fastigial nucleus and via that the vestibular nucleus and pontine nuclei. Thus they

will have an effect on the descending motor system.

2 Cells of the intermediate zone influence the interpositus nucleus and thence the red nucleus. It is presumed that the red nucleus affects the motor systems of the trunk.

3 Cells of the lateral cortical zone influence the dentate nucleus and via that the thalamus and thence the cerebral cortex. Clearly they will have an effect on the descending motor system.

As with sensory afferents, if the efferent pathways suffer lesions then the ability of the cerebellum to produce impulses useful to function are severely reduced.

ORGANIZATION OF CEREBELLAR FUNCTION

In order to facilitate the understanding of how the cerebellum might work it is easier to develop a series of steps through which the information passes. It should be noted that the 'whole story' is not yet clear and the subject of considerable research. Also, the system is not necessarily linear as this implies. In fact it is much more likely that a substantial number of parallel systems are simultaneously active.

Output from the Purkinje cells is onto the deep cerebellar nuclei. This output is a function of the inputs received. Also the nature of the combined output is precise as can be summarized by referring to Figure 3.14 and following the list below.

- Mossy fibres activate a small array of granule cells.
- Exciting a well defined array of parallel fibres.
- This *excites* a well defined array of Purkinje cells and *inhibits* surrounding Purkinje cells.
- After a short delay initiating input is inhibited by Golgi cells.

Figure 3.14   Cerebellar cortex. A, cell layers; B, afferent system; C, internuncial neurones; D, efferent system.

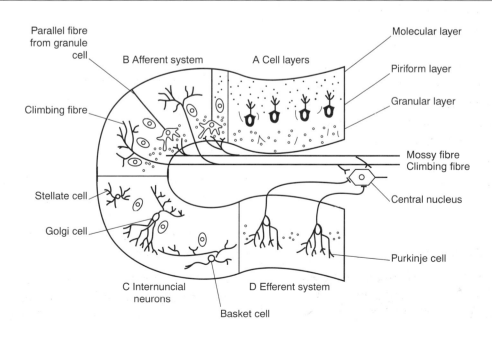

- At the same time climbing fibres are exciting Purkinje cells.
- Output from Purkinje cells onto deep cerebellar nuclei is inhibitory.
- Deep cerebellar nuclei show high levels of background activity.
- Thus the activity which is maintained is controlled by cerebellar cortex.
- Output from deep cerebellar nuclei on target nuclei is precisely controlled in response to changing environment and motor activation. Most granule cells respond to a single modality (touch, muscle length, muscle tension etc.) but there is considerable variation in the extent of their receptive field and the nature of their response (i.e. positive or negative).

The Purkinje cells, by virtue of their extensive input, respond to a wide receptive field but seem to respond particularly to stretch (i.e. particularly muscle spindles). It has been suggested that individual Purkinje cells might respond to particular joints and that the effect of joint displacement might alter the nature of the response.

Whichever way it turns out the output is a coordination of the input from motor and sensory centres and pathways .

The three major deep cerebellar nuclei each have their own output targets.

1 Dentate nucleus projects to the thalamus and from there affects the motor cortex and thus indirectly the corticospinal pathways.
2 Interpositus nucleus projects onto the red nucleus. It is presumed that in humans the red nucleus controls trunk stability.
3 Fastigial nucleus projects onto the vestibular nucleus thus affecting balance, and also onto the pontine reticular formation affecting general activation.

It is worth noting here that exactly when the pathways are activated is the subject of some debate. There is no point in having a coordinating system for movement that is not predictive. In caricature, for the cerebellum to 'tell' the cortex that it 'knew' all along that you were going to trip over the step after you have already fallen is useless. You need to be told beforehand so you could do something about it. Then learn for next time.

It appears that neurones in the dentate nucleus fire before a movement begins (their function is related to joint position and direction of movement) whereas the other nuclei fire after the movement has started (their function is related to force and rate of change). This indicates that the cerebellum can function in 'real time' to constantly improve the precision and quality of the movement.

CONCLUDING APPLICATIONS

It is clear that the cerebellum is essential in the coordination of the timing and force of movements. It does so via a complex series of pathways which integrate sensory and motor functions. That is, as the cerebral cortex and basal ganglia attempt to execute a motor plan (movement), the cerebellum first checks the programme (instruction) to ensure accuracy.

Lesions affecting these pathways either afferent to, efferent from or within the cerebellum are devastating to function. The timing of movements, and the force and response of movements to sensory input would not be correct. As a consequence the individual becomes uncoordinated. In the more profound states this may result in absence of any form of controlled synchronous movement.

How Does the Whole System Work Together?

So far we have established that for a motor plan to be executed there has to be a concept of where the body is starting from. Similarly as the movement progresses there has to be feedback on the speed and direction so that adherence to the plan can be judged.

We have also seen that there are reflexes which can be protective and used as feedback. We have seen that these need to be adaptive and adjusted through the range of movement to prevent unwanted reflex activity. We have also seen that not all sensations rise to consciousness nor are all movements controlled at a conscious level. So how does it all work?

The study of this is a huge topic but some of the principal concepts will be dealt with here in the form of questions.

1 *Are muscles contracted all the time?*
To a certain extent yes. This is muscle tone. Tone can be defined as the resistance a muscle has to passive stretch. This resistance comprises the physical length of the muscle due to the number of sarcomeres it has and the elasticity of its noncontractile parts and the degree of muscle contraction. The degree of contraction that occurs in response to the stretch is due to the contraction of the muscle spindle intrafusal fibres. If the level of gamma stimulation is low then the muscle will respond less to stretch and is said to be low toned. If the gamma stimulation is high then the response to stretch is high and the muscle is said to be high toned.

Disturbances of tone are common in neurological lesions. The treatment of abnormal tone can be by medication or physical therapy. There are many different concepts of physical therapy but you are advised to read the work of Davies (1994) and Carr and Sheppard (1991).

When we have hurt ourselves or when body parts are damaged the level of protection will rise. This shows itself as a rise in tone in the specific area. As a result the sensitivity to movement is greater as is the response to stimuli which are often perceived as painful. This is muscle spasm.

2 *Are reflexes important for functions other than protection?*
Yes. But how is more difficult to explain. The notion of the muscle spindle and Golgi tendon organs giving feedback should be clear. The muscle spindle can also act as a servo-assist. That is, if a reflex is set off at the same time as the alpha system contracts the extrafusal muscle fibres then the contraction will be enhanced.

In addition there are other reflexes which are present in infants which gradually disappear as the infant grows and movement becomes more complex. These do not reappear in adults except in pathological states. It appears that we need them as some sort of building block. But how is not yet explained. Why they return in pathological situations is also difficult to comprehend. An example would be the asymmetrical tonic neck reflex.

3 *How do we control movement we don't think about?*
This has been explained a bit already. The only part of our brain which has consciousness is the cerebral cortex. We know that movement is initiated there as a thought, but only the movement not all of its components. These are controlled by the basal ganglia and the cerebellum. Automatic movements such as synergistic and fixator components are initiated and controlled by the basal

ganglia. Similarly movements which we have learned can become fixed motor patterns within the motor system probably in the basal ganglia so that we initiate the movement pattern and only use our cerebral cortex when it becomes complicated. For instance once we have learned to walk it is easy but we need to pay attention to uneven paving slabs or to initiate stair-climbing.

4 Does this mean there is a hierarchy of movement?

Yes and no. Yes in that the cerebral cortex is the most complex and is able to control fine movements whereas the other centres control less complex movements. The cerebrum can affect the spinal cord directly and the cerebellum cannot. But by now it should be obvious that there is not a single linear sequence that has to be gone through. Instead there are very many parallel pathways to be activated for movement to occur.

5 Are there rhythms to movement?

There appear to be. We all have our natural walking pace for instance. This is possibly a function of our limb length, muscle length and tension as well as our nervous systems. There is evidence in lower animals of pattern generators. They are groups of nerves which act one upon another to execute patterns of rhythmic movement, for example swimming in fish. It seems that there is evidence of similar groups of nerves in humans that might control movements such as breathing, chewing or even walking. This is not without its contentious elements. Professor Sten Grillner has published a great deal of work in this area.

6 What are the clinical manifestations?

To ignore the central nervous system when considering people's ability to move would be a serious mistake. However, in movement terms to ignore the importance of muscle length, elasticity and pliancy of muscles and their tendons, range of movement, vision, balance and so on would be equally foolish. An holistic approach is required.

7 The major problems though are:

Paralysis The nerves to the muscles are cut or destroyed in some way. There is no way to stimulate the muscle to contract.

Alteration in muscle tone Hypertonia is when the tone is too high. This can be spasticity when the tone alters through range and tends to be in patterns, i.e. flexor or extensor spasticity. Or it can be rigidity when both the agonist and antagonist muscle are in the hypertonic state. It can be a relatively permanent state due to neurological disease, or as a result of altered biomechanics following orthopaedic injury. Or it could be temporary such as local muscle spasm.

Involuntary movements. These occur in basal ganglia disease leading to chorea, athetosis or tremor.

Ataxia This is incoordination of movement, most often as a result of cerebellar disease. But is it due to either inaccurate receipt of information, inappropriate processing of information, inappropriate recruitment of motor commands or a combination of all or any of these.

Altered sensation Obviously if any of the sensory pathways are interfered with or damaged then sensation will be affected adversely. This can be reduced or lost sensation or the presence of persistent sensations due to excessive stimulation. This too can be widespread as in conditions such as multiple sclerosis or local following peripheral nerve involvement in a bone injury for example. Clearly it is important to distinguish between the two.

Figure 3.15   Summary of the nervous system and motor control. The shaded areas indicate the principal sensory routes.

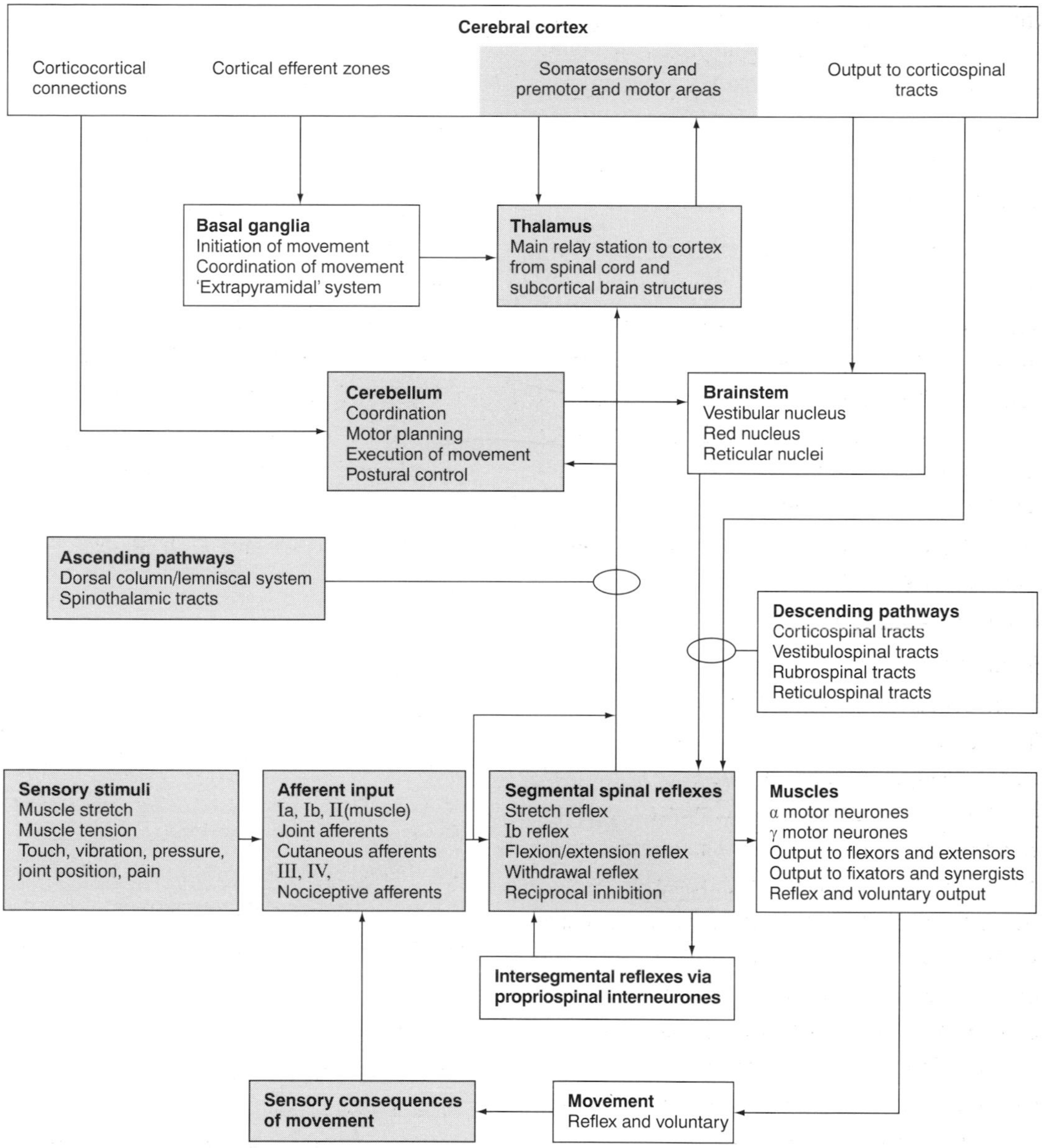

Cerebral cortex

| Corticocortical connections | Cortical efferent zones | Somatosensory and premotor and motor areas | Output to corticospinal tracts |

Basal ganglia
Initiation of movement
Coordination of movement
'Extrapyramidal' system

Thalamus
Main relay station to cortex from spinal cord and subcortical brain structures

Cerebellum
Coordination
Motor planning
Execution of movement
Postural control

Brainstem
Vestibular nucleus
Red nucleus
Reticular nuclei

Ascending pathways
Dorsal column/lemniscal system
Spinothalamic tracts

Descending pathways
Corticospinal tracts
Vestibulospinal tracts
Rubrospinal tracts
Reticulospinal tracts

Sensory stimuli
Muscle stretch
Muscle tension
Touch, vibration, pressure, joint position, pain

Afferent input
Ia, Ib, II(muscle)
Joint afferents
Cutaneous afferents
III, IV,
Nociceptive afferents

Segmental spinal reflexes
Stretch reflex
Ib reflex
Flexion/extension reflex
Withdrawal reflex
Reciprocal inhibition

Muscles
α motor neurones
γ motor neurones
Output to flexors and extensors
Output to fixators and synergists
Reflex and voluntary output

Intersegmental reflexes via propriospinal interneurones

Sensory consequences of movement

Movement
Reflex and voluntary

Summary

Refer to Figure 3.15 which summarizes the input and output systems to enable you to gain the most from the summary and also as a revision guide.

1 The nervous system is fundamental to the control of movement. This control is a function of the sensory input and its interpretation, the integration of sensations and the application of a motor programme.

2 The sensory system has important reflex functions in the form of protection (e.g. stretch reflex) but these are also incorporated into movement control. Thus the role of the muscle spindle is a length detector, the Golgi tendon organs are tension detectors and joint receptors are deformation detectors. With these three sensory types, speed, range and direction of movement can be detected accurately.

3 Interpretation of current position and movement can be used to predict the outcome subsequent to the implementation of motor commands. This is the function of the cerebellum. In this way movement can be smoothly coordinated and require minimal effort.

4 Planned movement will have automatic as well as precision elements. Automatic elements are the province of the basal ganglia, precision the cerebral cortex.

5 Errors in any part of the system will give rise to faulty movement. Faults or failings in specific areas give rise to specific symptoms. Thus diagnosis can be facilitated and treatment planned and focused.

Further Reading

Barr, M, Kiernan, J (1993) The Human Nervous System. Lippincott, London.

Bear, MF, Connors, BW, Paradiso, MA (1996) Neuroscience: Exploring the Brain. Williams & Wilkins, Baltimore.

Brooks, V (1986) The Neural Basis of Motor Control. Oxford University Press, Oxford.

Cody, F (1995) Neural Control of Skilled Human Movement. Physiological Society, London.

Lamb, JF, Ingram, CG, Johnston, IA, Pitman, RM (1991) Essentials of Physiology. Blackwell Scientific Publications, London.

References

Berne, R, Levy, M (1988) Physiology, 2nd Edition. CV Mosby Company, St Louis.

Brodal (1981) Neurological Anatomy, 3rd edn. Oxford University Press, Oxford.

Carr, J, Shepherd, R (1991) Physiotherapy in Disorders of the Brain. Butterworth Heinemann, Oxford.

Davies, P (1994) Steps to Follow. Springer-Verlag, Berlin.

Fitzgerald, F (1996) Neuroanatomy: Basic and Clinical. WB Saunders, London.

Fredericks, CM, Saladin, LK (1996) Pathophysiology of the Motor Systems: Principles and Clinical Presentations. FA Davis, Philadelphia.

Kidd, G, Lawes, I, Musa, I (1992) Understanding Neuroplasticity. A Basis for Clinical Rehabilitation. Edward Arnold, London.

Lemon, R (1995) Cortical control of skilled movements, in Cody F (ed.) Neural Control of Skilled Human Movement. Physiological Society, London.

Shumway-Cook, A, Woollacott, M (1995) Motor Control: Theory and Practical Applications. Williams and Wilkins, Baltimore.

Stein, J (1995) The posterior parietal cortex, the cerebellum and the visual guidance of movement. In Cody F (ed.) Neural Control of Skilled Human Movement. Physiological Society, London.

Williams, P, Warwick, R, Dyson, M, Bannister, L (1989) Gray's Anatomy 37th edn. Churchill Livingstone, London.

4

Neurodynamics

LOUIS GIFFORD

Chapter Objectives

Neurodynamics addresses the peripheral and central nervous systems in a unique way. Historically, the nervous system has been viewed as a communicating and coordinating organ for the rest of the body. Little attention has been focused on the fact that as the body moves so the nervous system has to accommodate and adapt to the movements it paradoxically produces.

After reading this chapter you should be able to:

1 Appreciate that the nervous system moves and has many design elements that allow this to happen. This includes both the central nervous system (CNS) and the peripheral nervous system (PNS);

2 Appreciate that joint movements in one area can have quite far-reaching mechanical effects on neural tissues;

3 Understand that neurodynamics looks at the effects of movement/posture on the nervous system. This includes both movements and postures that tend to compress neural tissue

and those that tend to elongate it. Most movements and postures are likely to produce combinations of compression and elongation effects;

4 Appreciate that neural compression and elongation produce physiological effects on neural tissue;

5 Appreciate that pathological processes in tissues that surround the nervous system may have detrimental consequences on its mechanical and physiological health and that alterations in compliance and sensitivity may be a consequence;

6 Appreciate that the nervous system in general is relatively insensitive, yet if it is injured or physiologically compromised in some way it has the potential to become an extremely hypersensitive tissue and a potent source of ongoing pain;

7 Have a good understanding of possible pathophysiological processes that can underlie enhanced neural sensitivity.

Introduction

That the nervous system moves is beyond doubt. In 1978 Alf Breig published a book called *Adverse Mechanical Tension in the Central Nervous System* which presented clear evidence that nerve trunks and roots, the spinal cord and its coverings, as well as the brain, are capable of quite remarkable movement. Professor Henk Verbeist, one of the world's leading neurosurgeons, wrote in the foreword to Breig's book:

> In my opinion his work should not only be read by specialists in neuroscience and orthopaedic surgery, but also by anaesthetists whose activities regularly involve the positioning of defenceless patients, and last but not least by physiotherapists for reasons which need no further precision. (Breig, 1978)

That was back in 1978. For physiotherapy it was not until the late 1980s and early 1990s that the notion that the nervous system has subtle design features that allow it to move, was more widely appreciated (Butler and Gifford, 1989; Butler, 1991).

The prime purpose of the nervous system is one of continuous communication, whatever the situation and whatever the body happens to be doing at the time. Thoughts about its anatomical design must take into account the need for vital electrical and chemical processes to be able to continue unhindered during movement. For instance, observe the highly coordinated yet extreme movements of gymnasts and dancers and consider the need for the nervous system to be able to physically adapt (Figure 4.1).

Figure 4.1 Extreme joint movement and muscle stretch requires considerable physical adaptation of the peripheral nervous system and the neuraxis. The elongation and compressive forces that the nervous system structures have to cope with in this gymnast are impressive.

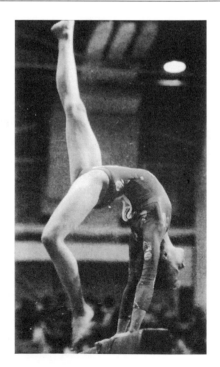

In terms of gross structure the nervous system appears as a well organized cord-like meshwork branching away from the core central nervous system (CNS) structures, the brain and spinal cord. The term 'neuraxis' (Bowsher, 1988) in place of CNS helps to focus us on this component of the nervous system from a biomechanical perspective. However, Butler (1991) introduced the idea that we should consider the nervous system as a continuum, in other words, get away from the traditional anatomical descriptive concepts of central, peripheral and autonomic nervous systems and move towards a view that the whole structure is closely linked. In this way, the nervous system is unique among organs and systems in that it has a pretty straightforward mechanical, electrical and chemical 'connectedness' (Butler, 1991). The implication is that mechanical, electrical and chemical changes in one part of the nervous system may have far-reaching effects for the rest of it.

Figure 4.2 The slump test: note how release of the head flexion allows greater knee extension range. The slump test is fully described in Maitland (1986), Butler (1991) and Butler and Gifford (1998). (Adapted, with permission, from Butler, 1991, *Mobilisation of the Nervous System*. Churchill Livingstone, Melbourne.)

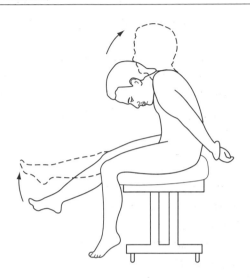

Clinical Example

Consider a subject who gets nasty calf pain in the full slump test position (see Figure 4.2). Lifting the head relieves the pain in the calf and allows the knee to be fully extended without any major discomfort. Putting the head flexion back on again causes a dramatic return of calf symptoms. Without knowledge of structural connections and sensitivity of the nervous system it would be difficult to explain such a clear-cut phenomenon in terms of other tissue systems.

In a grossly mechanical sense the nervous system can be seen as a massive ligament or tendon that just happens to contain a system of specialized conducting and communicating cells. In this extreme slump 'test' position (Maitland, 1986) (Figure 4.2) the loss of knee extension could be analysed in purely mechanical terms, thus, lift the head, put some slack into the neuraxis/sciatic system and allow the knee to extend. In some situations like this the nervous system *may* physically limit movement. The reality though, is that at any limit of range, noxious forces cause nociceptive messages that make most people call a halt to a movement as well as offering up an appropriate protective motor reflex that further prevents movement (Elvey, 1995; Hall *et al.*, 1995). Perhaps performing the slump test under a general anaesthetic would help clarify whether or not pure nerve mechanics/tension was the key limiting structure to this position.

Clinical reality forces us to consider both

Figure 4.3   Microanatomy of a peripheral nerve trunk and its components. (a) Fascicles surrounded by a multilaminated connective tissue perineurium (p) are embedded in a loose connective tissue, the epineurium (epi). The outer layers of the epineurium are condensed into a sheath. (b) and (c) illustrate the appearance of unmyelinated and myelinated fibres respectively. Nerve fibres are surrounded by the endoneurial connective tissue (end). Schw, Schwann cell; my, myelin sheath; ax, axon; nR, node of Ranvier. (Adapted, with permission, from Lundborg, G (1988) *Nerve Injury and Repair.* Churchill Livingstone, Edinburgh.)

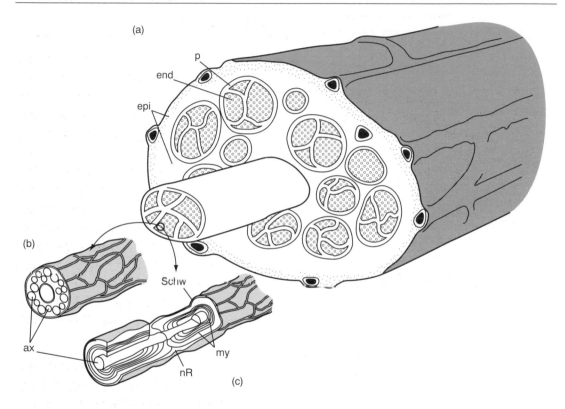

mechanics and sensitivity in parallel. In order to fully appreciate this we must recognize that the nervous system consists of four major tissue types, the first two of which are generally given most attention:

1 *Conducting nerve fibres, the neurones;*
2 *Collagenous connective tissues* whose important protective role is the major consideration;
3 Nonconducting *glial cells;*
4 The *vasculature.*

In the peripheral nervous system the conducting and connective tissue elements combine to form nerve trunks and nerve roots (Figure 4.3), whereas in the CNS the major protective connective tissues envelope and remain external to the neuraxis (Figure 4.4).

The existence of nonconducting cells in the CNS, the glial cells, was first recognized in the 1800s. For a long time these cells were considered as uninteresting putty that packs out spaces between the conducting cellular elements. What is now clear is that they have very important roles to play that include an immunological function, reabsorption of unused transmitters and providing the axons of conducting fibres with myelin (Streit and Kincaid-Colton, 1995).

Figure 4.4 Scanning electron micrograph of the lower spinal cord of a 15-month-old child. L, denticulate ligaments that suspend the cord within the sub arachnoid space. D, Dura; note the thickness and the layers. A, Arachnoid; note how it has come away from the dorsal dura in the preparation. S, dorsal septum. IL, intermediate leptomeningeal layer. Note the sectioned multifascicular nerve roots within the subarachnoid space. The pia can be seen adhering to and surrounding the cord. (From Nicholas, DS, Weller, RO, 1988, *Journal of Neurosurgery* **69**: 276–282, with permission.)

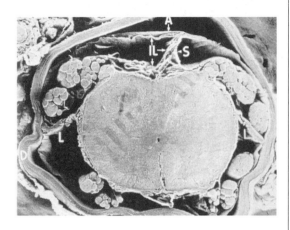

The last tissue type of importance is the vasculature. The recent upsurge in interest in the detrimental effects of ischaemia on nervous system structures means that more than passing attention should be paid to the whereabouts of feeder vessels and veins and, vitally, the important effects that movement and sustained posturing has on their patency. For now, consider that movements that compress or stretch blood vessels will tend to decrease the lumen size and hence deprive the local or regional tissues of blood.

It is clear that the nervous system moves and that its anatomy strongly reflects this to be a built-in feature of its design. In order to be complete, the nervous system has to be examined from all its functional perspectives, that is, in terms of its ability to conduct and its ability to move in a normal and symptom-free way.

The Nervous System Responds to Movement

Basic Concepts

1 *The relationship of nerve position to the axis of a joint helps establish the effect a movement may have on neural tissue*: Many of the modern neurodynamic tests have been developed as a result of the anatomical and biomechanical appraisal of nerve trunks in relation to their surrounding tissues. In particular, the relationship to joint axes of movement. It is a matter of mentally drawing the known position and course of a peripheral nerve on the body and then moving the various joint components that it traverses in a way that will exert increased tension on the nerve under consideration. There has also been much reflection on the literature (Butler and Gifford, 1989; Butler, 1991). For instance:

- From the work of Millesi (Millesi, 1986; Millesi *et al.*, 1990) it has been calculated that from wrist and elbow flexion to wrist and elbow extension, the 'bed' of the median nerve gets approximately 20% longer.
- Beith *et al.* (1995) have shown that the sciatic nerve bed increases in length by 8–12% during the straight leg raising (SLR) manoeuvre.
- As long as 100 years ago it was considered self-evident that the length of a nerve must undergo changes during joint movement and that these changes create intraneural tension when a nerve's length is increased (Dyck, 1984; Beith *et al.*, 1995).

A key consideration is the position of the nerve in relation to the axis of movement of

Louis Gifford

Figure 4.5 Diagram of a nerve as it traverses a joint while joint is in neutral position. Arrows indicate length of nerve bed at level of joint. (a) Neutral position – nerve is slack. (b) Angulated position – nerve bed has elongated, causing nerve to be lengthened and bent across joint. (Reproduced from Shacklock M, 1995, *Physiotherapy* **81** (1): 9–16, with permission.)

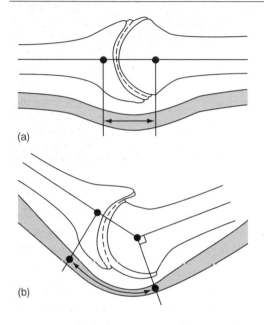

(a)

(b)

the adjacent joint (Figure 4.5). Thus during elbow flexion the ulnar nerve at the elbow will tend to elongate and the median and radial nerves on the ventral aspect of the joint will tend to shorten, buckle and be compressed. End range neurodynamic tests like the SLR and the upper limb tension tests (ULTT) must be considered in terms of rather gross elongation effects of whole nerve trunks, plexi and nerve roots with further possible repercussions in the neuraxis. What must be emphasized is that even localized joint movements will have quite marked effects on adjacent neural tissues.

2 *Sliding, elongation and compression*: In order to adapt to body movements the nervous system is known to slide over adjacent tissue, elongate and be compressed. For example:

- Normal nerve roots are known to be compressed by spinal extension due to the decrease in size of the intervertebral foramen (Yoo *et al.*, 1992; Farmer and Wisneski, 1994).
- At the wrist the median nerve can be simultaneously compressed and elongated in the carpal tunnel during wrist and finger extension (LaBan *et al.*, 1989; Yoshioka *et al.*, 1993).
- The median nerve in the upper limb of normal volunteers has been shown to slide an average of 7.4 mm during movements of the wrist alone (McLellan and Swash, 1976).

Key Point

The fundamental physiological effects of sliding, elongation and compression due to normal movements are that they will load the nervous system and hence cause an increase of pressure within it. Changes in pressure cause changes in circulation and prolonged changes in circulation are likely to have detrimental effects on a tissue that is relatively blood thirsty (see below).

3 *Anatomical and attachment considerations in neurodynamics*: Concepts of nervous system movement must embrace the fact that its structure, its attachments and the interfacing structures around it, are continuously changing and very variable from one site to the next. The implications of this are that simple movement of one part of it does not have a uniform spread of effects throughout the whole, as it would if one considered the peripheral nerves and neuraxis as a homogenous string-like structure of uniform thickness and

164

elasticity and having no attachments to neighbouring tissues. The reality is that the nervous system gets ever thinner and more branching as it reaches towards its target tissues and it has varying amounts of connective tissue within and around it. It has considerable attachments to adjacent tissues that may prevent dispersal of forces further proximally or distally and it has contracting and moving structures around it that may have varying effects on neural load dissemination (Sunderland, 1978).

Thus, the effects of joint movement have non-uniform effects on the nervous system (Shacklock, 1995). For example:

- Full spinal flexion induces a 15% dural strain at L1–2 whereas at L5, strain approaches 30% (Louis, 1981). Further, the load on the nervous system will be greatest in the neural tissue adjacent to the site of joint movement (Shacklock, 1995).
- Ankle plantar flexion – inversion will produce quite a marked effect on the tension and movement of the superficial peroneal nerve as it courses over the anterior aspect of the ankle and foot. This is very easy to demonstrate on a thin foot (Figure 4.6). Proximal movement and tension repercussions of ankle plantar flexion inversion on the peroneal nerve tract have been observed as far as the thigh (Borges *et al.*, 1981).
- Smith (1956) in monkeys and Breig and Troup (1979) observing fresh human cadavers, have demonstrated that ankle dorsiflexion with the leg and trunk in a neutral position can have mechanical influences as far afield as the lumbosacral nerve roots. Performing the same movement in a SLR may have tension repercussions as far as the cerebellum (Smith, 1956).

Figure 4.6   Demonstrating the superficial peroneal nerve on the dorsum of the foot. (From Butler and Gifford, 1998, *The Dynamic Nervous System.* Adelaide, NOI Press, with permission.)

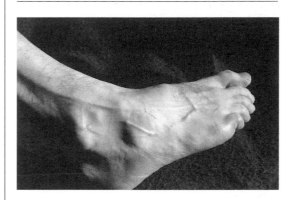

It seems that movements of one part of the body can have quite far-reaching repercussions for the nervous system elsewhere. This biomechanical consideration can be utilized in management approaches. For instance it may be desirable to physically influence nerve roots in a pain-free way post laminectomy. Moving the lumbar spine and hips as in performing SLR may be far too noxious, but moving the foot or knee may be tolerated well. One of the uses of this knowledge of the nervous system is that it can easily be influenced from a distance. It is also often worth giving some consideration to the order or sequence that tests and movements are performed in.

A key principle is that the greatest effect of a joint movement on a nerve will occur in the part of the nerve that is immediately adjacent to the joint being moved (Shacklock, 1995).

Thus ankle plantar flexion inversion will have most physical effect on the peroneal nerve over the dorsum of the ankle and less and less higher up the leg. Alterations of sequencing can be useful clinically when trying to localize tension to a particular segment of nerve trunk (Shacklock, 1995; Butler and Gifford, 1998).

It is now worth taking a more focused look at a few specific anatomical sites that illustrate some major neurodynamic principles and relate them to the pathological state.

The Effects of Movement and Sustained Posture on the Peripheral Nervous System

Trunk, head and limb movements and postures produce compression and elongation effects on the peripheral nervous system.

COMPRESSION

Nerves get relatively compressed when the cross-sectional area of the surrounding interface material diminishes in size. To demonstrate this, consider three anatomical zones that are commonly implicated in pain states associated with the nervous system. The first two zones relate to nerve roots, the third to a nerve trunk.

1 The L5–S1 nerve roots in the radicular canal;

2 The nerve roots generally in the intervertebral foramen (IVF);

3 The median nerve in the carpal tunnel.

L5–S1 Nerve Roots in the Radicular Canal

The L5–S1 roots are special because they cause a great many problems. It is not surprising that they have unique features and relationships that make them vulnerable to compressive distress and consequently the nerve root pain of sciatica.

Normal Anatomy / Biomechanics   Anatomically the lumbar spinal canal contains only the peripheral nerve roots of the cauda equina encased in their dural sac (Figure 4.7). (The cord terminates at approximately L1–2.) From the point at which they emerge from the spinal cord to their exit in the IVF the lumbosacral nerve roots may be as long as 16 cm (Grieve, 1988). The next important anatomical consideration is that nerve roots are positioned more centrally in the spinal canal when they emerge from the cord but, as they descend towards their exiting foramen, they course more and more laterally into less and less space (Figure 4.7) (Wall *et al.*, 1990).

Figure 4.7ab   Dural sac contents at L2–3 and L4–5 levels. (a) Diagrammatic representation of contents of lumbar dural sac at the L2–3 level. (b) Diagrammatic representation of contents of lumbar dural sac at the upper L4–5 level. (Adapted from Wall et al., 1990, *Spine* 15 (12): 1244–1247, with permission.)

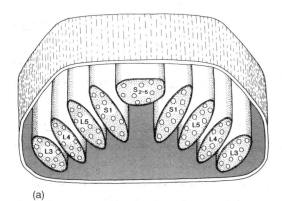

(a)

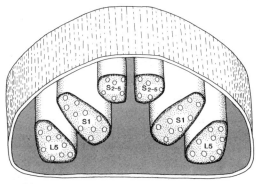

(b)

Figure 4.8   Diagrammatic representation of lumbar dural sac – nerve root anatomical relations and vulnerable zones. A, L4 root is less vulnerable to facet impingement here because the root exits the dural sac below the disc/facet level. B, L5 root vulnerable in standing/extension here – from superior facet of L5 coming down on it and from disc bulging backwards. C, S1 root vulnerable in standing/extension here – from superior facet of S1 coming down on it and from disc bulging backwards. D, L5 and S1 roots can both be influenced by movement-related compressive effects in this zone, especially if degenerate changes have caused narrowing of foramen and spinal canal. Line of section refers to Figures 4.9 and 4.10. (From Butler and Gifford, 1998, *The Dynamic Nervous System*, Adelaide, NOI Press, with permission.)

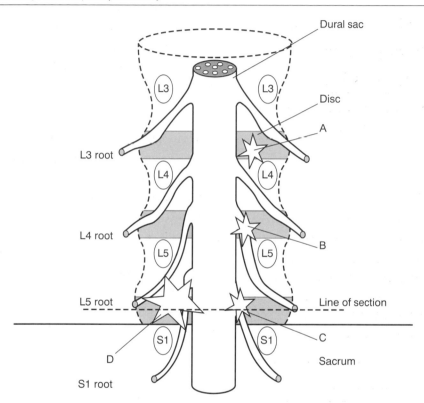

- Before emerging at the S1–2 intervertebral foramen the S1 nerve root lies in the lateral recess or 'radicular canal' medial to the articular pillar of S1 (Figure 4.8).
- Just above this it travels over the back of the L5 disc where it is in close relation to the overlying superior facet of S1.
- The salient feature is that the nerve root is isolated in its own dural sleeve having left the dural sac just above to the L5–S1 disc (Figure 4.8). A similar situation occurs with the L5 root at the L4–5 disc level.

- Note how the more rostral roots leave the dural sac just *below* the disc level.
- The significance of this is that the two 'isolated' roots (L5 and S1) are particularly vulnerable to compression effects within the lateral recesses of the spinal canal during movements of the spine.

Penning (1992) has convincingly shown that at the level of the disc/superior facet the size of the lateral recess is movement and posture dependent. For instance in standing, and increasingly in extension, the combined effects of the back-

Figure 4.9 (a) Horizontal section through L5–S1 disc in neutral position non-weight-bearing. (Line of section in Figure 4.8.) Image of vertebral arch of L5 is in background. (b) Horizontal section through L5–S1 disc in upright or extended position. (Line of section in Figure 4.8.) Image of vertebral arch of L5 is in background. Note how the contents of the spinal canal, the S1 facet and the L5–S1 disc move (arrows) to relatively compress the dural sac, the S1 root and surrounding tissues (adipose tissue and venous plexus). (From Butler and Gifford, 1998, *The Dynamic Nervous System*, Adelaide, NOI Press, with permission.)

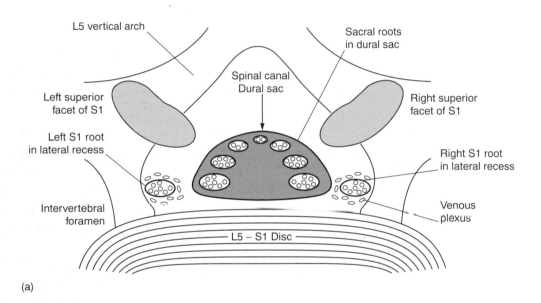

(a)

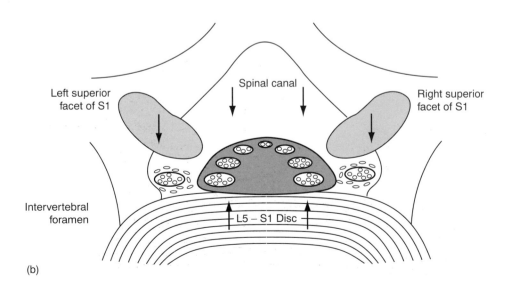

(b)

ward bulging disc and the forward-moving superior articular facet significantly reduces the size of the recess (Figure 4.9a,b). The major effects of this in the normal spine are a modest squashing of the dense venous plexus surrounding the root and a medial sliding of the root. However, it has been suggested that this medial sliding may be strongly curtailed due to ligamentous distal fixation of the root in the intervertebral foramen (Spencer et al., 1983).

Pathological Anatomy/Biomechanics Pathological encroachment of the radicular canal area by a protruding disc or as a result of degenerative facet enlargement and flaval ligament thickening may have dire compressive consequences in standing and extension (Figure 4.10). This may go a long way to explaining why so many patients with sciatic nerve root distribution symptoms so often dislike standing for long,

especially standing upright and extending, and prefer to be in varying degrees of flexion.

The important point is that we so often think of pathology affecting the root at the IVF, yet it should be apparent that if we follow the L5–S1 roots upwards there is a second zone where they are also vulnerable to compressive 'subarticular' forces (Vanderlinden, 1984).

Degenerative changes, congenitally limited radicular canal size and nerve root anomalies (Grieve, 1988) are important factors to consider when assessing any contributing factors to a disorder.

Nerve Roots and the Intervertebral Foramen
According to Hoyland et al. (1989) the roots of the lumbar spine occupy the upper pole of the foramen, *above the disc*, and occupy a maximum of 35% of the area of the IVF. These workers found that the average area occupied by the root was

Figure 4.10   Degenerate changes: horizontal section through L5–S1 disc in upright or extended position. (Line of section in Figure 4.8.) Image of vertebral arch of L5 is in background. Note how the thickened spinal canal contents, S1 facet and L5–S1 disc move (arrows) to compress the dural sac, the S1 root and surrounding tissues (venous plexus and adipose tissue). (From Butler and Gifford, 1998, *The Dynamic Nervous System*, Adelaide, NOI Press, with permission.)

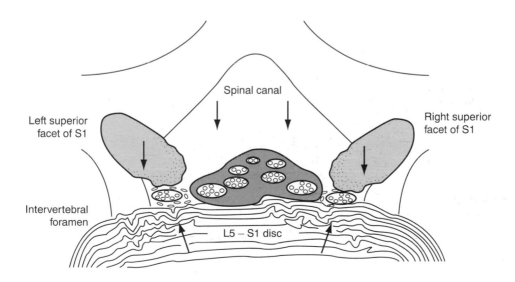

21% and that it ranged from as low as 2%. The rest of the apparently ample space is mainly occupied by adipose tissue, radicular arteries and a venous plexus meshwork. Hoyland *et al.* (1989) stressed that relatively few of the cadavers they studied showed evidence of direct compression of the nerve roots by the disc. They highlighted the fact that the disc protrusions they observed more frequently compressed and severely distorted the venous plexus situated predominantly in the lower pole of the IVF overlying the disc protrusion. The pathophysiological importance of this observation is supported by Jayson (1992) who noted that careful examination of radiculograms in patients with disc prolapse often showed dilated veins and swelling of the nerve root indicating the presence of oedema. Unfortunately observing dissected cadavers does not take into consideration the effect of posture and movement on the disc–superior facet–root structure relationship in this area.

Dorsal Root Ganglion   The position of the dorsal root ganglion (DRG) relative to the IVF is of some interest as this structure is recognized by some as a key player in the generation of radicular pain (Howe *et al.*, 1977; Devor and Rappaport, 1990; Devor, 1994). The reason for this is that the DRG is normally exquisitely mechanosensitive, yet the rest of the root tissue proximally and distally is relatively insensitive unless it is in an inflamed state (Garfin *et al.*, 1991; Kuslich *et al.*, 1991). The clinical implication of this is that symptoms of nerve root compression may only occur if the DRG gets compressed, or the adjacent insensitive areas of the root become inflamed – a process that does not invariably happen, and if it does, takes time to build up. It is very tempting to argue that sciatic pain that occurs at the instant of injury must be the result

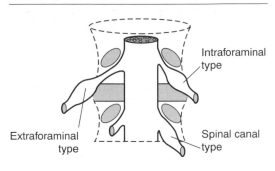

Figure 4.11   Variation in anatomical position of the dorsal root ganglion. Classification according to Sato and Kikuchi (1993). (Adapted from Sato and Kikuchi, 1993, *Spine* 18 (15): 2246–2251, with permission.)

of DRG compression since normal nerve root takes time to become inflamed and generate pain.

It seems likely that some people may be more prone to DRG compression. A recent cadaver study by Sato and Kikuchi (1993) revealed that the position of the ganglion relative to the foramen was remarkably variable. They classified the posiiton of the DRG as being either located medially (spinal canal type), within the foramen, or extraforaminal (see Figure 4.11) and found that the extraforaminal type was the least likely to suffer adverse pathological compression. As far as the L5 ganglion was concerned, it appeared more vulnerable if it was situated more proximally.

Sato and Kikuchi (1993) interestingly noted 'indentations' on the ganglia due to impingement by the disc and adjacent superior facet in elderly specimens which showed space encroaching pathology (enlarged degenerate facets and bulging disc material). The authors made no comment as to whether the ganglia were physically pinched by these structures when they dissected them (a dissected out lumbar spine is likely to be in a neutral position and not subjected to any compressive forces that would alter the relevant

Figure 4.12   Diagram of lumbar nerve root dynamics in the intervertebral foramen. (a) Flexion: posterior wall of disc annulus is stretched and tightened, the body of the vertebra above moves forwards and away from the root and the superior facet moves backwards in relation to the root. The intervertebral foramen area thus enlarges. (b) Extension: the opposite occurs; note how the disc bulges into the foramen, the facet tip and the posterior rim of the vertebra above come close together and the nerve gets relatively compressed by this pincer mechanism. (From Penning, 1992, *Clinical Biomechanics* 7 (1): 3–17, with permission.)

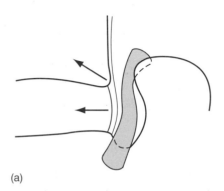

(a)

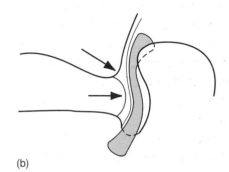

(b)

structures position and shape). According to Penning's (1992) findings, it is reasonable to assume that standing postures and extension movements would dramatically decrease the already pathologically limited space in the foramen and even physically pinch the ganglion/root there (Figure 4.12).

Thus the dorsal root ganglion/nerve root in the IVF can be compressed in the 'jaws' formed by the tip of the superior facet behind and the bulging disc and the inferior rim of the adjacent vertebral body in front. The fundamental movements to consider are those that tend to 'close' the IVF, i.e. going to standing (since erect standing compresses and causes the disc to bulge), extension and movements towards the side under consideration (Panjabi *et al.*, 1983). This principle also applies to the cervical spine (Yoo *et al.*, 1992; Farmer and Wisneski, 1994) and more than likely in the thoracic spine, judging by clinical findings.

The Carpal Tunnel

Since the carpal tunnel contains the median nerve to the hand, as well as nine flexor tendons, it has little room for intrusions. Thus any process that tends to cause narrowing of the space, or an increase in the size of the contents, will increase the tissue pressure in the tunnel.

Normal pressure in the carpal tunnel is around 2.5 mmHg, in wrist flexion the pressure increases to about 30 mmHg, a pressure which corresponds well to the critical pressure known to induce the first changes in intraneural microcirculation and axonal transport (see below) (Gelberman *et al.*, 1981).

Movements of the wrist alter the size of the carpal tunnel. For example, Yoshioka *et al.* (1993) have shown that in wrist flexion the carpal tunnel gets 16% smaller at the pisiform level. It is hardly surprising that sustained wrist flexion begins to cause hand paraesthesia in many who are otherwise normal.

SLIDING AND ELONGATION

Nerves get relatively elongated by limb and trunk movements that increase the length of their nerve

Figure 4.13 Anterolateral view of right sacral plexus and roots L4 and L5 as they emerge from their intervertebral foramen. Paper markers 1 cm long have been sutured to the nerves. In (a) with the trunk in neutral and hip in flexion the neural structures are relatively slack and the markers lie within (L4) and just distal (L5) to the intervertebral foramen. In (b) the right knee has been extended into the straight leg raise position and the amount of root movement relative to the foramen is clear. (From Breig, A, 1978, *Adverse Mechanical Tension in the Central Nervous System*, Almqvist and Wiksell, Stockholm, with permission.)

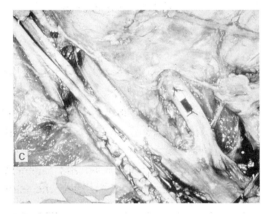

(a)

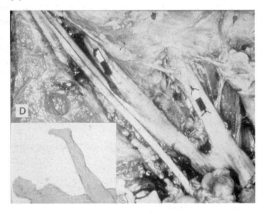

(b)

beds (i.e. the tissues which surround them and which they lie in). They adapt to this in two ways:

1 By sliding;
2 By elongation.

The remarkable movement of the L4 and L5 spinal nerves during the SLR manoeuvre is shown in Figure 4.13. The S1 nerve root complex has been reported to slide as much as 10 mm (Goddard and Reid, 1965) and tension transmitted as far rostrally as the mid brain (Smith, 1956). An important principle to consider with regard to neurodynamics is that in some situations more sliding of a nerve will occur, yet in others more tensioning and elongation will occur, and that what occurs when, is likely to be hugely variable between individuals.

Examination of fresh cadavers (Goddard and Reid, 1965) has revealed that during straight leg raising, when the heel is only 5 cm above the horizontal, movement/sliding of the nerve at the greater sciatic notch has already begun. The movement spreads proximally the more the leg is lifted and does not start to affect the nerve roots in the IVF until around 35° of SLR. As the leg raising continues so the sliding effect diminishes and the tension/elongation effects grow, so that by 70° there is little sliding and the adaptation has to be borne by the intrinsic elastic capabilities of the nerve. Considerable stresses are imparted on nerve roots during spinal movements. For instance, Louis (1981) calculated that during flexion greatest strain (16%) was taken by the S1 nerve root.

It should be noted, though, that cadaver observations must be interpreted with caution since close scrutiny of nerve trunks and roots reveals quite marked attachment tissues that often strongly anchor the nerve to the surrounding interfacing tissues (e.g. see Spencer et al., 1983). *These tissues may well be dissected away during exposure of the nerve and hence give a false representation of the amount of movement available* (Beith et al., 1995). For example, Lombardi et al. (1984) have criticized the notion that the L5 nerve root slips in and out of the IVF during SLR since it is securely bound to the side of the body of S1.

There is ample evidence that upper limb nerve trunks slide and move. For instance, the ulnar nerve migrates proximally during elbow flexion (Macnicol, 1980), extension of the index finger has been shown to move the median nerve in the carpal tunnel 4 mm distally (LaBan *et al.*, 1989) and wrist and finger extension will pull the median nerve in the upper arm downwards by an average of 7.4 mm (McLellan and Swash, 1976). This last result was achieved on normals by inserting fine needles into their median nerves that protruded out of the skin! The excursion of the nerve was calculated by observing the amount of movement produced by the tip of the needle.

In summary, the nervous system is capable of quite remarkable adaptations in response to the body's movement and postural demands. Peripheral nerve roots and nerve trunks are being continuously squashed and stretched and in situations where there is relatively little room or where they are anatomically tethered they are vulnerable to adverse forces and pathological tissue encroachment.

The Effect of Movement on the Neuraxis

EVIDENCE FOR DYNAMIC EFFECTS DUE TO SPINAL MOVEMENT

The neuraxis is housed in the spinal canal and cranium. Since the spinal canal increases in length by 5–9 cm from full extension to full flexion (Breig, 1978; Louis, 1981; Inman and Saunders, 1942) there are quite marked physical effects on

Figure 4.14   Normal deformation of the dura, cord and nerve roots in the cervical canal in the cadaver due to full extension (left) and flexion (right) of the cervical spine. A total laminectomy has been performed and the dura opened and retracted although still able to transmit tension. In cervical extension, the nervous system is slack, the root sleeves have lost contact with the pedicles (lower arrows) and the nerve roots with the inner surfaces of the dural sleeves (upper arrows). In flexion, the nervous system including the dura mater has been stretched and moved in relation to surrounding structures. Note change in shape of the blood vessels. (From Breig, A, 1978, *Adverse Mechanical Tension in the Central Nervous System.* Almqvist and Wiksell, Stockholm, with permission.)

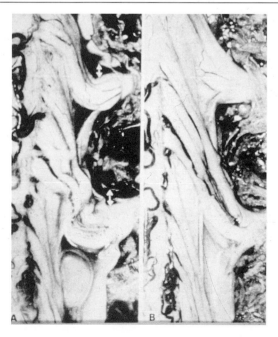

the connective tissue sheaths and the cord and brain structures themselves. Most lengthening occurs in the most mobile cervical and lumbar regions (28 mm each) and least in the thoracic region (3 mm) (Louis, 1981). The dynamic adaptations of the cervical cord and roots can be seen in the dissection photograph (Figure 4.14). Figure 4.15 illustrates the effects of flexion–extension on the brainstem. Further examples include:

- Neck flexion causing the floor of the fourth ventricle to elongate;
- The thoracic cord decreasing its diameter during spinal flexion (Breig, 1978);
- The folding and straightening of individual neurones in the dorsal column tracts of the cord during flexion and extension (Breig, 1978; Butler, 1991). This emphasizes the need for physical adaptations to movement right down to the cellular level.

- During spinal flexion the key considerations are that the whole neuraxis contained in the spinal canal tends to move anteriorly, elongate along its entire length and slide relative to the canal interface (see Shacklock *et al.*, 1994).

MOVEMENTS OF NEURAXIS RELATIVE TO THE SPINAL CANAL

Butler (1991) first brought more widespread attention to the fact that movements of the neuraxis *relative to the surrounding tissues* was not at all uniform and not necessarily in directions one would expect. For instance, during flexion of the monkey spine the dura at the level of L4 moves 3 mm caudally yet at L5 it moves 3 mm rostrally. In the neck the dura at C5 tends to move caudally and at C6–7 rostrally. In the thoracic region the dura above and below T6 tends to move away from it (Louis, 1981).

Figure 4.15   The remarkable movement of the brain stem in extension (a) and flexion (b) is illustrated by reference to the markers. Marked changes in tension of the eleventh cranial nerve (spinal accessory) can also be seen anterior to the cord/brainstem as it passes up from its origins on the cord to exit through the jugular foramen on the upper right of the picture. (From Breig, A, 1978, *Adverse Mechanical Tension in the Central Nervous System*. Almqvist and Wiksell, Stockholm, with permission.)

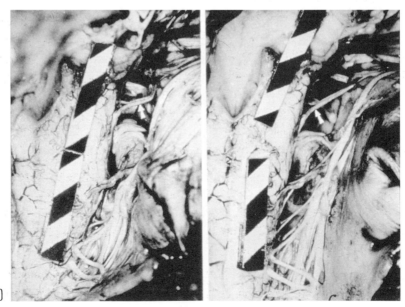

(a) (b)

Effects on Nerve Roots

These relative movements will have repercussions for the tension and angulation of the nerve roots as they leave the dura and as they exit in the IVF. For example, in flexion, nerve roots above L4 will tend to be angled more horizontally and those below more vertically. Further, any deviations from such 'normal' movement adaptations, due to for instance abnormal tethering following injury, may have serious mechanical overload repercussions at local and distant sites which may already be somewhat vulnerable. These thoughts have been used to hypothesize why symptoms often spread or jump to remote sites (Butler, 1991). For example, it is not uncommon for pain from whiplash injuries to appear in the midthoracic and lumbar regions long after the event.

EFFECTS OF SPINAL EXTENSION

- During spinal extension the whole canal shortens causing the neuraxis to slacken and increase in cross-sectional area. Observable folds can be seen in the cervical dural sac in extension.
- In the lumbar spine in particular, the spinal canal gets smaller in diameter in extension due to the posterior bulging of the discs and the forward bulging of the interflaval fat pad and the ligamentum flavum. This effect increases greatly in the presence of degenerative encroachment (Penning, 1992; Penning and Wilmink, 1981).
- This may be a reason why lumbar extension causes an increase in lumbar cerebrospinal fluid pressure (Hanai et al., 1985).

Zones of the spinal canal where there is relatively little space, like C5 compared to Cl or C2 (Figure 4.16), may be significantly more vulnerable to:

1 Pathological encroachment;
2 The addition of movements into extension.

Figure 4.16 The changing spaces available for the neuraxis and meninges in the cervical spinal canal at Cl(A), C2(B), C3(C) and C5(D). LF, ligamentum flavum; UJ, uncovertebral joint. (Reproduced from Parke, WW, 1988, *Spine* 13: 831–837, with permission. Lippincott Raven Publishers, Philadelphia.)

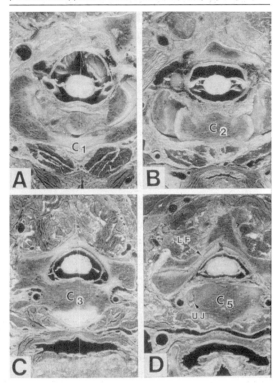

Think how common it is for the elderly degenerate spine to become relatively flexed. One way of viewing this is to see it as an adaptive process that helps maintain the least possible pressure on the threatened neuraxis and its peripheral roots and trunks.

SIDE FLEXION AND GRAVITY

Side flexion of the spine tends to produce slackening on the concave side and tightening on the convex side, and gravity displaces the spinal canal structures downwards (see Breig, 1978; Shacklock et al., 1994).

When interpreting symptom responses it is wise to consider the relative flexion / extension position of the spine as well as compression effects in the canal and IVF. It is apparent that it is not easy to find a position where there isn't some degree of mechanical impact on any one part of the nervous system. Knowledge of neurodynamic influences does help rationalize the difficulties patients have in finding relief when confronted by neurogenic pain.

Design Features and Nervous System Dynamics

Since it seems well established that movement of the nervous system occurs it is pertinent to highlight a few anatomical features that add weight to the notion of it having this dynamic capacity.

Neurones, Fascicles and Plexi

- Neurones, the individual nerve fibres, tend to run an undulatory course within the fascicles of peripheral nerves and within the tracts of the spinal cord (Breig, 1978).
- If a nerve fibre is stretched the myelin sheath lamellae slide on each other and little clefts (incisures of Schmidt–Lantermann) in the myelin part to accommodate the increased stress (Friede and Samorajski, 1969).
- The fascicles that contain the nerve fibres are capable of sliding within their epineurial sheaths

Figure 4.17   The fascicular branching in the musculocutaneous nerve. (Redrawn, with permission, from Sunderland, S, 1978, *Nerves and Nerve Injuries*. Churchill Livingstone, Edinburgh.)

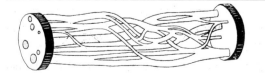

Figure 4.18   The brachial plexus as a force distributor. Tension on one trunk will be distributed throughout the whole plexus. (From Butler, DS, 1991, *Mobilisation of the Nervous System*, Churchill Livingstone, Melbourne, with permission.)

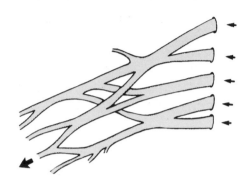

as well as following an undulating and branching course (Figure 4.17) that appears geared to a function of load dispersal.
- The reason for the complex branching of the various peripheral nerve plexi may relate to load dispersal (Figure 4.18) (Butler, 1991).

Connective Tissue

The peripheral and central nervous system contains connective tissue with viscoelastic properties, similar to ligaments and tendons (Bora *et al.*, 1980; Kwan *et al.*, 1992; Sunderland and Bradley 1961a,b). These tissues serve to allow and control nerve trunk motion in parallel with a protective role when forces reach physiological limits. It appears that in regions where the nervous system is more vulnerable to injury there is a higher density of connective tissue.

Clinical Example

The size of the superficial peroneal nerve over the top of the foot (Figure 4.6) is quite remarkable when one considers that it has only a relatively small dermal innervation field to reach that is very close by. Its size here has to be considered in terms of its obvious vulnerability to injury and therefore its need for a relatively large connective tissue protection component.

Other examples are the sciatic nerve at the buttock where it gets compressed in sitting. Here it contains in the region of 80% connective tissue (Sunderland, 1978). The peroneal nerve at the head of the fibula contains 17% more connective tissue than the same nerve a few centimetres proximally in the relatively sheltered area of the popliteal fossa (Sunderland and Bradley, 1949). Sunderland (1978) also demonstrated how the number of fascicles in vulnerable areas tends to increase in parallel with the increase in connective tissue, yet another mechanism thought to afford better protection to the nerve fibres from adverse compression.

Inside the spinal canal attention is focused on the tough dura mater connective tissue covering. This structure is particularly strong and well designed to cope with longitudinal forces (see Butler, 1991 and Shacklock *et al.*, 1994 for good overviews of the neuraxis connective tissues).

Blood Supply

There are many dynamic design features in the nervous system. It is designed to elongate and recoil and it is designed to cope with intermittent compression and distortion. During all this it must still continue to conduct and connect physiologically to its target organs and tissues — a condition only possible if adequate blood supply is provided. Although only accounting for 2% of the body mass the nervous system requires 20% of the available oxygen (Domisse, 1994).

Maintaining an adequate blood supply, whatever the posture or movement, is imperative for the metabolic demands of normal neural function. It is hardly surprising therefore that the blood vessels appear relatively slack and coiled, follow meandering courses along and within nerves, and enter the domain of the nervous system in zones where the system is relatively fixed in relationship to its adjacent structures (see Breig, 1978; Lundborg, 1988; Parke and Watanabe, 1985). For example, major feeder vessels enter the cervical cord between C5 and C7 — a region that does move in relation to the interface, but relatively little, due to the fixation effect of the brachial plexus and the strong tethering of these lower cervical nerve roots to the gutters on the transverse processes just distal to the IVF (Sunderland, 1974; Butler, 1991). Even though there is good design for continuous adequate blood supply, no matter what the posture or position, there are still plenty of opportunities that lead to its compromise (see below).

The Normal Nervous System as a Sensitive Tissue

Generally, tissues that are most likely to be exposed to extreme physical stress are likely to have a good sensory innervation — compare the mechanical sensitivity of the contents of the gut to the sensitivity of the skin or the musculoskeletal system for instance. Further, any tissue that is weakened or vulnerable following injury requires a greatly enhanced sensory mechanism to help protect it from further damage and to promote appropriate behaviour for it to recover (see Chapter 5). Coupled with a good sensory relay is a good reflex system, and in many higher

Louis Gifford

vertebrates, an active consciousness that provides the background for appropriate adaptive action/behaviour.

The normal nervous system copes with physiological movements in a remarkably silent way; however, extreme ranges of movement and direct forces often endanger neural tissue. The nervous system has the means to respond via its own sensory system. Just as the heart has its own blood supply so the nervous system has its own nerve supply. The innervation is specifically to the protective connective tissues of the peripheral and central nervous systems (see Butler, 1991, Shacklock et al., 1994, for good overviews).

It is well known that brain tissue itself is mechanically insensitive and that normal peripheral nerve fibres will only modestly respond to intense physical probing (Melzack and Wall, 1996). In fact there are many who report that peripheral nerve trunks are more or less insensitive to mechanical pressure and manipulation (e.g. Kuslich et al., 1991; Howe et al., 1977). However, anyone who has spent time learning to palpate peripheral nerves will know that some nerves are far more sensitive than others and that where any one nerve is sensitive depends on its anatomical site (Butler and Gifford, 1998). For example, a vulnerable nerve like the superficial peroneal on the foot (Figure 4.6), is pretty insensitive – you have to tap it or 'twang' it vigorously to get a modest tingling in its distal innervation field. Compare that to palpating the ulnar nerve at the elbow or the tibial nerve just behind the medial malleolus; in both cases gentle palpatory pressure reveals a rather sickening 'nervy' discomfort.

The important practical point is that peripheral nerves are variably sensitive – depending on the anatomic site and depending on the individual. Some people's nerves have great sensitivity over others.

Sensitivity to Stretch/Elongation

We should also consider sensitivity to stretch/elongation. Again there is great variability in sensitivity and some people have far more slack in their nervous systems than others.

Practical Task

Try this: place your arm down by your side, extend your elbow hard and keep it extended hard, extend your wrist with your fingers as straight as you can. Now depress your shoulder slowly and focus on what you feel in your hand and arm. Many of you will get a deep generalized ache vaguely in the elbow/forearm region plus or minus feelings of pulling and paraesthesia in the hand. Adding neck side flexion away normally increases the response still further, but go carefully. Those who have good mobility of their joints often have extreme mobility of their nervous systems and may get very little with a manoeuvre like this; others will easily get many of the symptoms described and more. Note that since the symptoms can be changed in the forearm/hand with scapular depression and neck movement, the assumption is that neural tissue is responsible (see Chapter 6). It is argued that fascia and vasculature that also traverse these regions are unlikely to produce such 'nervy' sensations as deep diffuse ache and paraesthesia in such a clearcut way.

Type of Sensitivity

There are two significant issues with regards to sensitivity:

1 Mechanical sensitivity;
2 Sensitivity to ischaemia.

Mechanical sensitivity
This exists through

- Mechanical stimulation of mechanically sensitive *nerve endings* in the protective connective tissue layers of the nerve;
- Mechanical sensitivity of the *nerve fibres* (neurones) themselves.

Nerve fibre axons are generally considered to be designed to convey impulses not generate them – nerve impulses traditionally originate from the ends of nerves that reside in target tissues, not mid-axon somewhere. Impulses that do originate mid-axon are said to be 'ectopic' (see Chapter 5) and if derived from afferent fibres may cause the generation of odd sensations – hence pins and needles are commonly felt when nerve trunks that supply cutaneous sensation are firmly tapped.

Sensitivity to ischaemia or to blood loss, i.e. 'Ischaemosensitivity' (Butler and Gifford, 1998). Falling asleep with your arms above your head and later waking up with a numb and tingling arm that does not respond to demands for movement is an extreme example that is not uncommon. Holding continuous pressure on the anterior wrist over the carpal tunnel produces a slowly building paraesthesia in many otherwise asymptomatic subjects. The fact that symptoms are not immediate suggests loss of blood supply to the underlying median nerve as a likely mechanism. Some people are more susceptible than others and they often find constant end-range positions in bed (wrist flexion for example) or

during the day (crossed leg sitting) a common source of irritation by way of numbness and pins and needles type sensations.

When individual nerve fibres are deprived of circulation their function is impaired and many of the large metabolically demanding Aβ sensory fibres begin to fire ectopically – hence pins and needles if they innervate skin. Ectopically firing sensory fibres (due to mechanical force or loss of blood) that innervate deeper tissues, like muscle, may produce incongruent sensations that relate to their innervated tissues. Thus persistent pressure over the radial nerve in the radial groove may produce deep aching sensations vaguely in the forearm muscles as well as paraesthesia in the skin over the back of the lateral hand. These areas relate to the muscles and skin innervated by the radial nerve.

Although not proven, it seems that nerve trunk mechanosensitivity in the normal physiological state depends firstly on vulnerability and secondly on design that includes connective tissue density as well as specialized local innervation characteristics, and the senstivity of the contained nerve fibres themselves (Lundborg, 1988). Thus, many nerves are in extremely vulnerable places near the surface of the skin, like the many little geniculate nerves on the side of the knee, the superficial peroneal nerve on top of the foot and the radial nerve in the radial groove on the lateral aspect of the humerus. These nerves seem particularly insensitive to palpation and are probably hugely adapted to cope by consisting of large quantities of protective connective tissue (Sunderland, 1978). By contrast, some superficially placed nerve trunks are remarkably mechanosensitive (Butler, 1991), the ulnar nerve at the elbow, the median nerve in the axilla and just distally, and the proximal cords of the brachial plexus in the supra clavicular fossa are examples. It appears that these nerves are less well endowed with connective tissue, have relatively exposed nerve fibres and are hence more sensitive (Butler, 1991). To a degree, these areas are situated in regions less likely to be directly injured in the rough and tumble of daily life. Deeper nerves often reside in zones prone to pressure changes with normal movements and postures, and seem to cope in a remarkably restrained and silent way. For example, nerve roots in the intervertebral foramen and the median nerve in the carpal tunnel get squashed and stretched all the time yet we are totally unaware of it unless pathological changes cause them to become acutely ischaemosensitive or mechano-sensitive.

Physiological Effects of Movement on Nervous Tissue

The Importance of Blood

The importance of an uninterrupted blood supply to the nervous system has already been discussed. Like all other cells, neurones require blood for their metabolic demands, but in particular for powering axoplasmic transport and impulse generation and conduction (Lundborg and Dahlin, 1996; Lundborg, 1988). Loss of conduction due to ischaemia is most notable by the appearance of paraesthesia, numbness and weakness as when you fall asleep with your arms above your head.

AXOPLASMIC FLOW OR TRANSPORT

Many neurones in the peripheral nervous system are unique in that they are extemely long cells, for example an individual nerve cell from the foot to the spinal cord may be 1 metre long. To put this in perspective, consider if this neurone's cell body was increased in size to 100 cm in diameter, it would have an axon diameter of 10 cm and a length of around 10 kilometres (Rydevik et al., 1984).

The viability of any cell is largely dependent on the activities of the nucleus and cell body and its ability to communicate with the rest of the cellular constituents.

In neurones the specialized flow of cytoplasm from the cell body to its distant peripheral sites and back is termed axoplasmic flow. This flow of neurochemicals and cellular structural components within the axoplasm is essential not only for the health and functioning of the cell itself, but also for the health of the tissues that the cell innervates. The nonmyelinated afferent C fibres are now thought to have a particularly important role to play in the maintenance of their target tissues' health and in aiding any healing process via a direct chemical contribution to the inflammatory cascade (see Chapter 5). Importantly, neurones are not just designated to an impulse-conducting role, many also have the ability to chemically sample the tissues they innervate and relay these chemicals as a type of 'messenger' back to their nucleus and cell bodies (Donnerer et al., 1992). The nucelus/cell body then alters its activity to produce a specific chemical response that is transported back to the target tissues in order to rebalance the trophic disturbance that was detected earlier (Donnerer et al., 1992; Heller et al., 1994; McMahon and Koltzenburg, 1994). In this way the nerve cell is constantly monitoring the health of its target tissues, responding to any abnormality and as a result helping to maintain tissue viability. The implications of this are that anything that disturbs the bidirectional axoplasmic flow between cell body and the axon and its terminals will have repercussions for the health of the nerve cell itself as well as the target tissues it supplies. If the loss of communication is severe enough the distal axon undergoes Wallerian degeneration or the whole cell may even die (Devor, 1994).

POSTURE AND MOVEMENT EFFECTS ON CIRCULATION TO NERVE

Axoplasmic flow is particularly sensitive to changes in circulation (Okabe and Hirokawa, 1989), and circulation to and within nerve tissues is influenced by changes in pressure produced by postures and movements of the interfacing tissues.

Circulation to a nerve, like any other tissue, is dependent on a pressure gradient existing between the incoming arterial supply and the outgoing venous return (Sunderland, 1978). Thus a greater pressure is required at the arterial side in order to push blood flow through the nerve and out into the veins. Further, any changes in pressure around the veins or nerve will upset this gradient and will cause back-pressures that lead to vascular stasis and ischaemia / hypoxia.

Pressure changes that influence circulation to nerve can be brought about by relative compression or elongation of nerve tissue. The influences of pressure changes produced by wrist flexion on the contents of the carpal tunnel have already been noted. Olmarker's group (Olmarker *et al.*, 1989) have found that pressures as low as 5–10 mmHg can stop venular blood flow in the lumbar nerve roots of pigs, pressures probably easily achieved at the IVF and radicular canal due to compression during normal extension or perhaps even during prolonged standing.

When *elongation* forces are applied to a peripheral nerve the supply vessels tend to straighten up and narrow; the intraneural vessels similarly unfold, stretch and reduce their lumens, and the intraneural pressure steadily increases the more the nerve is stretched (Pechan and Julis, 1975). In the rabbit peripheral nerve, venous return starts to decline at 8% elongation and by 15%, arterial, capillary and venous flow is completely occluded. If we consider that the length of the nerve bed of the median nerve can increase by as much as 20% in full arm, hand and finger extension, it is not surprising that many of us get building ischaemia-related neural responses when maintaining these positions.

> ### Key Points
>
> - *It is important to understand that the nervous system is designed to accommodate to continuous pressurizing and stretching forces and that recovery after short-term modest loading is normal.*
> - *What the nervous system does seem to find unacceptable is ongoing adverse physical stress – it far prefers movement. Long-term increased pressures and stretching that many of our relatively static lives foist upon the nervous system may well be quietly damaging it more than it otherwise should be.*
> - *Pechan and Julis (1975) showed that mere elbow flexion doubles the pressure in the ulnar nerve when compared to elbow extension.*
> - *Dahlin and McLean (1986) showed that modest prolonged pressures on rabbit vagus nerves will completely block axoplasmic flow and that its return to normal may take anything from 24 hours to 1 week depending on the amount and time of pressure.*

- *Axoplasm tends to increase its viscosity if nerves are not moved (Baker et al., 1977); it thus gets thicker, less fluid and its flow properties will be compromised at the expense of the health of the nerve and its target tissues. By contrast movement will enhance its flow properties and hence nerve and tissue health.*

Many of the features discussed may also be pertinent to the neuraxis. For example, the longitudinal stress imparted during spinal flexion may increase the pressure within the cord since it decreases its diameter in flexion (Breig, 1978). Longitudinal vessels may be narrowed (Figure 4.14) and movements of the limbs may influence feeder vessel lumens by directly or indirectly pulling or angulating them. Adequate cerebrospinal fluid circulation in the subarachnoid space of the cord and brain is maintained by movement and since much nutritional delivery is via this route it underlines yet again the importance of regular movement for adequate neural health and function.

The student is reminded that far more can be achieved in tissue physiological terms by the patient performing simple uncomplicated active movements than can be achieved by purely passive techniques.

Pathophysiology of Nerve and its Influence on Movement: 'Neural Pathodynamics'

Pathodynamics: Integrating Pathomechanics and Pathophysiology

So far the emphasis has been on the influence and interaction of mechanical forces on the physiology of the nervous system. Shacklock's (1995) timely introduction of the term 'neurodynamics' has helped focus attention away from pure mechanics (Butler and Gifford, 1989) and towards a perspective that powerfully includes the inseparable influences of mechanics and physiology on each other. Further, in order to emphasize thoughts of pathophysiology and pathomechanics when injury or disease occurs Shacklock has introduced the term 'neural pathodynamics' (Shacklock, 1995).

Many pain states that physiotherapists encounter are the result of some mechanical event which varies from the extreme of sudden insult to more minor sustained and prolonged adverse pressures or tensions of some kind. Adverse mechanical events lead to burgeoning pathophysiological responses, typically inflammation, healing and repair plus or minus a pain state, which taken as a whole, is the body's means of restoring function. That full or perfect repair in many of the more complex and metabolically sluggish tissues of the body can be achieved has to be questioned since most adult musculoskeletal tissues repair by scar tissue formation not regeneration (Butler and Gifford, 1998). Thus, it is to be expected that as a result of physiological reparative processes (pathophysiology / pathobiology), some mechanical dysfunction (pathomechanics) will inevitably occur during the later stages of healing and much may well remain permanently. Inevitably this means that tissues in the functional proximity of a given lesion will have to adapt accordingly and may well predispose the individual to further problems later on. It has to be assumed that if a repaired tissue is mechanically compromised it will also be physiologically compromised in some way too. For example, a tissue that remains scarred after healing may have a less than perfect vasculature and this could have futher negative consequences. In considering pain states local adverse physiology must be interpreted in terms of continued effects on the firing and sensitivity of sensory nerve endings in the neural connective tissues and on any local damaged nerve fibres.

Pain Mechanisms Relating to Injury of Nervous Tissue

The nervous system is a special tissue in that it must be considered as having two distinctly separate mechanisms that cause pain when it is physically injured (see Chapter 5 for review of mechanisms):

1 A nociceptive mechanism, which is due to injury and / or stimulation of the sensory endings of nerve fibres in its connective tissues; for example, injured and inflamed dura, in the spinal canal, or perineurium in a peripheral nerve trunk.
2 A neurogenic mechanism, which is due to injury and alteration of sensitivity of the conducting fibres themselves. *'Peripheral neurogenic mechanisms'* consider abnormal responsivity of peripheral neurones, and *'central neurogenic mechanisms'* consider lesions in the central nervous system as well as abnormalities of information processing (see Chapter 5 for expanded discussion) (Devor, 1996).

Clinically, the fact that several different mechanisms of pain production can operate when the nervous system is injured may in part account for the very complex pain patterns, pain qualities and pain behaviour that is so often seen.

Injuring Forces

Peripheral nerve trunks and roots can be injured and hence become pain sensitive as a result of direct mechanical force or as a result of alterations in pressure around the nerve. The key to understanding the influences of alterations in pressure (vascular factors) and direct mechanical injury really revolves around a consideration of length of time of the forces involved. As a generalization, sudden high forces cannot be tolerated well by the nervous system and, like any other tissue, lead to injury, inflammation, healing and repair plus or minus a pain state. More sustained forces can be tolerated surprisingly well, especially if the load is dispersed over a wide area. Long-term focal increases in pressure may not be tolerated without some expense. Alteration of normal circulation by pressure change may lead to degenerative changes in nerve tissue *without* necessarily any inflammation (Olmarker *et al.*, 1995) and more importantly *without* necessarily any pain. This is a rather 'occult' form of pathophysiology that is probably quietly accumulating in all of us as we progress through life.

SUDDEN MECHANICAL FORCE

Sudden mechanical force considers adverse stretching / compression of nerve, for example:

- Sudden twisting of an ankle which may injure the superficial peroneal nerve over the ankle (Nitz et al., 1985) or as far proximally as the lower part of the thigh (Nobel, 1966);
- Any sudden direct physical force on nerve, for example an injury to the radial nerve following a fracture dislocation of the radial head;
- A whiplash involves huge forces that may well rip and squash many major or minor nerve trunks and plexi (Jeffreys, 1980), as well as the cord (McMillan and Silver, 1987) and brain (La Rocca, 1978).

ONGOING MECHANICAL FORCE

As already discussed, ongoing mechanical forces result in the disruption of the subtle pressure gradient required to maintain adequate vascular supply to nerves. The spectrum of physical factors that can influence supply range from normal postural forces and ongoing inactivity to pathological intrusions such as disc protrusions, osteophytes, thickened ligamentous, muscular and tendinous tissues, scar tissue, oedema and inflammatory exudate and haematoma (Butler, 1991; Butler and Gifford, 1998).

Local pressure changes affecting the immediate nerve may not be the sole influencing factors. Thus, consideration of vascular 'control systems' focuses attention on sympathetic tone to supply vessels — if tone is increased the tissues in the supply field will suffer. There is also the possibility of pathologies in more remote regions adversely influencing the supply of blood to the area. This could range from heart disease (LaBan and Wesolowski, 1988) to localized adverse pressures on supply vessels due to for instance sustained postures, tight muscles, scar tissue, tumours or simple swelling.

The Repercussions of Neural Ischaemia

Loss of blood to a nerve results in local hypoxic or ischaemic conditions (Figure 4.19). This in itself may cause nerve fibres to start to fire ectopically and produce abnormal sensations that include paraesthesias, numbness and pain depending on the type of fibre affected and the central nervous system processing of the abnormal impulse discharges that are generated. Continuing hypoxia leads to plasma leakage from the endothelial walls of capillaries within the nerve itself (Lundborg, 1988; Lundborg and Dahlin, 1996). This intraneural oedema formation leads to a further increase in pressure within the nerve that adds to the problems of inadequate circulation. The nerve may even swell proximally or distally. The end result, originally proposed by Sunderland (1976), is that this protein-rich oedema promotes the formation of fibrosis both around the fascicles and within them. This must have detrimental affects on the normal mechanics and physiology of the connective tissue as well as on the health of the nerve fibres themselves.

It is easy to see how local loss of circulation can lead to dysfunction and damage to nerve fibres and even to their death (Jayson, 1992). Rather puzzlingly, this may or may not lead to a pain state. Examination of lumbar nerve roots post mortem often reveals quite severe nerve fibre damage and fibrosis yet the patients' medical records make no mention of back-related pain problems (Hoyland et al., 1989). On the other hand, conditions like those describe must surely be adequate to produce or predispose to a neurogenic pain state. Ultimately, or at least from a purely tissue-based perspective, it depends on whether the physiological changes are enough to sensitize and fire

Figure 4.19 Pathobiological effects of compression on nerve.

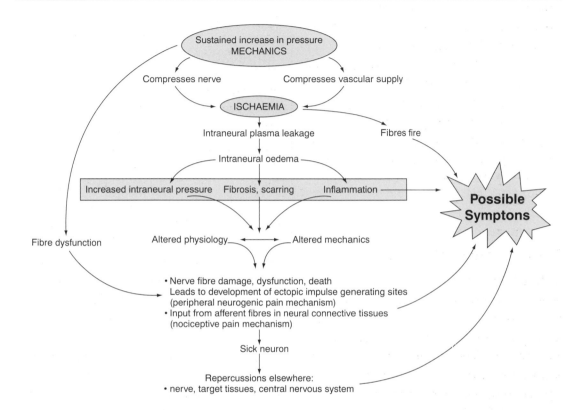

nociceptors or create ectopic impulse generating sites in damaged nerve fibres (Hasue, 1993). The other perspective to consider is that many of us may actually have many nociceptors and ectopic impulse-generating sites firing, but our CNS chooses to pay no attention to the activity.

The Importance of Inflammation

Inflammation, or at least the presence of irritative chemicals, may be a vital determinant as to whether or not a neuropathy is painful. There may be a marked difference in the chemical environment of a nerve that is being slowly compressed by developing degenerative invasion and one where inflammation has occurred due to a

more acute injury or where local interfacing tissue has been damaged and becomes inflamed.

Disc disruption is a powerful example of the many diverse influences on a nerve tissue.

- Any disc protrusion *may mechanically* damage the adjacent nerve root – compression of the dorsal root ganglion is likely to be immediately symptomatic since it is normallly mechanosensitive. Neural connective tissue may be damaged (perineurium, dura) which leads to an inflammatory response in this tissue and more than likely a pain state.
- The protrusion, even without contacting the nerve root tissue, may increase the pressure around the nerve and cause an increase in venous pressure. This may be sufficient to

produce ischaemic conditions both around and within the nerve — a situation that has the potential to lead to inflammation within the nerve (Hoyland *et al.*, 1989), or more likely to oedema and fibrosis in and around the nerve as described above (Cooper *et al.*, 1995).

- The disc injury itself may precipitate inflammation in the immediate environment of the nerve. Leakage of nuclear fluid is thought to create an inflammatory response (McCarron *et al.*, 1987; Saal, 1995), and chemicals so produced may get rapidly transported into the local nerve (Byrod *et al.*, 1995) and thus produce an intraneural pain-generating environment (Olmarker *et al.*, 1993, 1994).
- As a result of possibly profound intraneural physiological changes, nerve fibres become damaged and develop abnormal ectopic impulse generating sites that can be responsible for ongoing and often very disturbing pain states (see Hasue, 1993, for useful summary).

In summary,

- Acute disc injury has many potential repercussions when creating a pain state — from nociceptive mechanisms in damaged tissues of the disc and adjacent tissue, to peripheral neurogenic mechanisms as a result of direct or indirect nerve root irritation and damage (see Chapter 5). The mechanisms are complex and may develop over time which warns clinicians to progress cautiously with very early management of low back disorders.
- Physiotherapists should be aware that disc injury related pain and therapy is more complex than discs mechanically 'going out' and being 'put back'. Appreciation of the complexity and timing of the recovery process and the conditions that enhance the natural resolution arguably promote a rehabilitative physiotherapy approach coupled with a more rational use of the best that modern medicine can offer.

Implications of Peripheral Nerve Pathophysiology

The wider implications of any nerve injury seem quite daunting (Figure 4.19):

- Impulse barrages from ectopic impulse generating sites are potent modulators of central nervous system sensitivity (Chapter 5).
- Damage in one area of a nerve has been shown to influence the sensitivity and health of distal or proximal areas on the involved and related nerve trunks (Mackinnon, 1992). Thus healthy neurones effectively become 'sick neurones' and their seemingly malevolent influences can spread.
- Loss of, or poor communication, between the neurone nucleus and its target tissues may have dire consequences for target tissue health (see above).

Nerve contraction, loss of elasticity or any tethering as a result of pathophysiological processes may have far-reaching adverse mechanical influences on related tissues. For example, it is easy to visualize how a tethered, fibrous and inelastic segment of a peripheral nerve trunk would put more strain on its proximal and distal segments during movements that stretched it. Adverse mechanical tension in one area may thus lead to pathophysiological processes with the potential to become the source of symptoms at distant sites (Breig, 1978; Butler and Gifford, 1989, 1998; Butler, 1991). Thus, it is not uncommon to find that following a single neuropathy other pain states later crop up in 'neurally' related areas. For instance, carpal tunnel syndrome has been strongly related to nerve injury in the neck.

- Upton and McComas (1973) found approximately 80% of patients with carpal tunnel syndrome or lesions of the ulnar nerve at the elbow had neural lesions in the neck. These authors termed the phenomenon 'double crush' syndrome, i.e. where a proximal nerve compression predisposes a nerve to pathology distally.
- The literature also describes reversed double crush (Lundborg, 1988) and multiple crush syndromes (Mackinnon, 1992) that really highlight how the health of a whole nerve can be affected by modest forces that start in one area. Spreading of symptoms and signs is very common in chronic pain development.

Mechanical injury and changes in pressures and circulation to the spinal cord, brain and its lining connective tissues are less easy to study (Butler, 1991) than the peripheral nervous system. There is no reason not to assume that issues similar to those that influence peripheral nerves could operate in the CNS (see Butler, 1991; Butler and Gifford, 1998).

From Theory to Practice: Neural Sensitivity

Pathological Mechanosensitivity

Clinically, mechanosensitivity can be seen as an immediate symptom response that bears a direct relationship with a physical force. Nerves can be influenced mechanically by any movement, static muscular contractions, even the pulsating of arteries if extremely sensitive (Butler, 1991; Butler and Gifford, 1998).

It may make clinical analysis easier to think in terms of movements that mechanically stretch nerves — as in the neural tension or 'neurody-namic' tests (Shacklock, 1995), and those which compress nerves — as in the closing of the intervertebral foramina in spinal extension or ipsilateral rotation/side-flexion movements, or the compression of the median nerve in the carpal tunnel by wrist flexion or extension.

Butler (1996) has used the terms:

- 'Container dependent' for symptoms evoked by compressive effects;
- 'Neural dependent' for symptoms evoked by neural elongation/neurodynamic tests like the slump, SLR and ULTT (see Chapter 6).

Analysis of symptom-provocative postures and movements with these thoughts in mind is often very useful.

The frequent straightforward link between a performed movement or posture and symptom reproduction are often complicated by the fact that impulse discharges from ectopic impulse generators in mechanosensitive segments of nerve respond in a great variety of ways (Devor, 1994; Butler and Gifford, 1998). For example:

- You do a test, it hurts for a couple of seconds and then disappears, you repeat the test and nothing happens. Five minutes later you repeat the test and it responds again, and so on.
- A test may produce a fleeting symptom immediately tension or compression is applied and then again when the force is removed, there being no response when the force is maintained.
- A test may produce a response in parallel with the force applied but continue long after the test force is removed.

Odd and clinically frustrating reactivity like this makes one suspect a peripheral neurogenic pain mechanism (see Chapter 5).

Pathological Ischaemosensitivity

Further evidence of sensitivity is found when a delay and then a slow build-up and spread of symptoms is produced. This may be an indicator that the nerve is more ischaemosensitive than mechanosensitive, especially when the test performed could well be adversely influencing the pressure in the nerve or the circulation to it (Butler and Gifford, 1998).

- A classic example is an acute or subacute cervical or lumbar nerve root problem where sustained rotation towards the side of pain is at first symptom free but then after a few seconds a slow build-up of discomfort occurs that frequently spreads down the arm/leg to produce distal paraesthesia.
- Carpal tunnel syndrome symptoms are often heightened by Phalen's test. Here, sustained wrist flexion slowly produces an increase and spread of symptoms.

Further Considerations

Many peripheral nerve problems are far from predictable, are ongoing in nature or occur spontaneously often with agonizing ferocity that can be very worrying to the patient. There are many possible explanations that can be derived from current tissue pathophysiological knowledge. For example:

- A consideration of mechanisms that produce 'ectopic pacemaker' capability must be included (see Chapter 5).
- Ongoing normal or pathological pressures on sensitized nerve may be factors. Consider oedema, muscle tone, haematomas, or any pathology/defect/congenital defect that could occur adjacent to sensitized neural tissue

and that will put pressure on it or its vascular supply.

- Many ectopic impulse generating sites have increased sensitivity to circulating chemicals. Thus, anxiety and 'stress' may increase pain/symptoms since ectopic sites can become sensitive to adrenaline and noradrenaline released as a result of sympathetic nervous system activity (see Chapter 5 and Devor and Rappaport, 1990; Devor, 1994, 1996).

Neural mechanical sensitivity and ischaemosensitivity can be investigated by analysing pain quality and pain behaviour, pain response to normal movements, sustained movements and responses to tests that attempt to focus mechanical forces on neural tissues. These include tests that have a bias to elongation and tension (see Chapter 6) and to those that emphasize compression via joint movement or via direct 'palpatory' techniques (Butler and Slater, 1994; Butler and Gifford, 1998).

Restricted Range of Neurodynamic Tests – A Wise Stance?

Physiotherapists must consider the nervous system as capable of becoming a very mechanically sensitive system and rarely one that becomes so mechanically compromised that it is *physically* responsible for *major* losses of range of movement. It can be argued that in the majority of cases it limits range by producing pain/symptoms that then call a halt to movement via the active will of the patient and reflex protective muscular contraction in concert.

This now has support from current work reported by Elvey (1995) and Hall *et al.* (1995) that demonstrates increased muscle activity during straight leg raising in patients with sciatica.

They found that the electromyographic (EMG) activity of the hamstring muscle increases in parallel with the pain response felt by the patient.

The key point is that the nervous system, especially if it has become injured and hence sensitized, mobilizes adaptive motor protective mechanisms if it is physically challenged.

A blocked straight leg raise in a subject with chronic sciatica may be a point of argument for some, in that the block to movement can be seen as being due to tethered and noncompliant lumbosacral nerve roots, especially if sciatic pain is reproduced. The root may well be tethered and not moving as well as it once did, but can this tethering be responsible for as much as 30–40° of loss of SLR range?

Consider that:

- The amount of movement observed in fresh cadavers in the lumbar nerve roots is at best 10 mm (Goddard and Reid, 1965) (Figure 4.13), which is hardly enough to cause such a large loss of range.

It seems more likely that the nervous system may protect itself by:

- Becoming mechanically sensitive;
- Inducing powerful protective reflexes in the hamstrings/glutei when mechanically threatened;
- Later, more long-term protective processes may be added, e.g. adaptive physiological/mechanical changes in the hamstrings/glutei, the nerve root itself and other relevant tissues.

Thus, in the acute and subacute situation loss of range is related more to physiological processes and pain responses (sensitivity), and in the more chronic situation is related to both neural sensitivity and some mechanical compromise of multiple tissues that includes the nerve roots.

It is complex and often difficult to sort out clinically. The easiest way would be to place the patient under a general anaesthetic and observe the range devoid of any pain response or protective muscular activity. Although this is rarely feasible it does occasionally help to think when examining a patient, 'would this range be normal if there was no pain?' Ultimately, the nearest we can get to the answer comes from the highly skilled analysis of the 'end-feel', or the resistance felt during testing and the rate of improvement of range when attempts are made to mobilize it. However, Butler reports (1996) that he has had the opportunity to examine a few *apparently* mechanically 'blocked' straight leg raises under general anaesthetic and was surprised to find some quite normal in range and yet others that were indeed tight and blocked. Our thoughts must always be open.

The purpose of making these points about mechanical block and sensitivity is that there are great dangers in viewing disorders labelled as neural 'tension' solely in terms of mechanical compromise of the nerve, and that pushing hard into resistance at end of range is a necessary procedure to overcome a pain problem that presents with limited range of motion of a neruodynamic test.

Even if a nerve is mechanically compromised there are many inherent dangers in strongly mobilizing it since it is likely to be far more physically vulnerable and more easily resensitized than it was before injury.

Understanding Neurally Safe 'Stretching' or Mobilizing

It is possible to move into tissue resistance in 'neurally safe' ways.

Practical Task

Try this simple test observation on anyone who has difficulty reaching their ankles with straight knees in the standard forward-bending test and who has no symptom problems at all.

- *Perform a standard SLR test and ask carefully about their symptoms at a reasonably firm end-range position – the quality and distribution of the symptoms are important. In my experience there is commonly a deep diffuse aching sensation distributed anywhere from the back of the hip, back of thigh, back of knee into the calf and sometimes into the foot. Get the subject to focus on the symptoms and remember them so that they can be compared to the next test.*
- *On the same leg perform hip flexion to*
around 100°, add knee extension into modest resistance but do not allow it to go to full extension. If the knee does reach full extension take the hip into further hip flexion and add the knee extension again (see Figure 4.20).*
- *Keep the knee in exactly the same position while further flexing the hip and ask about the area and type of response in comparison to the first test. The classic response to this test is a well localized pulling sensation in the hamstring muscles – it 'feels' muscular.*

It seems that in the last position muscle tension and a muscle tension sensation come into play far earlier than neurally related tension and symptom response. The concept then is to use mobilization techniques that tend to produce more muscle tension feelings rather than neural ones.

Figure 20 Hip flexion test with knee short of full extension (see text for explanation). (Reproduced, with permission, from Butler and Gifford, 1998, *The Dynamic Nervous System*. NOI Press, Adelaide.)

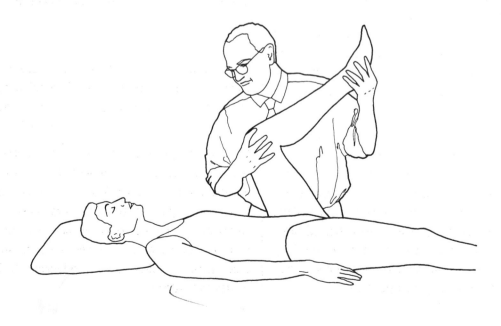

Practical Tips

It is quite often possible to mobilize a chronic or subacutely restricted SLR into resistance by going into flexion with hip abduction and external rotation and knee flexion as described above – the patient feels hamstring pulling, no discomforting neural symptoms and small progressive gains in range can be made. The patient can also perform home stretches utilizing similar components. For example, in sitting, symptomatic leg forward, heel on floor, foot in neutral, knee in 15–20° of flexion, hip in abduction and modest lateral rotation – perform gentle flexion movements from the back and hips.

In the SLR with the knee-flexed position described it is often possible to see the tibial division of the sciatic nerve standing out at the back of the popliteal fossa. It is certainly easy to palpate here even if it cannot be seen (Figure 4.21). The nerve in this position is very tight, and is a reasonable indication of quite marked dynamic changes along the length of the nerve that probably includes the nerve roots. However, in terms of symptom response, it seems that SLR with a fully extended knee is far more 'nerve provocative' than when the knee is flexed 15–20°.

Hopefully this illustrates one way of addressing resistance in a neurally safer way, i.e. perform the restricted movement into resistance so that a sensation of muscle stretch is produced (knee slightly flexed SLR) rather than one that produces strong neural symptoms (knee extended SLR). The essential element of safety is provided by focused symptom enquiry and analysis and cleverly adjusting starting positions.

Figure 4.21 The tibial and common peroneal nerve at the back of the knee are sometimes very visible in the position shown in Figure 4.20. The examiner's thumb is on the lateral aspect of the subject's right knee. The peroneal nerve lies medial to the biceps femoris tendon and the tibial nerve runs centrally into gastrocnemius. (Reproduced, with permission, from Butler and Gifford, 1998 *The Dynamic Nervous System*, NOI Press, Adelaide.)

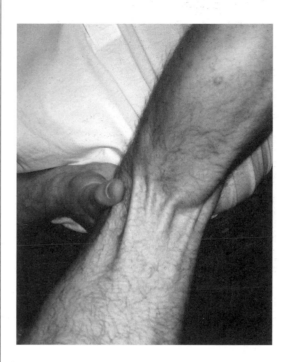

However, we should always be aware that symptoms reporting by consciousness is not always as accurate a reflection of what may be happening at tissue level as we would wish (see Chapter 5).

Restoring range of movement is an important tenet of physiotherapy that should be achieved in the safest possible way. Since it is argued here that in the majority of patients neural sensitivity issues are much more dominant than mechanical block to neural movement issues, it is suggested that physiotherapists use neurodynamic techniques and exercises:

1 With thoughts of promoting better physiology to help decrease sensitivity and restore range;

2 With thoughts of slowly stretching / elongating related musculature that may be reflexly more alert, or modestly mechanically shortened, due to the reasoning discussed above.

Final Comments

Butler and I published a paper in 1989 entitled 'The concept of adverse mechanical tension in the nervous system' (Butler and Gifford, 1989) which with hindsight viewed and addressed disorders of the nervous system in a predominantly mechanistic way — just as joints and muscles were examined at the time. Sensitivity of the nervous system was addressed by attempting to judge the irritability of the system as per Maitland (Maitland, 1986). This is no longer adequate. New biologically based knowledge now allows reasoned judgements to be made on the class of pain a patient may be suffering (see Chapter 5 and Butler and Gifford, 1998), and provides an understanding of the complex issues of sensitive neural tissues and their clinical correlates. For many patients, mobilizing neural tissue may well be as appropriate as mobilizing any tissue. However, under an expanded reasoning framework (see Chapters 5, 6 and Butler and Gifford, 1998) that pays due attention to the manual therapist's findings in relation to the pathobiological process involved in the patient, modern management now calls for better and gentler techniques, decisions on hands on or hands off, more patient self-management, empowering the patient with knowledge, and techniques and exercises done with the full understanding of the patient and therapist (see Chapter 15).

These are exciting times for physiotherapy. It is essential that clinicians take a forward step from the old mechanistic systems of manual therapy and integrate the pain-related sciences to provide a better and safer delivery of physiotherapy whose aims are to reduce pain, relieve suffering, restore range and enhance overall function.

Conclusions and Key Points

- The nervous system moves and this is reflected in many of its anatomical features.
- Movement of the nervous system is not at all simple. Over and above many fundamental gross movement features and principles there is great variability between one individual and the next.
- The nervous system is designed to cope with remarkable elongation and compression effects due to posture and movement. Sudden elongation or compression forces extend the nervous systems' safety adaptations to their limits and may easily cause injury. Long-term compression / elongation is detrimental too, but the system has time to adapt. Thus many pathological abnormalities are commonly found that *may* have no symptomatic sequelae.
- The nervous system has modest normal sensitivity in some areas, but if injured it can become the source of very disabling pain and hypersensitivity states.
- Treatment reasoning models based purely on mechanics of tissues without due respect for pathophysiology, enhanced sensitivity and a diagnostic framework that includes analysis of pain mechanisms, are arguably inadequate and incomplete.

FURTHER READING

Current texts

Butler, DS, Gifford, LS (1998) *The Dynamic Nervous System*. NOI Press, Adelaide.
Probably the most up-to-date in-depth examination of neurodynamics and pain relevant to clinical diagnosis and physiotherapy management.

Classic texts and chapters:

Breig, A (1978) *Adverse Mechanical Tension in the Central Nervous System*. Almqvist and Wiksell, Stockholm.
The classic pictorial atlas illustrating movement of the nervous system in freshly dissected cadavers.

Butler, DS (1991) *Mobilisation of the Nervous System*. Churchill Livingstone, Melbourne.

Butler, DS (1994) The upper limb tension test revisited, in Grant, R (ed) *Physical Therapy of the Cervical and Thoracic Spine. Clinics in Physical Therapy.* Churchill Livingstone, New York.

Butler, DS, Slater, H (1994) Neural injury in the thoracic spine. A conceptual basis to management, in Grant, R (ed) *Physical Therapy of the Cervical and Thoracic Spine*, 2nd edition. Churchill Livingstone, New York.

Shacklock, MO, Butler, DS, Slater, H (1994) The dynamic central nervous system: structure and clinical neurobiomechanics, in Boyling, JD, Palastanga, N (eds) *Grieve's Modern Manual Therapy*, 2nd edition, pp. 21–38. Churchill Livingstone, Edinburgh.

Classic papers

Butler, DS, Gifford, LS (1989) The concept of adverse mechanical tension in the nervous system. *Physiotherapy* 75: 622–636.

Elvey, RL (1986) Treatment of arm pain associated with abnormal brachial plexus tension. *Australian Journal of Physiotherapy* 32: 224–229.

Maitland, GD (1979) Negative disc exploration: positive canal signs. *Australian Journal of Physiotherapy* 25: 129–134.

Shacklock, M (1995) Neurodynamics. *Physiotherapy* 81: 9–16.

Troup, JDG (1986) Biomechanics of the lumbar spinal canal. *Clinical Biomechanics* 1: 31–43.

REFERENCES

Baker, P, Ladds, M, Rubinson, K (1977) Measurement of the flow properties of isolated axoplasm in a defined chemical environment. *Journal of Physiology* 269: 10P–11P.

Beith, ID, Robins, EJ, Richards, PR (1995) An assessment of the adaptive mechanisms within and surrounding the peripheral nervous system, during changes in nerve bed length resulting from underlying joint movement. In Shacklock MO (ed) *Moving in on Pain*, pp. 194–203. Butterworth–Heinemann, Australia.

Bora, FW, Richardson, S, Black, J (1980) The biomechanical responses to tension in a peripheral nerve. *The Journal of Hand Surgery* 5: 21–25.

Borges, LF, Hallett, M, Selkoe, DJ et al. (1981) The anterior tarsal tunnel syndrome. Report of two cases. *Journal of Neurosurgery* 54: 89–92.

Bowsher, D (1988) *Introduction to the Anatomy and Physiology of the Nervous System*. Blackwell, Oxford.

Breig, A (1978) *Adverse Mechanical Tension in the Central Nervous System*. Almqvist and Wiksell, Stockholm.

Breig, A, Troup, JDG (1979) Biomechanical considerations in the straight-leg-raising test: Cadaveric and clinical studies of the effects of medial hip rotation. *Spine* 4: 242–250.

Butler, DS (1991) *Mobilisation of the Nervous System*. Churchill Livingstone, Melbourne.

Butler, DS (1996) personal communication.

Butler, DS, Gifford, LS (1989) The concept of adverse mechanical tension in the nervous system. *Physiotherapy* 75: 622–636.

Butler, DS, Gifford LS (1998) *The Dynamic Nervous System*. NOI Press, Adelaide.

Butler, DS, Slater, H (1994) Neural injury in the thoracic spine. A conceptual basis to management. In Grant R (ed) *Physical Therapy of the Cervical and Thoracic Spine*, 2nd edn. Churchill Livingstone, New York.

Byrod, G, Olmarker, K, Konno, S et al. (1995) A rapid transport route between the epidural space and the intraneural capillaries of the nerve roots. *Spine* 20: 138–143.

Cooper, RG, Freemont, AJ, Hoyland, JA et al. (1995) Herniated intervertebral disc-associated periradicular fibrosis and vascular abnormalities occur without inflammatory cell infiltration. *Spine* 20: 591–598.

Dahlin, LB, McLean, WG (1986) Effects of graded experimental compression on slow and fast axonal transport in rabbit vagus nerve. *Journal of the Neurological Sciences* 72: 19–30.

Devor, M (1994) The pathophysiology of damaged peripheral nerves. In Wall, PD and Melzack, R (eds) *Textbook of Pain*, 3rd edn, pp. 79–100. Churchill Livingstone, Edinburgh.

Devor, M (1996) Pain mechanisms and pain syndromes. In Campbell, JN (ed) *Pain 1996 – An Updated Review. Refresher Course Syllabus*, pp. 103–112. IASP Press, Seattle.

Devor, M, Rappaport, ZH (1990) Pain and the pathophysiology of damaged nerve. In Fields, HL (ed) *Pain Syndromes in Neurology*, pp. 47–83. Butterworth–Heinemann, Oxford.

Domisse, GF (1994) The blood supply of the spinal cord and the consequences of failure. In Boyling, JD, Palastanga, N (eds) *Grieve's Modern Manual Therapy*, 2nd edn, pp. 3–20. Churchill Livingstone, Edinburgh.

Donnerer, J, Schuligoi, R, Stein, C (1992) Increased content and transport of substance P and calcitonin gene-related peptide in sensory nerves innervating inflamed tissue: evidence for a regulatory function of nerve growth factor in vivo. *Neuroscience* 49: 693–698.

Dyck, P (1984) Lumbar nerve root: The enigmatic eponyms. *Spine* 9: 3–6.

Elvey, RL (1995) Peripheral neuropathic disorders and neuromusculoskeletal pain. In Shacklock, MO (ed) *Moving in on Pain*, pp. 115–122. Butterworth–Heinemann, Australia.

Farmer, JC, Wisneski, RJ (1994) Cervical spine nerve root compression. An analysis of neuroforaminal pressures with varying head and arm positions. *Spine* 19: 1850–1855.

Friede, RL, Samorajski, T (1969) The clefts of Schmidt-Lantermann: a quantitative electron microscopic study of their study in developing and adult sciatic nerves of the rat. *Anatomical Record* 165: 89–92.

Garfin, S, Rydevik, B, Brown, R (1991) Compressive neuropathy of spinal nerve roots. A mechanical or biological problem? *Spine* 16: 162–6

Gelberman, RH, Hergenroeder, PT, Hargens, AR *et al.* (1981) The carpal tunnel syndrome – a study of carpal canal pressures. *Journal of Bone and Joint Surgery* 63A: 380–383.

Goddard, M, Reid, J (1965) Movements induced by straight leg raising in the lumbo-sacral roots, nerves and plexus, and in the intrapelvic section of the sciatic nerve. *Journal of Neurology, Neurosurgery and Psychiatry* 28: 12–18.

Grieve, GP (1988) *Common Vertebral Joint Problems*, 2nd edn. Churchill Livingstone, Edinburgh.

Hall, T, Zusman, M, Elvey, R (1995) Manually detected impediments during the straight leg raise test. In *Proceedings of Manipulative Physiotherapists Association of Australia 9th Biennial Conference: Clinical Solutions*, pp. 48–53. MPAA St Kilda, Gold Coast Queensland.

Hanai, K, Kawai, K, Itoh, Y (1985) Simultaneous measurement of intraosseous and cerebrospinal fluid pressures in lumbar region. *Spine* 10: 64–68.

Hasue, M (1993) Pain and the nerve root. An interdisciplinary approach. *Spine* 18: 2053–2058.

Heller, PH, Green, PG, Tanner, KD *et al.* (1994) Peripheral neural contributions to inflammation. In Fields, HL and Liebeskind, JC (eds) *Pharmacological Approaches to the Treatment of Chronic Pain: Concepts and Critical Issues*, pp. 31–42. IASP Press, Seattle.

Howe, JF, Loeser, JD, Calvin, WH (1977) Mechanosensitivity of dorsal root ganglia and chronically injured axons: a physiological basis for the radicular pain of nerve root compression. *Pain* 3: 25–41.

Hoyland, JA, Freemont, AJ, Jayson, MIV (1989) Intervertebral foramen venous obstruction: A cause of periradicular fibrosis. *Spine* 14: 558–568.

Inman, VT, Saunders, JB (1942) The clinico-anatomical aspects of the lumbosacral region. *Radiology* 38: 669–678.

Jayson, MIV (1992) Vascular damage fibrosis and chronic inflammation in low back pain and sciatica. In Jayson MIV (ed) *The Lumbar Spine and Back Pain*, 4th edn, pp. 101–109. Churchill Livingstone, Edinburgh.

Jeffreys, E (1980) Soft tissue injuries of the cervical spine. In *Disorders of the Cervical Spine*, pp. 81–89. Butterworth, London.

Kuslich, SD, Ulstrom, CL, Michael, CJ (1991) The tissue origin of low back pain and sciatica: a report of pain response to tissue stimulation during operations on the lumbar spine using local anesthesia. *Orthopaedic Clinics of North America* 22: 181.

Kwan, MK, Wall, EJ, Massie, J *et al.* (1992) Strain, stress and stretch of peripheral nerve. Rabbit experiments in vitro and in vivo. *Acta Orthopaedica Scandinavia* 63: 267–272.

La Rocca, H (1978) Acceleration injuries of the neck. *Clinical Neurosurgery* 25: 209–217.

LaBan, MM, Wesolowski, DF (1988) Night pain associated with diminished cardiopulmonary compliance. *Archives of Physical Medicine and Rehabilitation* 67: 155–160.

LaBan, MM, MacKenzie, JR, Zemenick, GA (1989) Anatomic observations in carpal tunnel syndrome as they relate to the tethered median nerve stress test. *Archives of Physical Medicine and Rehabilitation* 70: 44–46.

Lombardi, JS, Wiltse, LL, Porter, IS (1984) The ligaments surrounding and attaching to the L5 spinal nerve. In *Abstract of the Conference of the International Society for the study of lumbar spine*. Montreal.

Louis, R (1981) Vertebroradicular and vertebromedullar dynamics. *Anatomica Clinica* 3: 1–11.

Lundborg, G (1988) *Nerve Injury and Repair*. Churchill Livingstone, Edinburgh.

Lundborg, G, Dahlin, LB (1996) Anatomy, function and pathophysiology of peripheral nerves and nerve compression. *Hand Clinics* 12: 185–193.

McCarron, RF, Wimpee, MW, Hudgins, PG *et al.* (1987) The inflammatory effect of nucleus pulposus: a possible element in the pathogenesis of low back pain. *Spine* 12: 760–764.

Mackinnon, SE (1992) Double and multiple crush syndromes. Double and multiple entrapment neuropathies. *Hand Clinics* 8: 369–390.

McLellan, DL, Swash, M (1976) Longitudinal sliding of the median nerve during movements of the upper limb. *Journal of Neurology, Neurosurgery and Psychiatry* 39: 566–570.

McMahon SB, Koltzenburg, M (1994) Silent afferents and visceral pain. In Fields, HL and Liebeskind, JC (eds) *Progress in Pain Research and Management*, pp. 11–30. IASP Press, Seattle.

McMillan, BS, Silver, JR (1987) Extension injuries of the cervical spine resulting in tetraplegia. *Injury* 18: 224–233.

Macnicol, MF (1980) Mechanics of the ulnar nerve at the elbow. *Journal of Bone and Joint Surgery* 62B: 531–532.

Maitland, GDM (1986) *Vertebral Manipulation*, 5th edn. Butterworth, London.

Melzack, R, Wall, PD (1996) *The Challenge of Pain*, 2nd edn. Penguin, London.

Millesi, H (1986) The nerve gap. *Hand Clinics* 2: 651–663.

Millesi, H, Zock, G, Rath, T (1990) The gliding apparatus of peripheral nerve and its clinical significance. *Annals of Hand and Upper Limb Surgery* 9: 87–96.

Nicholas, DS, Weller, RO (1988) The fine anatomy of the human spinal meninges. *Journal of Neurosurgery* 69: 276–282.

Nitz, AJ, Dobner, JJ, Kersey, D (1985) Nerve injury and grade II and III ankle sprains. *The American Journal of Sports Medicine* 13: 177–182.

Nobel, W (1966) Peroneal palsy due to haematoma in the common peroneal nerve sheath after distal torsional fractures and inversion ankle sprains. *Journal of Bone and Joint Surgery* 48A: 1484–1495.

Okabe, S, Hirokawa, N (1989) Axonal transport. *Current Opinion in Cell Biology* 1: 91–97.

Olmarker, K, Rydevik, B, Holm, S *et al.* (1989) Effects of experimental graded compression on blood flow in spinal nerve roots. A vital microscopic study on the porcine cauda equina. *Journal of Orthopaedic Research* 7: 817–823.

Olmarker, K, Rydevik, B, Nordborg, C (1993) Autologous nucleus pulposus induces neurophysiologic and histologic changes in porcine cauda equina nerve roots. *Spine* 18: 1425–1432.

Olmarker, K, Byrod, G, Cornefjord, M *et al.* (1994) Effects of methylprednisolone on nucleus pulposus-induced nerve root injury. *Spine* 19: 1803–1808.

Olmarker, K, Blomquist, J, Stromber, J et al. (1995) Inflammatogenic properties of nucleus pulposus. Spine 25: 665–669.

Panjabi, MM, Takata, K, Goel, VK (1983) Kinematics of lumbar intervertebral foramen. Spine 8: 348–357.

Parke, WW, Watanabe, R (1985) The intrinsic vasculature of the lumbosacral spinal nerve roots. Spine 10: 508.

Parke, WW (1988) Correlative anatomy of cervical spondylotic myelopathy. Spine 13: 831–837.

Pechan, J, Julius, I (1975) The pressure measurement in the ulnar nerve. A contribution to the pathophysiology of the cubital tunnel syndrome. Journal of Biomechanics 8: 75–79.

Penning, L (1992) Functional pathology of lumbar spinal stenosis (review). Clinical Biomechanics 7: 3–17.

Penning, L, Wilmink, JT (1981) Biomechanics of lumbosacral dural sac. A study of flexion-extension myelography. Spine 6: 398.

Rydevik, B, Brown, MD, Lundborg, G (1984) Pathoanatomy and pathophysiology of nerve root compression. Spine 9: 7.

Saal, JS (1995) The role of inflammation in lumbar pain. Spine 20: 1821–1827.

Sato, K, Kikuchi, S (1993) An anatomic study of forminal nerve root lesions in the lumbar spine. Spine 18: 2246–2251.

Shacklock, M (1995) Neurodynamics. Physiotherapy 81: 9–16.

Shacklock, MO, Butler, DS, Slater, H (1994) The dynamic central nervous system: structure and clinical neurobiomechanics. In Boyling, JD and Palastanga, N (eds) Grieve's Modern Manual Therapy, 2nd edn, pp. 21–38. Churchill Livingstone, Edinburgh.

Smith, CG (1956) Changes in length and posture of the segments of the spinal cord with changes in posture in the monkey. Radiology 66: 259–265.

Spencer, D, Irwin, G, Miller, J (1983) Anatomy and significance of fixation of the lumbosacral nerve roots in sciatica. Spine 8: 672–679.

Streit, WJ, Kincaid-Colton, CA (1995) The brain's immune system. Scientific American November: 38–43.

Sunderland, S (1974) Meningeal-neural relationships in the intervertebral foramen. Journal of Neurosurgery 40: 756.

Sunderland, S (1976) The nerve lesion in carpal tunnel syndrome. Journal of Neurology Neurosurgery and Psychiatry 39: 615–626.

Sunderland, S (1978) Nerves and Nerve Injuries, 2nd edn. Churchill Livingstone, London.

Sunderland, S, Bradley, KC (1949) The cross-sectional area of peripheral nerve trunks devoted to nerve fibres. Brain 72: 428–439.

Sunderland, S, Bradley, K (1961a) Stress-strain phenomena in human peripheral nerve trunks. Brain 84: 102–119.

Sunderland, S, Bradley, K (1961b) Stress-strain phenomena in human spinal nerve roots. Brain 84: 125–127.

Upton, ARM, McComas, AJ (1973) The double crush in nerve intrapment syndromes. Lancet 2: 359–362.

Vanderlinden, RG (1984) Subarticular entrapment of the dorsal root ganglion as a cause of sciatic pain. Spine 9: 930–933.

Wall, EJ, Cohen, MS, Massie, JB et al. (1990) Cauda equina anatomy I: Intrathecal nerve root organization. Spine 15: 1244–1247.

Yoo, JU, Zou, D, Edwards, T et al. Effect of cervical spine motion on the neuroforaminal dimensions of human cervical spine. Spine 17: 1131.

Yoshioka, S, Okuda, Y, Tamai, K et al. (1993) Changes in carpal tunnel shape during wrist joint motion. MRI evaluation of normal volunteers. Journal of Hand Surgery 18B: 620–623.

5

Pain

LOUIS GIFFORD

Introduction

The main thrust of this chapter is to help the student understand the nature of pain and realize that the diagnosis of pain states is far from being an accurate and agreed upon science. Recent advances in our understanding of pain are powerfully challenging much of current medical practice. This includes the part played by physiotherapy and other closely allied professions that deal with noninvasive forms of pain therapy and management. If physiotherapy can take on pain, understand it more clearly and what it means for the individual and society, then the profession's future place in its management will be assured a very significant role.

Chapter Objectives

After reading this chapter you should be able to:

1 Understand and see the weaknesses of the terms organic/nonorganic.
2 Discuss and understand the three pain dimensions: the sensory dimension, the affective dimension and the cognitive dimension. The

student should be able to relate the pain dimensions to all pain experiences and understand that pain's primary purpose is to influence 'behaviour'.

3 Integrate pain into basic concepts of stress biology:

(a) Normal pain is generally an adaptive perceptual message generated by the brain in response to tissue damage. Pain does not necessarily occur at the time of injury.

(b) Ongoing pain is adaptive if it serves a protective function but maladaptive if healing is complete and the symptoms are way out of proportion to the stimuli that provoked it.

(c) Pain alters psychological/mental function and this markedly alters brain output systems.

4 Discuss the current controversies underlying the established pain pathways and the misguided notion that there is a single pain perception centre in the brain.

5 Appreciate the relevance of the pain dimensions to acute and chronic pain.

6 Understand the concept of dysfunction/altered function and relate it to:

(a) The patient in pain;

(b) The weakness of many modern therapy models.

7 Understand that there are multiple physiological mechanisms underlying the perception of any given pain and that the major ones in current clinical use by some physiotherapists are:

(a) Nociceptive mechanisms;

(b) Peripheral neurogenic mechanisms;

(c) Central mechanisms;

(d) Output mechanisms — sympathetic, motor, neuroendocrine;

(e) Affective/cognitive mechanisms.

8 Understand the biological principles underlying the pain mechanisms and relate the processes to clinical presentations.

9 Appreciate that there are many controversial issues in ascribing pain solely to a particular tissue or structure.

10 Understand the terms 'allodynia' and hyperalgesia and the difficulties of their clinical interpretation.

11 Understand the weaknesses of therapeutic approaches to pain that involve targeting a presumed 'source' of the pain and that use wholly passive techniques.

Organic and Nonorganic Pain?

The notion that pain is a pure sensation akin to taste and smell has received much derision in recent times (Wall, 1989; Melzack and Wall, 1996). Most of us tend to think of pain as an unpleasant, distressing sensation that originates in traumatized tissues and courses its way along neural pathways to the brain and consciousness. Thus, the amount of pain perceived fits with the amount of damage done and the pain happily recedes in direct relation to the pace of healing.

The problem is that our clinics and departments are full of patients who have ongoing pain with no clear trauma or disease process, or who have suffered trauma but the pain continues on long after a reasonable healing period. Often there is a huge discrepancy between the amount of pain perceived and evidence of any reasonable tissue abnormality with which to equate it. Time and again this very discrepancy has promoted the adoption of a two-tier diagnostic model that divides patients into 'organic', where observable pathology equates with the pain, and 'nonorganic' or 'psychosomatic' where no such relationship exists (Waddell et al., 1980; Waddell and Turk, 1992; Long, 1995). Put simply this often equates to: organic = 'we believe you, have an operation/pill/manipulation to fix it'; and nonorganic = 'you are making it up, you need to see the psychologist/psychiatrist'.

Since it is frequently noted that in only 15–25% of patients with low back pain an accurate diagnosis can be established (Nachemson and Bigos, 1984; Spitzer and LeBlanc, 1987; Deyo et al., 1992), the rather unsettling conclusion is that medicine is directly or indirectly denying the honesty of the vast majority of patients (Loeser, 1991). The tragedy of this attitude combined with the inadequacies of current diagnosis for pain, is that patients can become disillusioned and unhappy, often angry, and enter a rather forlorn pilgrimage that takes them from specialist to specialist and from therapy to therapy. They are given multiple diagnosis and get multiple forms of advice (Ochoa et al., 1994) that add to the confusion and which may

be a major factor in making their problem a lot worse (Morris, 1991; Loeser and Sullivan, 1995).

The Three Dimensions of Pain: Sensory, Cognitive and Affective

One of the key ways to understand pain and the patient's experience of pain is to view it in three interrelated dimensions (Melzack and Casey, 1968; Melzack, 1986) and never as a single 'sensory' one (Figure 5.1).

Unless we are under fairly severe physical threat or extremely focused on something, most of us, if we twist our ankle or sprain a finger, generally feel some pain at the time of the incident which goes on for some time afterwards. We very quickly become aware of where the pain is coming from, how intense the pain is, how the pain is behaving over time and the type or quality of the pain. This is the 'sensory' dimension of pain and the dimension which most physiotherapy assessments focus

Figure 5.1 Three dimensions of pain (see text for details). (Reproduced, with permission, from Butler and Gifford 1998 The Dynamic Nervous System. NOI Press, Adelaide)

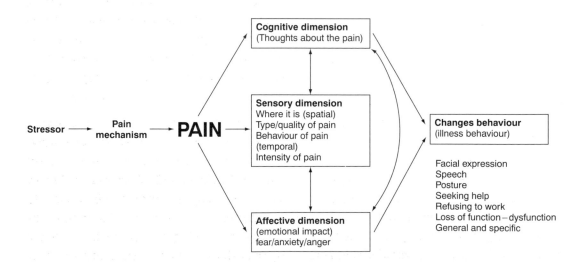

on when filling in our body charts and asking questions during the subjective examination. However, pain to a lesser or greater degree alters the way we think, the 'cognitive' dimension of pain, and the way we feel, the emotional or 'affective' dimension of pain.

Thoughts (the *cognitive dimension*) might involve some assessment of how bad the damage is, what to do about it and alterations of planning for work and recreation, for example. Individual thoughts vary greatly, for example: 'I better seek help from my nearest physiotherapist / acupuncturist / healer'; 'I better go to bed for two weeks'; 'I'll ignore it and get on with my plans and see how it goes'; 'I think I have broken it, I'm not going to move until the ambulance arrives'; 'Last time I did this it took 4 months: this isn't looking good at all'; 'Oh great I can take a week off work'. Even in acute pain there is a great variability in individual thought processes that may have marked repercussions on outcome. A simple cognitive spectrum has at one end a stoical attitude that ignores the problem and makes light of it and at the other extreme the catastrophizer who just sees the downside of it all and appears, at least to some, to rather revel in the drama.

The *affective dimension* of pain recognizes that for every pain we have, an emotional reaction is expressed that is fundamental to the pain experience and not just a reaction to the sensory appreciation of pain (Chapman, 1995). If you strike a dog it will either yelp and run, or bare its teeth and possibly even bite you. In biological terms threat and the pain message generally produce very powerful aversive behaviours that adaptively serve to protect the threatened organism. In human terms (and probably in higher vertebrates too; Dawkins, 1993), threat is strongly associated with aversive *feelings* of fear and anger which promote

adaptive behaviours that are ultimately protective in function and powerfully serve to enhance individual and species survival (Gray, 1987; Panksepp *et al.*, 1991; Chapman, 1995). The immediate discomfort of a twisted ankle is likely to produce some sort of emotional response like anger, mild annoyance, worry and anxiety. Most responses to pain involve some kind of unpleasant emotion that is encompassed in the terms 'psychological distress' (Main *et al.*, 1992) and 'suffering' (Cassell, 1991).

A simple spectrum way of viewing often complex affective dimensions is a scale of emotional impact that has at one end modest psychological distress and at the other extreme a status of clinical depression. Thus, a twisted ankle may invoke mild concern or moderate anxiety while a sudden sciatic pain for no apparent reason may be far more distressing. Ongoing severe pain combined with marked disability and loss of function may be a severe test of an individual's coping capability and may easily lead to ongoing maladaptive emotional states. Just as thoughts about pain alter our behaviour so too do the emotions compel action – we shout, we moan, we grimace, we chastise, we change our posture often in quite dramatic ways, all of which conveys powerful meaning to others in that it summons assistance and support, in particular from those who are closely related. For instance, witness the powerful support given by a parent to their injured and emotional child.

Figure 5.1 illustrates the three pain dimensions and highlights their main objective, that is, to change our behaviour in order to promote restoration of function (MacLean, 1990). What we are ultimately looking at is a coping strategy that is as unique to an individual as his or her physical features are. Biologically, the injury message can be viewed as a signal of threatened homeostasis that kickstarts adaptive *physiological* and *behavioural* coping mechanisms in order to promote survival.

Behavioural changes involve alterations in movement patterns and great vigilance for the part concerned. The idea is to care for the part that is injured and hurting as well as to keep others who are likely to damage it further well away from it. Thus the pain of a twisted ankle may compel limping and restricted range of movement as well as extreme guarding involving verbal and physical demonstration to nearby others. So often a patient can happily touch an acutely injured area themselves, but note the change of facial expression, the protective reactions and the enhanced tissue sensitivity when under physical examination, especially when the examiner has done little to gain the trust of the patient. Everyone's behaviour in a given situation is a unique interaction of innate reactions modified by the experiences our upbringing and culture imposes upon us (Gray, 1987; Gross, 1992). Everyone behaves differently and we must be prepared to try and adapt to each individual.

Pain and Stress Biology

While the three dimensions of pain are seen as part and parcel of every pain experience it should also be clear that each dimension must interact with the others (Figure 5.1). For example, negative or 'unhelpful' thoughts about the injury and the pain promote unhelpful emotional responses that then promote the arousal of the autonomic and neuroendocrine axes which in turn promote noxious sensory responses from the tissues and neurones responsible for the mechanisms of the pain (Figure 5.2).

Figure 5.2 is an attempt to simplify the main input,

or afferent systems, and the main output, or efferent systems, involved in the central 'processing' of stressors associated with pain and to demonstrate their powerful interactions. The term 'stressor' is used in the sense of any real or perceived threat to homeostasis, and 'stress reaction' or 'stress response' as the body's adaptive counterresponse to it (Levine and Holger, 1991). Stressors, like a twisted ankle, may be seen as resulting from environmental factors outside the body, i.e. exogenous stressors, or, like some disease processes, resulting from endogenous factors that originate from within the body. Endogenous stressors must include mental/cognitive 'stress' since negative thoughts and emotions very powerfully influence the activity of the stress response (Goldberger and Shlomo, 1993; Sapolsky, 1994).

Witness how you feel when you see something disturbing on the television, or think of something that has upset you in the past, or have ongoing unexplained pain. Typical signals of anxiety like pounding of the heart, a queasy stomach and a loss of appetite are powerful examples of how the 'psyche' can influence the body — this is termed a 'psychosomatic' reaction in the stress literature (Weiner, 1991). Note how the proper biological use of this term is *not* in the derogatory sense that it is so common.

The crucial message here is that our thoughts and feelings strongly influence biological processes in the tissues of the body. This has powerful repercussions for the way in which we manage the patient in pain, especially chronic pain where negative/unhelpful thoughts and feelings often dominate the patient's lives.

At the present time it seems that the scientific disciplines of stress and pain biology have hardly met each other, yet the links are fairly clear and

Figure 5.2   The afferent and efferent systems related to physical stressors. (Reproduced, with permission, from Butler and Gifford 1998 The Dynamic Nervous System. NOI Press, Adelaide)

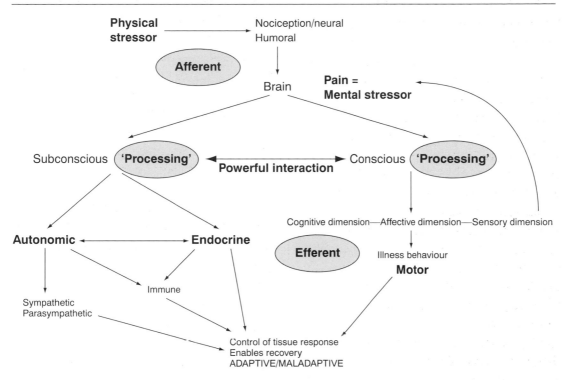

help greatly in providing a much needed reinterpretation of our thoughts about pain and pain management.

Let us overview the afferent and efferent systems using the sprained ankle as an example. The primary stressor consists of the physical forces acting on the ankle joint and its associated structures. The first adaptive reaction is flexor withdrawal response brought on by an impressively quick and complex sensory/afferent — motor/efferent reflex neural response (see Chapter 3). At the same time tissue trauma afferent messages are relayed via nociceptive systems to the brain whose processing may invoke a conscious appreciation of the stressor (as pain) as well as activating complex 'subconscious' brain

compartments that invoke appropriate outputs to counter the stressor.

The three major output systems are:

1 The autonomic (sympathetic and parasympathetic nervous systems);
2 The neuroendocrine systems;
3 The motor systems.

All three are influenced by the way we are thinking and feeling. The degree to which these systems are activated vary greatly and depend to a large extent on the degree of perceived threat. Thus, their activation is greatly enhanced if the twisted ankle occurred at the same time as a loud and unusual noise compared to just quietly walking along a street. This again emphasizes the powerful link between the way we are thinking and feeling —

the mind/our cognition – and the activity of systems that powerfully influence the tissues of the body. These two situations also serve to demonstrate how the stress response may activate the very powerful stress-induced analgesic systems. Injury in the presence of acute threat (such as at the same time as a very loud noise) may not produce any feeling of pain at the time, as pain would merely hinder any physical activity needed to escape the threat (McCubbin, 1993; Blank, 1994; Fields and Basbaum, 1994).

Note how input to the brian involves two routes, one via the nervous system which is fast (and hence evolutionary advanced), and the other more primitive route via the bloodstream (humoral) which is far slower. Damaged tissues produce chemical messengers like the cytokines and other inflammatory mediators that are thought to communicate with the brain via the bloodstream (De Souza, 1993; Rivier, 1993; Udelsman and Holbrook, 1994; Watkins et al., 1995). Input about injury also involves the ears, eyes and occasionally smell, and their afferent pathways to the brain.

Nociceptive pathways or wiring diagrams have been described in great detail and the reader is directed elsewhere for fuller information (see Willis, 1985; Charman, 1994). However, there are two interesting aspects that arise from the pioneering work of Ronald Melzack (Melzack and Casey, 1968) and the comments of his long time associate, Patrick Wall (Wall, 1996a). Melzack and Casey (1968) assigned two separate anatomical pathways to the sensory and affective dimensions of pain; that is, the lateral neospinothalamic (neo = biologically 'new' and hence fast) pathway that relays from the nociceptor terminal synapses in the dorsal horn, across the cord and ascends to nuclei in the thalamus before being relayed on to the somatosensory projection areas of the cortex. This pathway was assigned to the sensory dimension of pain described earlier.

The affective dimension was assigned to a more medial multisynaptic pathway that courses from the dorsal horn up to the brainstem reticular formation and on to the limbic nuclei that perfuse the brainstem and areas of the more primitive cortex. These areas of the brain are powerfully linked to centres involved in emotional feelings and to the activation of their associated reflex behaviours (Damasio, 1995). In parallel there are also links to seats of sympathetic efferent activity, like the locus coeruleus nucleus in the brainstem, and to seats of endocrine hormone activity via the hypothalamus and its links to the pituitary gland (Chrousos and Gold, 1992; Johnson et al., 1992; Valentino et al., 1993). These subconscious nuclei/ regions of the brain not only output to the body but are also capable of exerting a remarkably global influence on brain activity in general. There are thus very powerful links to and from higher centres associated with consciousness.

The key concept to hold on to is that any form of threat activates conscious and subconscious systems that are bidirectionally linked by known pathways and that each can influence the other (Chapman, 1995). Changes in behaviour and tissue repair processes require a coordinated physiological response to be successful.

The second issue, raised frequently by Wall (see Wall, 1996a, b), relates to the problems of viewing the nervous system and brain as a computer-like creature that is given its wiring diagram during development and from then on never changes. Wall tends to balk at the concept of dedicated pathways and regions in the brain (Wall, 1996b), like one each for sensory and affective component of pain. No one has managed to perform a surgical lesion or focal application of a drug to a specific tract or area of the brain that can produce an isolated loss of affect or sensation with regard to pain (Wall, 1996a). Further, neurosurgical lesions along presumed pain pathways only produce temporary relief that is later followed by the ability to again generate a pain state. Tragically, cutting the so-called pain pathway or destroying a presumed pain 'centre' in the brain, just does not work and may often make the pain worse later on (Melzack and Wall, 1996). What this highlights is the complexity of the 'thing' we call pain and that there is not a simple dedicated pain pathway and pain appreciation centre. We are really looking at a hugely distributed system that involves the integration of many subsystems whose ultimate goal is the coordinated restoration of a homeostatic equilibrium sufficient to allow survival.

Basically it looks as if the whole of the brain is involved in pain. This makes sense if one views the brain as the primary 'stress control centre' and that injury and pain require the activation of many systems in order to promote survival. In viewing the pain as a component of a stress system/response, it is worth drawing attention to the fact that pain itself is a stressor, and on its own, without any necessary tissue damage or nociceptive activity (think of things like ongoing migraine headaches here), will activate a stress response to a greater or lesser degree depending on the significance our thoughts give to the pain.

The stress response thus has two components that are influential in determining its activity, a mental component and physical component, and they are inseparable (Figure 5.3).

Figure 5.3   Adaptive and maladaptive stress responses. (Reproduced, with permission, from Butler and Gifford 1998 The Dynamic Nervous System. NOI Press, Adelaide)

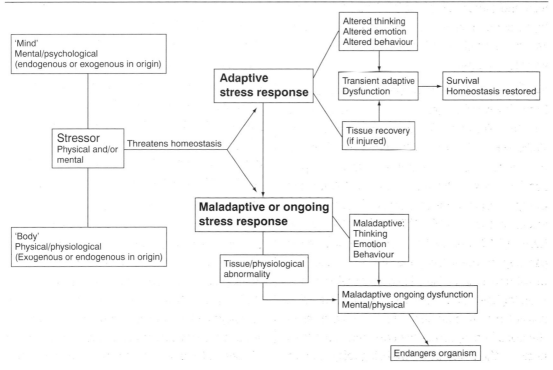

Figure 5.4   Demonstrating the relative importance of the dimensions of pain in the acute and chronic situation. All dimensions are variable. (Reproduced, with permission, from Butler and Gifford 1998 The Dynamic Nervous System. NOI Press, Adelaide)

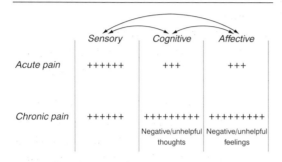

Before discussing Figure 5.3, the reader's attention is drawn to Figure 5.4 because it highlights some of the great differences between acute and chronic pain in relation to the three dimensions of pain discussed. In acute pain the sensory dimension is fairly dominant – patients in acute pain visit our clinics and describe the pain in precise terms, can often easily identify physical factors that make it better or worse and in addition simply and quickly state their feelings and thoughts about it if given the opportunity. By contrast, in chronic pain the dominance of cognitive and emotional dimensions is profound when compared to the acute problem (Figure 5.4). Chronic pain sufferers can often keep talking for hours about the problems that they encounter, in themselves, in their family, at work and with medicine and their management. If you ask a chronic pain patient if they are upset or angry – the answer is invariably yes (see Fernandez and Turk (1995) for an excellent review).

The great mistake is to view pain, especially chronic pain, from the perspective of an isolated sensory dimension that sees all pain as an adaptive warning that damage is being done.

Much chronic pain is largely maladaptive and results in far-reaching disability. What it really needs is a rehabilitative approach whose primary aim is to restore physical function and at the same time addresses both the cognitive and affective dimensions of the patient's disorder (see Chapter 15; Gatchel and Turk, 1996; Turk *et al.*, 1983).

Briefly, this means educating the patient about the underlying mechanisms of their pain (see Chapter 15) and the influences their thoughts, emotions, attitudes and physical behaviour can have on it. Having then established a sound basis of knowledge that the patient can understand and relate to, the phase of 'mental', behavioural and physical rehabilitation can go ahead.

Figure 5.3 represents two hypothetical routes that can be taken as a result of some sort of event that can be deemed stressful and may include pain as one of the mental or psychological stressors. The two routes are:

1 The adaptive one, where function and homeostasis are happily restored;
2 The maladaptive one, where an ongoing problem occurs and which is ultimately a threat to the viability of the organism.

The adaptive stress-response route is the one most of us take when confronted with minor injuries and aches and pains. However, it is common for some maladaptive issues to creep in, especially with regard to our thoughts and feelings.

Pain and Altered Function: 'Dysfunction'

The interaction of our thoughts and feelings about a problem combine to promote altered behaviour while tissue recovery proceeds. During this time we generally adopt a state of adaptive or maladaptive altered function which for the purposes here is loosely described as 'dysfunction' and divided into three subcategories (see Butler and Gifford, 1998). It is the author's view that along with pathobiological mechanisms (see below), dysfunction should be added and integrated into the five hypothesis categories put forward in the clinical reasoning model proposed by Jones (Butler, 1991; Jones, 1992) and further developed to include the pain mechanisms suggested by Butler (Butler, 1994). (Clinical reasoning is discussed at length in Chapter 6, but see also the proposals in Butler and Gifford, 1998.)

The three subcategories proposed are:

1 General physical dysfunction;
2 Specific physical dysfunction;
3 Psychological/mental dysfunction.

General Physical Dysfunction

This refers to limping, hobbling, stereotyped patterns of movement and posture, difficulty/inability to perform simple tasks like negotiate stairs, sit comfortably etc. It is anything a good subjective and objective functional physiotherapy assessment reveals and which by the World Health Organization definition would be termed 'disability' (WHO, 1980).

Specific Physical Dysfunction

This includes:

- a loss of range of joints, muscles and nerves as a result of increased tissue sensitivity, mechanical block/tightness, pure spasm, fear or a combination of these;
- Weakness due to neurological deficit, disuse, pain inhibition, fear and so forth;

- Symptoms/abnormal responses, e.g. excessive tissue tenderness to palpation (allodynia, hyperalgesia, see below), pain provoked at end of range, pain provoked in specific test positions;
- Instability/muscle imbalance;
- 'Other', e.g. deformity, leg length discrepancy, tissue thickening, tissue thinning/wasting.

This is the area where physiotherapy excels, i.e. finding specific dysfunction. However, we should be cautious and a little wary of adopting what may be a pseudo-diagnostic approach. Pain has generated many very enthusiastic specialists in specific techniques of treatment and analysis. Manual therapy is one such approach. If you look closely, there are subspecialities within manual therapy — some practitioners focus on the cranial sutures, others on reflex areas on the feet, or the sacroiliac joint position, or muscle imbalance and tightness, for example. The list could spread to include electrotherapy and many different surgical approaches. The statement 'if you look you will find' should alert us to the dangers of dogmatic single-model approaches to pain states. This is especially true in the analysis of specific physical dysfunction in chronic pain (see Loeser, 1991).

It is important to note that we are all full of dysfunctions whether or not we are in pain. If we are in pain it is easy to find something wrong relevant to a precise tissue model but which may not be relevant at all to the patient's pain state. While everyone wants to know what is wrong, there are dangers from those who obsessively bias their models.

Pain science forces the broadening of our views about pain states. A good example is a patient with a 4-month-old sciatica who goes to see five or six different therapists and comes away from each with a different diagnosis and different advice. He may well have 'cranial suture abnormalities', 'leg length discrepancies' and 'sacro-iliac upslip', problems with 'lymph drainage', loss of 'passive accessory movements' in his lumbar spine, 'adverse neural tension', 'muscle imbalance', and so on. But this is just a list of specific, and rather equivocal, physical dysfunctions which may or may not be relevant to the underlying pathobiological mechanisms that are giving rise to the pain state.

Psychological / Mental Dysfunction

This category of dysfunction recognizes the importance of the cognitive and affective dimensions of pain and their fundamental role in the production of suffering and maladaptive physical dysfunction. Current stress biology and the relatively new scientific disciplines like psycho-neuroimmunology are demonstrating and emphasizing the powerful links between negative or unhelpful thoughts and feelings and negative tissue physiological effects (Ader et al., 1991). If we can helpfully change patients' beliefs, thoughts and feelings about their problems the recovery will be vitally enhanced. Although traditionally this area is the domain of clinical psychology, physiotherapists who specialize in managing pain can with guidance and proper training effectively help these components of many patients' disorders. If pain is multidimensional then so should its management be — whether we are dealing with chronic or acute pain. The majority of patients in pain need more information about their problem and what to do about it. A good deal of patients' needs are met when they are given understandable answers to the following fundamental questions (see Butler and Gifford (1998) for full discussion):

1 What is wrong with me?
2 How long will it take to get better?
3 Is there anything that I can do to help?
4 Is there anything that you can do to me or give me that will help me?

Pathobiological Mechanisms: Pain Mechanisms

In the rest of this chapter the focus will be on some of the pathophysiological or pathobiological mechanisms that can give rise to pain and produce physical and psychological / mental dysfunction. This is important since most current diagnostic systems in medicine and physiotherapy are based on ill-founded anatomic or mechanistic labels that focus the patient's and clinician's attention on a damaged structure which is in need of some kind of passive therapy or passive intervention to fix it (Loeser, 1991; Loeser and Sullivan, 1995). As noted earlier there is little pathological / structural / anatomical evidence to be found that equates with the degree of pain in the great majority of patients suffering with ongoing pain. There is also plenty of evidence to show the continued presence of apparently blameworthy anatomical abnormality long after the resolution of pain (for example see Garfin et al., 1991). Current pain biology draws our attention to the need for an inclusion and analysis of pain mechanisms into a diagnostic clinical reasoning hypothesis.

The refreshing aspect of this approach is that the inclusion of maladaptive central nervous system afferent and efferent processing as a means of generating pain independently of any tissue or peripheral nerve abnormality, means that many of our patients' more atypical pains and pain behaviours can more easily be explained. This is helpful to those of us who deal with them and hence to the poor patient who up to now has been largely denied a reasonable organic basis for their very real pain. At long last many complex regional pain syndromes that have previously been considered as hysterical 'conversion' disorders are now rightly being considered as neurological disease states (Janig, 1996). The answers to understanding pain surely lie in a far broader understanding of pathobiological mechanisms that emphasize the significance of the central nervous system rather than the anatomical aberrations of its target tissues.

Pain Mechanisms

There are five recognized pain mechanism categories in the clinical reasoning model used by some manual therapy systems today (Butler, 1994; Jones, 1995).

These are:

1 Nociceptive mechanism;
2 Peripheral neurogenic mechanism;
3 Central mechanism;
4 Sympathetic/motor mechanism;
5 Affective mechanism.

Each term relates to a physiological process that can give rise to pain jointly or in isolation. Some mechanisms stand out as being far more dominant in a pain presentation than others.

NOCICEPTIVE MECHANISM

This mechanism represents pain at its physiologically simplest. The pain is coming from roughly where it is felt, or at least from where tissue damage and inflammation are stimulating and provoking nociceptors to transmit impulses that produce the perception of pain in the brain. Prevent the nociceptive messages from reaching the cen-

tral nervous system by inhibiting inflammation, or by blocking the nerves supplying the injured area and the pain slowly or rapidly vanishes. Nociceptors are specialized afferent neurones of two basic types, fast myelinated Aδ fibres and smaller, slower unmyleinated C fibres (Fields, 1987). It is the Aδ fibres that are responsible for the flexor withdrawal reflex, the C fibres are much too slow. In fact, if one were to stick a pin in the foot of a horse a C fibre would relay the event to the spinal cord in about 8 seconds (Wall, 1989) – an event which is much too slow to prevent injury.

In the normal state nociceptors will only fire if noxious or near noxious stimuli are presented to them. They are thus said to be 'high threshold' afferents. This means that if a therapist performs an end-range stretch on a normal tissue, nociceptors will begin to fire and the recipient will start to frown and become ever more vigilant as the therapist slowly pushes harder and harder. In most people, the amount of discomfort/pain is consistent and in proportion to the force. Some people are obviously more sensitive than others but there is a recognizable limit to what one would expect under normal conditions before thinking that something may be wrong. It could be useful to put people on a pain-response scale with feeble at one extreme and stoical at the other – *so long as it does not colour your view of that person.* Appreciate that everyone is different because their sensitivity is a result of interaction of genes and environment.

A further consistent feature of normal nociception is that once the pressure is released the noxious sensation immediately diminishes. Nociceptors in this non-injury, or 'physiological', state only fire at a set point, increase their firing as the stimulus gets more noxious and stop firing very quickly once the stimulus terminates (Woolf,

1991). But, while what we feel does equate with nociceptor activity in many situations, there are times when nociceptor activity may be intense, yet we feel no pain at all. How often have you noticed being covered in bruises yet were unaware of the exact incident that caused the injury? Lack of pain at the time of injury is surprisingly common — it depends on whether or not the central nervous system is in a pain-permitting mode (Woolf, 1994), or put another way, whether the *pain gates* are being held firmly closed by powerful inhibitory currents (Melzack and Wall, 1965, 1996). Our central nervous system contains incredibly powerful pain-inhibiting circuitry that is kickstarted in threatening circumstances or when our attention is focused elsewhere (Fields and Basbaum, 1994).

So far it has been suggested that nociceptors only fire in response to noxious events in the tissues. This is not strictly true, since a small percentage do fire a little all the time and in parallel with other fibres (Schmidt *et al.*, 1994). This includes the very large myelinated, fast-conducting Aβ fibres. Aβ fibres, in the physiological state, send impulses that relate to non-noxious stimuli such as joint position, pressure and stretch on tissues and so forth. They inform us of our body's position and its actions, and provide the sensory information necessary for an adequate body image (Melzack, 1991) (see Chapter 3). Thus, there is a constant background barrage of impulses from the tissues of the body involved in locomotion which includes a modicum of nociceptive activity.

It has been found that in the knee joint of a normal resting cat there is a continuous afferent neural activity of about 1800 impulses every 30 seconds. When the joint is slowly moved in mid-range this increases to 4400 impulses every 30 seconds (see Schmidt *et al.* (1994) for an excellent overview). If the joint is then experimentally inflamed to mimic a nociceptive event, there is a quite remarkable increase in afferent activity. At rest, the barrage increases to 11 100 impulses every 30 seconds and when gently moved it increases to a 30 900 impulse rate. Here we have a seven-fold increase in afferent activity with gentle movement, so no wonder we don't want to move an acutely inflamed joint! Hanesch *et al.* (1992) have noted a 100-fold increase in some fibres. It appears that the afferent fibre population, in particular the nociceptors, actually change their response properties in the presence of injury. There is a dynamic or 'plastic' change in their function which is the result of chemical activity at the site of injury (Perl, 1992; Levine and Taiwo, 1994; Meyer *et al.*, 1994). What is interesting is when observed over time there is a steady increase of activity in parallel with the growing inflammatory chemical cascade.

Practical Example

Think about some of the features of a twisted ankle. After the immediate pain of injury subsides there is a period of modest constant ache in the absence of any clear stimulus, which often steadily builds up over the following few hours and into the night. Some tissues give very little pain until the next morning. Ongoing background ache is probably the result of the ongoing afferent fibre barrage dramatically increasing. Nociceptors — Aδ and C fibres, as well as Aβ fibres — increase their spontaneous firing rate in the presence of inflammation (Schmidt et al., 1994). Further, many nociceptors that were silent before the injury now wake up and begin firing too (McMahon and Koltzenburg, 1990). Some fibres take several hours to wake up and keep increasing their activity for many hours after this (Schaible and Schmidt, 1988). This all fits nicely with the fairly predictable time course of pain in relation to ligament, muscle and tendon injury. The fact that some injuries may not become painfully apparent until the next day may be due to such factors as their poor metabolic turnover (slow to inflame and swell), lack of a good blood supply, a feeble nerve supply (think of a disc's innervation) and one which contains mainly those of the sleeping variety. An injured disc may react very slowly, may be injured in an area that has no nerve or blood supply and those nerves which do eventually get to know about the injury may take a long while to wake up (Gifford, 1995). Additionally, a slow build-up of fluid may in part account for increasing discomfort over time (See Gifford (1995) for an overview of possible disc pain mechanisms). Constant background aching may not always be a feature, but check and double check with the acute pain patient, for as is so often the case, the background ache may be of little concern compared to the horrible sharp pain experienced with pressure and movement.

Over a similar time-frame the ankle becomes acutely sensitive to touch, and minor movements that would not normally hurt become acutely painful. The quality of pain, in contrast to the 'ache' just described, is sharp in nature and quite often it continues for some moments after the stimulus has stopped. This clinically reactive state is beautifully mirrored by the dynamic changes in responsiveness of damaged tissue nociceptor populations

that have been observed in the laboratory (Handwerker and Reeh, 1991; Meyer et al., 1994). Nociceptors which typically only fired at a set high threshold in the non-injury state, now fire at considerably lower thresholds, and when they are stimulated they fire far more as well as tending to go on firing long after the stimulus is removed (Woolf, 1991; McMahon and Koltzenburg, 1994).

Hyperalgesia

Tenderness and increased sensitivity to mechanical testing for most of us is a sure sign that the area and underlying tissues that produce the tenderness are injured in some way. This is especially true if the tenderness can easily be associated with some injuring activity. Tissue tenderness is generally termed 'hyperalgesia'. However, the International Association for the Study of Pain (IASP) defines hyperalgesia as 'an increased response to a stimulus which is normally painful' (Merskey and Bogduk, 1994). Broadly, this means that if you twist your ankle and it hurts, and then later twist it again, it hurts a great deal more than it did the first time.

Clinical Examples of Hyperalgesia

With a non-injured tissue, in physiotherapy terms, if you perform a firm unilateral postero-anterior pressure in the L5–S1 region of a normal back, it is likely to produce some local discomfort. If the tissues are in a hyperalgesic state, due to some form of injury somewhere, and you repeat the procedure with exactly the same force, an increased response will occur – i.e. pain rather than mere discomfort.

> *Another example would be the early normal perception of discomfort when a physiotherapist passively tests a SLR, upper limb tension test or simple wrist extension into the first few degrees of resistance. If the tissues being gently mechanically stressed in these tests were hyperalgesic this modest awareness of onset of discomfort would be signalled with increased intensity, as pain.*

Allodynia

Unfortunately the term hyperalgesia is rarely used in this strict IASP definitional sense in much of the pain literature. It is additionally used to encompass pain that is produced in response to a stimulus which does not normally provoke pain, for which the IASP uses the term 'Allodynia' (Merskey and Bogduk, 1994). Thus, as already described, if you twist your ankle, some hours later movements and tests that would not normally cause pain will now start to do so. Modest attempts at inversion will hurt, very gentle palpation of the area will elicit pain and so on.

Clinical Examples of Allodynia

In the examples used above, unilateral postero-anterior pressures over L5–S1 will hurt with very gentle pressures, and straight leg raise, upper limb tension testing and wrist extension will begin to hurt very early in range where no symptoms would normally be elicited. Extreme examples of allodynia can be seen in ghastly neuropathic (peripheral neurogenic) conditions like trigeminal neuralgia and Herpes Zoster (shingles), where pain can

be elicted by gently blowing on the skin in the affected area.

Although the two terms *hyperalgesia*, and *allodynia* may initially be a bit confusing we must all persevere as they need to become the words of choice in physiotherapy assessment of pain.

It is probably most useful to view hyperalgesia as an umbrella term to refer to enhanced sensitivity in general (Campbell *et al.*, 1993).

Primary and Secondary Hyperalgesia

Hyperalgesia, enhanced sensitivity of tissues, may be an honest reflection of underlying tissue damage. 'The damage is where it hurts when I press on it or mechanically stress it or test it in some way' is a justifiable statement in many acute injury states, especially if the tenderness is in an area that fits with the injury history. Hyperalgesia at the site of injury is termed *primary hyperalgesia*. The best way of understanding this is to think of the exaggerated response as a 'true positive' — the thing that hurts is damaged or diseased in some way, it is the tissue responsible for this patient's pain.

It seems easy, but the overzealous readiness of most of us to jump to a conclusion of 'this is the tissue at fault because it is tender when I press on it and it produces pain when I mechanically stress it with this test and this test' may be one of the biggest clinical errors to be unmasked by pain science.

It is becoming more obvious that many tissues that hurt when they are physically stressed may be perfectly normal (Wall, 1993; Quintner and Cohen, 1994; Cohen, 1995). This phenomenon of normal tissues being abnormally mechanically sensitive is termed *secondary hyperalgesia*. In contrast to primary hyperalgesia, here we are clearly dealing with a 'false positive' in terms of the tissues under test. Thus, a positive upper limb tension test in a patient with a chronic repetitive strain injury or a chronic whiplash may not be a reflection of anything wrong at all with the nerves being tested, it is just that *normal inputs* to the central nervous system induced by the test are processed in terms of pain rather than innocuous sensation. The source of the mechanism for this type of sensitivity is in the circuitry of the central nervous system – not in the tissues under duress (Dubner, 1991a; Dubner and Basbaum, 1994; Price *et al.*, 1994).

The brunt of the understanding of this biologial mechanism is that the huge injury and inflammatory related increase in impulse delivery to the dorsal horn of the spinal cord (the afferent barrage) is thought to be largely responsible for setting up sensitivity changes in second-order neurones that relay rostrally. It turns out that specific populations of second-order dorsal horn cells (nociceptive specific (NS) cells), which normally only respond to impulses arriving via nociceptors (Aδ and C fibres), actually change their response characteristics to becoming responsive to innocuous Aβ fibre input (Cook *et al.*, 1987). Further, cells that normally respond to both nociceptive and Aβ input (wide dynamic range (WDR) cells) now increase their sensitivity so as to fire far more dramatically and for far longer (Dubner and Basbaum, 1994). This is quite dramatic 'plasticity', because what in effect has happened is that the wiring and circuitry normally dedicated to the transmission of innocuous peripheral sensations has now become diverted into a pain transmitting one, and that dedicated to noxious information transmission has been upregulated to a highly sensitive status.

The view that the nervous system is a hard-wired unchanging computer-like organ has to be revised. As will be further discussed, the nervous system has an in-built and remarkable flexibility that widely accounts for our ability to adapt to the ever changing circumstances our lives and the environment we live in impose upon it.

Inflammation and Nociception

Inflammation is currently regarded as one of the key initial processes leading to increases in sensitivity and the clinical pain state (Levine and Taiwo, 1994). It is not simple, but it needs our attention in the sense that it should be seen as a benign event that, apart from frequently leading to pain, is vital in initiating the recovery of damaged tissues and setting the stage from which the later phases of healing evolve. Inflammation has to be seen as an adaptive response and therefore something which should be tolerated better perhaps. Chronic inflammation and pathological inflammation are maladaptive and a different matter in that they may adversely contribute to tissue damage and the general well-being of the patient.

Inflammation can be seen as having two major components, one that involves chemicals released from the terminals of nerve fibres in the damaged area, *the neurogenic component*, and the rest, *the non-neurogenic component*.

The non-neurogenic components of inflammation broadly encompass:

1 The first aid/damage limitation aspects that include the clotting and laying down of fibrin lattices.
2 The physical activity of cells of the immune system, such as the polymorphonuclear leukocytes and macrophages involved in removing 'debris' and any threatening micro-organisms.

Importantly, the immune system is not only involved in fighting invading organisms but also in initiating and controlling healing, and in chemically signalling to the central nervous system (Abbas *et al.*, 1994). For instance, mast cells at the site of injury release chemical messengers called cytokines into the tissues as well as into the general circulation. Cytokines, such as the interleukins, are thought to be transported to the brain via the circulation and help mobilize systems involved in the control of inflammation. They also appear to have a role to play in producing hyperalgesia — both at the nerve terminals and in the central nervous system (Watkins *et al.*, 1995).

3 The flow of fluid into the area, so-called plasma extravasation that gives rise to oedema (Coderre *et al.*, 1989, 1991).

4 The release of chemicals from cell membranes that have been damaged and from specialized inflammatory cells themselves. The prostaglandins and leukotrienes are important chemicals that are produced as the result of cell wall breakdown with the subsequent release of membrane phospholipids (Pettipher *et al.*, 1992). Phospholipids are the precursors to a complex cascade of chemical reactions that result in leukotriene and prostaglandin formation. The whole cascade is inhibited by corticosteroids. Non-steroidal anti-inflammatory drugs only inhibit the so-called cyclo-oxygenase pathways that give rise to the prostaglandins (Velo and Franco, 1993).

5 The release of chemicals synthesized within specialized inflammatory cells and from plasma, for example mast cell degranulation and release of histamine, or the infiltration of fibrin from plasma (Rang *et al.*, 1991, 1994).

The neurogenic components of inflammation can be described as follows.

Neurones are traditionally thought of as solely having an impulse-conducting function. Recently there has been an upsurge in interest in the secretory function of peripheral nerve fibres, in particular the C fibres (Levine *et al.*, 1988; Sluka *et al.*, 1995). As already mentioned, C fibres are unmyelinated slow conductors and, at face value, pretty useless at warning of acute injury. Thankfully Aδ fibres fulfil this function.

The question has arisen as to what all the C fibres are for. In some cutaneous nerves over 90% of the afferent fibres found are C fibres (Melzack and Wall, 1996). It appears that their major role is to help maintain the health of the tissues they supply. C fibres actually sample the tissues, take up chemicals, actively transport them to their cell bodies in the dorsal root ganglia where appropriate responses are instigated and relayed back to the tissues (Moskowitz and Cutrer, 1994). If a tissue is damaged the nucleus in the cell body and cells in the dorsal horn of the spinal cord gets to know about it via these slow chemical channels of communication as well as via impulse activity (Donnerer *et al.*, 1992). Not only do they get to know, they also do something about it. C fibres become highly active in secreting chemicals in damaged tissues. They add to the inflammatory soup that is already forming and influence the secretion of chemicals, the local circulation and plasma extravasation (Levine *et al.*, 1986a).

The active chemicals that C fibres secrete are neuropeptides such as substance P and CGRP (calcitonin gene related peptide) (Walsh *et al.*, 1992). C fibres release neuropeptides experimentally when impulses travel down their axons and dendrites in the 'wrong direction' — so-called antidromic impulses. These impulses may be

Figure 5.5   Simplification of injury events leading to activation of a C fibre. Direct activation by intense pressure and consequent cell damage. Cell damage leads to release of potassium (K+) and hydrogen (H+) ions, adenosine triphosphate (ATP) and protaglandins (PG). Bradykinin (BK) is released into the area via the plasma 'kinin' system. (Adapted from Fields, HL, 1987, *Pain*, McGraw-Hill, New York, with permission.)

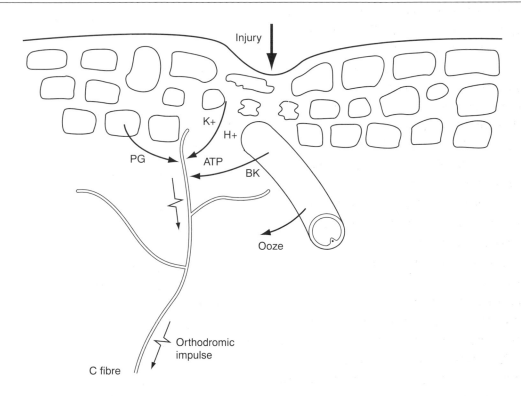

propagated from the dorsal horn terminals of the C fibres as well as locally where orthodromic (correct direction) impulses travelling proximally along dendrites may actually pass back down an adjacent dendrite in the 'wrong' direction (Sluka *et al.*, 1995).

Sympathetic postganglionic fibres, in addition to their motor function on the smooth muscle of blood vessels, also have a secretory role when tissues are injured and when we are under stress. They are known to release noradrenaline (nor-epinephrine, USA), which enhances the vascular response and may cause pain if the nociceptors become sensitized to it (Janig and McLachlan, 1994).

So the combined effect of neurogenic and non-neurogenic components seems to be a rather daunting and massively angry soup of noxious chemicals. Figures 5.5 and 5.6 highlight a few important aspects. The injuring force damages the tissues and causes nociceptive nerve impulses to be transmitted. Prostaglandins, hydrogen ions (inflammatory soup is acidic), potassium ions and adenosine triphosphate are among the early chemicals released from the damaged tissues and bradykinin and fluid enters the area from the circulation (Fields, 1987; Levine and Taiwo, 1994). All these chemicals are known to have sensitizing effects on nociceptors, in other words they lower

Figure 5.6   Simplification of some of the post-injury events leading to C fibre sensitization and propagation of impulses. Antidromic impulses lead to release of neuropeptide substance P (SP). Substance P produces vascular effects and facilitates 5HT and histamine (His) release from mast cells and prostaglandin and histamine release from platelets. Sympathetic efferent terminals secrete norepinephrine (nor) which only acts to excite C fibres directly if alpha-L-adrenergic receptors have been expressed. Norepinephrine acts to enhance the vascular response in 'normal' inflammation. (Adapted from Fields, HL, 1987, *Pain*, Mcgraw-Hill, New York, with permission.)

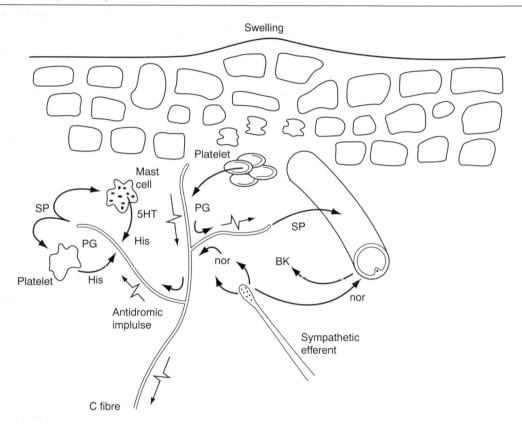

their thresholds and thus become more sensitive, i.e. they account for primary hyperalgesia.

Some of the chemicals, like bradykinin, promote firing of nociceptors – hence ongoing ache/awareness. As time goes on, the soup becomes more complex, mast cells and platelets appear and are activated to release further sensitizing and pain-producing chemicals; the sympathetic efferents secrete noradrenaline, the C fibres secrete substance P and CGRP and the whole area becomes a swollen sensitized mass of interacting chemicals. Most of the literature cited focuses on the rather explosive and self-enhancing nature of inflammation. Little is mentioned about mechanisms that actually inhibit and control the events.

PERIPHERAL NEUROGENIC MECHANISM

Pain can derive from damage to peripheral nerve trunks and roots, hence the neuralgias, sciatica, brachialgias and many nerve entrapment syndromes that are well documented. The discussion here involves a consideration of nerve fibre (neurone) injury alone, not the consequences of injury to nerve trunk and root connective tissue (see Chapter 4).

Normal afferent neurones basically report what is happening in the tissues they innervate — the target tissues. An afferent sensory neurone is thus seen as an independent sensory channel. Impulses start at the nerve end (encoded), then travel along the axon (transmission) into the dorsal horn of the spinal cord to form the first synapse with second-order neurones and interneurones. The impulse 'message' is normally contained within the fibre. If anything goes wrong at any level along this pathway, abnormal impulse discharges, in abnormal patterns, which may begin in abnormal places along the axon, will give rise to the input of false and rather strange information (Devor and Rappaport, 1990; Devor, 1994). When nerve fibres are injured and responding like this the patient tends to perceive rather odd pain and symptoms that are in odd places. Symptoms often appear to have a mind of their own and are therefore rather worrying to the patient. Further, the pain generated can be out of all proportion to events that caused it, and it can be very nasty, unremitting and very hard to alleviate (Tanelian and Victory, 1995).

If impulses start somewhere along an axon the source of this abnormal impulse activity is said to be 'ectopic'. This is easily demonstrated if you briskly tap the ulnar nerve at the elbow and get a shower of pins and needles in your little finger. Thus, ectopic impulses can be demonstrated on a normal nerve, but as a generalization, normal nerve fibres are relatively insensitive and we go about our daily lives quite unaware that our nerves are being stretched, pinched and distorted in some way all the time. The only region of a nerve which is known to have enhanced mechanosensitivity under normal conditions is the dorsal root ganglion (Devor and Rappaport, 1990; Wall and Devor, 1983).

The pathophysiological mechanisms which can lead to ectopic impulse generator sites in nerve fibres have already been discussed (Chapter 4). It is highly likely that many of us house injured and regrowing nerve fibres that are of no consequence whatsoever. The fact that some of us succumb to peripheral neurogenic pain and symptoms may be simply down to the expression and installation of protein receptors and ion channels in the regrowing and damaged cell walls of nerve fibres which then render them mechanically and chemically hypersensitive (Devor et al., 1994; Devor, 1995).

In order for normal afferent nerve fibre terminals in target tissues to be mechanically sensitive they have to contain active receptors in their cell walls that are sensitive to mechanical forces. A normal fibre does not contain large populations of active mechanoreceptors along the length of its axon, nor does it contain large populations of ion channels other than those essential for impulse propagation.

When a nerve is injured there may be loss of continuity of many individual fibres with subsequent Wallerian degeneration distally accompanied by attempted regrowth of the proximal axon (Devor and Rappaport, 1990). If a fibre is damaged but remains in continuity there may be loss of myelin and modest disruption of the axon membrane.

In any region of nerve damage there is usually a massive proliferation of Schwann cells, fibroblasts and macrophages into the area (Devor et al., 1994; Wong and Crumley, 1995). Subsequent to this is the release of bioactive molecules like nerve growth factor that are absorbed by the axons and transported to their cell bodies in the dorsal root ganglion where the production of membrane receptors and ion channels is upregulated (Devor *et al.*, 1994). These receptors and channels are protein molecules which are actively transported back to the damaged areas and installed in the membranes, hence changing their sensitivity (Devor *et al.*, 1994). Receptors may be mechano-receptors (stretch-activated ion channels) making the area more mechanically sensitive, but may also be adrenoreceptors (sensitive to adrenaline and noradrenaline) or receptors that are sensitive to hypoxia or inflammatory chemicals. Thus the area can not only become more sensitive to movement – stretches and pressures – it can also become more sensitive to chemicals like adrenaline and noradrenaline that arrive via the general circulation or are secreted from sympathetic nerve terminals in the area.

Additionally, these sites of damage can start to produce sustained impulse volleys that are *self-generated*, may go on and on or come in continuously repeating bursts and waves, and which are thought largely responsible for some of the devastating ongoing and uncontrollable pains that nerve injury sometimes produces. These sites are termed 'ectopic pacemaker sites' because they have this independent ability to produce ongoing trains of impulses (Devor, 1994). Clinically all this stands for ongoing pain which waxes and wanes for no apparent reason. Pain that is produced in response to movement may continue on and on long after the movement is stopped. This type of pain may be influenced by fluctuations of adrenaline and noradrenaline secretion due to mental and physical stress, and it is pain that is often of bizarre qualities which happens in odd places with strange referrals.

It is often a great relief for the patient to have this knowledge explained to them in simple terms, just because pain that comes and goes for no apparent reason is worrying to most people. For example, neurogenic pain that gets worse at rest, or during the night may be due to a nerve's abnormal sensitivity resulting from ischaemia/hypoxia — blood pressure is lower at night and the circulation is relatively sluggish. Getting up, moving around, shaking a hand that has carpal tunnel syndrome may often be enough to restore peace to a nerve that has started firing as result of building ischaemia. This sort of information is helpful for the patient and focuses us on the need to include strategies that improve circulation to the area.

There are a few important issues.

1 Nerve injury that develops ectopic pacemaker ability will barrage the central nervous system with massive impulse activity. This has far-reaching implications for possibly permanent changes in central cell sensitivity and 'rewiring' of the nervous system (see central mechanisms below) (Woolf *et al.*, 1992; Woolf and Doubell, 1994).

2 This activity is not mandatory in every nerve injury. In the laboratory, rats can be bred that have a high or low propensity to developing pacemaker capability, some nerves are more vulnerable than others and some sites on individual nerves are more prone than others (Devor and Raber, 1990). The genetic aspect is intriguing, especially if you consider that the receptors and ion channels are produced as a result of specific genes in the cell bodies of the affected nerve being 'switched on' to express the proteins required. Some of us may be innately more prone to being 'switched on' than others.

3 Ectopic pacemaker capability may take a while to occur after injury. For instance, Aδ fibres that are injured may remain totally silent for

the first day or two after injury, but then slowly increase their spontaneous activity over the following two weeks. C fibres tend to increase activity as the A fibres decrease theirs (Devor, 1994). Think of the unfortunate whiplash patient who for the first few days feels stiff and sore but some days or weeks later develops weird symptoms in odd places. Not only is it strange and worrying to the patient, it also tends to be seen as the first signs of malingering by many health professionals. It is hardly surprising that people with odd neurogenic pain develop a fear of moving and adapt to movement patterns and postures in strange and unnatural ways, but they are often confronted with undertones of disbelief and frustration by those who have to deal with them. It should also be appreciated that lesions to nerves that are capable of producing such devastating pains are best seen as pathophysiological in nature; the anatomical evidence for them is at a molecular level on the membranes of individual neurones, something that cannot be picked up on radiographs, modern imaging techniques or nerve conduction studies.

CENTRAL MECHANISMS

Some mention has already been made of plastic changes in the response properties of dorsal horn cells when they are subjected to nociceptive-derived impulse barrages. These cells clearly shift their properties to an enhanced excitability state in order to accommodate damaging events in the periphery (Woolf, 1994). The adaptive value of this is seen in terms of increased and spreading pain as well as a spread of tenderness in order to promote tissue protective behaviour during the first stages of healing when tissues are at their weakest and most vulnerable. A corollary of this is that

enhanced sensivity should drift back to normal as healing progresses.

What is intriguing is that in some circumstances increased excitability may remain long after healing has taken place and that ongoing pain — generated by abnormal and spontaneous discharges of dorsal horn neurones, and tissue hypersensitivity (wholly secondary hyperalgesia), as a result of normal input from the periphery activating these hyperactive cells — may be a major mechanism in many chronic pain states. While the pain and tenderness are blatantly perceived in the tissues, the dominant mechanism that is creating the pain and sensitivity state is in the central nervous system (Wall, 1988; Pennisi, 1996).

Unfortunately, hyperexcitable dorsal horn cells cannot be blamed for all chronic pain states. Although its understanding is crucial to new concepts about pain, it has to be taken as just one tiny fraction of the many possibilities the central nervous system holds. Knowledge of the dorsal horn is gratefully accepted. It would be very handy indeed for the many who suffer chronic and disabling pain to blame a small population of highly excitable dorsal horn cells as being responsible for producing an ongoing illusion that the peripheral tissues are still in a damaged state. Unfortunately the complexity of the CNS is unlikely to allow such a simple concept to be much more than a late twentieth century notion that will ultimately be superseded as yet more knowledge of the brain unfolds. However, it is worth speculating with regard to possible repercussions of central mechanisms for chronic pain states and their management. What we are really looking for are analogies and metaphors that help us to understand and explain the crazy chronic pain states to our patients and to then give them confidence that their tissues are no longer primarily responsible. Confidence in being able to work through pain, work *with the pain*, or nudge *slowly* into it without fear, is one of the most powerful ways of starting chronic pain rehabilitation (see Chapter 15).

This concept of prolonged 'hyperexcitability' can be taken a stage further if one considers phantom limb pain. If a patient who has ongoing pain without having had an amputation then decides to have an amputation in a radical effort to be rid of the pain, the exact same pain would unfortunately remain (or return a short while later) in the form of a phantom (see Dielissen *et al.*, 1995). In effect, what this is saying is that any ongoing nociceptive input into the central nervous system may give rise to an 'imprint', 'memory' or 'central representation' of the pain. Thus, this pain 'imprint' or 'memory' may ultimately be unresponsive to anything therapeutic that is done to the tissues where the pain originated and where the pain and tenderness are still felt, or that is done to the peripheral nervous system that innervates the tissues that are painful – even an amputation. Clearly the mechanism responsible for the pain has moved from a nociceptive tissue dominant one, to one being housed in central nervous system pathways. Chronic pain sufferers are mutilated daily by operations that purport to correct 'relevant' anatomical abnormalities, that denervate the affected zones, that block the pain pathway etc., but careful scrutiny shows that the outcomes, although initially very good, are in reality very poor (see Melzack and Wall, 1996, p. 222; Wall, 1996b). The repercussions of this for physiotherapy pain treatments are clear.

The concept of a somatosensory memory for pain in amputees and spinal cord injured patients who suffer ongoing pain has been put forward by Katz and Melzack (1990). It seems likely that this concept may be relevant to many chronic pain sufferers who have not undergone any form of amputation or surgery. At the synaptic level, the biological processes involved in memory are considered in terms of an increasing and strengthening 'bond' between chains of neurones (Dudai, 1989; Rose, 1992). If one considers that one neurone may synapse with up to 20 000 others in the central nervous system it is quite easy to see that many of the 10 million million or more synapses (Rose, 1992) and possible pathways may be quite ineffective or 'silent' and that there are huge potentials for new unique pathways forming that have specific meaning. Thus, when something new happens, such as an ongoing pain experience, previously dormant synapses are woken up and new pathways are formed, weakly at first, but as the process is repeated during 'learning', the synaptic efficacy becomes ever stronger until eventually permanent synaptic relationships are formed. This is a situation considered to be analogous with the establishment of a long-term memory (Pockett, 1995). In short-term memory links are strengthened but only short-lived (Rose, 1992; Kandel *et al.*, 1995). The biological and biochemical processes involved in synaptic efficacy are very complex but crucially involve the pre-synaptic neurone being able to have greater and greater influence on the post-synaptic neurone. In other words, the post-synaptic, neurone becomes more excitable in relationship to the special messages received presynaptically.

During injury, this is the very state of the relationship between the primary afferent fibres arriving from the peripheral tissues and the second-order dorsal horn cells that relay up the spinal cord to the brainstem and higher centres. Similar processes occur at higher level synapses in the brain and go on to include enhanced efferent (output) response patterns due to whole input–output circuits becoming more effective (Dougherty and Lenz, 1994; Flor and Turk, 1996; Galea and Darian-Smith, 1995). Thus we get enhanced motor responses in the form of antalgic postures, protective movement patterns and reflexes and emotionally generated feelings and behavioural responses (crying, anger, frustration etc.), as well as enhanced sympathetic and neuroendocrine activity via output from the limbic and reticular formation relays (Chapman, 1995).

Since there are such stereotyped responses to most acute injuries it does suggest that some pathways may be innately ready-to-run. Indeed, any threat to an organism requires a sophisticated and well coordinated reaction and recovery operation. However, if inputs carry on for long enough in conditions where normal inhibitory influences fail to keep a check on neurone excitability, these well established input–output pathways may run amok — maladaptively providing abnormal inputs and outputs that may help maintain abnormal and often unique physical and psychological/mental dysfunctions (for expanded discussion, see Butler and Gifford, 1998).

If this analogy with memory is true it suggests that chronic pain, its behaviour and the physically reactive movement patterns we so often see, are stubbornly implanted 'habits' in the nervous system. Further, they would require immense efforts to overcome, perhaps equivalent to an 'unlearning' or 'relearning' process. It may help if one considers how relatively easy it is to influence acute pain or ongoing nociceptive pain with drugs, yet how difficult it is to alter the pain of many chronic sufferers with drugs or anything else. It perhaps could be likened to finding a drug that could ablate long-term memories with the proviso that we remain conscious.

In order to understand some of the conditions that give rise to ongoing excitability it is necessary to journey back to the dorsal horn cells.

Synaptic efficacy and enhanced excitability, like the biology of the peripheral neurogenic mechanisms, is all about receptors. In particular, the barrage of impulses in concert with increased central delivery of neuropeptides by primary afferent C fibres is thought largely responsible for the observed changes in the second-order neurones of the dorsal horn (Pockett, 1995; Yaksh and Malmberg, 1994). Thus, dormant receptors become effective and the cells' nuclear machinery is activated to produce more receptors that are transported to and then planted in the dendritic cell wall. Luckily, the excitability of these second-order cells does not inexorably tumble on — there are inhibitory currents and neurochemicals that control and dampen down these events (gate control — see Melzack and Wall, 1996). Thus lifting of inhibitory currents, or the loss of pertinent inhibitory neurones may have far-reaching consequences. Three clinically relevant examples of how changes in inhibitory checks may lead to abnormally enhanced second order cell sensitivity are given below. All would theoretically interact.

1 There are continuous (tonic) descending inhibitory currents going on all the time which can be hugely influenced by our attention (Melzack and Wall, 1996). What is also known is that this descending inhibitory current is actually enhanced during and immediately after tissue injury (Schaible and Grubb, 1993). It seems that there is a reflex pathway that tries to adaptively limit the hyperexcitability and the consequent expansion of receptive fields of second-order neurones. It could be argued that these inhibitory currents may be lifted or overridden by

consciously over-focusing attention on pain (see Butler and Gifford, 1998).

While everyone does tend to focus on pain there are circumstances when excessive attention may occur. Consider the situation of a keyboard operator who begins to get discomfort and odd pins and needles in her arm. She knows of others in the same office who have been off work for months, she gets slightly anxious, she discusses it with them, the bosses increase the work load, there are financial worries and other pressures at home, she consults the doctor who listens quietly but is unhelpful and not overly concerned, and so on.

There are plenty of situations in modern life that can be translated into cumulative and rather malevolent, adverse biological reactions. Note that the intention here is to speculate on the mechanisms, not insist, as none of this has been tested. However, the concept of pain as a memory and the issues of enhancing of a pain imprint by maladaptively focusing on a problem, have received some interest and support from Wall (1995b), a pain scientist, and Rose (1995), a memory scientist. Importantly, some people may simply be born with, and/or develop, via the mental and physical rough and tumble of life, relatively weak inhibitory controls.

2 Inhibitory interneurones can actually be killed by large afferent barrages from damaged tissues and nerves in animal experiments where descending inhibitory currents are lifted (see Dubner and Basbaum, 1994). Massive and ongoing volleys of C fibre impulse activity cause a marked build-up of the excitatory amino acid neurotransmitter chemicals glutamate and aspartate. Both have been shown to cause neurone death and it is believed that dorsal horn inhibitory interneurones are par-

ticularly vulnerable (Dubner, 1991a, b, 1992; Dubner and Basbaum, 1994). Loss of inhibition means loss of control of excitability of second-order neurones and hence the threat of chronic pain.

The important clinical element here is that barrages from ectopic pacemaker sites in damaged nerves are particularly spiteful since they generate such massive barrages that go on for such a long time. Additionally, nerve damage invariably causes some death of afferent fibres, and the central nervous system, realizing that it has lost sensory input, upregulates its sensitivity in an attempt to seek out and recover the missing input. In some cases damaged neurones may actually grow new dendritic sprouts that wander into neighbouring dorsal horn zones and make further and often inappropriate synapses (Shortland and Woolf, 1993; Woolf and Doubell, 1994). The potential for ongoing pain, misinformation and abnormal processing is almost frightening.

3 Melzack and Wall's pain gate theory (Melzack and Wall, 1965) very strongly considered the inhibitory influence of Aβ fibres on second-order neurones (see Melzack and Casey, 1968; Melzack and Wall, 1996). It was the basis on which transcutaneous nerve stimulation (TENS) was developed for pain control. Modern pain science, as we have seen, has shown that Aβ fibre input can *enhance* pain once a dorsal horn cell has become sensitized. However, there is no doubt that Aβ input in the early stages of injury does inhibit and hence reduce potential for enhanced excitability. Any peripheral loss of Aβ fibres may therefore be an important factor. Aβ fibres, being large, myelinated and fast conducting, are metabolically demanding and therefore very prone to

damage and degeneration in conditions that enhance peripheral nerve ischaemic conditions (see Chapter 4). Minor and ongoing peripheral nerve damage that causes loss of Aβ fibres and hence its central inhibitory function may be a contributing factor in the injury-induced prolonged enhanced sensitivity state of dorsal horn cells.

Maladaptive central mechanism recognition in chronic pain is as yet only an assumption; there is no physical diagnostic test that unequivocally identifies it and there probably won't be for a long time. In fact, most standard clinical diagnostic tests reveal little (see Ochoa et al., 1994) despite the fact that our physical assessments can be very lengthy when pain response is focused on. The key to understanding central mechanisms and many chronic pains is to view the problem as a hyperalgesic one — excessive abnormal and ongoing hypersensitivity of tissues such as muscle, joint, nerve, skin etc; remember the 'If you look you will find' statement earlier. There are often abnormal movement patterns and gross restrictions in ranges if pain is focused on, yet if you really look there is little evidence of true mechanically blocked loss of range any more than in most normal people.

Below are some of the features of pain related to a maladaptive central mechanism (Butler and Gifford, 1998).

- There is lack of symptom consistency.
- Symptoms do not fit within the normal boundaries set out in textbooks.
- Symptoms are often weird.
- All examining movements tend to hurt. It is rare for the patient to report a decrease in pain with examining movements.
- Patients have excessive 'reactivity' or inappropriate reactivity. In manual therapy terms they are often designated as having a highly irritable pain state and the pain treated with great respect. Unfortunately, focusing on the pain like this for therapeutic reasons may well be a factor in enhancing the pain for the patient.
- They have atypical movement patterns — compare the movement patterns of a typical acute or subacute shoulder with a chronic maladaptive one for example; often there are odd writhing movements of the body, odd shakes and contortions of the arm with plenty of facial grimacing, yet patients are quite capable of normal movement patterns when distracted from the pain.
- Response to treatment is unpredictable — one treatment may help immensely, but repeat the exact treatment again another time and the pain gets much worse.
- The patients are not happy, are often angry and have many maladaptive thoughts and emotions about their lives, their bodies, their medical management and the society and workplace they are in.

The central pain mechanisms category provides us and the patient with a developing organic basis with which to explain much maladaptive or 'enigmatic' pain (Pennisi, 1996). The description and stance taken here is my own interpretation of modern pain and memory science that many of my patients have found immensely helpful in understanding, validating and coming to terms with their chronic pain problems (see Butler and Gifford, 1998 for fuller discussion).

SYMPATHETIC AND MOTOR MECHANISMS: EFFERENT/OUTPUT MECHANISMS

The sympathetic nervous system (SNS) has received a mass of attention with respect to pain states that are said to be maintained by or dependent on its activity, for example causalgia, reflex sympathetic dystrophy, sympathetically maintained pain (SMP), algodystrophy and many more. The classic justification for pinning blame on the sympathetic nervous system has always been the successful alleviation of symptoms following sympathetic block techniques (Wallin *et al.*, 1976, but see Bonica, 1990).

The truth of the matter is that there is no key set of signs and symptoms that enable one to distinguish whether or not a given pain state is 'sympathetically maintained'. It is rather a hit and miss affair. Thus a patient may have a classic 'sympathetically maintained' pattern – of ongoing pain in the distal extremity of an arm or leg, obvious oedema, cold extremities and discolouration of the skin, marked hyperalgesia / allodynia and perhaps dramatic joint loss of range and stiffness – yet be totally unresponsive to a sympathetic block technique. This has led to the current use of the term 'SIP', or sympathetically independent pain (Campbell *et al.*, 1994), to help classify a group of pain patients who have an apparently 'sympathetic' syndrome and yet are not helped by sympathetic blocking techniques.

Classifying these complex pain presentations using presumed pathology as the guiding principle was extremely difficult and has recently been acknowledged as being unworkable (Janig, 1996; Stanton-Hicks *et al.*, 1995). The current proposal is that the term 'Complex regional pain syndrome' (CRPS) Types I and II now be used (Janig and Stanton-Hicks, 1996). These two categories broadly encompass all pain syndromes which have similar features to those mentioned above but which may or may not have a component that is relieved by sympathectomy or sympathetic block:

1 Type I encompasses those that are sympa-

thetic, dystrophy-like and are initiated by some sort of noxious event.
2 The Type II grouping is more causalgia-like in that the constellation of symptoms develops after a nerve injury (see Janig and Stanton-Hicks, 1996; Stanton-Hicks *et al.*, 1995).

Many of the chronic pain syndromes seen by physiotherapists, such as chronic whiplash pain and 'repetitive strain injury', at times, can come under this classification. To think of them in terms of simple aberrations of the sympathetic nervous system is a serious oversimplification. Ongoing pain states have multiple sources and multiple pathobiological mechanisms. Sometimes the SNS just happens to play a part that is amenable to invasive or pharmaceutical therapy.

The SNS needs to be viewed as a compartment of a complex system, albeit relatively primitive, that helps integrate general and specific responses to challenges to our homeostasis.

Its function as part of the autonomic nervous system is paramount to survival and it therefore has to be activated in any pain state. Nociception, and hence pain, is thus a kick-starter of the sympathetic nervous system in terms of general survival responses, e.g. increased heart rate and a more alert brain, as well as more tissue-specific responses, e.g. local vasolidation and chemical influences on inflammation in tissues (Levine *et al.*, 1986b).

The SNS responses are hugely influenced by the way we are thinking – think about a nice cup of coffee and you will start salivating, dream about a romantic night out with a friend and all sorts of amazing things start happening, be slightly anxious about something and your body starts to think it's being physically threatened and so forth. The autonomic nervous system responds to tissue input as well as conscious input. This is a very powerful mind—body, body—mind link, and it is an area which we must acknowledge in every single dealing with our patients. If you can influence the way a person is thinking and feeling you may influence physiology in the tissues and nerves that serve the body.

The sympathetic nervous system is involved in all pain states. For instance:

- It moderates the local circulation and chemical environment.
- It innervates lymphoid and thymus tissue and therefore plays a part in controlling the immune responses (Arnason, 1993; Smith and Cuzner, 1994).
- It helps regulate endocrine hormone functions such as those that control the release of the powerful anti-inflammatory corticosterones via pathways to the hypothalamus and pituitary (Chrousos and Gold, 1992; Valentino et al., 1993).

Pain, healing, recovery and our general organ responses are all under the influence of the SNS. The fact that a pain may be sympathetically maintained focuses on the fact that sympathetic secretions of adrenaline and noradrenaline can:

1 Initiate nociceptive impulses from the terminals of nociceptors that have become sensitized to these chemicals (Sato et al., 1993); and/or
2 Initiate impulses from damaged nerve axons and/or regrowing endbulbs of nerve fibres that have undergone Wallerian degeneration and become similarly sensitized (Devor, 1994). (These are the ectopic sites mentioned earlier.)
3 It is also known that dorsal root gangion cell bodies increase their sensitivity to adrenaline when their axons are damaged (Wall and Devor, 1983) or there is chronic inflammation persisting at their nerve terminals (see Janig and McLachlan, 1994).

The SNS to the limbs and nonvisceral tissues of the body does not contain any sensory fibres – it only contains sensory fibres from visceral nerves. There are no sympathetic afferents in the somatic nerves. Thus, sympathetically maintained pain has to be a result of the secretory, efferent function of this system (Walker and Nulsen, 1948). Post-ganglionic sympathetic fibres innervate most tissues of the body. They travel in somatic nerves or accompany vascular plexi and have two basic functions:

1 Control of smooth muscle and hence peripheral circulation;
2 Secretory – secretion of noradrenaline and prostaglandins.

It is important to incorporate the knowledge that the adrenal medulla powerfully secretes the catecholamines adrenaline and noradrenaline and that this is controlled by SNS activity (Sapolsky, 1994). Thus any increase in anxiety, any emotional response or any excitement will powerfully influence plasma and hence tissue levels of these catecholamines.

The reader may start to see that through knowledge of this mechanism, there are multiple facets to take into account when considering the often bizarre patterns of many pain states. The difficulties do not stop here; for instance, it has recently been shown that commensurate with the fact that pain mechanisms change and move with time (Butler and Gifford, 1998; Melzack and Wall, 1996), SMP may with time become SIP (Torebjork et al., 1995). Thus, even though the symptoms for the patient feel the same, the mechanism may change over time. In some patients SMP may thus be a transient phenomenon. This is certainly the case in the animal models used by pain scientists (Wall, 1995a).

Similar to the peripheral neurogenic and central mechanisms discussed, the common feature is sensitivity due to the presence of relevant receptors. In SMP the receptor thought responsible for enhanced catecholamine sensitivity in damaged nerve fibres and in nociceptors, is called the alpha-2 adrenoreceptor (Bennet and Roberts, 1996). If it is absent there is no sensitivity; if present there is potential for a pain state. It rather begs the question, 'why shouldn't the DNA that is ultimately responsible for producing these receptor proteins be able to shut down its maladaptive production of these malevolent little chemicals ... and does our multidimensional therapeutic interaction with our patients help bring this about?' Maybe?

The current literature on SMP makes fascinating reading and is as good as any starting point to get into the science of pain in relation to those chronic pain patients we try to 'fix' in our day-to-day dealings with patients (see for example, Janig and Stanton-Hicks, 1996).

Lastly, it is important to consider all efferent systems in the maintenance of any given pain state: somatic motor, neuroendocrine and even the immune system can be considered here (see Butler and Gifford, 1998).

Muscle itself can be a primary source of pain if it has been injured, but this has to be considered in terms of a nociceptive pain mechanism. In terms of pain and all pain mechanisms generally, there has to be a highly efficient link of afferent input — to central processing, to rapid efferent output, in order to provide an appropriate response. Clearly, screwing up one's face and screaming, tears, jumping out of the way, running away, limping, antalgic postures, abnormal movement patterns, getting into a hot bath, and going to the doctor are all motor reactions in response to pain. Prolonged maladaptive muscle activity should be considered as a mechanism that can add to the discomfort of the tissues and hence an increased nociceptive drive (Ohrbach and McCall, 1996).

The following is an interesting example of how pain behaves and the sorts of indirect influences that there can be on its behaviour. Herta Flor and colleagues (Flor et al., 1991, 1992; Birbaumer et al., 1995), using electromyographic (EMG) measures, have shown that subgroups of chronic pain patients show markedly increased muscular activity and tension when they are in pain and when they are exposed to personally relevant stressful situations. The increase in muscular response was found to be localized to the site of pain and maintained for a prolonged period when compared to healthy controls. They also noted that patients with pain exhibit a reduced capacity to consciously perceive and voluntarily regulate their levels of muscular tension. In any pain state, whatever the mechanism, there is likely to be an increased muscle response which may well add to the barrage of afferent impulses that help maintain the pain state, the often multiple pain mechanisms responsible, and the levels of perceived pain (see Ohrbach and McCall, 1996, and Flor and Turk, 1996, for excellent critical overview of current theories).

AFFECTIVE MECHANISMS

This pain mechanism 'hypothesis category' was introduced by Butler (1994) for manual therapy and was an attempt to incorporate the notion that 'affect' or emotion influences our perception of pain and that this is a vital consideration in all pain states. The reader should take into account that bringing the emotions and the brain into the 'hard-wired' and strongly tissue-based manual therapy philosophy back in 1993–1994 was quite a bold step by Butler.

There are many problems with misguided day-to-day clinical application of psychological and psychiatric theory and pain states, in particular when a patient's thoughts and feelings are over-focused on *as the reason for their pain problems.* The stance proffered here is that:

1 Low or depressed mood and other maladaptive alterations in psychological function that are commonly found in ongoing pain states are largely *the result of the pain state* rather than the cause of pain (see psychological / mental dysfunction earlier in chapter and see Chapter 15). (For a review of psychological factors in chronic pain see Gamsa, 1994a, b, and Banks and Kerns, 1996.) Patients happily accept this; what they cannot accept, and what most rational investigative science cannot accept either, is that their emotions are causative or blameworthy for their pain state from the very beginning (for good overview see Mendelson, 1995; Banks and Kerns, 1996).

2 Low or depressed mood and other maladaptive alterations in psychological function power-fully influence the health of the body and the perception of pain.

The affective 'pain mechanism' still stands and is in use today to help manual therapy clinicians in their evaluation of factors involved in their patients pain states. It is by no means perfect for two reasons:

1 The affective 'pain' mechanism, in isolation, implies that the emotions are a *primary* source of pain. This is obviously dangerous in the evaluation of pain that is 'physical' in character, in history and in nature. However, to most open-minded people, it is reasonable to link

pain with emotions like sadness, grief, anger, disgust, extreme anxiety, and even love, for it can 'physically' and 'mentally' hurt when you are deeply emotional (see Cassell, 1991; Damasio, 1995; Morris, 1991, for example). Problems arise when a psychological component is used and viewed in terms that disparage and suggest hysteria or even dishonesty and malingering.

2 By only using the word 'affective' it unfortunately omits the 'cognitive' dimensions and factors discussed earlier. Thoughts influence feelings and the interaction of thoughts and feelings influence the perception of pain and the health of the body.

It may be a wise and open-minded step to rename this category 'psychological / mental processing mechanisms' and leave it at that (see Butler and Gifford, 1998).

A Proposal Of How We Should Be Thinking?

Pain is a regular companion to impaired movement. It follows that in order to understand fully the altered movement patterns and loss of range that accompany pain, we need to understand pain in its broadest sense.

Hopefully the reader will realize that pain diagnosis and the management of the patient in pain is not that easy and therefore being unable to help or understand a patient in pain should not be attributed to personal failure by the therapist. We have to face many difficulties, not just in advancing our knowledge about pain, but more importantly in making it useful to the patients we see. In this chapter an attempt has been made to highlight the importance of the cognitive and emotional dimensions of pain as well as attempt to demystify some of the complexities of pain mechanism biology.

One message should be that the continuing search for a passive technique or therapy for pain relief may need re-evaluating. It certainly seems as if the current medical model, that evaluates a disorder in terms of a 'disease' and then targets a therapeutic intervention on it, is not living up to its promise for many patients in pain (Loeser and Sullivan, 1995).

The great irony of this latter part of the twentieth century is that we now know more about pain than ever before, yet the problem is getting mark edly worse. More and more people are *complaining* about ongoing pain and medicine is clearly losing the battle to contain it (CSAG, 1994; Fordyce, 1995; Morris, 1991).

On physiotherapy courses, the question that so often arises is, 'we have identified the mechanism and the source of the problem, now what technique do we use to fix it?' The effect of any successful therapeutic intervention involves a complex interaction of components like personal interaction, security, trust, warmth, interest, empathy, knowledge, faith in the therapist and the technique, expectations, therapist reputation, expense, touch, novelty, technique and the impressiveness of the technique, exercise, planning of goals and coping strategies, restoration of range and strength and so forth. A given patient may respond powerfully to a specific technique done by a specific practitioner. The same technique given in exactly the same physical way by anyone else may be quite impotent. This does not denigrate the power of the physical technique if it is seen as an important physical part that may be essential to the whole atmosphere of 'therapy' or restoration of function. As a Gestalt psychologist would put it, the key is that the whole is not the same as the sum of its individual parts, it is something far greater. Thus, trying to evaluate or scientifically prove the power of a technique on its own, without including the whole atmosphere of 'therapy', is problematic.

The recent Clinical Standards Advisory Group that investigated the current management of back pain recommended an 'increased role and resources for physical therapy for back pain, but this is contingent on resources being used to provide interventions of proven value' (CSAG, 1994, p. 46). Consider how we currently 'prove' the value of an intervention — it is often by attempting, to the best of our scientific ability, to cut out the most powerful dimensions of human suffering — the mental dimensions and their so-called placebo effect. Perhaps what we should be proving is the power of the whole and encouraging therapists to recognize that the atmosphere they create during therapy (including what they physically do) is biological and is the key to successful outcome. It is important with your patients to use the physical and communicative techniques which you feel most comfortable and confident with for that particular patient. It may be with a bias to manual therapy, electrotherapy or simply explaining, advising, setting goals and giving a simple exercise. I imagine that they are the ones that would be shown to be scientifically effective for me with that particular patient, but they could be a total waste of time for the next therapist with the same patient.

Measuring Success in Therapeutic Pain Relief

The last message is that we must be more aware of how we measure our therapy successes and perhaps question whether the fact that the patient walked out with less pain and more range is a real advance or just a timely positive blip that polishes our egos yet is of no real advantage to the overall functional result. What we perceive we are doing may be quite different from reality. For instance, Howe *et al.* (1985) tabulated surgical results for the same patients, using different definitions of satisfactory results. By some definitions the success rate was 50%; by other definitions, almost 100%. The same could probably just as easily apply to physiotherapy interventions if they were measured in different ways and scrutinized. Ultimately, successful outcome has to be seen in terms of restoration of mental and physical function and the re-establishment of a positive role in the family and society – and not wholly contingent on the relief of pain.

Currently there is an underlying and very powerful body of literature that requires us to pay less attention to pain focused and pain relief directed therapy and more to functional recovery and active rehabilitation, especially where problems are beyond the early acute stage (see Fordyce, 1995). What is largely criticized, and is the most important message, is that if patients perceive that they are attending therapy *for it to cure them*, if they have surrendered to the authority and power of medicine/physiotherapy, then we may be inadvertently reinforcing their problem (Pither and Nicholas, 1991) and helping it to become chronic. Physiotherapy is all about providing information, restoring confidence and restoring function by empowering the patient in an optimistic and happy atmosphere.

Conclusions and Key Points

1 Pain is a perception. In this sense its source is always in the brain (Backonja, 1996).

2 Pain is multidimensional; it is more than just hurt, it alters the way we think and feel, it changes our behaviour and it alters our lives and the lives of those around us.

3 Clinicians are urged to have a better understanding of pain mechanisms and to bring the knowledge into the clinic. There are many patients who have pain that their physiotherapists, their doctors and their family and friends cannot understand. The patient is left with a bewildering condition whose validity is often tacitly and cruelly challenged by those around them and society in general. If some steps can be taken to improve our understanding of pain, and our ability to diagnose and explain it to our patients, we will surely emerge with a more constructive approach to its management than we have at present.

4 Much of the current literature on pain is upholding the principles of rehabilitation proposed by the psychology driven cognitive–behavioural approach to pain states (see Chapter 15) (Gatchel and Turk, 1996; Turk *et al.*, 1983). The integration of these principles into the current physiotherapeutic-driven physical assessment and management skills used in primary care holds considerable promise for the future of the patient with pain (Butler and Gifford, 1998).

5 This chapter, although critical of some current therapy systems, is not suggesting we reject anything physiotherapy has so far evolved. However, it is stongly demanding (as pain science is of us: see Loeser and Sullivan, 1995 and Waddell, 1996) that we question what we

now have in order to move forward. Physiotherapy must continue to develop approaches empowered by hindsight in tandem with open-minded speculation based on up-to-date scientific knowledge. Good science is about making hypotheses but at the same time framing them so they are open to being challenged and capable of being disproved. Contrast this with a 'pseudoscience' approach where the systems and hypotheses are often framed so that they are invulnerable to any experiment that offers a prospect of disproof and where sceptical scrutiny or criticism is often powerfully opposed (see Sagan, 1997).

Further Reading

Butler, DS, Gifford, LS (1998) *The Dynamic Nervous System.* NOI Press, Adelaide. This book represents a distillation and integration of the biology of pain and stress into a clinical model for physiotherapists. It takes many of the theoretical and clinical issues raised here and in the chapter on neurodynamics to a greater breadth and depth and has large practical sections and clinical examples.

Sapolsky, RM (1994) *Why Zebras don't get Ulcers. A Guide to Stress, Stress-related Diseases, and Coping.* Freeman, New York. An ideal start to understanding the biology of stress as it relates to humans!

Melzack, R, Wall, PD (1996) *The Challenge of Pain,* 2nd edition. Penguin, London. The most readable and profound book on pain.

Wall, PD, and Melzack, R (1994) *Textbook of Pain,* 3rd edition. Churchill Livingstone, Edinburgh. The ultimate reference book on pain.

References

Abbas, AK, Lichtman, AH, Pober, JS (1994) *Cellular and Molecular Immunology,* 2nd edition. WB Saunders, Philadelphia.

Ader, R, Felten, DL, Cohen, N (eds) (1991) *Psychoneuroimmunology,* 2nd edition. Academic Press, San Diego.

Arnason, BGW (1993) The sympathetic nervous system and the immune response, in Low, P (ed) *Clinical Autonomic Disorders,* pp. 143–154. Little Brown and Co, Boston.

Backonja, MM (1996) Primary somatosensory cortex and pain perception. Yes sir, your pain is in your head (part 1). *Pain Forum* 5: 171–180.

Banks, SM, Kerns, RD (1996) Explaining high rates of depression in chronic pain: A diathesis–stress framework. *Psychological Bulletin* 119: 95–110.

Bennett, GJ, Roberts, WJ (1996) Animal models and their contribution to our understanding of complex regional pain syndromes I and II, in Janig, W, and Stanton-Hicks, M (eds) *Reflex Sympathetic Dystrophy: A Reappraisal,* pp. 107–122. IASP Press, Seattle.

Birbaumer, N, Flor, H, Lutzenberger, W et al. (1995) The corticalization of chronic pain. In Bromm, B and Desmedt, JE (eds) *Pain and the brain: From nociception to cognition,* pp. 331–343. Raven Press, New York.

Blank, JW (1994) Pain in men wounded in battle: Beecher revisited. *IASP Newsletter* Jan/Feb: 2–4.

Bonica, JJ (1990) Causalgia and other reflex sympathetic dystrophies. In Bonica, JJ (ed) *The Management of Pain,* 2nd edition, pp. 220–243. Lea & Febiger, Philadelphia.

Butler, DS (1991) *Mobilisation of the Nervous System,* Churchill Livingstone, Melbourne.

Butler, DS (1994) The upper limb tension test revisited. In: Grant, R (ed) *Physical therapy of the cervical and thoracic spine. Clinics in Physical Therapy,* Churchill Livingstone, New York.

Butler, DS, Gifford, LS (1998) *The Dynamic Nervous System,* NOI Press, Adelaide.

Campbell, JN, Raja, SN, Meyer, RA (1993) Pain and the sympathetic nervous system: connecting the loop. In Vecchiet, L, Albe-Fessard, D, Lindblom, U et al. (eds) *New Trends in Referred Pain and Hyperalgesia,* pp. 99–108. Elsevier, Amsterdam.

Campbell, JN, Raja, SN, Selig, DK et al. (1994) Diagnosis and management of sympathetically maintained pain. In Fields, HL and Liebeskind, JC (eds) *Progress in Pain Research and Management,* pp. 85–100. IASP Press, Seattle.

Cassell, EJ (1991) *The nature of suffering and the goals of medicine,* Oxford University Press, New York.

Chapman, CR (1995) The affective dimension of pain: A Model, In Bromm, B, and Desmedt, JE (eds) *Pain and the Brain: From nociception to cognition,* pp. 283–301. Raven Press, New York.

Charman, RA (1994) Pain and nociception: mechanisms and modulation in sensory context. In Boyling, JD, Palastanga, N (eds) *Grieve's Modern Manual Therapy,* 2nd edition, pp. 253–270. Churchill Livingstone, Edinburgh.

Chrousos, GP, Gold, PW (1992) The concepts of stress and stress system disorders. Overview of physical and behavioral homeostasis [published erratum appears in JAMA 1992 Jul 8; 268(2): 200]. *Jama* 267: 1244–52.

Coderre, TJ, Basbaum, AI, Levine, JD (1989) Neural control of vascular permeability: interactions between primary afferents, as cells, and sympathetic efferents. *Journal of Neurophysiology* 62: 48–58.

Coderre, T, Chan, AK, Helms, C et al. (1991) Increasing sympathetic nerve terminal-dependent plasma extravasation correlates with decreased arthritic joint injury in rats. *Neuroscience* 40: 185–189.

Cohen, ML (1995) The clinical challenge of secondary hyperalgesia. In Shacklock MO (ed) *Moving in on Pain,* pp. 21–26. Butterworth–Heinemann, Australia.

Cook, AJ, Woolf, CF, Wall, PD et al. (1987) Dynamic receptive field plasticity in rat spinal cord dorsal horn following C primary afferent input. *Nature* 325: 151–153.

CSAG (1994) *Report of a Clinical Standards Advisory Group Committee on back pain.* HMSO, London.

Damasio, AR (1995) *Descartes' Error,* Picador, London.

Dawkins, MS (1993) *Through our eyes only? The search for animal consciousness,* WH Freeman, London.

De Souza, EB (1993) Corticotropin-releasing factor and interleukin-1 receptors in the brain-endocrine-immune axis. Role in stress response and infection. *Annals of the New York Academy of Science* 9–27.

Devor, M (1994) The pathophysiology of damaged peripheral nerves. In Wall, PD, Melzack, R (eds) *Textbook of Pain*, 3rd edition, pp. 79–100. Churchill Livingstone, Edinburgh.

Devor, M (1995) Neurobiological basis for selectivity of NA$^+$ channel blockers in neuropathic pain. *Pain Forum* 4: 83–86.

Devor, M, Raber, P (1990) Heritability of symptoms in an experimental model of neuropathic pain. *Pain* 42: 51–67.

Devor, M, Rappaport, ZH (1990) Pain and the pathophysiology of damaged nerve. In Fields, HL (ed) *Pain Syndromes in Neurology*, pp. 47–83. Butterworth-Heinemann: Oxford.

Devor, M, Lomazov, P, Matzner, O (1994) Sodium channel accumulation in injured axons as a substrate for neuropathic pain. In Boivie, J, Hansson, P, Lindblom, U (eds) *Touch, Temperature and Pain in Health and Disease: Mechanisms and Assessments*, pp. 207–230. IASP Press, Seattle.

Deyo, RA, Rainville, J, Kent, DE (1992) What can the history and physical tell us about low back pain? *JAMA* 268: 760–765.

Dielissen, PW, Claassen, ATPM, Veldman, PHJM et al. (1995) Amputation for reflex sympathetic dystrophy. *Journal of Bone and Joint Surgery* 77B: 270–273.

Donnerer, J, Schuligoi, R, Stein, C (1992) Increased content and transport of substance P and calcitonin gene-related peptide in sensory nerves innervating inflamed tissue: evidence for a regulatory function of nerve growth factor in vivo. *Neuroscience* 49: 693–8.

Dougherty, PM, Lenz, FA (1994) Plasticity of the somatosensory system following neural injury. In Boivie, J, Hansson, P, Lindblom, U (eds) *Touch, temperature, and pain in health and disease: Mechanisms and assessments*, pp. 439–460. IASP Press, Seattle.

Dubner, R (1991a) Neuronal plasticity and pain following peripheral tissue inflammation or nerve injury. In Bond, MR, Charlton, JE, Woolf, CJ (eds) *Proceedings of the VIth World Congress on Pain*, pp. 263–276: Elsevier.

Dubner, R (1991b) Neuronal plasticity in the spinal and medullary dorsal horns: A possible role in central pain mechanisms. In Casey, KL (ed) *Pain and Central Nervous System Disease: The Central Pain Syndromes*, pp. 143–155. Raven Press, New York.

Dubner, R (1992) Hyperalgesia and expanded receptive fields. *Pain* 48: 3–4.

Dubner, R, Basbaum, AI (1994) Spinal dorsal horn plasticity following tissue or nerve injury. In Wall, PD, Melzack, R (eds) *Textbook of Pain*, 3rd edition, pp. 225–241. Churchill Livingstone, Edinburgh.

Dudai, Y (1989) *The neurobiology of memory*, Oxford University Press, Oxford.

Fernandez, E, Turk, DC (1995) The scope and significance of anger in the experience of chronic pain. *Pain* 61: 165–175.

Fields, HL (1987) *Pain*, McGraw-Hill, New York.

Fields, HL, Basbaum, AI (1994) Central nervous system mechanisms of pain modulation. In Wall, PD, and Melzack, R (eds) *Textbook of Pain*, 3rd edition, pp. 243–257. Churchill Livingstone, Edinburgh.

Flor, H, Turk, DC (1996) Integrating central and peripheral mechanisms in chronic muscular pain. An initial step on a long road. *Pain Forum* 5: 74–76.

Flor, H, Birbaumer, N, Schulte, W et al. (1991) Stress-related EMG responses in patients with chronic temporomandibular pain. *Pain* 46: 145–152.

Flor, H, Schugens, MM, Birbaumer, N (1992) Discrimination of muscle tension in chronic pain patients and healthy controls. *Biofeedback and Self Regulation* 17: 165–177.

Fordyce, WE (1995) *Back pain in the workplace. Management of disability in nonspecific conditions. A report of the task force on pain in the workplace of the International Association for the study of pain*, IASP Press, Seattle.

Galea, MP, Darian-Smith, I (1995) Voluntary movement and pain: Focussing on action rather than perception. In Shacklock, MO (ed) *Moving in on Pain*, pp. 40–52. Butterworth-Heinemann, Chatswood.

Gamsa, A (1994a) The role of psychological factors in chronic pain I. A half century of study. *Pain* 57: 5–15.

Gamsa, A (1994b) The role of psychological factors in chronic pain. II. A critical appraisal. *Pain* 57: 17–29.

Garfin, S, Rydevik, B, Brown, R (1991) Compressive neuropathy of spinal nerve roots. A mechanical or biological problem? *Spine* 16: 162–6.

Gatchel, RJ, Turk, DC (eds) (1996) *Psychological Approaches to Pain Management: A Practitioner's Handbook*, Guildford Press, New York.

Gifford, LS (1995) Fluid Movement may partially account for the behaviour of symptoms associated with nociception in disc injury and disease. In Shacklock, MO (ed) *Moving in on Pain*, pp. 32–39. Butterworth-Heinemann, Chatswood, Australia.

Goldberger, L, Shlomo, B (1993) *Handbook of stress. Theoretical and Clinical Aspects*, 2nd edition, The Free Press, New York.

Gray, JA (1987) *The psychology of fear and stress*, 2nd edition, Cambridge University Press, Cambridge.

Gross, RD (1992) *Psychology. The Science of Mind and Behaviour*, Hodder & Stoughton, London.

Hadler, NM (1996) If you have to prove you are ill, you can't get well. The object lesson of fibromyalgia. *Spine* 21: 2397–2400.

Handwerker, HO, Reeh, PW (1991) Pain and Inflammation. In Bond, MR, Charlton, JE, and Woolf, CJ (eds) *Proceedings of the VIth World Congress on Pain*, pp. 59–70. Elsevier, Adelaide.

Hanesch, U, Heppelmann, B, Messlinger, K et al. (1992) Nociception in normal and arthritic joints. Structural and functional aspects. In Willis, WDJ (ed) *Hyperalgesia and Allodynia*, pp. 81–106. Raven Press, New York.

Howe, J, Fryomer, JW (1985) Effects of questionnaire design on determination of end results in lumbar spine surgery. *Spine* 10: 804–805.

Janig, W (1996) The puzzle of 'reflex sympathetic dystrophy': Mechanisms, hypotheses, open questions. In Janig, W, and Stanton-Hicks, M (eds) *Reflex Sympathetic Dystrophy: A Reappraisal*, pp. 1–24. IASP Press, Seattle.

Janig, W, McLachlan, EM (1994) The role of modifications in noradrenergic peripheral pathways after nerve lesions in the generation of pain. In Fields, HL, and Liebeskind, JC (eds) *Pharmacological approaches to the treatment of chronic pain: Concepts and critical issues. Progress in pain research and management*, pp. 101–128. IASP Press, Seattle.

Janig, W, Stanton-Hicks, M (1996) *Reflex Sympathetic Dystrophy: A reappraisal*, IASP Press, Seattle.

Johnson, EO, Kamilaris, TC, Chrousos, GP et al. (1992) Mechanisms of stress: a dynamic overview of hormonal and behavioral homeostatis. *Neurosci Biobehav Rev* 16: 115–30.

Jones, M (1995) Clinical reasoning and pain. *Manual Therapy* 1: 17–24.

Jones, MA (1992) Clinical Reasoning in Manual Therapy. *Physical Therapy* 72: 875–884.

Kandel, ER, Schwartz, JH, Jessell, TM (eds) (1995) *Essential of neural science and behavior*, Prentice Hall, London.

Katz, J, Melzack, R (1990) Pain 'memories' in phantom limbs: review and clinical observations. *Pain* 43: 319–336.

LeShan, L (1964) The world of the patient in severe pain of long duration. *Journal of Chronic Diseases* 17: 119–126.

Levine, J, Taiwo, Y (1994) Inflammatory pain. In Wall, PD, and Melzack, R (eds) *Textbook of Pain*, 3rd edition, pp. 45–56. Churchill Livingstone, Edinburgh.

Levine, JD, Dardick, SJ, Roizen, MF et al. (1986a) Contribution of sensory afferents and sympathetic efferents to joint injury in experimental arthritis. *J Neurosci* 6: 3423–3429.

Levine, JD, Taiwo, YO, Collins, SD et al. (1986b) Noradrenaline hyperalgesia is mediated through interaction with sympathetic postganglionic neurone terminals rather than activation of primary afferent nociceptors. *Nature* 323: 158–160.

Levine, JD, Coderre, TJ, Basbaum, AI (1988) The peripheral nervous system and the inflammatory process. In Dubner, R, Gebhart, GF, and Bond, MR (eds) *Proceedings of the Vth World Congress on Pain*, pp. 33–43.: Elsevier Science Publishers.

Levine, S, and Holger, U (1991) What is stress? In Brown, MR, Koob, GF, and Rivier, C (eds) *Stress, neurobiology and neuroendocrinology*, pp. 3–21. Marcel Dekker, New York.

Loeser, JD (1991) What is chronic pain? *Theoretical Medicine* 12: 213–225.

Loeser, JD, Sullivan, M (1995) Disability in the chronic low back pain patient may be iatrogenic. *Pain Forum* 4: 114–121.

Long, DM (1995) Effectiveness of therapies currently employed for persistent low back and leg pain. *Pain Forum* 4: 122–125.

MacLean, PD (1990) *The triune brain in evolution: Role in paleocerebral functions*, Plenum Press, New York.

Main, CJ, Wood, PLR, Hollis, S et al. (1992) The distress and risk assessment method. A simple patient classification to identify distress and evaluate the risk of poor outcome. *Spine* 17: 42–52.

McCubbin, JA (1993) Stress and endogenous opioids: Behavioral and circulatory interactions. *Biological Psychology* 35: 91–122.

McMahon, S, Koltzenburg, M (1990) The Changing role of primary afferent neurones in pain. *Pain* 43: 269–272.

McMahon, SB, Koltzenburg, M (1994) Silent Afferents and Visceral Pain. In Fields, HL, and Liebeskind, JC (eds) *Progress in Pain Research and Management*, pp. 11–30. IASP Press, Seattle.

Melzack, R (1986) Neurophysiological foundations of pain. In Sternbach, RA (ed) *The Psychology of Pain*, 2nd edition, pp. 1–24. Raven Press, New York.

Melzack, R (1991) The gate control theory 25 years later: new perspectives on phantom limb pain. In Bond, MR, Charlton, JE, and Woolf, CF (eds) *Proceedings of the Seventh World Congress on Pain*, pp. 9–21. Elsevier, Amsterdam.

Melzack, R, Casey, KL (1968) Sensory, motivational, and central control determinants of pain: A new conceptual mode. In Kenshalo, D (ed) *The Skin Senses*, pp. 423–443. C C Thomas, Springfield.

Melzack, R, Wall, PD (1965) Pain mechanisms: a new theory. *Science* 150: 971–979.

Melzack, R, Wall, PD (1996) *The Challenge of Pain*, 2nd edition, Penguin, London.

Mendelson, G (1995) Psychological and Psychiatric aspects of pain. In Shacklock, M (ed) *Moving in on Pain*, pp. 66–89. Butterworh-Heinemann, Chatswood.

Merskey, H, Bogduk, N (1994) *Classification of chronic pain*, IASP Press, Seattle.

Meyer, RA, Campbell, JN, Srinivasa, NR (1994) Peripheral neural mechanisms of nocicepetion. In Wall, PD, and Melzack, R (eds) *Textbook of Pain*, 3rd edition, pp. 13–44. Churchill Livingstone, Edinburgh.

Morris, DB (1991) *The Culture of Pain*, University of California Press, Berkeley.

Moskowitz, MA, Cutrer, FM (1994) Possible importance of neurogenic inflammation within the meninges to migraine headaches. In Fields, HL, and Libeskind, JC (eds) *Progress in Pain Research and Management*, pp. 43–49, IASP Press, Seattle.

Nachemson, AL, Bigos, SJ (1984) The Low Back. In Cruess, J, and Rennie, WJR (eds) *Adult Orthopaedics*, pp. 843–937. Churchill Livingstone, New York.

Ochoa, JL, Verdugo, RJ, Campero, M (1994) Pathophysiological spectrum of organic and psychogenic disorders in neuropathic pain patients fitting the description of causalgia or reflex sympathetic dystrophy. In Gebhart, GF, Hammond, DL, and Jensen, TS (eds) *Proceedings of the Seventh World Congress on Pain, Progress in Pain Research and Management*, pp. 483–494. IASP Press, Seattle.

Ohrbach, R, McCall, WD (1996) The stress-hyperactivity pain theory of myogenic pain. Proposal for a revised theory. *Pain Forum* 5: 51–66.

Panksepp, J, Sacks, DS, Crepeau, LJ et al. (1991) The psycho- and neurobiology of fear systems in the brain. In: Denny, MR (ed) *Fear, Avoidance and Phobias: a Fundamental Analysis*, pp. 7–59. Lawrence Erlbaum, Hillsdale, NJ.

Pennisi, E (1996) Racked with pain. *New Scientist* 9 March: 27–29.

Perl, ER (1992) Alterations in the responsiveness of cutaneous nociceptors. Sensitization by noxious stimuli and the induction of adrenergic responsiveness by nerve injury. In Willis, WDJ (ed) *Hyperalgesia and Allodynia*, pp. 59–79. Raven Press, New York.

Pettipher, ER, Higgs, GA, Salmon, JA (1992) Eicosanoids (prostaglandins and leukotrienes). In Whicher, JT, and Evans, SW (eds) *Biochemistry of Inflammation*, pp. 91–108. Kluwer, Dordrecht.

Pither, CE, Nicholas, MK (1991) The identification of iatrogenic factors in the development of chronic pain syndromes: abnormal treatment behaviour? In Bond, MR, Charlton, JE, and Woolf, CJ (eds) *Proceedings of the Seventh World Congress on Pain*, pp. 429–433. Elsevier, Amsterdam.

Pockett, S (1995) Spinal cord synaptic plasticity and chronic pain. *Anesthesia and Analgesia* 80: 173–179.

Price, DD, Mao, J, Mayer, DJ (1994) Central neural mechanisms of normal and abnormal pain states. In Fields, HL, and Liebeskind, JC (eds) *Progress in Pain Research and Management*, pp. 61–84. IASP Press, Seattle.

Quintner, JL, Cohen, ML (1994) Referred pain of peripheral nerve origin: An alternative to the 'myofascial pain' construct. *The Clinical Journal of Pain* 10: 243–251.

Rang, HP, Bevan, S, Dray, A (1991) Chemical activation of nociceptive peripheral neurones. *British Medical Bulletin* 47: 534–548.

Rang, HP, Bevan, S, Dray, A (1994) Nociceptive peripheral neurons: cellular properties. In Wall, PD, and Melzack, R (eds) *Textbook of Pain*, 3rd edition, pp. 57–78. Churchill Livingstone, Edinburgh.

Rivier, C (1993) Effect of peripheral and central cytokines on the hypothalamic-pituitary-adrenal axis of the rat. *Annals of the New York Academy of Sciences* 697: 97–105.

Rose, S (1992) *The making of memory: From molecules to mind*, Bantam Press, London.

Rose, S (1995) Personal Communication.

Sagan, C (1997) *The Demon-Haunted World. Science as a Candle in the Dark*, Headline, London.

Sapolsky, RM (1994) *Why Zebras don't get Ulcers. A Guide to Stress, Stress-related Diseases, and Coping*, Freeman, New York.

Sato, J, Suzuki, SI, Kumazawa, T (1993) Adrenergic excitation of cutaneous nociceptors in chronically inflamed rats. *Neuroscience Letters* 164: 225–228.

Schaible HG, Grubb, BD (1993) Afferent and spinal mechanisms of joint pain. *Pain* 55: 5–54.

Schaible, HG, Schmidt, RF (1988) Time course of mechanosensitivity changes in articular afferents during a developing experimental arthritis. *Journal of Neurophysiology* 60: 2180–2195.

Schmidt, RF, Schaible, KM, Heppelmann, B et al. (1994) Silent and active nociceptors: structure, functions and clinical implications. In Gebhart, GF, Hammond, DL, and Jensen, TS (eds) *Proceedings of the Seventh World Congress on Pain, Progress in Pain Research and Management*, pp. 213–250. IASP Press, Seattle.

Shortland, P, Woolf, CJ (1993) Chronic peripheral nerve section results in a rearrangement of the central axonal arborizations of axotomized A Beta primary afferent neurons in the rat spinal cord. *Journal of Comparative Neurology* 330: 65–82.

Sluka, KA, Willis, WD, Westlund, KN (1995) The role of dorsal root reflexes in neurogenic inflammation. *Pain Forum* 4: 141–149.

Smith, T, Cuzner, ML (1994) Neuroendocrine-immune interactions in homeostasis and autoimmunity. *Neuropathology and Applied Neurobiology* 20: 413–422.

Spitzer, W, LeBlanc, Fea (1987) Scientific approach to the assessment and management of activity-related spinal disorders, Report of the Quebec Task Force on Spinal Disorders. *Spine* 12: S1–S59.

Stanton-Hicks, M, Janig, W, Hassenbusch, S et al. (1995) Reflex sympathetic dystrophy: changing concepts and taxonomy. *Pain* 63: 127–133.

Tanelian, DL, Victory, RA (1995) Sodium channel-blocking agents. Their use in neuropathic pain conditions. *Pain Forum* 4: 75–80.

Torebjork, E, Wahren, L, Wallin, G et al. (1995) Noradrenaline-evoked pain in neuralgia. *Pain* 63: 11–20.

Turk, DC, Meichenbaum, D, Genest, M (1983) *Pain and behavioral medicine. A cognitive–behavioral perspective*, The Guildford Press, New York.

Udelsman, R, Holbrook, NJ (1994) Endocrine and molecular responses to surgical stress. *Current Problems in Surgery* 31: 653–720.

Valentino, RJ, Foote, SL, Page, ME (1993) The locus coeruleus as a site for integrating corticotropin-releasing factor and noradrenergic mediation of stress response. *Annals of the New York Academy of Sciences* 697: 173–188.

Velo, GP, Franco, L (1993) Non-steroidal anti-inflammatory drugs and pain. In Vecchiet, L, Albe-Fessard, D, Lindblom, U et al. (eds) *New trends in referred pain and hyperalgesia*, pp. 409–415. Elsevier, Amsterdam.

Waddell, G, Turk, DC (1992) Clinical assessment of low back pain. In Turk, DC, and Melzack, R (eds) *Handbook of Pain Assessment*, pp. 15–36. Guildford Press, New York.

Waddell, G, McCulloch, JA, Kummel, E et al. (1980) Nonorganic physical signs in low-back pain. *Spine* 5: 117–125.

Walker, AE, Nulsen, F (1948) Electrical stimulation of the upper thoracic portion of the sympathetic chain in man. *Archives of Neurology and Psychiatry* 59: 559–560.

Wall, PD (1988) Stability and instability of central pain mechanisms. In Dubner, R, Gebhart, GF, and Bond, MR (eds) *Proceedings of the Fifth World Congress on Pain*, pp. 13–24. Elsevier, Amsterdam.

Wall, PD (1989) Introduction. In Wall, PD, and Melzack, R (eds) *Textbook of Pain*, 2nd edition, Churchill Livingstone, Edinburgh.

Wall, PD (1993) The mechanisms of fibromyalgia: a critical essay. In: Voeroy, H, and Merskey, H (eds) *Progress in Fibromyalgia and Myofascial Pain*, pp. 53–59. Elsevier, Amsterdam.

Wall, PD (1995a) Noradrenaline-evoked pain in neuralgia. *Pain* 63: 1–2.

Wall, PD (1995b) Personal Communication.

Wall, PD (1996a) Comments after 30 years of the gate control theory. *Pain Forum* 5: 12–22.

Wall, PD (1996b) The mechanisms by which tissue damage and pain are related. In Campbell, JN (ed) *Pain 1996 – An updated review. Refresher course syllabus*, pp. 123–126. IASP Press, Seattle.

Wall, PD, Devor, M (1983) Sensory afferent impulses originate from dorsal root ganglia and chronically injured axons: A physiological basis for the radicular pain of nerve root compression. *Pain* 17: 321–339.

Wallin, BG, Torebjork, E, Hallin, RG (1976) Preliminary observations on the pathophysiology of hyperalgesia in the causalgic pain syndrome. In Zotterman, Y (ed) *Sensory functions of the skin in primates*, pp. 489–499. Pergamon Press, Oxford.

Walsh, DA, Wharton, J, Blake, DR et al. (1992) Neural and endothelial regulatory peptides, their possible involvement in inflammation. *International Journal of Tissue Reactions* 14: 101–111.

Watkins, LR, Maier, SF, Goehler, LE (1995) Immune activation: the role of pro-inflammatory cytokines in inflammation, illness responses and pathological pain states. *Pain* 63: 289–302.

Weiner, H (1991) Behavioural biology of stress and psychosomatic medicine. In Brown, MR, Koob, GF, and Rivier, C (eds) *Stress. Neurobiology and neuroendocrinology,* pp. 23–51. Marcel Dekker, New York.

WHO (1980) *International classification of impairments, disabilities, and handicaps,* World Health Organization, Geneva.

Willis, WD (1985) *The pain system: the neurobasis of nociceptive transmission in the mammalian nervous system,* Karger, New York.

Wong, BJ, Crumley, RL (1995) Nerve wound healing. An overview. *Otolaryngologic Clinics of North America* 28: 881–895.

Woolf, CJ (1991) Central Mechanisms of acute pain. I: Bond, MR, Charlton, JE, and Woolf, CJ (eds) *Proceedings of the Seventh World Congress on Pain,* pp. 25–34. Elsevier, Amsterdam.

Woolf, CJ (1994) The dorsal horn: state-dependent sensory processing and the generation of pain. In Wall, PD, and Melzack, R (eds) *Textbook of Pain,* 3rd edition, pp. 101–112. Churchill Livingstone, Edinburgh.

Woolf, CJ, Doubell, TP (1994) The pathophysiology of chronic pain — increased sensitivity to low threshold Aβ-fibre inputs. *Current Opinion in Neurobiology* 4: 525–534.

Woolf, CJ, Shortland, P, Coggeshall, RE (1992) Peripheral nerve injury triggers central sprouting of myelinated afferents. *Nature* 355: 75–78.

Yaksh, TL, Malmberg, AB (1994) Central pharmacology of nociceptive transmission. In Wall, PD, and Melzack, R (eds) *Textbook of Pain,* 3rd edition, pp. 165–200. Churchill Livingstone, Edinburgh.

B

Examination, Assessment and Measurement Techniques

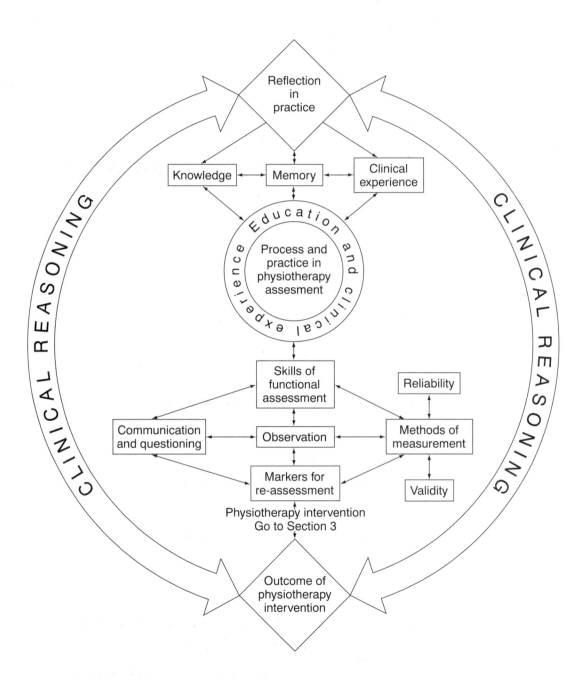

6

Clinical Reasoning:
Basic Principles of Examination and Assessment

HEATHER REID

Introduction

Definition of Clinical Reasoning: The Cornerstone of Clinical Practice

In order to solve the problems that challenge us every day in our lives we use a process of reasoning. This process requires relevant knowledge, experience and reflection.

Clinical reasoning in physiotherapy is the cornerstone of clinical practice (Maitland, 1986) and is dependent upon a process of cognition (reflective inquiry). The specialist knowledge and experience required by physiotherapists, for the purpose of clinical reasoning, relate to the function of human movement.

> The clinical reasoning process is a description of the actions and evolving thoughts used by a clinician to arrive at a diagnostic and management decision and subsequently administer and advance the patient's treatment. (Jones, 1994)

The process of clinical reasoning is used throughout the assessment and subsequent treatment of the patient. It allows us to make professional decisions and helps to justify our therapeutic interventions.

This chapter aims to highlight the keys to examination and assessment by clinical reasoning. Clinical examples are used throughout to illustrate the process.

Chapter Objectives

After reading this chapter you should be able to:

- Understand the major components of the clinical reasoning process;
- Appreciate the key elements required for successful clinical reasoning;
- Create opportunities in your own clinical practice to help develop your reasoning skills;
- Demonstrate (and reflect upon) your ability to reason during the assessment and ongoing treatment of your patients;
- Demonstrate (and reflect upon) your ability to actively communicate with your patients;
- Recognize problems that can occur during communication;
- Conduct a focused and informative subjective assessment;
- Use the information retrieved constructively to help direct your physical examination;

- Justify your assessment procedure and subsequent treatment by analysing the outcome;
- Reflect on your management effectiveness.

Models on which Clinical Reasoning is Based

There are a number of models from which the clinical reasoning process has developed. Perhaps the most commonly referred to are discussed by Higgs and Jones (1995). They describe clinical reasoning in the context of three conceptual approaches:

1 Hypothetico-deductive reasoning, which originated mainly in medical research;
2 Pattern recognition or inductive reasoning, otherwise known as intuitive reasoning;
3 Knowledge—reasoning integration. The view within this conceptual approach is that reasoning cannot occur independently of relevant professional knowledge.

Hypothetico-deductive Reasoning

This type of reasoning relates to how we respond to the clues given to us by the patient. As soon as you meet a patient you will perceive a huge amount of relevant information such as age, posture, ability or reluctance to move, willingness to confide information etc. You will make an initial judgement of the patient's problem based on these clues (induction or hypotheses generation) and will then go on to test this (deduction).

Clinical Example

A patient enters the department and may be reluctant to weight-bear on the right leg, which is also held in lateral rotation at the hip throughout the gait cycle. From initial observation you note that there is a problem with the right lower limb and question whether this is the reason the patient has sought treatment. You then test this broad based hypothesis: bearing in mind all the possibilities that might cause this type of posture and gait.

So the data collection exercise continues (it has already begun with your initial observations). In other words you conduct a subjective and a physical examination.

You must remember that the data collection exercise is an *active process* in which you constantly modify your working hypothesis (metacognition). Both the questions you ask and the tests you perform in the physical examination are not just retrieved from a pre-prepared list. Each stage must remain unique in response to the previous information you gained (see Table 6.1).

Pattern Recognition

Part of clinical reasoning includes a process of categorization. Categorization requires the process of grouping or recognizing the similarity between a set of signs and symptoms. You could come across this when dealing with a patient with a specific, single incident — for instance a sprained ankle. You might categorize the severity of the injury in a particular way. This will be done in relation to the familiarity of the injury (expert knowledge/past experience). You may then go on to prescribe treatment according to the category. This is called *forward or inductive reasoning* (Cox, 1988).

Clinical Example

A patient explains the symptoms of his low back pain to you. During the questioning he admits that he was having a problem controlling his bladder and bowel function and that his saddle area felt numb.

Table 6.1
The hypothetico-deductive model highlights the use of the experimental design in clinical reasoning

Hypothesis	With each patient you will formulate a working hypothesis or a presumptive diagnosis
Method	You will then use the method of assessment and subsequent treatment to test out the hypothesis
Materials	Observation, Questioning and functional measurement
Results	The initial and post-treatment (outcome) measurements are recorded and compared
Discussion	The results are considered with regard to your working hypotheses and clusters of clinical relevance deduced
Conclusion	The outcome can be used to strengthen/or challenge outcomes/evidence of effectiveness from past experience and knowledge
Recommendations	These might include either to repeat the experience or consider an alternative should a similar clinical situation arise

You recognize that these are the classic features of a cauda equina nerve entrapment and refer him to the appropriate medical colleague immediately.

Simple uncomplicated problems where the clinical features point to a certain problem/diagnosis rather than a probability/hypothesis allow quick and efficient management (often acceptable with diseases that are of predictable outcome, course and duration).

Let us go back to the patient with the ankle injury. Consider what you might do if the injury does not resolve according to plan, and goes on to become a chronic problem despite early treatment. You may ask yourself what else could be responsible (other than the musculo/skeletal structures at the site) and wish to consider other structures within the region. The superficial peroneal nerve could be a possible source of the problem. Performing a neurodynamic test will clarify this possibility (Butler, 1992). This type of pattern recognition is highlighted by Higgs and Jones (1994) as *backward reasoning* (who cite Patel and Groen (1986) and Arocha (1993)). It relates to how we recognize an ill-fitting pattern and our subsequent strategy to 'make features fit' (Maitland, 1986).

When dealing with a problem of supposedly predictable pathology you might find that treatment may need to be modified to allow for the patient's expectations, motivation and requirements and the possible pre-existence of dysfunction.

Most physiotherapy problems tend to require more complex activity than categorization and pattern recognition. In fact, you should find yourself *always considering the alternatives* whenever you are posed with a clinical problem despite how much the features suggest one particular pathology and treatment protocol.

Knowledge–Reasoning Integration

Without the relevant professional knowledge, the ability to reason clinically would be negligible. Throughout your professional development the emphasis of your knowledge will shift from that of basic sciences (anatomy, pathophysiology, biomechanics and psychology) to clinical sciences which incorporate signs and symptoms.

As a student you exploit your recently acquired skills of basic assessment when presented with a patient. You observe and measure certain movement anomalies by drawing on your basic science knowledge to generate and test multiple hypotheses regarding the cause of the problem. Don't be alarmed if this takes time. With clinical experience you will tend to restructure how this information is stored and will create 'clinical concept clusters' based on abstract clinical categories. It is these abstract categories that form the basis of clinical reasoning. Your ongoing clinical experience will allow you to acquire or accumulate multiple scripts which you recognize more readily and test out; this also helps you to draw conclusions more quickly with experience!

Clinical reasoning is the marrying of the hypothetico-deductive concept with pattern recognition. Higgs and Jones cite the suggestion made by Simon in 1980, that it takes at least ten years to become proficient in this process, as well as the other skills related to professional competence and expertise.

Practical Example
An Analogy: The Kitchen Pantry

How often do people decide to prepare a particular meal from a recipe only to find a supposed vital ingredient is unavailable?

If the person intending to do the cooking is inexperienced s/he will probably have no alternative but to either abandon the project or quickly pop out to the shop for the ingredient.

A more experienced cook might have a closer look at what is available as an alternative to the ingredient and use this instead.

The even more experienced cook might approach the cooking differently: in the first place 'Let's have a look in the pantry first, see what is available, and then decide what to cook'.

The first cook is rather like the novice student hanging on to a set 'recipe' due to lack of experience.

The second cook is more experienced and although still perhaps conscious of a possible set regime is able to consider alternatives.

The third cook is much more adept at the practicalities of assessment, reasoning and dealing with what is found. In other words is able to use the cues from the pantry and his/her knowledge and experience to decide on a line of management.

Keys to Clinical Reasoning

Knowledge

> Recent research in the health sciences has demonstrated that clinical reasoning is not a separate skill that can be developed independently of relevant professional knowledge (Higgs and Jones, 1995)

As an inexperienced clinician, you store an immense amount of basic knowledge such as anatomy, pathophysiology and biomechanics. You need to draw upon this knowledge store when attempting to deduce the patient's problem. Your initial experience of clinical problems will probably be second-hand (case studies) and you use this information to incorporate some degree of pattern recognition. However, with personal experience of a clinical problem you will begin to alter how you structure your knowledge. The knowledge you have already acquired will become more relevant and meaningful and you will begin to store details in the long-term memory in clusters of clinical relevance. This is why you feel you learn so much whilst out of college on clinical experience.

Long-Term Memory

Long-term memory is a database which you access when attempting to analyse a clinical problem. The long-term memory is made up of knowledge (stored in semantic memory) and experiences (stored in episodic memory).

As a student you tend to rely on semantic memory to solve the clinical problem. With experience you will gradually access the more readily available episodic memory (i.e. rely on past experiences of similar patients presenting).

The interaction between the two types of memory needs to be high during problem solving In order to either confirm or modify previous knowledge. It is important for you to cross-reference any clinical information coming from the patient with the knowledge held in semantic memory. Equally when armed with recently acquired knowledge it is important to challenge the reasoning behind present management strategies.

Artistic / Innateness / Natural Feel of the Therapist

It is true to say that some therapists may assess and treat a patient according to their 'gut feeling' and if successful will store the success along with the clinical features (probably in their episodic memory). It is important to try to reason why such an outcome might have occurred and if a logical reason is unavailable (due to lack of current available knowledge) it may be necessary to repeat the experience when faced with a similar clinical problem and record the outcome. If success is repeated it strengthens the link between a set of clinical data and the management of a condition. When this situation occurs you will also probably generate a hypothesis as to the treatment success. Further acquisition of knowledge might reveal why the outcome was successful.

Manual Skills

Without adequate manual skill you will not be able to test out your working hypotheses. This will result in inadequate information retrieval and weaken your ability to progress through the clinical reasoning process effectively.

Manual skills are developed with practice. The use of clinical reasoning will allow you to develop and create manual techniques according to your patients' functional requirements.

Communication Skills With Patients and Colleagues

Whilst reasoning through a clinical problem, it is difficult to access another persons thoughts – or indeed fully bring one's own thoughts to consciousness. You may find it helpful if either your mentor or another colleague interrupts you during a clinical session and asks for your working hypothesis. The thought of this may fill you with dread. The facilitator will need to be selective so as not to disrupt the proceedings, but it may act as a catalyst to the process. Interruption in front of the patient requires considerable sensitivity from the facilitator so that you do not feel undermined. It may be possible to utilize a 'clinical reasoning analysis form' (metacognition form) as part of your assessment and management. This may allow discussion at a less threatening, more convenient time (e.g. at the end of the subjective, physical examination, each treatment or discharge). It provides a script from which you can discuss your findings, perceptions and justify your treatment plan. It also provides you with a record of your thoughts which can easily be accessed in the future. For an example of clinical reasoning form refer to the Appendix at the end of the chapter.

Successful communication with patients in the clinical setting, demands the ability to make sense of the information they give you. Asking pertinent questions means you must actively listen and have made some sense of the previous answers (working hypotheses). This will allow you to access deeper information. This subject will be discussed in detail in the section on looking for clues: Questioning.

Education and Training

It has been argued that clinical reasoning cannot in fact be 'taught'. However, it is possible to accept that teachers or facilitators could help you to develop your reasoning skills by encouraging you to learn in a purposeful manner.

Teaching methods often incorporate clinical reasoning as an integral aspect of the subject area. A case study may be used to illustrate a clinical problem allowing you to reason at each stage of the assessment and ongoing treatment. You may be asked to assess or treat a patient in front of an audience (mentor or peer) or you might be a member of an audience yourself.

Whatever the method utilized, it is imperative that the experience integrates theory and reflection and includes practice and experience; this is often termed 'praxis'. It is also important for you to gain in confidence by reasoning problems that reflect your present abilities and experience (i.e. you do not try to utilize these skills with a clinical problem that is too complex).

Opportunities to encourage reflection need to be created prior, during and after learning activities in order to develop the skills of a 'reflective practitioner' (Schon, 1987). Practical ways of creating these opportunities include:

1 *Metacognition sheets* These are designed to help you to reason the stages of assessment and treatment throughout the procedure (reflection in action) (see example at end of chapter).

2 *Use of a diary* These allow you to record your experiences on a weekly/daily basis (reflection about action).

3 *Learning contracts* You can utilize these to reflect on past experiences and help negotiate opportunities for learning.

4 *Group discussions* These create a forum for you to share experiences with fellow colleagues. It is in this forum that you can discuss a critical incident that you have experienced.

5 *Case studies* This allows the opportunity to present a reasoned problem. Also presenting a problem to others helps to clarify it in your own mind.

6 *Observation* Having the opportunity to observe and question an experienced clinician is extremely valuable; it gives you confidence to question and try out demonstrated procedures. Being observed by an experienced clinician allows you to discuss/reason the present procedure (reflection in practice).

Looking for Clues: Reasoning in Relation to Assessment and Treatment

The first works in clinical reasoning related to medical diagnosis. Clinical reasoning in physiotherapy aims to identify both a diagnostic hypothesis and plan an appropriate treatment strategy.

Remember that clinical reasoning is an ongoing process and does not stop when a working diagnosis has been reached. The patient's problem must be continually reviewed (metacognition) and the result of each intervention analysed to verify its worth.

The methodological and involved approach of

clinical reasoning in relation to assessment is difficult to describe without the liberal use of clinical examples. The following section therefore aims to use clinical examples to illustrate and provoke understanding of the key issues to this concept.

The clinical reasoning approach in the examination of every patient aims to consider the following questions (Jones and Butler, 1991):

- What is/are the source/s of the symptoms and/or dysfunction?
- Are there any contributing factors?
- Are there any precautions/contraindications to physical examination and treatment?
- What is the prognosis?
- What treatment should be selected and what progression is likely?

You will find that each patient assessment becomes a unique experience. Some similarities will emerge from patients examined in the past (pattern recognition) and some clinical symptoms and signs you will encounter for the first time.

It is usual to start the examination by asking the patient a few pertinent questions about their symptoms.

Questioning

The patient will have either been referred by a medical practitioner (if NHS hospital or community sector) or will have made an appointment themselves (if private sector). Whatever the initial route the patient will arrive at the department with some sort of global 'diagnostic label' (e.g. right hip pain/LBP). It will be your task to question the patient in order to gain some initial insight into the features of, and possible cause of, the problem.

Questioning is an extremely important and difficult skill, requiring a high level of personal commitment to every patient. You will need to be able to actively communicate and listen — without prejudice. The better you are at inspiring confidence, the greater the probability of conducting a successful and thorough examination and treatment.

Clinical Example

A stoical patient from whom the therapist did not fully appreciate the irritability and severity of the condition. The physical examination conducted was therefore too vigorous and severely stirred up the patient's symptoms. The patient took days to recover and was reluctant to attend for physiotherapy again.

This happens probably more often than we care to admit. The instances when patients decline to attend following examination are not all related to spontaneous recovery !

Clinical Examples of Problems That Can Occur With Communication

- Asking closed questions

Clinical Example

You are questioning an elderly patient about the behaviour of his stiff and painful ankle in the mornings.

You ask, 'Is your ankle stiff in the mornings?' and the patient replies 'Oh yes —

very' You decide you need to know more about this problem, for instance the duration of the symptoms, so you ask, 'How long for?' and the patient replies, 'For about half an hour until after breakfast.'

You then make the mistake of supposing that the morning **stiffness** is the main problem and do not allow the patient to express what she considers the main problem to be. Much useful information will therefore be lost.

Clinical Example

You are questioning the same patient, as in the previous example, but alternatively you ask, 'What are your ankle symptoms in the morning?' The patient replies, 'Well fine until I put my foot to the floor. I then feel an achy stiffness for about 20 paces which seems to gradually ease.'

You think you must follow this up further and ask, 'What happens then?'

You have covered more options than in the previous example and you can hypothesize that the symptoms could be related to weight bearing possibly following prolonged rest. This you will need to test further.

- Asking leading questions

Clinical Example

You are asking a patient whether he gets any pain in his cervical spine during functional activities. He has replied that he gets no pain during all the activities involving rotation that you mention. You then say, 'So you don't have any problem with driving then?' The patient actually does find turning his head to the right at a T-junction difficult, i.e. a sustained rotational position but your initial questions did not cover this. The patient is reluctant to say, 'Well actually yes' as he assumes this will be an incorrect answer due to the phrasing of your question.

Much useful information will therefore be lost.

- The body's capacity to inform / not reading the clues from body postures

Clinical Example

Your patient has been given a 'global diagnosis of tennis elbow'. He certainly complains of pain over the insertion of the right common extensor tendon and is tender on palpation. You fail to notice that the patient is also tending to hold his right shoulder girdle in some degree of elevation and is reluctant to abduct the same shoulder. You treat the patient locally with ultrasound and for a number of treatments with minimal success. Eventually you consider the possibility of a neurodynamic component and test the radial nerve. The patient announces a very comparable replication of his pain and you go on to treat this problem successfully.

- Nonverbal communication — Not inviting information through closed body posture of the therapist
- Not pursuing a throwaway line or broad comment to seek out the specific information required

Clinical Example

You are questioning a patient about her cervical spine symptoms and she has given much information about her neck and shoulder pain. She then remarks aside that her neck pain is almost as bad as the headaches she has had for the past year. You omit to consider this comment as an **underlying primary source** *of her lower cervical spine problem due to altered movement patterns or muscle imbalance.*

- Not allowing the patient to use his own words or the physiotherapist rephrases for the patient until he begins to feel awkward/confused about his use of language.

Clinical Example

As clinicians we learn a whole new language and sometimes forget how to speak in lay terms. You are asking a patient about his ankle pain. n.b. he is keen on keep fit and gym work. He refers to the pain occurring during 'flexion' of his foot. What he actually means is extension (dorsiflexion) of his ankle. You correct him and he becomes irritated and confused with the terminology.

- Making assumptions (also refer to asking leading questions)

Clinical Example

A patient complains of shoulder pain. You conduct a specific shoulder examination rather than also considering the possibility of cervical spine involvement.

- Not allowing the patient time to explain their problem

Clinical Example

You are behind time due to unforeseen circumstances whilst examining your patient. You are aware that your next patient has arrived. Because of this you start to rush and do not allow the patient to explain their problem. Much information will not be retrieved and the patient will become irritated.

- Attempting to gain sensitive information in an unsuitable environment

Clinical Example

You are examining a woman with backache. You are in a cubicle situation with a curtain around you. Next door a man is being asked about his knee pain and his voice carries in such a way that every answer is audible. You want to retrieve some information regarding your patient's back pain and her menstrual cycle. She is clearly embarrassed by the question and declines to respond to the question openly.

- Biasing

Clinical Example

You are treating a patient for knee pain and are questioning her following the first treatment. You ask, 'Were you any better following yesterday's treatment? The patient feels a postive response is being sought and although her symptoms remain unchanged she answers, 'Yes, just a little.'

Perhaps a better way of phrasing the question might be 'Has there been any change in your symptoms since yesterday?'

The Subjective Element

The patient questioning that takes place is called 'the subjective element'. This is what our medical colleagues refer to as 'history taking'. You are concerned with the patient's history and any predisposing factors that might have led to or influenced the functional problem. However it is useful to establish the patient's symptoms first at the actual time of examination. Informing the patient of this at the beginning of the questioning will prevent the patient from becoming enmeshed in a long tortuous history.

Clinical Example

Suggestion for your opening comments: greeting and exchange niceties. 'Mrs. Brown I see you have come to see me with right hip pain. What I am going to do is ask a few questions about your hip.

*But what I would like to do first is get an initial picture of how your hip is **now** and **then** ask you some questions about your past history.*

The aim of the subjective history is to discover the possible *sources, severity, irritability and contributing factors* that may be responsible for the patient's *symptoms*. These are used to formulate an initial hypothesis (induced) which is then tested in the physical examination (deduced).

The emphasis of the subjective element is not to mindlessly ask questions from a pre-prepared list. Each patient response should focus you as to what to ask next. There are, however, broad templates to which you can refer, depending on the type of patient you are dealing with.

The following section will relate to a patient with disorder of the neuromusculoskeletal system (excluding pathology of the central nervous system).

General Questions

General questions are designed to provide background information and might give you clues to the possible contributing factors of the patient's problem. The main areas you might seek information about are age (gender you will hopefully determine!), occupation, hobbies, home situation and referring physician (see Table 6.2).

Specific Questions about Symptoms

Specific questions about the patient's symptoms will give you the information required to formulate an initial working hypothesis. This will help

Heather Reid

Table 6.2
General questions to ask during the subjective element

Question	Reason for asking
Age?	Will give some idea as to the healing state of tissues
Gender?	Useful for recording/data collection/trends
Occupation?	Might give some insight as to the functioning mechanisms required on a daily basis. If you are unfamiliar with the work it is useful to inquire what the job entails
Is the patient able to work?	Ability to work or effect of work will give some insight regarding the magnitude of the condition.
Does the problem affect the ability to do the job or does work make the problem worse? Useful to ask also how long the patient has been in the job and any previous jobs.	This information may also give clues to the patient's motivation/happiness at work
Hobbies?	Gives some insight into the patient's lifestyle
Does the problem affect the ability to continue with hobbies or make the problem worse? Has the hobby caused the injury?	Gives insight into the magnitude of the condition
Home situation	Gives insight in the level of care/home situation. Particularly relevant if either the condition makes the patient dependent on others or the patient has dependants and is now unable to fulfil this role.
Referring physician	Important to know whom to communicate with regarding the working diagnosis, prognosis, management and outcome (especially important for professional promotion)

you to decide what to test in the physical examination. Symptoms relate to a loss or decrease in functional movement, whatever the reason:

- Pain;
- Altered sensation;
- Weakness;
- Stiffness;
- Depression/anxiety.

The information you need to acquire about the symptoms include: *what* they feel like, *where* they are (site), how *severe* they are, and how they *behave* (including what exacerbates/alleviates the symptoms).

DESCRIPTION AND SITE OF THE SYMPTOMS

You need to obtain a description of the symptoms and where they occur. There may be more

Figure 6.1 Clinical example of a body chart

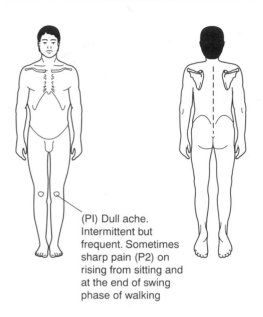

(P1) Dull ache. Intermittent but frequent. Sometimes sharp pain (P2) on rising from sitting and at the end of swing phase of walking

You then need to use your knowledge of anatomy to consider the structures that lie immediately under the site and the structures that could refer symptoms (pain, altered sensation, weakness) to that site (see Table 6.3).

Reason for acquiring information: The description of the symptoms will give you further clues as to their possible source. For instance a 'tingling feeling' is suggestive of nerve involvement, 'weakness' could involve muscle, nerve or joint instability, a 'deep ache' suggests an inflammatory element.

than one site. It is important for you to establish where all symptoms occur and record them in the order in which the patient reports them. It might be useful to give each symptom a number. The usual way of recording the site and description of the symptoms is by use of a body chart (Figure 6.1).

Remember that the symptoms might not always be present so it is also important to establish if the symptoms are intermittent or constant.

SEVERITY OF THE SYMPTOMS

Reason for acquiring information: This will give you an idea of the magnitude of the problem and might indicate caution during the physical examination. There are a number of ways of recording this. The visual analogue scale (VAS) may be utilized to record pain in clinical practice. The severity of weakness or stiffness needs to be physically assessed (see Chapter 6).

Note that severity of pain can be variable depending on the activity etc. It is therefore useful to establish what it is like now, when it is at its best and when it is at its worst (Figure 6.2).

Table 6.3
Structures that refer symptoms to the recorded area, e.g. antero/medial aspect of the knee

Type of structure	Possible offending structure
Muscle	Vastus medialis, semitendinosis, semimembranosis, gracilis, sartorious, adductor magnus
Joint (intra/extra articular)	Tibio-femoral, patello-femoral, hip, sacro-iliac and lumbar spine
Nerve	Saphenous, obturator
Other	Popliteal artery, bursa

Figure 6.2   Body chart with scale of severity of pain

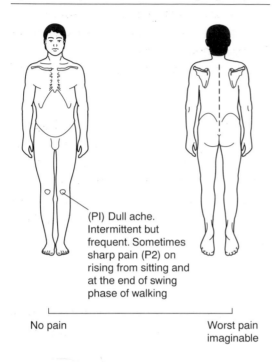

(PI) Dull ache. Intermittent but frequent. Sometimes sharp pain (P2) on rising from sitting and at the end of swing phase of walking

No pain   Worst pain
                                          imaginable

BEHAVIOUR OF THE SYMPTOMS

Irritability of Pain (Table 6.4)

This is an indication of how acute the problem is; in other words what stage in the inflammatory process has been reached. It is a ratio between how easily a symptom is stirred up (exacerbated) with how easily the symptom goes away (alleviated). The word 'easily' includes reference both to time and to the magnitude (aggressiveness) of the *offending functional movement*. For example, throwing a javelin is a more aggressive activity than combing one's hair! Remember you also need to know what the patient does to reduce the symptoms and for how long.

Reason for acquiring information: Establishing the irritability of the pain (along with the severity) will help you to decide the degree of caution required during the physical examination. Indeed the irritability might appear to be so great that you will choose to avoid testing a particular movement altogether.

There are instances when the patient is suffering with a condition that occurs infrequently or momentarily.

Clinical Example

A bowler gets shoulder pain every third over as he releases the ball. It goes away immediately but when it occurs it causes his delivery to be interfered with. This pain is of low irritability due to the on/off nature and the aggressive action required to reproduce his pain. This pain will require more aggressive investigation. If the therapist does not push to limit

Table 6.4
Establishing the irritability of the pain / condition. Example: shoulder pain

Aggravating factor	Easing factor	Irritability	Degree of caution
Lift shoulder joint to 90° 1 s	Hold arm in neutral 2 h	Very high	Extreme? avoid
as above	as above 20 min	High	With care painfree
as above	as above 2 min	Moderate	? examine to pain
as above	as above 2 s	Mod / low	? examine to pain
as above 20 min	as above 2 s	Low	? examine to limit

and consider the combination of movements required in the bowling action she may not reproduce his symptoms on physical examination.

Diurnal and Functional Variation

Symptom behaviour throughout the day and night will give some indication as to the nature of the patient's pain. It is helpful if you establish the change in symptoms: on rising, throughout the day (in relation to functional activity), evening and through the night (see Chapters 4 and 5).

Clinical Example

The presenting functional symptoms of a patient with knee pain and stiffness cause you to suspect he is suffering from early degenerative knee joint pathology. He complains of a dull ache at night (possible venous congestion). He also gets early morning stiffness, eased by moderate activity, which then returns and persists (especially with activities involving weight bearing). Pain symptoms are eased when weight bearing ceases but the stiffness returns.

Specific Questions about the History

You might find it useful to wait until this part of the subjective examination before asking specific history questions. These will include questions about:

- Onset;
- Predisposing factors;

- Duration of the problem;
- Previous incidents and treatment sought;
- Management/treatment to date including any investigations undertaken;
- General health and treatment for medical conditions.

Reason for acquiring the information at this point: It allows you and the patient to remain focused on the problem that initiated the consultation. In retrospect you might require some further information, but often too much information without a useful time reference or basic picture might be impossible to interpret.

ONSET

You will need to know how and when the problem began. Was the onset *insidious or traumatic?*

Insidious Onset

If the condition came on insidiously you will need to establish if there are any predisposing factors that might have caused the condition. You need to establish whether the patient feels the problem is related to **work** or **lifestyle** and if there have been any previous incidents. You need to view the problem from both a physical and a psychosocial perspective (see Chapter 5).

Reason for acquiring this information: This might give insight into the mechanism of injury/tissues involved.

Is the problem work-related?

- Long-term effects of a particular job (e.g. midwifery poor working postures and back pain);
- Recent change of job or change of work environment (e.g. a typist with neck pain has recently moved offices and finds herself answering the telephone more frequently. She

tends to continue to type whilst talking on the phone);

- Stress in the workplace (threat of redundancy, lack of empowerment, shortage of staff).

Could the problem be related to lifestyle?

- Long-term effects of a particular activity (e.g. postural effects of gardening on LBP);
- Recent change in lifestyle or activities (e.g. take up a new sport);
- Unusual activity (e.g. move house, decorate, lay patio);
- Stressful change in home situation (e.g. arrival of new baby, divorce, dependent relative requiring physical and / or emotional care).

Has the patient had any previous incident/s or injury?

- Possibly a related injury or incident in the past (whiplash and neck pain − possible impact of impending litigation, fractured femur and LBP);
- If the patient has had previous incidents, are they getting any more frequent? (susceptibility of tissues over time).

Traumatic Onset

When you deal with an initial incident of traumatic onset you must also consider *all the predisposing factors* that might have primed the patients tissues to be vulnerable at the moment of injury.

An injury of traumatic onset is usually easier to untangle, and careful questioning should expose the possible mechanism of injury. It is very important to *establish at exactly what point in the activity* the injury occurred.

Reason for acquiring this information: It is necessary to be specific so that you can identify the actual body posture, load and velocity of an activity. This may give some indication of the struc-

tures involved. It will also help you to identify the specific pattern of movement you will need to assess in the physical examination.

Clinical Example

Right-handed bowler with left SI joint pain. Injuring posture occurred after heel strike of left foot and just after delivery of ball. You will need to analyse this movement and get the patient to recreate this movement pattern in the physical examination (if the irritability allows).

DURATION OF THE PROBLEM

You will need to consider how long the patient has suffered from the problem and reflect upon this along with its features. It is important to establish whether the problem is resolving, getting worse or remaining the same and what the patient has done (or had done!) so far and whether the intervention has been successful.

Reason for acquiring this information: This will give clues as to the point in the pathological process, the body's natural healing mechanisms and the patient's motivation and / or understanding of the condition. If the patient has sought treatment it is usually helpful to establish whether the treatment was helpful or not.

PREVIOUS INCIDENTS AND TREATMENT SOUGHT

If the patient has suffered from previous incidents it will be helpful if you establish when and how often. As mentioned above, it is useful to gain information as to the success or failure of any previous treatment.

Reason for acquiring this information: Previous incidents may indicate an underlying biomechanical or ergonomic fault. Questioning about treatment may give information regarding the cause of the problem or give you some starting point for your initial treatment. On occasion you may find that a previous treatment could have contributed to the condition. This has been well documented with regard to back pain and the prescription of bed rest (Fast, 1988; Deyo, 1991).

MANAGEMENT/TREATMENT TO DATE INCLUDING ANY INVESTIGATIONS UNDERTAKEN

It is always helpful to establish the management and investigations undertaken for the patient with this incident. Points to consider include:

- Drugs prescribed;
- Blood tests;
- X-rays;
- Other body scans, e.g. magnetic resonance imaging (MRI).

Sometimes the treatment already undertaken may indicate caution or contraindicate treatment (or indeed give further general information).

Drugs

Certain drugs may affect the treatment. For instance NSAIDs indicate that the patient is being treated for an inflammatory condition. They reduce the effects of inflammation. The therapist would take this into consideration if wishing to utilize ultrasound in the treatment of this patient, as ultrasound is thought to promote the inflammatory response.

Steroids are drugs that can effect bone matrix and long-term consumption can lead to osteoporosis. Therefore rigorous manipulative procedures would be contraindicated.

Blood tests

Blood Tests can give some indication as to whether there is an inflammatory element to the patient's condition.

Radiographs (X-rays)

These can give information about the joint structure of the patient and might lead the therapist to make a particular clinical decision. However *a word of warning*: radiographs cannot illustrate soft tissue pathology and whilst it may be possible to diagnose an osteoarthritic joint from a radiograph, this might not be the offending structure causing the patient's symptoms.

> Clinical Example
>
> *Osteoarthritic cervical spine where the painful joint was C56 and the osteoarthritic changes were detected at C7 and T1. This could be as a result of stiffness at the level C7 and T1 and thus the level C56 was overcompensating for the movement loss creating an inflammatory incident. In other words the radiograph is unable to detect inflammatory changes.*

Magnetic Resonance Imaging (MRI) Scans

These generally will give information about more of the tissues within the offending area. They are however expensive and therefore sparingly requested.

GENERAL HEALTH AND TREATMENT FOR MEDICAL CONDITIONS

It is useful to ask general questions about the patient's health and past medical history. You might find a specific link between the reason for the patient's referral to you for treatment and their general health. It is unfair to expect the GP to always make the association. Remember some patients will seek your advice directly or have been referred from Accident and Emergency departments. The following list includes examples and is not exhaustive.

Weight Loss for no Apparent Reason
If the patient describes significant weight loss (and they have not been on a reducing diet) you should be suspicious of serious pathology (e.g. carcinoma) and the patient should be referred to a medical practitioner.

Intractable Night Pain
This also might be an indication of serious pathology and the same management as above should be taken (see Chapter 5)

A Past History of Serious Illness
It may be that the patient has suffered in the past from carcinoma of the breast, for example, and is now seeking help for back pain. If the patient describes the two factors mentioned above (weight loss and/or intractable night pain) even to a lesser degree, *be suspicious* and contact the GP with your thoughts.

Bladder and Bowel Dysfunction
You may find that questioning your patient with back pain about their bladder and bowel function reveals a lack of control and some saddle anaesthesia. This is indicative of a cauda equina lesion and requires urgent surgical intervention. You must refer the patient to the appropriate medical colleague.

Long-term Drug Therapy
You will need to establish whether long-term drug therapy has had any relevant effects. For example, a patient who has been on long-term steroids may have osteoporotic changes and care will be required with any manual handling.

Other Medical Conditions
A patient may have a condition which will require care in positioning the patient (e.g. a patient with a heart condition may not be able to lie flat).

Summary: Reasoning Behind the Subjective Assessment

All the activity so far has been related to formulating the initial working hypothesis. This hypothesis has already probably been modified a number of times with respect to the patient's response to questions. However, a summary of the findings so far creates a basic framework from which you can conduct your physical examination. The functional movements to be tested will relate to the structures under suspicion, and the vigour of the examination will relate to the magnitude/irritability/susceptibility of the problem.

The Physical Examination

As already mentioned the subjective assessment formulates the clues/hypotheses that are tested in the physical examination. Like the subjective examination, the physical examination is tailored for every patient and is not a set of mindlessly conducted tests. However, there remain some broad templates to which the therapist can refer.

The physical examination also aims to highlight repeatable measures from which the effects of treatment can be analysed. Of course one can argue that this also will be catered for by symptomatic relief (see section on markers for reassessment below).

The physical examination should be conducted in the same way as the subjective examination. The initial working hypothesis should be constantly modified with respect to the patient's response.

Observation

At the beginning of the chapter we referred to the initial observation you will make of the patient when they first walk into the department. Posture, gait, how they may move, undress, sit, use their body for expression etc. are all noted.

Posture

Further investigation or differentiation is required to discover the reason why a posture has been adopted. Has it been adopted to relieve pain (antalgic posture), is it habitual, or is it due to structural adaptation?

Clinical Example

A patient complaining of neck and right arm pain holds the right shoulder girdle in elevation and the cervical spine in left rotation. Bringing the head back to neutral reproduced the pain (antalgic posture). The right shoulder girdle was higher due to the upper fibres of trapezius becoming shortened (structural? possibly due to long-term protection of the brachial plexus? working hypothesis).

Measurement of Gait / Functional Movement

The subjective examination will lead you to test particular functional movements. The actual sequence of the physical examination (movement testing) will relate specifically to the particular movement problem the patient has. More detail about the patient's movement disorder needs to be established by testing out your initial hypothesis. The outcome of each test will either strengthen or challenge your suspicions.

Remember you have already gone to some lengths to ensure the vigour of the physical examination is appropriate to the patient's condition. It would be unwise to disregard the information you have gained.

During the physical examination, you will need to ask yourself the following questions and refer to the relevant chapters within this book for more specific information about the actual testing procedures.

- Is the range of movement full?
- What does the end of range feel like? (soft? hard?)
- What is limiting range? (weakness, pain, stiffness, obstruction, poor coordination)
- Is the pattern of movement within normal limits?
- Are there any specific conditions I need to implement whilst testing this movement? (weight bearing / loading, repetition, sustained position, time)
- What is the patient's balance like?
- Is the patient's general fitness adding to the problem?
- Is the patient's muscle strength length and power acceptable?
- What do I need to palpate for? (swelling,

Table 6.5

Testing a patient with a movement disorder for sources of problem

1 Source of pain or stiffness	Test movement
Muscles, joint structures, or nerve	Active test
Joint structures, tight muscles or nerve involvement	Passive test
Intra-articular structures	Add joint compression
Peri-articular structures	Add joint distraction
Nerve structures or fascia	Add a remote movement
2 Source of weakness	
Muscles, nerve supply	Active test

temperature changes, muscle spasm, muscle length, bony/joint changes, joint position, stiffness)

You might find it useful to refer to the diagrammatic summaries at the beginning of each section of this book.

When you observe a functional movement disorder you need to test specific movements and attempt to differentiate the possible structures and pathology responsible for the dysfunction. You must always bear in mind the irritability and nature of the problem. Table 6.5 summarizes the possible sources related to a movement disorder.

You might be unsuccessful if you try to reproduce the patient's symptoms when the structure being tested is subjected to an entirely different set of circumstances.

The example below shows that the functional circumstances needed to be recreated.

Clinical Example

A patient complains of a sharp pain on the medial border of the foot during the push-off phase of the gait cycle. You are unable to reproduce the patient's pain on accessory movements of posteroanterior and anteroposterior to the joints along this aspect of the foot. You then add compression and extension to the first metatarsophalangeal (MTP) joint and repeat the accessory movements to this joint – the pain is reproduced.

MEASUREMENT

Where indicated (and possible) you will use the variety of measuring tools available. This is in order to attempt to bring objectivity to the examination and thus create a reliable base from which to reassess. There has been an increasing trend towards 'evidence-based practice' within health care. Thus objective measurement is an area of physiotherapy that has gained much attention in recent years (see Chapters 7 and 8). More research is still required, in order to prove the worth of the various assessment tools available. This in turn could help to provide physiotherapy with measurable evidence for patient intervention.

Markers for Use in Reassessment of the Dominant Features of the Problem

You may find it useful to mark any particularly significant findings that apply to the dominant features of the problem (Maitland suggested the use of an asterisk *). You can then reassess that actual component (muscle strength, range of movement, antalgic posture) following and before any intervention (along with a similar marker related to the symptoms). This will allow you to assess the efficacy of the treatment strategy and analyse whether you were correct in your hypothesis. If you were correct, this in turn will be stored and commented upon as a successful intervention, and will add weight to similar clinical experiences of the past. If the patient does not respond as anticipated it will allow you to take stock of the situation, question your thinking (or possible error in judgement) and consider another line of management. The latter experience should not be considered as a failure on your part but as an opportunity for you to learn and respond to further clues. You will only have failed if you 'plod on regardless, in the hope it will turn out okay in the end'. (Clinical Example opposite.)

Clinical Reasoning: the Future for Physiotherapy

The need for clinical reasoning to be the norm is crucial to the development of the physiotherapy profession. Clinical reasoning in physiotherapy cannot occur without a detailed, relevant knowledge regarding the function of human movement.

Clinical Example

Continuation notes of a patient (teacher) with right shoulder pain.

Date

S *Patient can write on the chalkboard for 1 min before onset of P2.*

O *Elevation through abduction (passive) = 105° before onset of P2.*

A *Subacromial impingement due to poor stabilization of scapular muscles.*

P *PNF (rhythmical stabilizations) to encourage contraction of lower trapezius.*

Following treatment or on reassessment

O *elevation through abduction = 120° before onset of P2.*

Date

S *Patient can write on the chalkboard for 10 min before onset of P2.*

O *Elevation through abduction (passive) = 130° before onset of P2.*

A *Subacromial impingement due to poor stabilization of scapular muscles.*

P *PNF (rhythmical stabilizations) to encourage contraction of lower trapezius.*

Following treatment

O *elevation through abduction = 150° before onset of P2.*

S = Subjective marker, O = Objective marker, A = Analysis of assessment data, P = Plan of treatment.

The development of reasoning skills within the profession will give rise to an increase in clinically related knowledge and thus greater independence. It is important that through this process, a more research-orientated approach leads to the publication of outcomes from both single case studies and the more sophisticated methods of evaluation, such as randomized controlled trials. This will create a more soundly justified, evidence-based approach within physiotherapy.

Of course this chapter has already highlighted how human dysfunction is often multifactorial and unique to the individual involved. This is why every patient can be considered as an experiment.

In essence you would be doing a disservice to your patients if you treat them according to pre-prepared protocols. We should accept that trends may occur and we should always take account of this. However, physiotherapists are usually treating conditions of unpredictable outcome to some degree, which makes working all the more exciting and challenging.

Key Points

- Clinical reasoning cannot be 'taught' as such, but it can be developed by learning in a purposeful manner.
- Clinical reasoning requires both an in-depth specialist knowledge of human function and relevant clinical experience.
- Assessment and treatment of human dysfunction is an active process and requires the ability to reason clinically at all stages.
- Patients often present with problems which are multifactorial in nature. The unravelling of these problems requires the skill of the phy-

siotherapist whose ability lies in dealing with complex problems.
- Given the multifactorial nature of the problems physiotherapists deal with there is a need to create a method by which outcomes can appropriately be assessed. This is an issue for the research underpinning the profession of physiotherapy.

Further Reading

Becker, HS (1962) The nature of a profession: education for professions, in *The Sixty First Yearbook of the National Society for the Study of Education*, part III, pp. 27–46. University of Chicago Press, Chicago.

Edwards, BC (1994) Clinical assessment. The use of combined movements in assessment and treatment. In Twomey, LT and Taylor, JR (eds) *Physical Therapy of the Low Back*. 2nd edn, pp 197–220. Churchill Livingstone, New York.

Gifford, LS (1995) *The Clinical Biology of Aches and Pains*. Course notes. Neuro-Orthopaedic Institute, UK.

Grieve, GP (1981) Clinical features. In *Common Vertebral Joint Problems*, pp. 161–196. Churchill Livingstone, Edinburgh.

Jones, MA (1994) Clinical reasoning process in manipulative therapy. In Boyling, JD, Palastanga, N (eds) *Modern Manual Therapy*, 2nd edn, Churchill Livingstone, Edinburgh.

Jones, MA, Butler, DS (1991) Clinical reasoning. In Jones, DS (ed) *Mobilisation of the Nervous System*. Churchill Livingstone, Melbourne.

Jull, G, Treleaven, Versace, G (1994) Manual examination. Is pain provocation a major cue for spinal dysfunction? *Australian Journal of Physiotherapy* 40: 159–165.

Kendall, FP, McCreary, EK, Provance, PG (1993) *Muscles Testing and Function*, 4th edn. Williams and Wilkins, Baltimore.

Maitland, GD (1994) The Maitland concept: assessment, examination, and treatment by passive movement, in Twomey, LT, Taylor, JR (eds). *Physical Therapy of the Low Back*, 2nd edition. Churchill Livingstone.

Norris, CM (1995) Spinal stabilisation, muscle imbalance and the low back. *Physiotherapy* 81: 61–79, 127–138.

Shacklock, M (1995) Neurodynamics. *Physiotherapy* 81: 9–16.

Terry, W, Higgs, J (1993) Educational programmes to develop clinical reasoning skills. *Australian Journal of Physiotherapy* 39: 47–51.

References

Butler, DS (1991) *Mobilisation of the Nervous System*. Churchill Livingstone, Melbourne.

Cox, K (1988) How to teach clinical reasoning, in *The Medical Teacher*, 2nd edition, pp. 102–107. Churchill Livingstone.

Deyo, RA (1991) Fads in the treatment of low back pain. *New England Journal of Medicine* 325: 1039–1040.

Fast, A, (1988) Low back disorders, conservative management. *Archives of Physical and Medical Rehabilitation* 69: 880–891.

Higgs, J, Jones, M (1995) Clinical reasoning. In *Clinical Reasoning in the Health Professions*, 1st edn, pp. 3–23. Butterworth Heinemann, Oxford.

Jones, MA (1994) Clinical reasoning process in manipulative therapy. In Boyling, JD, Palastanga, N (eds) *Modern Manual Therapy*, 2nd edn, Churchill Livingstone, Edinburgh.

Jones, MA, Butler, DS (1991) Clinical reasoning. In Jones, DS (ed) *Mobilisation of the Nervous System*. Churchill Livingstone, Melbourne.

Maitland, GD (1986) *Vertebral Manipulation*. 5th edn. Butterworths, London.

McKenzie, R (1994) Mechanical diagnosis and therapy for disorders of the low back. In Twomey, LT, Taylor, JR (eds) *Physical Therapy of the Low Back*. 2nd edn, Churchill Livingstone, New York.

Schon, DA (1987) *Educating the Reflective Practitioner*. Jossey-Bass, San Francisco.

APPENDIX: CLINICAL REASONING FORM

(Adapted from Jones, 1994, in *Modern Manual Therapy*, 2nd edn., Churchill Livingstone, Edinburgh, with permission.)

Patient's name _____ Date _____ Physiotherapist _____

For Consideration Following/During Subjective Assessment

Mechanisms of symptoms

Peripherally provoked	Centrally provoked	Autonomic	Affective

Sources of symptoms (ie. possible structures at fault)

Structures directly under the symptomatic area	Structures that can refer into the symptomatic area

Are there any structures that I must ensure to examine on day one?

Is there any commonly associated disorder/syndrome which the above features fit?

Are there any contributing features of note?

Symptom Behaviour

How do you interpret the symptom behaviour?

- Severity

  |_____|_____|

  Low   High

- Irritability

  |_____|_____|

  Non-irritable   Very irritable

Why have you interpreted the above as such?

- Nature

  |_____|_____|

  Inflammatory   Mechanical

What facts support / challenge your initial hypothesis?

Support	Challenge

History

How have you interpreted the symptomatic history?

- Nature of the onset?
- Extent of tissue damage / change
- Progression since onset (stage, rate and stability of the disorder)

Precautions and Contraindications to Physical Examination

Will the disorder be easy / hard to find?

- Do you need to be cautious? _____ If yes, why?
- Do you need to specifically test any structure?
- At what point will you limit your physical examination? Circle appropriate description.

Point of onset / increase in resting symptoms
Partial reproduction of symptoms
Total reproduction of symptoms

- Do you need to consider both active and passive components of movement?
- What is the pattern of the functional movement disorder?
- Are there any clues as to the possible treatment techniques you might employ?

You may now undertake the physical examination

For Consideration Following / During Physical Assessment

The Sources and / or Physical Contributing Factors to the Symptoms

Component	Possible structure at fault	Supporting evidence	Negating evidence

Mechanism of symptoms	Supporting evidence	Negating evidence

- Indicate your principle hypothesis
- Briefly note the key features of the underlying pathophysiology of the disorder

Prognosis
- Note your thoughts regarding prognosis (i.e. favourable and unfavourable features)

7

Clinical Measurement

FRAN POLAK

Chapter Objectives
•
Inroduction
•
Why Measure?
•
Levels of Measurement
•
Measurement Reliability and Validity
•
Errors of Measurement
•
Clinical Measurements Commonly Used in Clinical Practice
•
Summary

Measurement is an essential process for all physiotherapy practitioners in both the clinical field and research practice. Measurements are used during a clinical examination to establish a diagnosis/hypothesis, monitor the progress of the patient, and provide information for the generation of treatment plans. An understanding of measurement techniques and measurement standards allows us to convey information among fellow workers, and evaluate clinical practice and research.

In recent legislation entitled *The Health of the Nation* (Department of Health) there was a call for effective measures of health care, and as providers of health care services we are currently being asked to demonstrate the effectiveness of our interventions to satisfy both purchasers and patients. As we move towards a more rigorous evaluation of our practice we need to incorporate sound measurement techniques, thus adding professional credibility by providing evidence of the efficacy of our work.

Chapter Objectives

This chapter focuses on the theory underlying our measurements. After completing this chapter the reader will have gained an understanding of the following:

- The merits and suitability of subjective and objective data in clinical decision-making;
- The scale/level of measurement used in clinical practice, with reference to appropriate analysis;
- Reliability and validity of measurements with reference to physiotherapy practice;
- Errors involved in clinical measurement.

Introduction

Measurement has been defined as 'the procedure of attributing qualities or quantities to specific characteristics of objects, persons or events' (Polgar and Thomas 1991). Currently in our clinical practice we may make judgements based on well recognized clinical measurements, which are often recorded as numerical data. There are quantitative data, e.g. degrees of joint motion. However, we may also need to measure quantities/qualities other than physical measures which may be less amenable to direct numerical representation. We may be interested in the patient's self-esteem, depression, or level of motivation and we cannot just give these psychological phenomena numbers (see Chapter 15). The method of measurement we choose will depend on the clinical situation, but the measurement technique must be clearly stated and fully explained so that others may judge the appropriateness and adequacy of the measure selected. In addition the measurement procedure should be able to be replicated by others if it is to be of any clinical value, for example a measurement made by one clinician should be able to be repeated by another clinician and a very similar value obtained, assuming the variable measured is unchanged. As therapists we must avoid measurement inadequacies which may lead us to question the validity of the diagnosis given to the patient.

Why Measure?

The main reason why we measure is to communicate our findings between practitioners. For example, rather than simply saying the patient cannot fully extend their right knee, we are able to describe the right knee range of motion as lacking 20° extension. By using more formal measurement we have increased the precision of a visual observation and enabled fellow colleagues to understand our assessment.

It is important to recognize that as soon as we meet a patient, evaluation of that patient commences. This is firstly through personal judgement, experience and intuition. We usually then formally measure some specific characteristics of the patient's movements. This allows us to be more objective.

Rothstein (1985) defines an objective measurement as one that is not affected by the person taking the measurement (assuming that the measurement procedure is carried out correctly), e.g. the limitation of joint range of motion. A subjective measurement may be defined as a measurement that is affected by the measurer, e.g. our patient/therapist relationship. Often it is incorrectly assumed that all objective measures are better than subjective measures. When we assess our patients and use instrumentation we may think we are performing a worthwhile objective measurement yet if it is neither reliable nor valid it may be a waste of valuable clinical time. Whether you adopt objective or subjective measurements will depend on many factors. These may include the variable to be measured, the patient, the degree of privacy and the resources available. However, it is the quality of the measurement undertaken and knowledge of its limitations which are important. These are based on the following:

- The correct level of measurement;
- The application of appropriate analysis;
- Elimination of error.

These issues are addressed in the following sections.

Levels of Measurement

Throughout all the specialist areas of physiotherapy there are measurements that need to be recorded, e.g. range of motion, the distance a patient can walk, peak flow, repetitions completed of an exercise etc. which are then recorded in our treatment notes. Although all the above measurements are in different units they all belong to one of four levels or scales of measurement. It is important to understand which level of measurement you are using, as statistical analysis subsequently performed on the data depends on the measurement level utilized. The classification system for categorizing different measurement falls into four levels. These are:

1 Nominal level;
2 Ordinal level;
3 Interval level and;
4 Ratio level.

Nominal Level

This is the lowest or most basic level of data collected and thus we get least information from it. An example is the number of female and male patients who attend the hospital physiotherapy outpatient department each year. We could collect this patient information on a computer soft-

ware programme by coding the information, for example when entering patient details you could assign 1 for male patients and 2 for female patients. Although numbers have been assigned to the groups they are purely labels and do not represent quantity. In our example we do not imply that 2 'means more' than 1, as the coding could easily be reversed. This is nominal level data and each patient is allocated to a single 'named' group. Assignment must be to one group only and the groups must be mutually exclusive (i.e. a patient cannot belong to more than one group!). The groups must be exhaustive, i.e. there is a group for everyone attending the physiotherapy department. Nominal data do not allow us to imply order or relative merits of belonging to any of the groups. The use we can make of these data is limited to frequency counts, in this example enumerating the number of female and male referrals.

Ordinal Level

The next level of measurement in the hierarchy is the ordinal level. In many ways this is a similar measurement to nominal level in that it has the same operational definitions, i.e. assignments are mutually exclusive and exhaustive. However, an ordinal scale allows us to rank order the data. For example, patients that attend for treatment may answer a questionnaire relating to their first impressions of the service offered (see Figure 7.1).

With ordinal measurements we cannot make any statements regarding the relative size differences between the categories. The difference between fair and good may not be the same as between good and excellent. Ordinal data does, however, tell us the relative ranking of the data, such that we know more information than just asking if first impressions of the department were good or not. As with nominal data the mathematical options

Figure 7.1 Example of a patient questionnaire.

	Excellent	Good	Fair	Poor	Not applicable
Information sent prior to appointment					
Parking facilities					
Directions to department					
Access to department					
Waiting time to see therapist					
Helpfulness of receptionist					

with the data are limited. Statistical tests for use with nominal and ordinal level data are discussed in detail elsewhere (see Clegg, 1991) but it is worth noting that many statistical tests are not permissible with ordinal level data. The best known physiotherapy measurement of ordinal level is the Oxford manual muscle scale (MRC, 1976). Another example encountered in the clinical field is the visual analogue scale of pain, where the intervals between the graduations may vary. These types of scale are often incorrectly used as higher level measurements (interval and ratio).

Interval Level

With an interval level scale there are numerically equal intervals between the measurements. With interval level data there is no absolute zero, rather one is arbitrarily assigned. An example is measurement of temperature with either Fahrenheit or Celsius. 0°C or 0°F does not mean there is no heat at all although 0°C does represent the freezing point of water. Thus interval levels of measurement are more informative than ordinal levels as there are equal intervals between the values and further mathematical computations can be employed.

Ratio Level

This is the highest level of measurement and top of the hierarchy. The ratio level is similar to the interval level of measurement except that it does have a meaningful zero, i.e. zero point on the scale represents a total lack of the quantity being measured. Interval level of measurements because of their lack of a rational zero fail to provide information about the absolute magnitude of the attribute. The classic measurement of temperature illustrates this point. When measuring temperature on a Fahrenheit or Celsius scale an arbitrary zero is applied, which signifies a total absence of heat. However, it is incorrect to conclude that 30°C is twice as hot as 15°C. This difficulty of inappropriate ratios at interval level data can be overcome if we change our data into degrees Kelvin (scale with absolute zero). Then we may correctly work out differences between our measurements.

Many physical measures have a rational zero and are therefore ratio level data, e.g. weight and height. It is permissible to say that a patient who weighs 70 kg is twice as heavy as one who weighs 35 kg. All mathematical computations are permissible with ratio level data, and ratio level data are usually preferable when gathering measurements for research purposes. Another important note is that in the hierarchy of measurement levels, one may manipulate the data into one of a lower level, but the reverse is not possible.

Measurement Reliability and Validity

Definitions

The adequacy or usefulness of a measurement is determined by its reliability and validity.

Reliability is the extent to which a measurement varies under identical conditions, i.e. how repeatable or consistent the measure is.

Validity refers to the degree to which the measurement measures what it is intended to measure.

Each of these terms is expanded below in relation to clinical practice.

Reliability

INTEROBSERVER AND INTRAOBSERVER RELIABILITY

As stated above, a reliable measure is one that produces consistent results when measured repeatedly. In the clinical situation sometimes the *same* observer will repeatedly measure the same measurement (e.g. joint angles following joint replacement) and the variation in these measurements is noted (known as *intraobserver reliability*). Sometimes measurements may be undertaken by two or more observers (known as *interobserver reliability*). This refers to the extent of the variation between *different* observers making the same measurement. Generally the greater the number of observers the greater the opportunity for differences to occur between them. In the busy hospital situation it is not always possible to ensure that a patient is measured by the same observer on different visits, and interobserver reliability should be known. This is important, so that differences in the variable noted can be appropriately attributed either to real change or to errors in measurement.

If change is inappropriately attributed to therapy this is known as a type I error, and if a change is present but not measured it is known as a type II error. These types of error are important in research. Further explanation is beyond the scope of this section except to emphasize that knowledge of the variation and reliability of measurements undertaken enable the therapist to ascertain if the results fall within a clinically acceptable limit, and if clinical judgements can be made from these measurements.

ASSESSING THE REPEATABILITY OF CLINICAL MEASURES

As stated above, a reliable measure is one that produces consistent results when measured repeatedly. This may be referred to as test–retest reliability and is often measured by correlation coefficient. Correlation's describe how closely related one measure is to a second measurement. Correlation coefficients have a range of possible values between +1.0 and −1.0. If a test–retest reliability is reported as 0.95 this would generally indicate that the measurement technique was good, although the interpretation of this depends on the clinical situation to which it is being applied. Two variables which are often thought to be related to each other are height and weight. If these two variables were perfectly related such that the tallest person in your physiotherapy department was the heaviest, and the smallest person in your department was the lightest, we would expect the correlation coefficient to be 1.0. However, in reality we know this perfect correlation does not exist and for example is more likely to be a correlation of 0.6. If two variables are totally unrelated, the correlation coefficient is zero. Correlation's between 0 and −1.0 express a negative relationship. This occurs when increments of one variable are associated with decrements of the other variable. Let us suppose there is a negative relationship between a nurse's age and number of cigarettes smoked. This means that, the older the nurse generally the less she smokes.

The most commonly used correlation index is the product moment correlation coefficient, also referred to as the Pearson's r. The coefficient is computed when measurements are made on interval or ratio data. An important point to stress is that a strongly positive or negative correlation does not mean there is a causal link between the variables.

Despite their popularity in medical journals it is argued by many that correlation coefficients are inappropriate for assessing reliability, or the comparison between an established measurement technique with a new one. The argument is based on several factors:

- Correlation coefficients assess the tendency of two variables to co-vary without respect to scaling differences – one physiotherapist may consistently measure twice the joint angle measured by another physiotherapist during a measurement session yet the correlation would still be high, suggesting good reliability.
- Correlations measure the strength of a relation between variables, not the agreement between them.
- Correlations depend on the range of the quantity in the sample. Generally the wider the range the greater the correlation.
- A statistical test of significance showing two methods of measurement are related is irrelevant to the question of agreement.

An alternative technique described by Bland and Altman (1986) is widely accepted as an appropriate method for assessing the reliability of measurement techniques. Their approach, which is based on graphical techniques and simple calculations, is described together with the relation between this analysis and the assessment of repeatability. The reader is referred to this paper.

Validity

A valid test is one which measures what it is intended to measure!

How do we find out if our measures are valid? If we measure a patient several times and get the same result we know the test is reliable, but this does not imply the test is valid. To help us to consider whether a measure is valid we can approach the issue from a number of different angles.

1 We can consider the content of the measurement, or its *content validity*;
2 We may consider the relationship between the measurement and an external criterion: *criterion-related validity*.
3 We can establish *construct validity*.

CONTENT VALIDITY

Content validity is used mostly in the design of tests of knowledge in specific content areas. Consider the exams at the end of your first year of physiotherapy training. These may have been the only measure of student performance thus determining the grades attained. For the examinations to have been valid they needed to reflect adequate sampling from the entire first year course content. For example, the anatomy exam should have included questions on joints, nerves and muscles. If, however, the examination only included questions relating to muscle action the exam would not have content validity. If there has been adequate sampling of the content area, these exams are then said to be valid. This is based on the examiner's judgement and not an objective method of assessing adequate content coverage. So content validity describes the sampling adequacy of the content area being measured. This kind of validity may be important to consider in clinical situations where questionnaires are being devised to gain clinical information.

CRITERION-RELATED VALIDITY

Whereas content validity relied on judgements and expert opinions, criterion-related validity compares the relationship between the obtained measurement and some external criterion. Validity is established if the scores correlate highly.

Sometimes a distinction is made between the types of criterion-related validity.

Predictive Validity
Predictive validity refers to the adequacy of a measurement and infers something about some future criterion. For example, when the physiotherapy school correlates incoming students' 'A' level results with the subsequent degree level attained, the predictive validity of the 'A' level grade for physiotherapy degree performance is being evaluated.

Concurrent Validity
Concurrent validity deals with whether an inference is acceptable at the present time. When measurements are made of muscle strength after spinal injury, we can say something about the patient at the time of the test, but this does not allow us to predict their future muscle strength and to what extent recovery will occur.

CONSTRUCT VALIDITY

Construct validity is an important concept in the research and psychology fields. It is difficult to have objective criterion for concepts such as anxiety, grief, or empathy yet we often deal with these issues daily. Construct validity helps us tackle these difficult issues. However, it is beyond the scope of this text to describe construct validity in detail. The reader is referred to Rothstein (1985).

Errors of Measurement

Measurements always contain error, as all our measuring tools are fallible. Therefore,

Measurement score obtained
= real score ± error

The error of measurement is the difference between the true (hypothetical perfect measurement) and the obtained score. The difference results from a number of extraneous factors including the following.

Incorrect Use of Equipment If the directions for obtaining a measure are not clearly understood by the therapist or patient this will introduce more error into the measurement. For example, when obtaining a peak flow measurement if the therapist does not give the correct instructions and the patient gently exhales for a short period the scores obtained would reflect this ambiguity and misunderstanding.

Situational Factors Measurements obtained from patients are often affected by the conditions under which they are taken. Patients may be reluctant to demonstrate their disability in front of other relatives or carers, if the examination area is not private etc. There may be gender issues of a male therapist treating a female patient. Patients are sometimes swayed in their answers to questions (often not knowingly), to try to please the therapist. Environmental factors may also influence certain measurements, e.g. temperature, humidity, lighting, time of the day measurement is recorded. All these factors need careful consideration when obtaining measurements.

Administrative Differences There may be an alteration in the method of collecting data from one patient to the next. This may create variation in the scores obtained which does not reflect the true variations. For example, one therapist may measure a joint range of motion as soon as the patient arrives, and another therapist may measure the same patient on a different occasion at the end of an exercise session.

Response Bias e.g. Extreme Responses Patients often feel inhibited from giving extreme responses and, are a potential source of error especially in self-reported scores (e.g. questionnaires). If patients have felt unhappy about the treatment they have received they may not feel they can complain, as they may be dependent on therapists again in the future.

Temporary Personal Factors, e.g. Hunger, Fatigue, Mood Many of these factors will influence a patient's measurement as they directly influence the patient's motivation. We all encounter the poorly motivated patient whom we feel could obtain a better functional level yet refuses to cooperate fully.

This list is only intended to illustrate that data collected is susceptible to measurement error. It is not exhaustive. The reader may be able to think of other examples and is referred to Pollit and Hungler (1989) for further discussion.

Key Points

It is important to consider the value of any clinical measurement technique both in terms of its reliability and its validity.

1 *Is the measure reliable — i.e. how repeatable are measures taken by the same tester (intratester reliability) or different testers (intertester reliablity)?*

2 *Is the measure valid — i.e. does it measure what it is intended to measure?*

3 *Have all potential measurement errors been eliminated? If the error margin has been found to be small (through research) compared to change in response to treatment, the measurement may be used confidently.*

Clinical Measurement Commonly Used in Clinical Practice

In clinical practice it is important to recognize the value of the information detailed above. This allows us to assess the worth of the clinical measures upon which we base our hypotheses/diagnosis of a patient's signs and symptoms.

Joint Range of Motion

Assessment of joint range of motion (ROM) is the most commonly used evaluative technique of the physiotherapist (Gajdosik and Bohannon, 1987). This may be by visual observation or by instrumentation. Clinical measurement of joint range of motion allows us to record the present state of the joint motion. It may assist us in diagnosis and the formulation of treatment plans. For example, in rotator cuff impairments during the acute phase, the degree of shoulder joint rotational mobility provides vital information for an accurate diagnosis. In more chronic conditions information about joint mobility may indicate the severity of the disease (e.g. limitation of range of motion in the arthritic joint) and even a guide to the prognosis. Accurate assessment of joint range of motion indicates how treatment is progressing and the efficacy of the treatment. Actual restoration of joint range of motion may in itself be the primary treatment goal. It therefore requires accurate measurement.

GONIOMETRY

Universal Goniometer
The simplest method of measuring joint range of motion is goniometry, the universal goniometer being the simplest tool. It is popular and widely

Figure 7.2   Universal goniometer.

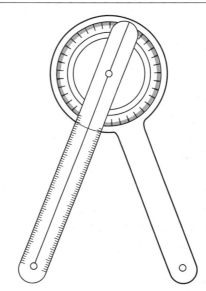

used in clinical practice. The universal goniometer consists of a protractor (usually 360°) with two arms. One is fixed, and the other mobile which rotates about a central axis (Figure 7.2). One arm of the goniometer should be aligned with the axis of the proximal segment and the other arm aligned with the axis of the distal segment. It is usual to hold the fixed arm proximally and in place whilst the joint is moved, and then the distal portion of the goniometer is rotated. After completion of the range of motion the reading is taken from the goniometer. In the treatment notes it is imperative to record if the joint range is passive (therapist moving limb) or active (patient moving limb).

Plastic goniometers have generally replaced the older metal models, being cheap and lightweight. The transparency also allows the arms to be more accurately placed over the bony landmarks. Smaller goniometers are often carried in therapists' pockets despite published work stating the larger ones are more accurate (Robin, 1966).

Whereas the larger universal goniometer is more useful in measuring joint motion at the knee, hip, elbow and shoulder, the smaller goniometers have a role in joint measurement of finger motion. It is worth checking the accuracy of the goniometer against known angles of 0°, 45° and 90°. The author was once given a pocket-sized goniometer by a drugs company that had 5° inaccuracy against known angles – excellent as promotional material, but worthless to the clinician!

Greene and Heckman (1993) write:

> although joint motion can be usually estimated, a goniometer enhances accuracy of measurement and is preferred at the elbow, wrist, finger, knee, ankle and hallux. These joints allow palpation of bony landmarks and reasonable consistent alignment of the goniometer. A goniometer may be used for measuring hip and shoulder motion. The overlying soft tissue, however, does not allow the same degree of repeatability when aligning the goniometer in these areas.

There has been some debate about the importance of the goniometer placement in relation to the joint axis. Accurate placement of the goniometer's axis of rotation has been thought to be essential for accurate measurement. Miller (1985) points out that this argument suggests that the goniometer axis should be aligned with the joint axis, i.e. congruency with the joint axis is absolutely essential for accurate measurement. However, Miller also states that this assumption may be incorrect since most joints have no single identifiable axis. The axes of rotation of joints change as limb segments move through range of motion (e.g. at the knee joint during the gait cycle).

In clinical practice the two goniometer arms are lined up with bony landmarks, and we do aim at placement of the axis of the goniometer with the centre of rotation of the joint. However, if the arms are correctly aligned often the axis of the goniometer is not. We are left with a dilemma that needs a compromise. Most authors suggest we ignore the placement of the goniometer axis after accurately aligning the movement arms, as more consistent placement may be achieved according to the bony landmarks (Miller, 1985).

Fluid-filled Goniometers

Fluid-filled goniometers (or inclinometers) also measure joint motion. They are more expensive than the universal goniometer but have some distinct advantages. They are useful in measuring spinal motion, spinal deformity (rib hump in scoliosis) and motion of the hindfoot. They consist of a 360° protractor in a flat fluid-filled container, which also contains an air bubble. Working on a similar principle to a spirit level, the ROM is read when the fluid is stationary on the protractor (Figure 7.3). They are however less robust than the universal goniometer, being prone to breakage when dropped. Placement on the limb is a large potential source of error, particularly if they are not correctly aligned to a bony landmark. As motion takes place the inclinometer may slip as it is merely strapped to the limb. Another

Figure 7.3   Fluid-filled goniometer. As the joint moves the fluid is inclined and the degree of motion can be measured.

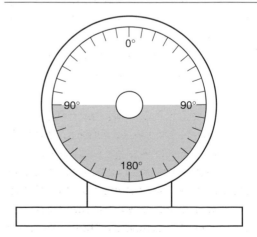

consideration is movement of underlying soft tissues which introduces additional error. A combination of joint motion and soft tissue motion is often mistakenly recorded.

Pendulum Goniometers

Pendulum goniometers consist of a 360° scale to which is attached a weighted pointer. Pendulum goniometers are often strapped to the limb or body segment, and therefore like the inclinometer may be prone to slipping. They seem to be most commonly used for cervical spine motion. The scale and the pointer are both influenced by gravity but operate independently. The dial is locked at the extreme range of motion and after motion has occurred the ROM is registered under the pointer. It is thought the pendulum goniometer is at its most accurate when the patient is upright, otherwise the scale will need adjustment.

Electrogoniometers

An electrogoniometer converts angular motion into an electrical signal. It consists of a potentiometer attached to two arms, with a resistance which varies theoretically linearly with a change in motion of the two arms. The arms of the device are strapped to the limb segments, so the electrical resistance will vary as the joint moves. The device is calibrated to represent joint angles in degrees. Many gait laboratories have constructed their own electrogoniometers, and some are commercially available.

To ensure maximum accuracy the position of the potentiometer is adjusted so that it is as close to the joint axis as possible. A single electrogoniometer will only record measurements in one axis. If joint motion is to be fully monitored, three electrogoniometers need to be worn in the three orthogonal planes. Unfortunately, these may prove cumbersome to the patient, and the trailing straps and cables may inhibit the patient. The fitting and aligning of the electrogoniometers may also be a time-consuming procedure (Pratt, 1991).

The main advantage of electrogoniometers is that they measure dynamic joint motion and they have a role in more sophiticated gait analysis. Electrogoniometers are relatively easy to manufacture and therefore fairly inexpensive. The output signal is immediately available from the device, and from consecutive gait cycles. However, they do take time to attach to the patient and require calibration. Furthermore, as the output from the electrogoniometer is the relative angle between the two arms, when used in a patient with a fixed flexion deformity it may be difficult to decide which angle is taken as zero.

Electrogoniometers are becoming increasingly popular in the clinical setting where measurement of limb segments is not related to other equipment, and the high degree of accuracy found in gait laboratories is not needed.

Strain Gauge Goniometers

A flexible strain-gauge electrogoniometer consists of a flat thin strip of metal which is fixed by endplates to limb segments, either side of the joint to be monitored. The bending of the metal as the joint moves is monitored by strain gauges, with the output from the device depending on the angle between the two endplates. As with electrogoniometers, to record motion in more than one plane additional strain gauges will need to be fixed to the patient.

Standards in Recording Goniometry Measurement

Having obtained the joint range of motion it is usual to compare it against some standard. The most widely used standards, describing both technique and normal joint range, were first published in 1965 by the American Academy of Orthopaedic Surgeons, entitled *Joint Motion: Method of Measuring and Recording*. An updated version of this book is now available and should be a reference text in all physiotherapy departments.

The new version, *The Clinical Measurement of Joint Motion* (AAOS, 1993), advocates that wherever possible the motion of the affected extremity should be judged against that of the opposite side. This is acceptable practice for unilateral acute involvement, but care needs to be taken with measurement in more chronic conditions where adopted patterns of use may have evolved which may alter values on the uninvolved side. Many studies have confirmed that joint motion in healthy subjects is equivalent on the right and left extremity (Boone *et al.*, 1979; Murray *et al.*, 1985).

Figure 7.4   Measurement of knee joint range. Zero starting position: Patient supine with knee extended. Flexion is measured from the zero starting position. Extension/ hyperextension is measured in degrees opposite to flexion from the zero starting position. (Adapted from Greene and Heckman, 1993, *The Clinical Measurement of Joint Motion*, American Academy of Orthopaedic Surgeons, Chicago.)

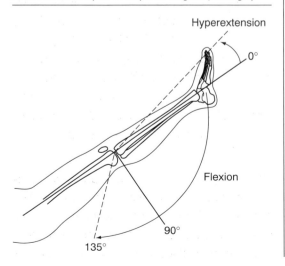

Defining the starting position or zero position for measurement is critical. The most widely used notation system is the 0–180 system (see below). The neutral zero position (Cave and Roberts, 1936), is the extended 'anatomical position' of the extremity and to avoid confusion this position is described as 0° rather than 180°. For example (Figure 7.4) at the knee joint the zero starting position is with the knee extended (straight) with the patient supine. Flexion is measured in degrees of motion towards 180°. Hyperextension may be measured in degrees opposite to flexion from a zero starting position. In an arthritic patient the knee ROM may be from 20° to 100° of flexion actively and from 10° to 115° passively. The usual notation for this would be 20–100 AROM and 10–115 PROM, respectively.

Age and Sex Differences in Joint Range of Motion

Many authors have presented data on 'normal' ROM with considerable variation in their results. Some of the differences may be attributable to variables such as age, gender, cultural differences, and even occupation which all influence joint range of motion. When looking through the literature consider the sample size being reported, and whether it represents a true diversity of backgrounds or a more homogeneous sample. Cheng *et al.* (1991) report that range of motion is slightly greater in children than in adults, probably associated with increased joint laxity that decreases with age. Roach and Miles (1991) evaluated hip and knee motion in healthy adults and reported the difference in motion between the 25- to 39-year-old group and the 60- to 74-year-old group ranged from 3° to 5° in each plane. In the elderly substantial loss of joint range of motion (with or without pain) is abnormal and may not be attributed to age alone.

Practical Note

Whilst reflecting on these issues it is also worth thinking about why we are measuring our patients' range of motion and against what standard we are to compare their performance. Does your patient need full range of motion and do you need to treat him until it is obtained? For example, are you being over-zealous in attempting to rehabilitate shoulder flexion to 170° when your elderly patient has no cupboards that require them to have more than 140° shoulder flexion? Ascertaining how much range of motion a patient functionally needs rather than aiming treatment at 'normal' values is advisable. Remember, range of motion is a contributory factor in functional level and must be considered in relation to balance, muscle strength and posture.

Reliability of Goniometry

Greene and Heckman (1993) report that the variability of joint measurement is greater when a patient is measured by different therapists (intratester variability). Boone *et al.* (1978) report that intratester variability accounted for half the variability recorded when different therapists made measurements. The importance of this observation is that small differences in joint ROM should not be mistakenly interpreted as real change. Boone *et al.* recommend that joint motion measured by goniometry should differ by at least 5° before a real increase or decrease in joint motion has occurred.

Klaber Moffet *et al.* (1989) report on the reliability of an inclinometer for cervical spine movements. They conclude that there were no significant statistical differences in either intraobserver or interobserver measurements. However, they recommend that a change of less than 10° in ROM should not be considered evidence of patient progress or regression.

Goodwin *et al.* (1992) found that the electrogoniometer produced the best results in terms of intertester reliability when compared with the universal goniometer and the fluid goniometer, with Clapper and Wolf (1988) reporting the electrogoniometer as no more accurate than the standard goniometer.

As the reader can see, there is insufficient evidence to promote the use of one type of goniometer above another. In practice, clinical therapists develop preferences depending upon experience, availability of equipment and the area of the body to be measured.

Validity of Goniometry

It is important to consider whether the goniometer can measure the angle formed between the limb segments accurately and whether this represents joint motion. Early studies reporting on joint range of motion have ignored this issue, assuming the validity of goniometry. Gogia *et al.* (1987) compare universal goniometer measurements by therapists with X-rays and found good agreement. Nicol (1989) states that the only method of testing the accuracy / validity of goniometric measures is to refer to skeletal positions using X-rays.

The latter procedure is clearly impractical in clinical practice and clinicians must recognize the limitations of their measurements. It is equally important to find a balance between the requirement for more objective methods of assessment of joint motion and the practical difficulties encountered before discarding methods too quickly.

LINEAR MEASUREMENTS

Linear measurements (i.e. distances) rather than angular measurements may be the technique of choice when motion involves several joints moving simultaneously. For example, measuring the floor to fingertip distance for forward flexion and lateral flexion of the spine are methods occasionally seen in clinical practice. Tape measurement of lateral flexion of the spine was found to be acceptable both for intratester reliability and intertester reliability by Mellin (1986). He reports this measurement as a reliable indicator of spinal mobility for patients with low-back pain (Figure 7.5).

Similarly the modified Schober test for lumbar

flexion may more commonly be used. The modified Schober test is performed by surface marking the midline between the Dimples of Venus on the pelvis. The skin is then marked 5 cm below and 10 cm above this point (Figure 7.6). The patient is instructed to flex fully and the distance between the upper and lower marks is measured by a tape measure. The increased distance (>15 cm) is recorded as lumbar flexion. Clinical studies have shown intratester and intertester reliability to be satisfactory with this method (Fitzgerald *et al.*, 1983).

VISUAL ESTIMATION

Visual estimation of joint range of motion is an easy and cheap technique as no equipment is needed. Every clinician 'eyeballs' joint motion as soon as they encounter the patient. However, when observing rapid motion at more than one joint (e.g. gait) details escape even the most experienced observer. It is important to recognize these limitations.

NOTATION

One of the main aims of measurement is to communicate with other practitioners, so notation and recording of joint range of motion need to be clear, concise, understandable and unambiguous. Notation is *how* motion is described and recording refers to which table, chart or form is used. Most clinicians use the 0–180 system of notation as recommended by the American Academy of Orthopaedic Surgeons (1993). Other notation systems that can be used are the 180–0 system and the 360 system. The latter two systems are not in common usage in the clinical field and further details can be found in Rothstein (1985).

Figure 7.5 Tape measurement of lateral bending to the right. Measurement marks in starting position (A) and the maximum lateral bend (B) position. (Adapted from Mellin, 1986, *Clinical Biomechanics*, 1: 85–89.)

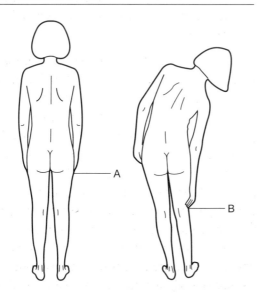

Figure 7.6   Modified Schober Test: start position. A 15 cm span is measured from 10 cm above a line connecting the Dimples of Venus to 5 cm below this line. (Adapted from Greene and Heckman, 1993, *The Clinical Measurement of Joint Motion*, American Academy of Orthopaedic Surgeons, Chicago.)

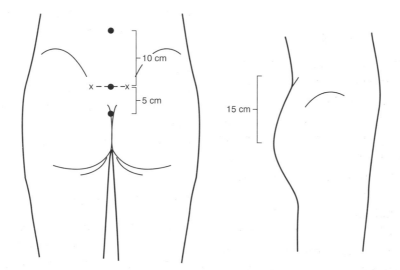

RECORDING

Joint motion is often recorded in the form of tables in the clinical setting. Pre-formatted tables guide the busy clinician to measurements needed to examine the patient.

In more sophisticated movement analysis, for example joint motion during the gait cycle, measurements are often presented in graphical form, which becomes easy to interpret once a basic knowledge of the graphs is obtained. Although this form of measurement is mainly used in research at present, it is becoming increasingly accessible to clinical therapists for their patients.

A system worth noting is the sagittal/frontal/transverse/rotational (SFTR) recording system developed by Gerhardt and Russe (1975) (see Table 7.1). It records motion in each plane, and shortens the recording process. Three numbers are recorded for each plane of motion. The first and last number represent the extreme range of motion, whilst the middle number represents the

starting position (0 for normal motion). Extension, movements away from the trunk, lateral flexion and rotation to the left are recorded first, the reciprocal motion recorded last. For example, fixed flexion of the knee in the sagittal plane of 20 to 100 maximum flexion would be recorded as S 0–20–100. Hyper extension of the knee as opposed to fixed flexion would be recorded as S 10–0–100.

The usage of this system allows clear concise recording of the starting position, as well as joint range. Clinically this is important as a fixed position at one joint will influence motion at both proximal and distal joints. Fixed deformity is recorded as two digits, e.g. a fixed valgus knee deformity would be described by F 20–0 (frontal plane). If the motion occurring was not fixed, i.e. due to ligamentous laxity (20° passive valgus from the neutral position) this would be recorded as (F 20–0–0). If the middle number of the notation is not zero this indicates that the starting position was not neutral, i.e. a contracture. Although this

Table 7.1
An example of recording of ROM by the SFTR notation of shoulder joint motion

Shoulder joint	Degrees	
S	60–0–170	Extension/flexion in sagittal plane
F	184–0–0	Abduction in frontal plane
T	45–0–135	Horizontal abduction/adduction
R (90 frontal plane)	90–0–90	Rotation

notation is not in common usage it does have some advantages, particularly clarity and brevity. However, for it to be widely adopted it requires all clinicians and students to become familiar with the notation.

Muscle Strength

The principle of muscle strength testing makes use of gravity, plus an applied external force to determine the strength of muscles at their maximum voluntary contraction. Muscle strength testing is an integral part of the examination of the patient, remaining a useful assessment tool for both prognostic and diagnostic purposes.

The term muscle strength has various connotations amongst different health care professionals, which often causes confusion. Lamb (1985) has described muscle strength as 'a function of the ability of muscles to develop tension through its long axis'.

MUSCLE TORQUE/MOMENT

It is important to stress that there is no direct measure of muscle tension, so for practical measurement purposes muscle tension is divided into two forces: firstly, the force along the axis of the bone, and secondly the perpendicular force acting to rotate the body segment about an axis (i.e. joint centre). This second force is known as the rotating component, with the rotational effect termed *muscle moment* or *muscle torque*. A muscle moment must overcome the weight of the body segment and any applied forces to maintain the position of the body segment. When testing for muscle strength these variables are critical, with muscle torque varying depending on the muscle length and moment arm. For any useful clinical measure to be derived, there needs to be consistency in the distance the force is applied from the joint axis, and whether gravity is being negated or resisted. Another factor which has to be determined is whether motion is allowed during the strength tests (muscles can generate force isometrically or isotonically) with this being directly related to the role of the muscle being tested, e.g. prime mover, synergist, or antagonist. To test a muscle fully you must test the performance of the muscle in all of these roles. Therefore good clinical muscle strength testing depends on a comprehensive anatomical knowledge, i.e. muscle function and its actions in different starting positions.

MANUAL MUSCLE TESTING

The success of manual muscle testing (MMT) is entirely dependent on rigorous attention to detail during testing. This must include consideration of the patient's position, stabilization of the limb to be tested (and other parts of the body) and the consistent application of the external force to the body segment. The skill and consistency with which the clinician applies the external force is crucial. Resistance must be applied at the same location, with smooth application of the external force in the correct direction. Much relies on the clinician's skill and subjective judgements. A skilled clinician has the ability to ensure the patient is permitted to exert the optimal response. This may come more intuitively to some and through experience to others.

It is evident from the literature that there is a lack of consistency in methodology for many manual muscle tests, with varying starting positions, differing constraints to the patient, differing types of muscle action and points of application of applied resistance. These differences inevitably lead to variations in reported results. Therefore when testing muscle strength it is advisable to record accurately every detail of the test undertaken as well as the result obtained.

In clinical practice the most commonly used method of grading muscle strength is the Medical Research Council (MRC) scale. This is an 0–5 scale:

0 = No active contraction can be detected.

1 = A flicker of muscle contraction can be seen, or found by palpation over the muscle, but the activity is insufficient to cause any joint movement.

2 = Active movement through full range with gravity counterbalanced, by careful positioning of the limb.

3 = Active movement through full range against gravitational resistance.

4 = Active movement through full range against gravity with some added resistance.

5 = Normal power.

This is a useful clinical standard but in practice there are two common errors in its use. Firstly, the scale is intended for use with assessment of concentric muscle activity and not isometric activity. A muscle cannot be tested through range if it is working isometrically! Secondly, there is some ambiguity with regard to the meaning of the term 'through full range'. Most patients who are being assessed in physiotherapy clinics are there because of movement problems. These problems are usually associated with limitation of range of motion as well as muscle dysfunction. It is therefore sensible to interpret the term 'through full range' as 'full available range'. Otherwise, strictly speaking most patients would rarely score more than a grade 1.

For a muscle to attain a grade 5 it must be equal to the contralateral limb if the condition is unilateral, or judged to be the same as that of a person of same age, build and sex as the patient. Often in clinical practice clinicians subdivide the grades further into plus or minus grades (e.g. 4+ or 4−) which adds further subjectivity to the grades. The scale may be useful clinically but it is important to recognize its limitations. Oldham and Howe (1995) suggest that the scales as a whole are insensitive and are not accurate enough for research projects. In fact, in practice, the muscle strength of most patients is covered by only one or two grades (Munsat, 1990). These are usually grades 4 and 5.

Despite the shortcomings of this scale, it remains widely used in clinical practice, as there are no other widely available, more reliable alternatives.

Another scale less commonly used in Britain is one advocated by Kendal and McCreary (1983) based on percentages:

100% Hold against maximum applied force.

80% Hold against gravity and less than maximum applied force.

50% Hold against gravity.

20% Move through small arc of motion with gravity eliminated.

5% Palpable contraction but no movement.

0% No palpable contraction.

This scale can be more easily adapted for use with isometric testing. Like the MRC scale, it is quite specific for the lower grades whereas higher grades require a more subjective judgement.

A problem common to all manual muscle tests is that in order to accurately assess muscle strength at the lower end of the scales the tester requires considerable skill and sensitivity. Without this the tests can be very unreliable.

Reliability of MMT

Due to the increasing demand for objectivity in our clinical measurements, and the widespread use of MMT, there are concerns about the reliability, both as intraobserver (between testers) and interobserver (repeated measures by same therapist) measures. As discussed above the literature is full of conflicting methodology and it is not perhaps surprising that there is generally a lack of agreement on its reliability. Frese *et al.* (1987) report on the reliability of MMT of gluteus medius and the middle fibres of trapezius by 11 physiotherapists. They report that the interobserver reliability was low, with the percentage of physiotherapists obtaining a rating of the same grade (or within one third of a grade) ranging from 50 to 60%. However, Silver *et al.* (1970) standardized testing methods whilst training the physiotherapists on normal subjects. The same physiotherapists then muscle tested patients with 97% agreement, within plus or minus half a grade

over 12 muscle groups. Overall the literature seems to suggest that exact agreement is low, whereas if agreement is considered to be acceptable at plus or minus one grade then percentage agreement rises.

HAND HELD DYNAMOMETERS

Another method of assessing muscle strength which is becoming increasingly available to therapists in the clinical field is that of hand held dynamometry. Dynamometers aim to provide objective data regarding the amount of force used during manual muscle testing. The patient applies a force against the dynamometer which is translated via a strain gauge to give a reading. However, the problems of standardization, stabilization etc., identified above still apply.

Most dynamometers only measure perpendicular force in one plane, with slight angulation of the dynamometer altering the readings. For example, when testing for dorsiflexion it is difficult to place the dynamometer on the dorsum of the foot at exactly the same angle for each repeated test. With hand held dynamometers there are additional concerns relating to the interface between the part being tested and the surface of the dynamometer. As therapists our hands adapt to the surface being tested and experience tells us how much resistance to apply in a smooth consistent manner. If the dynamometer is not correctly positioned on body segment, the patient may experience some discomfort and this makes it unlikely that they will exert optimal force. Difficulties also arise with dynamometer placement when the patient is stronger than you!

Reliability of Hand Held Dynamometers
Again, the literature indicates some conflict in determining reliability of hand held dynamome-

try. Lennon and Ashburn (1993) report large error rates in the inexperienced user, whilst Bohannon and Endemann (1989) report more favourably claiming good intra- and intertester reliability.

Increasing demand for accurate documentation to demonstrate treatment efficacy is leading therapists towards instrument measures of muscle testing. With many types of commercial dynamometers, contradictory reports on the reliability of its use, the feasibility of routine use of a dynamometer remains difficult to judge. From personal experience, reliability is only acceptable when measurements are made in accordance with a strict protocol to which the therapist must rigidly adhere.

ISOKINETICS

A more sensitive mechanical measure of muscle performance may be obtained from isokinetic dynamometers. These provide objective, quantitative measures of both isometric and isotonic muscle strength.

The older isokinetic systems were only capable of measuring the moment generated during concentric and isometric contractions. The latest isokinetic dynamometers have the capacity to drive the limb segment at a pre-set speed during an eccentric contraction. This capability is sometimes termed the 'active' capability of the equipment.

Figure 7.7   Isokinetic system.

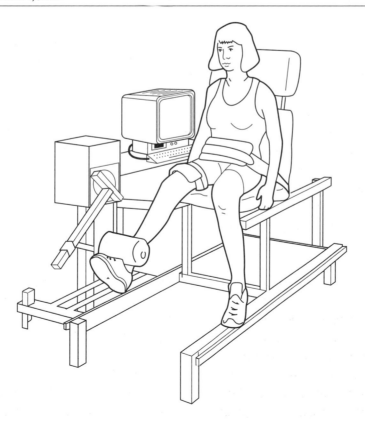

The principles of isokinetic exercise allow the muscle to work at a constant velocity ranging from 1° to 500° per second. The resistance is variable depending on the ability of the muscle to generate force to keep pace with the selected speed. The isokinetic devices measure muscular torque generated during the testing, i.e. when the patient attempts to accelerate past the pre-set instrument speed, the machine resists the movement with accommodating resistance.

An hydraulic load cell measures the torque which is registered on the display. Torque measurements are derived by multiplying the force by the perpendicular distance from the axis of rotation. Usually with isokinetic devices the axis of rotation of the limb is aligned with the mechanical axis of the instrument and the limb and machine act upon each other with the same moment arm (Figure 7.7).

Most studies to date have focused on the lower limb, in particular the knee, but more recently specialized isokinetic machines to study trunk muscle strength have been introduced (Marras and Mirka, 1989). The use of isokinetic devices is increasing in the clinical field, although they are still not commonly found in the physiotherapy department due to the prohibitive costs.

A point worth considering before using isokinetic devices is the level of measurement during isokinetic muscle testing. Torque measurements are often considered of ratio scale (zero indicates an absence of the quantity being measured). Yet, when the patient moves the limb at a slower speed than the device is set, no torque will be recorded (only resistive force is recorded). When the limb speed is below the device speed, the muscles are still developing tension and creating moments which cause the limb to move. However, the isokinetic device only records when critical values are exceeded with these depending on the limb weight, length and velocity settings. Therefore zero measurements do not reflect a total absence of muscle torque, and so the level of measurement should really be considered an interval scale.

Reliability of Isokinetic Devices

As isokinetic devices were the first instruments to measure dynamic muscular activity they have created much interest with several early studies on reliability. More recently with more advanced equipment Walmsley and Pentland (1993) report good reliability when the therapist is familiar with the equipment, the testing procedure and patient instructions. From studies highlighted in other parts of this section it is not surprising that intraobserver reliability is reported to be higher than interobserver reliability (Walmsley and Pentland, 1993).

As with many other physiotherapy measurements the reliability of results is dependent on many factors both physical and psychological, e.g. correct machine calibration, stabilization of the joint to be tested, patient starting position, the degree of other body segment stabilization, the therapist's commands, encouragement, visual feedback to the patient, patient cooperation, patient fatigue etc. All of these variables need consideration and elimination as far as possible from assessments which are undertaken.

Validity

Often two approaches to validity of hardware instruments are used: face validity and criterion-related validity. Face validity is based on subjective opinion and there is little doubt that the isokinetic devices demonstrate face validity. The patient would appreciate this form of validity and participate fully.

Regarding criterion-related validity, i.e. the use of an established instrument for measuring the known phenomenon, and comparison of measure (degree of agreement) between the new instrument and the established instrument, good validity has also been documented. Bodie *et al.* (1990) reported excellent validity when comparing the results obtained from their isokinetic device against known weights suspended from the instrument and calculating the forces applied.

Many early studies have been heavily criticized due to failure to take into account the effect of gravity, with measurements taken in a study with gravity eliminated being higher than those with the effects of gravity included (Winter *et al.* 1981). This has led to some incorrect assumptions regarding muscle strength. The recent generation of isokinetic machines is capable of correcting for the effect of gravity and therefore these difficulties have been addressed.

Another area of controversy remains in the level of measurement obtained. Published papers have expressed maximum torque values in terms of ratios between agonist and antagonist, or comparisons between the different contraction types (concentric/eccentric) within the same muscle. As the isokinetic machines are strictly measuring values of interval scale data these are not suitable for creating ratios.

Outcome Measures

Increasingly, within clinical practice, more evidence is required of the effectiveness of interventions in patient care. This has led to the development of a number of measurements of the 'outcomes' of care.

An outcome measure attempts to assess the effect of the care on the patient. These effects may be both physical and psychological, and can be assessed in individual patients or many patients in specific settings or geographical areas. The issue of outcome measures is a large subject and of increasing interest to those involved in producing evidence to support therapeutic intervention. It can only be covered briefly within this text. However, Ellis and Worthington (1993) provide a good overview of the issues and difficulties of the various approaches to measurement.

Good techniques for the measurement of outcome are difficult to produce. There are differences of opinion as to which are the appropriate indicators of good or bad outcome, and the problem of disentangling the result of the health care variable from the confounding effects of other variables such as socioeconomic and psychosocial factors. Another difficulty is examining the relationship between the care process and the related outcome.

Some outcome studies look specifically at local outcomes deemed as important by clinicians, e.g. follow-up procedures for women with abnormal cervical smears. These outcome measures are clinically focused and quite specific. In this section, techniques will be discussed which include a number of instruments for the measurement of general health care outcomes.

GENERAL HEALTH INDICATORS

These scales are generally self-report questionnaires and measure general health and well-being. Measurement of general health has become more significant as it reflects the aims of care described by the World Health Organization (1958) as 'physical, mental and social well-being and not merely the absence of disease and infirmity'.

One of the best established scales is the Nottingham Health Profile (Hunt *et al.*, 1981), which has 38 questions grouped into six sections on energy level, pain, emotional reaction, sleep, social isolation and physical ability. A large number of general health scales exist, and are used more in the health research context than quality assurance. McDowell and Newell (1987) provide a good review of the scales for readers who wish to pursue further references.

DISABILITY MEASURES

Measures of disability fall into two main groups: firstly indirect measures such as the number of days off work, and secondly scales and questionnaires that measure functional impairment. Earlier tests tended to be based on a description of the impairment, whereas more recent tests are based on the patient's capacity to perform activities of daily living. The most frequently used scale in the UK is the Barthel Index (Mahoney and Barthel, 1965). This is a rating scale, and produces an overall score of between 0 and 100, where 0 denotes complete dependence for the ten aspects of daily living reviewed, and 100 denotes complete independence. The ten aspects of daily living reviewed include, feeding, transfers, toileting, bathing, mobility, dressing and continence. Some clinicians have commented that the Barthel Index lacks sensitivity, but the reliability and validity of the scale are well documented. It is important to note that most of scales used are rating scales and therefore the scoring procedure used and subsequent analysis must relate to that level of the measurement.

PATIENT SATISFACTION MEASURES

Patient satisfaction measures are being used increasingly in health care quality assurance. Difficulties still remain in collecting useful information from these measures. A prime example in patient satisfaction studies is that patients still receiving care may not wish to offend their carers by criticism. Although these measures do have a role, Evason and Whittington (1991) suggest that patient satisfaction surveys are superficial exercises and avoid the harder issues surrounding treatment priorities, quality of life and equity of access.

Summary

Each patient is unique. They have individual characteristics and these affect their suitability for different clinical measurements. It is more important to aim to take measurements in some form rather than disregard the value of a measurement because of a patient's particular characteristics. The therapist should measure appropriately and accurately record the results. In order to accomplish this, it is important to recognize the limitations of measurement and establish the reliability and validity of measurements undertaken.

- Therapists measure to communicate findings between practitioners, provide information for diagnosis and to assess the efficacy of treatment.
- It is important to understand which level of measurement is used as statistical analysis subsequently performed on the data is dependent on the measurement level utilized.
- Its reliability and validity determine the usefulness of a clinical measure.
- The reliability of a measure is the extent to which a measurement varies under identical conditions, i.e. how repeatable the measure is.
- The validity of a measure refers to the degree to which the measurement measures what it is intended to measure.
- Joint range is often measured by goniometry.

The various types of goniometer available in the clinical field, their reliability and clinical use are discussed.

- Recording of joint range measurements can be by the conventional 0–180° system in widespread clinical use, or the SFTR system.

- Muscle strength can be measured by manual muscle tests, or via equipment such as hand held dynamometers or isokinetic dynamometers. The different techniques, their reliability and validity are highlighted.

- Measurement of general health care outcomes is increasingly common, and of great interest to those involved in producing evidence to support therapeutic intervention.

Our profession (as well as others) has been laden with unproven techniques, so as we move forward carefully scrutinizing our own and others' clinical practice, we must have useful measurements. 'A science is only as good as the measurement on which it is based' (Rothstein, 1985).

References

AAOS (1965) *Joint Motion: Method of Measuring and Recording*. American Academy of Orthopaedic Surgeons, Chicago.

AAOS (1993) *The Clinical Measurement of Joint Motion*, Greene, WB, Heckman, JD (eds). American Academy of Orthopaedic Surgeons, Chicago.

Bland, MJ, Altman, DG (1986) Statistical methods for assessing agreement between two methods of clinical measurement. *The Lancet*, 8 February, 307–310.

Bodie, D, Callaghan, M, Green, A (1990) Ergo test 200. A new device for muscle testing and rehabilitation. *Physiotherapy* 76, (7): 412–414.

Bohannon, RW, Endemann, N (1989) Magnitude and reliability of hand held dynamometer measurements within and between days. *Physical Practice* 5 (4), 177–181.

Boone, DC, Azen, SP (1979) Normal range of joints in male subjects. *Journal of Bone and Joint Surgery* 61A: 756–759.

Boone, DC, Azen, SP, Lin, C-M, et al. (1978) Reliability of goniometric measurements. *Physical Therapy* 58: 1355–1390.

Cave, EF, Roberts, SM (1936) A method for measuring and recording joint function. *Journal of Bone and Joint Surgery* 18: 455–465.

Cheng, JC, Chan, PS, Hui, PW (1991) Joint laxity in children. *Journal Paediatric Orthopaedics* 11: 752–756.

Clapper, MP, Wolf, SL (1988) Comparison of the reliability of the Orthoranger and the standard goniometer for assessing active lower extremity range of motion. *Physical Therapy* 68: 214–218.

Clegg, F (1991) *Simple Statistics*. A course book for the social sciences. Cambridge University Press, Cambridge.

Ellis, R, Worthington, D (1993) *Quality Assurance in Health Care. A Handbook*. Edward Arnold, London.

Evason, E, Whittington, D (1991) Patient satisfaction Studies: Problems and Implications Explored in a Pilot Study in Northern Ireland. *Health Education Journal* 50 (2): 73–97.

Fitzgerald, GK, Wynveen, KJ, Rheault, W, et al. (1983) Objective assessment with establishment of normal values for lumbar spinal range of motion. *Physical Therapy* 63: 1776–1781.

Frese, E., Brown, M and Norton B.J. (1987) Clinical reliability of manual muscle testing. *Physical Therapy* 67 1072–1076.

Gajdosik, RL, Bohannon, RW (1987) Clinical measurement of range of motion: review of goniometry emphasising reliability and validity. *Physical Therapeutics* 67: 1867–1872.

Gerhardt, JJ, Russe, OA (1975) *International SFTR Method of Measuring and Recording Joint Motion*. Huber, Bern.

Goodwin, J, Clark, C, Deakes, J. et al. (1992). Clinical methods of goniometry: a comparative study. *Disability and Rehabilitation* 14 (1): 10–15.

Greene, WB, Heckman, JD (eds) (1993) *The Clinical Measurement of Joint Motion*. American Academy of Orthopaedic Surgeons, Chicago.

Gogia, PP, Braatz, JH, Rose, SJ et al. (1987) Reliability and validity of goniometric measurements at the knee. *Physical Therapy* 67: 192–195.

Hunt, SM et al. (1981) The Nottingham Health Profile: subjective health status and medical consultations. *Social Science and Medicine* 15A: 221–229.

Kendall, FP, McCreary, EK (1983) *Muscles. Testing and Function*, 3rd edn. Williams & Wilkins, Baltimore.

Klaber Moffett, JA, Hughes, I, Griffiths, P (1989). Measurement of Cervical Spine Movements Using a Simple Inclinometer. *Physiotherapy* 75 (6): 309–312.

Lamb, RL (1985) Manual muscle testing, in JM Rothstein (ed) *Measurement in Physical Therapy*. Churchill Livingstone, New York.

Lennon, SM, Ashburn, A (1993) Use of myometry in the assessment of neuropathic weakness: testing for reliability in clinical practice. *Clinical Rehabilitation* 7 (2): 125–133.

McDowell, I, Newell, C (1987). *Measuring Health: A Guide to Rating Scales and Questionnaires*. Oxford University Press, New York.

Mahoney, FI, Barthel, DW (1965). Functional evaluation: The Barthel Index. *Maryland State Medical Journal* 14: 61–65.

Mellin, GP (1986) Accuracy of measuring lateral flexion of the spine with a tape. *Clinical Biomechanics* 1: 85–89.

Miller, PJ (1985) Assessment of joint motion. In Rothstein, JM (ed.), *Measurement in Physical Therapy*. Churchill Livingstone, New York.

Mirka, GA, Marra, WS (1989) Trunk Strength during Asymmetrical Trunk Motion. *Human Factors* 31 (6): 1–11.

MRC (1976) *Aids to the Examination of the Peripheral Nervous System*. Medical Research Council, Memorandum No.45. HMSO, London.

Munsat, TL (1990) Clinical trials in neuromuscular disease. *Muscle and Nerve* 13 (suppl): S3–S5.

Murray, MP, Gore, DR, Gardner, GM, *et al.* (1985) Shoulder motion and muscle strength of normal men and women in two age groups. *Clinical Orthopaedics* 192: 268–273.

Nicol, AC (1989) Measurement of joint motion. *Clinical Rehabilitation* 3: 1–9.

Oldham, JA, Howe, TE (1995). Reliability of isometric quadriceps muscle strength testing in young subjects and elderly osteo-arthritic subjects. *Physiotherapy* 81 (7): 399–404.

Pratt, DJ (1991) Three dimensional electrogoniometric study of selected knee orthoses. *Clinical Biomechanics* 6: 67–72.

Polgar, S Thomas, SA (1991). *Introduction to Research in Health Sciences.* Churchill Livingstone, London.

Pollit, DF Hungler, BP (1989) *Essentials of Nursing Research. Methods, Appraisals and Utilisation.* 2nd edn. Lippincott Company, London.

Roach, KBE, Miles, TAP (1991) Normal hip and knee active range of motion: The relationship to age. *Physical Therapy* 71: 656–665.

Robin, P (1966) A method to reduce the variable error in joint range measurement. *Ann Med* 8: 262.

Rothstein, JM (ed.) (1985) *Measurement in Physical Therapy.* Churchill Livingstone, London.

Silver, M, McElroy, A, Morrow, L, Heafer, K (1970) Further stabilisation of manual muscle test for clinical study. Applied in chronic renal disease. *Physical Therapy* 50: 1456.

Walmsley, RP, Pentland, W (1993) An overview of isokinetic dynamometry with specific reference to the upper limb. *Clinical Rehabilitation* 7: 239–247.

Wilnes, CM Karni, Y (1983). The measurement of muscle strength in patients with peripheral neuromuscular disorders. *Journal of Neurology, Neurosurgery and Psychiatry* 46: 1006–1013.

Winter, DS, Wells, RP, Orr, GW (1981) Errors in the use of isokinetic dynamometers. *European Journal of Applied Physiology* 46: 397–408.

8

Gait Analysis

FRAN POLAK

Introduction

Historically gait analysis has often been considered to be performed in two distinct settings, the research laboratory and the clinical setting. Although both have similar aims the approaches used have differed. Traditionally clinicians have often performed gait analysis by simple visual observation, whilst research laboratories have used sophisticated, expensive equipment. However, the distinction between these two activities is lessening due to the very rapid development of instrumentation suitable for routine clinical use. This in turn has resulted in an increasing number of gait laboratories in the UK, which are available both for routine clinical use and for clinically based research. The physiotherapist needs to be aware of these new developments, and appreciate the theory, methods and level of accuracy, of the equipment available. This chapter addresses these issues and describes the various techniques for studying gait. These range from the simple to the very complex. Beside the obvious financial differences, the advantages and disadvantages of each technique will be highlighted.

As both purchasers and providers of health care require increasing evidence of the cost justification of treatments, the discussion will help the reader to evaluate the potential usefulness of gait analysis and help the unwary avoid the many pitfalls. Enthusiasts claim gait analysis quantifies movement, assisting in the selection of appropriate treatment options with the ability to evaluate treatment outcomes objectively (Gage, 1994). Others dispute the application of gait analysis in a clinical setting and regard it as a pure research tool (Watts, 1994).

Chapter Objectives

After reading this chapter you should have an understanding of the following:

1 The gait cycle, and features of an efficient gait;
2 Gait measurement techniques, including observational analysis, footfall measurements, kinematics, kinetics and electromyography;
3 The effect of gait on energy consumption, and ways of calculating energy expenditure;
4 Maturational changes in gait;
5 The impact of musculoskeletal impairments on gait, and how to distinguish between the primary impairment and secondary 'coping mechanisms';
6 The different walking aids and gait patterns used with walking aids;
7 Gait re-education.

Background

Human gait has been a subject of interest as part of medical diagnosis for a long time, yet it is only during the last twenty years that the 'science' of gait analysis has been more widely applied in the clinical setting. Gait analysis is reported to have begun in 1872 when Muybridge developed the technique of using a series of stationary cameras to study the Governor of California's horse running at full speed. Since then there have been many developments in gait analysis technology, not least due to the explosion in the capabilities of computer hardware and user-friendly software. Pioneering work by Vern Inman, David Sutherland, Jacquelin Perry and James Gage in the USA has stimulated interest in clinical gait analysis in the UK. Several gait laboratories now exist in the UK investigating clinical problems in addition to carrying out clinically based research.

Three-dimensional (3D) gait analysis has radically changed the treatment for some neuromuscular diseases, yet gait analysis assessments are still not commonly carried out on patients with walking difficulties. Patrick (1991) suggests the reasons for the unpopularity is complex rather than financial. He states 'technology and applied mechanics are subjects which are anathema to many doctors, so the methods are ill understood'. He further suggests that some research writers of gait analysis reports produce a mass of unintelligible figures and take hours to provide an understandable clinical result. The clinician meanwhile has moved onto the next problem. Indeed, for gait analysis to be successful and to have an impact in the clinical field there needs to be clearly identifiable and measurable objectives, and the derived information needs to be presented to the clinicians in a palatable format.

Proponents of gait analysis claim that with a precise gait assessment all the pathological components of gait are identified, and selection of the appropriate treatment follows, which saves time, money, and unnecessary pain and inconvenience to the patient. Firm scientific evidence supporting these views has yet to be established. There has been no randomized prospective study comparing the outcome of surgery decided by the gait laboratory compared to the outcome decided by observation and interpretation by a clinician without a gait laboratory (Watts, 1994). For the patient gait analysis offers no new treatment options and can be very time consuming – it can even prove intolerable to the patient who tires rapidly. However, the study of a patient's gait is a skill all therapists utilize, through which many treatment and functional outcome measures are planned. A thorough understanding of normal gait provides the background for assessing pathological gait and the successful planning of treatment goals.

The Basic Parameters of Normal Gait

The walking pattern is studied with reference to the gait cycle, which begins when one foot makes contact with the floor and ends when the same foot contacts the floor again. Figure 8.1 shows the gait cycle is divided into a period of stance (ground contact) and a period of swing (no ground contact). The stance phase consists of

Figure 8.1 The subdivisions of the gait cycle.

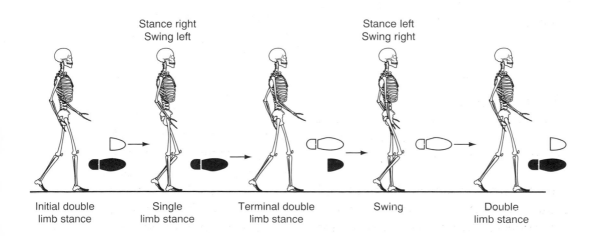

Stance right Swing left   Stance left Swing right

Initial double limb stance   Single limb stance   Terminal double limb stance   Swing   Double limb stance

two periods of double support when both feet make ground contact, plus a period of single support when only one foot is on the ground. Thus in each gait cycle there are two periods of double support and two periods of single support. The complete stance phase usually lasts about 60% of the gait cycle (40% single support phase plus two periods of 10% double support phase), and the swing phase 40% of the gait cycle. The proportion of time spent in each phase varies with walking speed. As speed increases the swing phase becomes proportionally longer, and the single stance and double stance phases shorter (see section on velocity).

Familiarity with the subdivisions or phases of the gait cycle is necessary for the understanding of gait analysis. The gait cycle will only be summarized here as it is described comprehensively by others; see Inman *et al.* (1981), Gage (1991), and Perry (1992).

Some workers divide the gait cycle into actions separating the phases of the normal gait cycle. Whilst this terminology is easily applicable to normal gait, there are difficulties for pathological gait. For example, the action of heel strike denotes the onset of the stance phase in normal gait, yet in pathological gait it may not exist, heel strike being replaced by whole foot contact or forefoot contact. Consequently Perry (1992) has advocated a generic terminology of 'descriptors' for the functional phases of the gait cycle (both normal and pathological) the titles of which will be used in this section. The use of the functional phases of the gait cycle helps identify the integration of movements occurring at individual joints and gives a totality of function of the limb.

The gait cycle is now described in periods of stance and swing. The stance period is further broken down into tasks of weight acceptance and single limb support, with the swing period task comprising limb advancement (Figure 8.2).

Figure 8.2 Divisions of the gait cycle. (Adapted from Perry, 1992, *Gait Analysis, Normal and Pathological Function*, Slack Inc., New Jersey, with permission.)

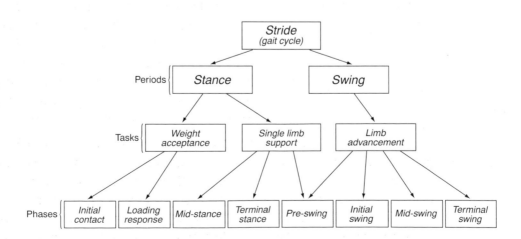

Stance Phase

WEIGHT ACCEPTANCE: INITIAL CONTACT AND LOADING RESPONSE

Initial contact commences the moment the foot touches the floor (0–2% of gait cycle) and the loading response corresponds to the first period of double support (2–10%). Loading response finishes as the contralateral limb is lifted for the swing phase. At initial contact the ankle is in minimal dorsiflexion. The heel is used as the 'first rocker' to lower the foot to the floor, the ankle moves into plantarflexion and forward momentum of the body is maintained. The hip is in approximately 30° flexion. The knee has 7° flexion at initial contact, the knee flexes further to 20° during weight acceptance. In the frontal plane about 5° of adduction occurs and in the transverse plane the knee internally rotates at heel strike. At the hip in the frontal plane transfer of the body weight to the single limb requires lateral stabilization of the pelvis, the abductors contracting stabilize the pelvis and trunk.

SINGLE LIMB SUPPORT: MID-STANCE, TERMINAL STANCE AND PRE-SWING

Mid-stance (10–30%) commences as the contralateral foot is lifted. The body starts to advance over the stationary foot and therefore the ankle dorsiflexes to maintain momentum (the 'second rocker'). Soleus acts eccentrically to control the rate of dorsiflexion. The knee extends to 3° flexion through the mid-stance phase and hip motion is towards extension. The body's centre of mass now reaches its maximum vertical height. The lateral displacement of the pelvis is also at its maximum, about 25 mm from its central position. Trunk rotation is neutral over the pelvis. As the stance phase progresses, the tibia externally rotate, and the subtalar joint causes the midfoot to pronate.

Terminal stance phase (30–50%) commences with heel rise ('third rocker' action) and continues until the contralateral limb makes ground contact. The need for abductor power now dimishes, as the lateral displacement over the single support limb reduces. The body's centre of mass now passes ahead of the forefoot and the foot progresses with the body causing further heel rise. As the heel rises it inverts and the foot then supinates. Maximum hip extension occurs and the knee joint commences rapid flexion.

Swing Phase

Pre-swing (50–60%) corresponds to the second period of double support and final phase of the stance phase. It is a period when the limb prepares for the rest of the swing phase. It commences with ground contact by the contralateral limb and ends with toe-off of the ipsilateral limb. With the onset of double support the body weight is transferred to the other limb, and the ankle plantarflexes to 20°. The power generated by the plantarflexors propels the swing limb forwards. The need for strong stabilization of the limb during stance phase has passed and the knee flexes rapidly to 40° flexion by the end of pre-swing. Hip flexion increases in response to knee flexion having moved quickly from maximum extension into flexion denoting a period of limb acceleration.

Initial swing (60–73%) commences at toe-off and finishes as the advancing limb is level with the stance limb. The swing limb is unloaded and lifted from the ground, acting as a compound pendulum. The ankle moves into dorsiflexion to facilitate foot clearance and the knee joint continues to flex rapidly, reaching a maximum of 60° flexion. Continuation of hip flexion assists the limb in progressing forwards.

Mid-swing (73–87%) starts when the swing limb is opposite the stance limb and finishes when the swing limb is forward of the stance limb and the tibia vertical. The ankle remains dorsiflexed and the hip in flexion to ensure foot clearance; the knee flexion reduces to 30°.

Terminal swing (87–100%) completes the gait cycle. The thigh advancement is curtailed, while the knee continues to extend, reaching maximal extension of 0–5°. The ankle reduces the amount of dorsiflexion and may even go into a few degrees of plantarflexion. The limb is then poised for initial ground contact again.

Spatial and Temporal Gait Parameters

Spatial parameters are a spatial measure (usually in metres) of foot contact during the gait cycle. Figure 8.3 shows the basic spatial parameters.

- *Stride length* is the distance between two successive foot placements. Footwear and a person's height have a direct influence on stride length.

- *Step length* is the distance by which one foot moves in front of the other foot.
- *Stride width* is the perpendicular distance between the midpoints of the heel for consecutive steps.
- *Angle of foot progression* is the angle between a reference line along the midline of the foot and the direction of progression.

The *temporal parameters* reflect the timing of events in the gait cycle and include stance time, swing time, single support stance time, double support stance time, and the entire gait cycle time.

The *combined temporal and spatial parameters* allow the calculation of cadence and walking velocity.

- *Cadence* is the number of steps in a given time, i.e. steps per minute.
- *Velocity* is step length $\times$ cadence, or $\dfrac{\text{stride length}}{2} \times$ cadence, measured in distance travelled per unit time, usually metres per minute.

It is important to remember that velocity of gait will alter the dynamic joint ranges recorded and when comparing two gait cycles velocity should be matched as closely as possible. Always consider the timing of motion, which is crucial for

Figure 8.3   Spatial parameters of gait. (Reproduced from Whittle, 1991, *Gait Analysis, An Introduction*, Butterworth-Heinemann, Oxford, with permission.)

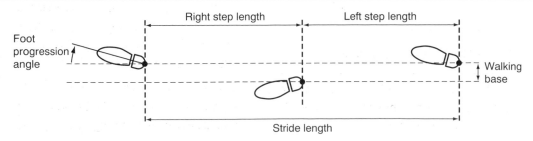

efficient gait. If the patient has minimal knee flexion (e.g. 15°) at the pre-swing phase of gait, and rapid knee flexion occurs only when the limb is unloaded (during swing phase), although the patient may have the correct range of knee motion the gait will be affected by the incorrect phasing of the knee flexion. Loss of joint range and loss of muscle power does not automatically mean that gait will be affected. There is an excess of capacity of both. Perry (1992) observed that the hip abductors only required 40% of full strength for the subject to walk without a limp, and that full knee joint range of motion is 140°, whereas only 60° of motion is needed for an efficient gait pattern.

Key Points

A gait cycle consists of a period of stance (60%) and a period of swing (40%).

Stance phase is further subdivided into two periods of double support (2 × 10%) and one period of single support (40%).

Proportion of time spent in each phase varies with velocity.

Velocity alters joint range.

Footwear influences stride length.

Gait does not require full joint range or full muscle power.

Features of an Efficient Gait

Gage (1991) states that normal gait has five major attributes which are frequently lost in pathological gait (in order of priority):

1 Stability in stance;
2 Sufficient foot clearance during swing;
3 Appropriate swing phase pre-positioning of the foot;
4 Adequate step length;
5 Energy conservation.

Loss of any of these attributes will decrease the efficiency of gait, resulting in an increased energy demand for the patient. The spastic diplegic child who has minimal knee excursion caused by co-spasticity of knee extensors and hamstrings has a very tiring and energy-draining gait. To minimize the additional energy costs the patient may develop secondary or 'coping' mechanisms (e.g. the hemiplegic patient who circumducts the leg to obtain foot clearance in swing). Gait analysis helps identify the loss of the prerequisites for normal gait and assists in separating primary causal gait deviations from secondary deviations. Wasted clinical time is avoided if treatment is aimed at the primary cause of gait deviation and not directed at a secondary response. Permanent harm would be done to the patient if an operative technique eliminated the coping mechanism adopted during gait.

Practical Task

Try walking with fixed plantarflexion at one ankle. Notice how difficult it is to maintain a stable base during stance, and the gait deviations you make during the swing phase. Did you use excessive hip and knee flexion during the gait cycle? Now try walking with limited hip flexion and fixed plantarflexion.

Did you circumduct the swing leg to advance it forwards? Maybe you went into plantarflexion during stance phase with the sound limb (known as vaulting). The difficulty of the task is to recognize which of these gait deviations is primary and which secondary when observed in your patient's gait pattern.

In their classic paper, 'The major determinants of normal gait', Saunders *et al.* (1953) describe human locomotion as 'the translation of the centre of gravity through space requiring the least energy expenditure'. They refer to six determinants for an efficient gait, described as pelvic rotation, pelvic tilt and knee flexion during the stance phase which minimizes the need to lift the head, arms and trunk against gravity. The fourth and fifth determinants are the interaction of the knee and hip during the stance phase ensuring the centre of gravity proceeds in a sinusoidal pathway. The sixth determinant is the lateral displacement of the pelvis, also minimizing the displacement of the

centre of gravity and avoiding sharp inflexions to its pathway. In normal gait the lateral and vertical displacement of the centre of masses is kept to 2.5 mm in each direction, and many of the mechanisms involved in walking are devoted to this task (Figure 8.4). Dec *et al.* (1958) consider that with loss of any one of the major determinants compensation may be reasonably effective (loss of knee determinant most costly) and that the loss of two determinants would make effective compensation impossible and energy costs must be increased. In pathological gait where there is often larger motion of the centre of mass of the body the energy expenditure involved may increase drastically. Butler *et al.* (1984) report the energy requirements for cerebral palsy patients can be three to four times the normal value using the physiological cost index (PCI) as an indicator of energy consumption (described more fully later in this chapter).

Figure 8.4   Centre of mass displacement during the normal gait cycle. (Adapted from Perry, 1992, *Gait Analysis, Normal and Pathological Function*. Slack Inc., New Jersey.)

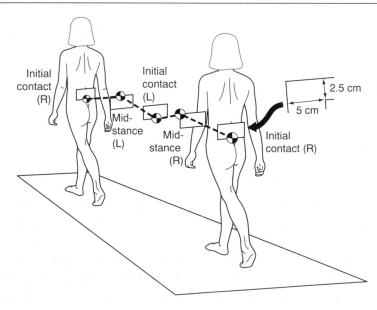

Try walking with very long strides. Note how during the double support stance phase your centre of mass is very low, and this has to be raised more than during your normal gait to its highest point during mid-stance phase (single stance phase). Which is the most tiring — long strides or your normal stride length?

Gage (1991) states that in addition to the three-dimensional excursion of the centre of mass being minimized, two other mechanisms conserve energy: firstly the ability to control momentum by eccentric muscle action, e.g. heel rocker controlling forward momentum; secondly the ability of two joint muscles to transfer energy from one segment to another, e.g. during terminal swing the hamstrings act as decelerators of knee extension prior to ground contact. The forward momentum of the swinging leg is transferred by the hamstrings to forward propulsion of the pelvis.

Measurement Principles and Techniques

In the context of instrumented clinical gait analysis we need to measure force acting on the body, the body position, energy consumption and how these vary over time. To make full use of the data gathered, we need an understanding of the limitations of each measurement system utilized and to ensure that measurements from any of our systems are as good as they can be. We must know if the differences noted in the data are due to the natural phenomenon of human gait (e.g. stride variability) or due to differences/error in the recording system, or the impact of our therapy.

Measurement of gait is never perfect — there is always error (see section on clinical measurement error). Error is introduced not only via the hardware capabilities of the measurement system, but also as a result of the actual measurement influencing the patient's gait and thus altering the very information we seek to collect, e.g. trailing wires attached to the patient may encumber the patient which alters their customary gait pattern. The signals generated in gait analysis are continuous in time, yet digital computers have finite storage capacities; therefore sampling must be performed at discrete time intervals. The sampling rate should be optimal — over-sampling can give rise to data storage and handling problems whilst under-sampling may cause crucial events in the gait cycle to be missed.

Practical Task

Try observing a friend walking along whilst slowly blinking your eyes. Note how certain points of the gait cycle are not seen. Information from these times may be crucial. Now observe your partner without blinking. Your sampling rate has increased and information about the gait cycle improved.

With all gait analysis techniques the reliability and validity of measurements are also limited by the resolution of the instrumentation (minimal distance or time by which two measurements may differ), and the frequency response (ability of the system to respond to time-varying inputs). The next section looks more closely at different measurement systems and highlights the advantages and limitations of each technique.

Observational Gait Analysis

This is a qualitative method of assessing gait, and is the commonest form of gait analysis in the clinical field. The aim is to identify gait deviations in patients by visual observation. This identification depends on the clinician's skills and a good knowledge of normal gait. Although observational gait analysis is used on a daily basis, no standardized observational gait analysis system is in universal use (see Moulin, 1995). Clinicians tend to develop their personal approach even though systematic gait evaluation forms are available. The best known of these is the Rancho Los Amigos Observational Gait Analysis System, developed by Perry (1992). It is in the form of a handbook including instructional comments, information on normal gait and highlights main gait deviations (see Figure 8.5).

It is important for the clinician to be aware that the reliability and validity of observational gait analysis have yet to be fully established. Studies of interobserver reliability show variable results. Goodwin and Diller (1973) reported percentage agreement as 60–93%, whereas Miyakaki and Kubota (1984) showed the agreement to be only 67% (using videotaping). In a more recent study, whilst acknowledging the convenience of observational gait analysis, the reliability was only classed as moderate (Krebbs *et al.*, 1985). Validation work against instrumental gait analysis equipment has been reported. Salch *et al.* (1985) claim the ability of clinicians to detect gait abnormalities is low (22%), but with the elimination of time–distance variables detection increases to 65%. Although observational gait analysis techniques will remain popular in the clinic due to the minimal cost, as well as rapid and easy use, clinicians need to recognize their own limitations in this technique.

> Key Points
>
> *Observational gait analysis has minimal cost and is rapidly performed by experienced clinicians.*
>
> *In routine clinical practice no standardization of technique is used.*
>
> *Clinicians need to be aware of the limitations of the technique.*

VIDEOTAPING

The use of video cameras to record gait has grown in popularity over the last few years. Human eyes sample at 24 frames per second whereas most video cameras have a sampling rate of 50 Hz (European countries, 60 Hz in the USA) which is adequate for recording normal gait. Rapid movements (running) require a faster sampling rate. As video equipment is relatively inexpensive and easy to use many physiotherapy departments have purchased this equipment. Advantages include the immediate viewing of patient data and as there are no external attachments to the patient there should be no modification to their normal gait pattern. If data are recorded over several treatment sessions it makes sequential comparison of gait easier, rather than relying on memory or a previous assessment notes. Most video decks have slow play-back facilities and freeze frame capabilities which allow repeated viewing of data without patient fatigue, and video recordings can allow other professional opinions to be sought without asking the patient to walk before a large audience. Bi-planar or tri-planar

Figure 8.5 Full body observational gait analysis (Rancho system). Rows = gait deviations: columns = gait phases. Gait dysfunction is tabulated by studying the white boxes. White boxes = major gait deviations; stippled boxes = minor gait deviations; black boxes = not applicable. (Reproduced from Perry, 1992, *Gait Analysis, Normal and Pathological Functions*, Slack Inc., New Jersey, with permission.)

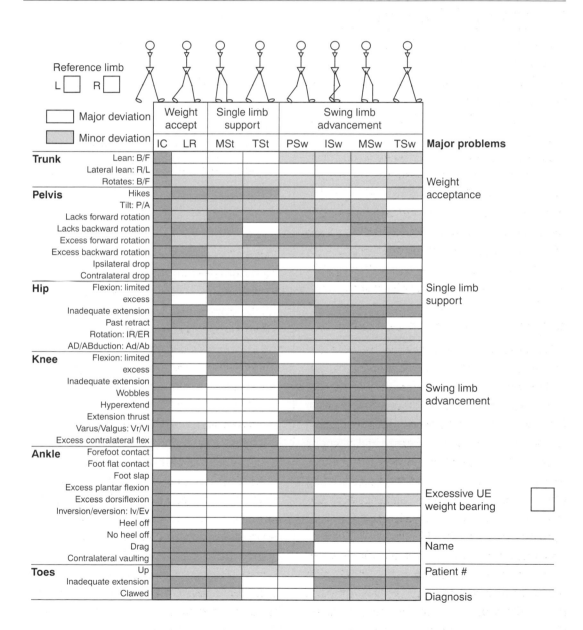

video recording aids the visual detection of out-of-plane movement.

Quantification of video recording is possible by digitization, but without any fully automated systems available on the market there remains the tedious task of working through the data frame by frame.

> ### Key Points
>
> *Video equipment is relatively inexpensive and easy to use.*
>
> *Video taping allows immediate and repeated viewing if patient data without patient fatigue.*
>
> *Video taping allows sequential recordings to be reviewed to assess patient progress.*

Foot Fall Measurements

The techniques available will measure spatial parameters (stride length, step length, base of support), temporal parameters (stance and swing phase, periods of single and double support) and a combination of both spatial and temporal parameters (cadence and velocity). The methods range from the very simple (chalk, dark mat, ruler and stopwatch) to more complex walkways incorporating electrical pressure switches. Most make use of an imprint of the patient's foot. Footfall parameters may be useful indicators of function but do not provide information on causal factors or the interaction of other segments of the body. Many of the measurements outlined below allow the collection of data from several strides rather than a single step, but it is worth noting that any attachment to the patient's shoe or foot can cause an unintentional alteration of customary walking

pattern. For foot fall parameters the size and the spacing of the sensors is crucial for quality data collection. The effect of walking aids and whether systems can accommodate their use during data collection is another factor when considering the potential use of a particular piece of equipment.

The methods of data collection fall into four main groups:

1 Walkways constructed of electrical circuits with electrical strip conductors on the patient's shoe. The metal strips allow a current to flow to a measurement circuit.

2 Pressure-sensitive switches attached to the patient's foot or footwear. Microswitches sensitive to pressure are attached to the foot or on a flexible insole in the shoe. Unless the foot switches encompass the whole foot surface, floor contact may be made by a part of the foot where no switches are situated. Placement is the key to data quality. The transducers do have a finite thickness, and with many systems having trailing wires there may be modification of patient's gait so the validity of some methods is uncertain. Telemetry methods may offer a solution to this problem, with signals being sent to a host computer via radio waves.

3 Walkways covered with pressure-sensitive switches (e.g. Gaitmat II). These walkways cause minimal interference with gait, enhancing their validity. The Gaitmat II software allows for the use of sticks, crutches, and frames without loss of footfall data.

4 Pressure-sensitive footplates (e.g. Musgrave footprint system). The patient walks on a walkway containing two pressure-sensitive plates. The position of the plates can be adapted for the patient's step length, but they must remain as unobtrusive as possible to avoid a 'stepping

stone' effect. The patient may try to please you by deliberately stepping onto the footplates rather than walking normally over their surface. The size of the sensor and good system calibration is crucial for quality data.

Kinematics

Kinematics is the term used to describe movement in terms of range, angle, angular velocity and angular acceleration. Kinematic data describe movement with no information as to the causal mechanisms. There are many types of commercially available 3D systems, and detailed information on each is beyond the scope of this chapter (see Whittle (1991) for a full description). All systems have strengths and weaknesses but there remain various difficulties encountered by all kinematic systems and these will be discussed.

Common to all kinematic systems is some sort of reference system and the use of markers. The reference systems are used to estimate body segment orientation in space and to define joint movement. A common clinical approach is for the pelvis and foot progression line to be plotted relative to laboratory coordinates (absolute spatial reference) whilst other movements are relative to another part of the body (relative spatial reference). Even within this reference system variation between laboratories exists. As yet there is no standardized convention for the collection of data, although a European initiative, CAMARC (Computer Aided Movement Analysis in a Rehabilitation Context II), has recently been published to address the lack of standardization. Therefore, when examining gait data it is essential to know the convention being plotted and to be wary of comparison of data between laboratories that may be of dubious value. Similar caution is needed when comparing pathological gait data with 'nor-

mative' data. Both sets of data need to have been collected by the same instrumentation, with the same marker placements.

All systems use a marker system. These markers are either active, e.g. LEDs tracked by special cameras (e.g. Coda, Charnwood Dynamics; Selspot, Molndal, Sweden) or passive reflective markers illuminated by CCTV camera strobing infrared light (e.g. Elite, BTS; Vicon, Oxford Metrics). Three markers are placed on each body segment so that a local coordinate system to each body segment can be calculated mathematically.

One of the major sources of error during the collection of kinematic data is marker placement on the anatomical landmarks of the patient. The relationship between these markers and the underlying bony structures remains a quandary, due to the difficulty in quantifying the movement of the skin and muscle (and thus markers) over the underlying bony structures during gait. In reality the gait analysis kinematic hardware system error may be classed as small compared to the human error during marker placement. Most kinematic systems have additional software that approximates the centre of rotation for each joint. These calculations are derived after various assumptions are made from anthropometric data and marker placements, and thus may be erroneous. Error may be introduced by poorly positioned markers or by incorrect anthropometric assumptions. For example, the patient with a malformation of the pelvis may not have his hip joint centre located in the same anthropometric relationship as the healthy subject, and software algorithms do not allow for anthropometric anomalies. Although sophisticated kinematic systems provide a wealth of data, it needs to be interpreted within a knowledge of the limitations and constraints of the system.

During the interpretation of the kinematic gait data the emphasis is mainly on the overall functional ability of the patient, without focusing on any single joint movement. With the CCTV systems there is a calibrated volume for data capture, usually set to cover the height of the patient and two stride lengths. It can be a time-consuming process to alter the capture volume being used. However, this may be necessary if very detailed information about a single joint or single body segment is required. For example, the foot is often considered as a rigid body segment with 'standard' marker placements on the lateral malleoli and fifth metatarsal head. Clearly this is not a true functional representation of foot motion with true motion occurring at ankle, hind foot, mid foot and fore foot. In pathological gait these movements can be of great importance. Recent studies (Abuzzahab *et al.*, 1996) have been published on the relative motion between the hind-foot, midfoot and forefoot, by increasing the number of markers on the foot, and it seems certain that further studies in this area will follow.

Most kinematic systems on the market are true 3D which helps eliminate the error associated with the 2D systems. Davis (1995) states that 'utilization of 2D gait analysis strategies in clinical settings where the pathology can result in significant out-of-plane motion is inappropriate and ill-advised'.

Although kinematic systems have difficulties outlined above they also have many advantages. Their markers do not encumber the patient and this increases the validity of the data. Most systems have a sampling rate of between 100 Hz and 200 Hz, thus a considerable improvement on the video camera and human eye. Systems have a high resolution and accuracy across the data capture area, with rapid processing of the data. The kinematic data is often linked to other measurements (kinetic data and EMG) of the same subject via software options, producing a thorough integrated movement analysis. The data generated allow comparison across the joints and through the three planes of motion. A typical example is shown in Figure 8.6. This shows how overlaying the pathological gait kinematic profile on a normal profile allows visual inspection to judge the relative nature of the gait deviation.

Figure 8.6　Gait analysis sagittal plane data from Elite BTS system. The patient's data are shown in the solid line and the normative comparative data in the dotted line.

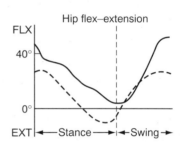

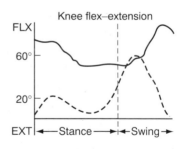

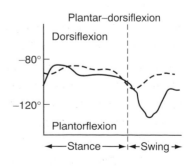

Kinetics

Kinetic analysis of gait is based on the study of ground reaction forces (GRF). These forces are equal in intensity and opposite in direction to those forces experienced by the supporting limb. From this information the forces acting on the joints and the body's response to control these forces are identified. Measurement of the GRF is made by a force platform, e.g. Kistler force platform (Kistler Instruments, Switzerland). Force platforms consist of a flat plate suspended on piezoelectric or strain gauge transducers, fitted at each corner. Although both strain gauges and piezoelectric crystals produce electrical output signals, their methods of operation are different. Strain gauges are bonded to the surface of the transducer, and as the transducer deforms under the applied force, the gauge deforms with it, changing the electrical resistance. Force platforms utilizing the piezoelectric transducers work on the principle that an electrical charge develops on the surface of the crystal when stressed. When a constant load is applied the signal decays and therefore piezoelectrical transducers are not suitable for measuring static forces. However, during gait the loads applied to the forceplate are constantly changing and the transducers detect the force in orthogonal directions (transverse, horizontal and vertical load). By further calculations the GRF vector, its magnitude and its point of application are determined.

A typical display of GRF vectors in the sagittal plane during normal gait is shown in Figure 8.7. Note the characteristic double bump of the vertical force, commencing and finishing above body weight, whilst dipping below body weight during mid-stance. Longer steps exaggerate this double peak pattern (related to the task described in features of an efficient gait) as body mass excur-

Figure 8.7   Typical kinetic data in sagittal plane.

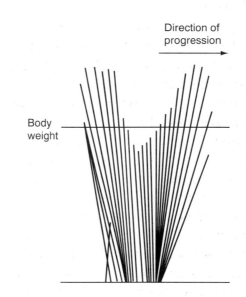

sion is greater than normal. These diagrams known as 'butterfly' diagrams can be used alone as a gait assessment tool, but more often they are used in conjunction with kinematic data (Figure 8.8).

There are several difficulties in obtaining reliable kinetic data:

1 A single full footfall per plate should be recorded. Gait aberrations can make the calculation of kinetic data impossible. For example, toe-drag on the forceplate, or the swing limb hitting the stance limb can invalidate data. As partial footfalls are unacceptable, some consideration to the patient's stride length and walking base is needed. Often with pathological gait insufficient step length prevents the use of the forceplate.

2 The patient may deliberately 'target' the forceplate — the strike recorded is therefore unrepresentative of the patient's usual gait pattern.

3 The positioning of the forceplate should be unobtrusive, and in the centre of the walkway.

Fran Polak

Figure 8.8   The Derby Gait Laboratory. (Adapted from Whittle, 1991, *Gait Analysis, An Introduction*, Butterworth-Heinemann, Oxford, with permission.)

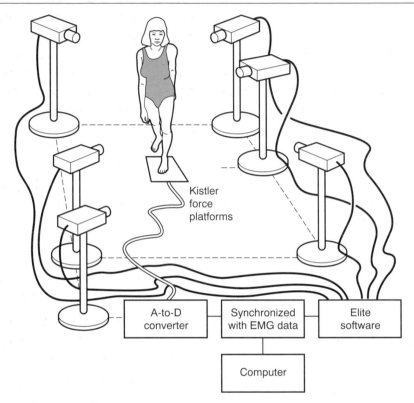

Kistler force platforms

| A-to-D converter | Synchronized with EMG data | Elite software |

Computer

The patient should be neither accelerating nor decelerating when they strike the forceplate. If two or more forceplates are used it becomes increasingly complex to obtain a single footfall per plate. Repositioning of the forceplates in relation to the patient's stride pattern is not possible due to the rigid mounting of the forceplate in the floor.

4 Changes in walking velocity can lead to misinterpretation of the data (Davis, 1995). The relationship between velocity, peak moments and powers is established in normal gait (i.e. increased velocity causes increase in peak moment and power) but this is not established for pathological gait. Kinetic plots alter with velocity and this needs to be matched when

comparing right/left data over single or multiple trials, pre/post treatment trials or trials barefoot and shod.

Having collected kinetic data from the force platform this then allows us to calculate joint moments (see section 1, Chapter 2). There are two basic methods for calculating joint moments. The first is the 'external' moment – the perpendicular distance from the joint centre (determined from kinematic coordinates) multiplied by the resultant ground reaction force. This method (f × d) is simple yet has limitations (Winter, 1990). The error associated with calculation increases more proximally (knee and hip). In this simple calculation the effects of gravity and inertia are not included, and calculations in the swing phase are not possible (GRF acting on contralateral leg). The second method of calculating joint moments is often termed 'inverse dynamics' or 'internal' moments. These represent the body's response to the external load, and include the GRF, segment mass and inertia. The segment inertial characteristics are estimated from anthropometric tables based on simple measurements of the patient's stature. It is worth noting that data obtained from these tables are often based on the healthy population and certainly not the disabled or elderly frail population, many of whom have noticeable asymmetrical segment mass (e.g. hemiplegic patient). As such their segment mass will vary considerably from the normal healthy individual.

During normal gait the moments calculated refer primarily to muscular forces that act to control segment rotation, with the influence of soft tissues being minimal (see Rose *et al.*, 1991). As a result the net joint moment indicates the dominant muscle group controlling the joint moment, without indicating the contribution of the muscles on the other side of the joint, or the role of the soft tissues which may be increased in pathological gait. For example, the hemiplegic patient who strikes the ground with their toe, and rapidly extends, or hyper extends the knee during midstance phase (a plantarflexion–knee extensor moment) will be keeping the GRF anterior to the knee. The knee is stabilized during stance by the position of the GRF, but it may be the posterior capsular structures and not the knee extensors controlling the joint position and resisting further motion. Additional electromyography (EMG) information may help determine whether the forces produced are soft tissue or muscular. This information is of great clinical significance if the joint is at risk of damage due to absence of muscular support.

Further computations of the gait data are possible to determine joint power, using both kinetic and kinematic data. Power is defined as work done per unit time, and in gait analysis is derived from multiplying the resultant joint moment by the joint angular velocity. Joint power generation is often associated with concentric muscle contraction (shortening under tension) and joint power absorption with eccentric muscle contraction (lengthening under tension). Key points in the gait cycle show periods of joint power generation, which have great clinical significance when studying pathological gait.

> ### Key Points
>
> *As we walk force is generated on the floor and can be measured by a forceplate.*
>
> *The ground reaction force is equal in magnitude and opposite in direction to the force acting on the body.*
>
> *Kinetic data allows further computation of the force acting at the joints, and magnitude of joint power.*

Electromyography

Electromyography (EMG) involves detecting, amplifying and recording the myoelectrical changes during muscle activity. It has become an important tool in gait analysis, providing an indirect measure of the timing and relative intensity of muscle contraction. Electromyography has been employed by several researchers to study gait and is well documented (see Sutherland, 1978). General agreement about the timing and level of activity of muscles exists, yet differences are present in the literature due to results being

Figure 8.9   Temporal EMG patterns for adult lower limb extremity muscles. (From Craik and Oatis who reprinted it by kind permission of San Francisco Shriners Hospital for Crippled Children.)

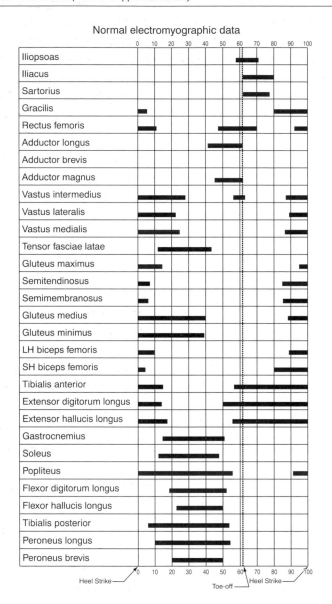

Normal electromyographic data

obtained using different data collection methods (Figure 8.9).

Data obtained by EMG provides information about the timing or phasic activity of muscles. The phasic data reveal whether the muscle activity is normal, out of phase, premature, prolonged, curtailed, delayed, absent, continuous or clonic. Phasic information may be useful clinically for determining primary muscles responsible for gait deviations. For the patient with an inverted foot in stance and/or swing phase, EMG recordings from both tibialis posterior and tibialis anterior could determine which muscle is chiefly contributing to the gait deviation. For full interpretation EMG data should be coupled with kinematic and kinetic data whenever these are available. This will assist in determining whether muscle activity recorded is abnormal or is in response to the demands placed on a joint (Rose et al., 1991).

Practical Task

Try walking around the room in a crouched position (continual hip and knee flexion). Besides noticing how tiring it is, also palpate your quadriceps muscles. These are working throughout the stance phase to prevent you slipping into a deeper crouch position. An EMG trace would show the continuous activity of these muscles in the stance phase, which is not their usual pattern of activity during gait.

Before deciding whether treatment should be aimed at these overactive muscles, we can interpret this activity in relation to our other gait data to show the quadriceps activity is in response to the demands placed upon it, and is not the primary cause of the gait deviation.

Muscles are normally active through very short time periods (<0.7 s), and there are periods in the gait cycle when only minimal activity is noted, revealing that much of lower limb motion is governed by inertia and momentum (Craik, 1985). For example in relation to kinematics, from terminal stance through to initial swing phase, knee flexion increases from 35° to 60° of flexion without this

increase being actively generated by hamstring activity. Studies using EMG show that hamstring activity commences during the late swing phase to temper the rate of knee extension. Thus EMG studies have shown that muscles are primarily the controlling rather than the propulsive factors during gait, and muscle function is primarily that of protection and control against movement occurring in the opposite direction.

A further characteristic of the EMG signal studied is the amplitude of the signal. Caution is needed when studying the amplitude of the EMG, as this is not the same as muscle force. Studies of the relationship between EMG and force are limited to isometric muscle contractions; therefore quantification of the dynamic EMG signal is difficult. The amplitude of the EMG signal is affected by many factors including the diameter of the muscle fibre, the filtering properties of the electrode and the distance between the electrode and the active muscle fibre (i.e. different constituencies of body tissue). An obese patient will have a greater distance between a surface electrode and the active muscle than a thin patient. Therefore direct comparison of EMG amplitude is precluded on the basis of individual differences in subjects and differences between muscles.

It is suggested that EMG comparisons are possible if normalized in some fashion against a maximum voluntary effort. This normalization technique involves treating the data from each electrode as a ratio of a reference generated with the same electrode. For subjects without pathology this is an EMG registered during maximum effort. This can be generated by manual grading (percentage of manual muscle test [% MMT], see Chapter 7) or measurement with a dynamometer (percentage maximum voluntary contraction (% MVC), see Chapter 7). The latter is more accurate, although it is more time-consuming (Perry, 1992). However, this criterion for normalization must be questioned for certain patient groups. Many patients may be unable to isolate movement or generate a maximum voluntary effort.

Further care is needed with the interpretation of data, as the actual acquisition techniques will influence the EMG results. Electrode type, i.e. surface or fine wire, is one potential source of variation. Detailed reviews of each are available (Kadaba *et al.*, 1985). These authors report that surface electrode recordings produce higher reliability than those from fine wire electrodes for the gait cycle, in run-to-run and day-to-day comparisons. Young *et al.* (1989) showed that the temporal–distance characteristics were affected in 36 cerebral palsy children by the encumbrance of 'wearing' EMG electrodes. The greatest change occurred with fine wire electrodes, but alteration of cadence was also evident with surface electrodes. Surface electrodes are noninvasive, generally well tolerated by the patient and more reproducible, but they do have limitations. Some have a large pick-up area with an increased risk of 'cross-talk' (picking up signals from neighbouring muscles). Fine wire electrodes are more definitive, as they are better able to detect defined EMG signals due to sampling a larger range of frequencies. With accurate placement they can record specific, deep and small muscles. The disadvantages include discomfort, which can promote cramping, tightness and spasticity. When isolated movements are not possible electrical stimulation is necessary to check electrode placement. Thus fine wire electrodes are not suitable for every patient group.

An improved insight into muscle activity during gait can be gained from EMG studies, with greater potential for interpretation if linked with kinematic and kinetic data. However artefacts are always present in the data. Electrical noise, skin surface conditions, electrode spacing and movement all influence the recording. Most systems use telemetry (radio signals) to send the data back to a host computer, but some systems are still using trailing wires that introduce additional mechanical artefacts. When reviewing EMG data you must carefully question the reliability and reproducibility of the data obtained, and know the limitations of the interpretations.

Key Points

EMG is the study of myoelectric changes during muscle activity.

Electrodes used may be surface or fine wire (indwelling).

The amplitude of the signal is not the same as muscle force.

Comparisons between patients or within different muscles of the same patient are not possible unless the recording is 'normalized'.

Energy Expenditure

For therapists it can be important to know the patient's energy expenditure during gait when assessing the overall impact of treatment. If, after treatment, the patient's energy requirement for walking has increased, even if the gait pattern has improved, one may question the usefulness of the intervention. If an elderly patient now walks with increased hip and knee flexion, but can only manage a few tiring steps, have we helped them, or hindered them?

Two basic methods of energy expenditure measurement have been described:

1 Mechanical energy levels; and
2 Metabolic energy costs.

Mechanical energy levels refer to work and power both of the whole body and individual segments. Information from kinetics, both internal and external moments, powers, kinematic data plus anthropometric measurements is used. Using this data calculations of the energy requirements of individual joints are derived. A complete review of muscle physiology and energy transfer between segments is beyond the scope of this text but is well described by Perry (1992).

The metabolic energy costs provide an overall measure of effort involved, without indication as to why gait has a particular level of efficiency. Methods for calculating the energy expenditure may be through oxygen consumption measures. One such measure is oxygen cost. This is the amount of oxygen consumed per kilogram body weight per unit distance travelled (ml/kg/m). Measurement of oxygen consumed and carbon dioxide expired requires relatively expensive and cumbersome equipment and is therefore not suitable for all patients. These factors have led to the development of a simpler technique – the physiological cost index (PCI). This equates change of heart rate from a steady resting state to distance travelled. As such the PCI is independent of velocity. Physiologists have shown that oxygen uptake and heart rate are linearly related at submaximal levels (Astrand and Rodhal, 1970), and the use of telemetry makes it possible to monitor ambulatory heart rate in addition to walking speed without causing additional stress to the patient (Stallard *et al.*, 1978). The PCI was first described by McGregor (1981) and provides a single number which quantifies walking performance. It is calculated as follows:

$$PCI = \frac{\text{Walking heart rate (WHR)} - \text{Resting heart rate (RHR)}}{\text{Walking speed (WS)}}$$

WHR and RHR units are heartbeats per minute; WS units are metres per minute; therefore units of PCI are heartbeats per metre walked.

The use of PCI has increased in recent years, both in research and as a clinical tool. The technique has been used to study both children and adults, and the reliability and validity have been established (see Butler *et al.*, 1984; and Rose *et al.*, 1990).

> **Key Points**
>
> *PCI is directly proportional to energy expenditure.*
>
> *PCI is an easy, acceptable noninvasive technique.*
>
> *Oxygen consumption (as an indicator of energy expenditure) requires expensive, often cumbersome equipment and thus it is not suitable for all patient groups.*

Maturation of Gait

Age is an important consideration affecting both kinetic and kinematic patterns. With ageing there are changes in the musculoskeletal and neurological systems of the body, and these are expressed as biomechanical changes in gait. We all recognize that the gait of a young child is different from an elderly person.

Children

Sutherland *et al.* (1980) studied normal children between the ages of 1 and 7 years. They observed similar sagittal plane joint rotations in children by the age of 2 years. However, gait of children less than 2 years old exhibited greater knee flexion and dorsiflexion during stance, a reduced knee flexion arc and more pronounced external rotation of the hip. Reciprocal arm swing and heel strike was well established by the age of 18 months. They concluded from the criteria used (duration of stance, walking velocity, cadence, step length and ratio of pelvic span to ankle spread) that mature gait was well established at the age of 3 years.

Marion and McDonald (1986) reported on running patterns in 63 children aged between 6 and 12 years of age. They concluded that most characteristics of the running pattern are established by the age of 6 years, with no significant differences between 6 and 12 years of age. However, shorter stride lengths and a slower running velocity were noted in the children aged between 6 and 7 years of age.

Elderly People

Murray *et al.* (1969) report kinematic gait patterns in elderly men and Finley *et al.* (1969) report on elderly women. Both authors report age-related changes occurring, with Murray stating that these occur as early as 60 years of age. Most studies agree that the elderly have a shorter step and stride length, a broader walking base, reduced swing phase and slower cadence. The hypothesis that these changes are due solely to age is a tentative one, as studies do not report the medical background of these patients. Often studies only include volunteers, i.e. the 'elite elderly' who are able to come to the laboratory and do not reflect the range of capabilities of the whole elderly population.

Velocity

It is well established from the literature that lower limb kinematics are dependent on walking speed. Perry (1992) states that normal customary free gait velocity on a smooth surface averages at 82 m/min for adults. Men are 5% faster (86 m/min) than the group mean and women 6% slower (77 m/min). These reported values are similar to Murray *et al.* (1964) and Finley and Cody (1970). The latter is a study of 1106 pedestrians walking in an urban environment.

When walking faster the stride length increases. An increase in velocity proportionally lengthens single stance and shortens the two periods of double stance. When double stance period is omitted and replaced by double float running has commenced.

The biomechanics of running are well described by Cavanagh (1990) and detail of any depth is beyond the scope of this text. Stride length, sagittal plane kinematics, muscle activity, rearfoot motion are all presented with some useful information about running injuries. Large databases of asymptomatic distance runners do not as yet exist; neither do clear indications of patterns of motion that may be expected from specific pathologies. Cavanagh (1987) states that 'many mechanical changes that represent the difference between running "in pain" and running "pain free" may be at a level of subtlety that we have not yet explored'. However, as technology advances and centres of sporting excellence develop these issues will be addressed. Successful treatment of running injuries should embrace both biomechanical evaluation and clinical judgement.

Briefly, during running the hip joint motion is increased, except for the movement of hip hyperextension, which is greater in walking due to the increased time in stance phase. At the knee there is an increased in flexion in both the swing and stance phase, and at the ankle there is increased dorsiflexion prior to initial ground contact, increased dorsiflexion during the stance phase, and rapid plantarflexion during terminal stance. As running velocity increase the amount of plantarflexion decreases.

Lastly a final reminder that caution is advised when reviewing both kinematic and kinetic data, where velocity is not identified. Information about footwear, the number of subjects studied, free walking or treadmill walking should all be noted. If unilateral data or comparisons against a normal database are being used, velocity remains crucial for data interpretation.

Stairs

For patients the ability to walk around the house and climb the stairs is often considered the most important functional requirement. A review of stair-climbing can be found in Hamil and Knutzen (1995). In stair-climbing the higher leg produces the greatest effort both ascending and descending. At the hip the muscles contribute less than the muscles acting at the knee and ankle.

Ascent is initiated by the hip flexors, which lift the leg up against gravity to the next stair. Rectus femoris becomes active to assist hip flexion and works eccentrically to slow the rate of knee flexion. During weight acceptance and pull-up the majority of extension is generated at the knee joint, whilst the contralateral ankle generates power to push the subject up to the next step.

Descending requires minimal hip muscular activity. As the contralateral leg is lowered to the stair there is hamstring activity to control the motion. During weight acceptance the weight is controlled by eccentric work at the knee and ankle. The controlled lowering is primarily controlled at the knee, and during weight acceptance the contralateral ankle eccentrically absorbs contact via eccentric action of the plantarflexors. The dorsiflexors then co-contract to stabilize the ankle on the lower stair. The knee extensors thus have a vital role during stair ascent and descent; a reduction of their full power makes stair-climbing difficult (see following section on pathological gait—knee extensor weakness).

Pathological Gait

Following the sections on 'normal gait' in which identifiable parts of the gait cycle have been described, we now consider the impact on gait of some muscloskeletal impairments. We are able to predict some of these impacts if the patient has intact sensory and proprioceptive feedbacks. Often compensatory actions or 'coping' mechanisms are adopted by the patient in the light of the muscloskeletal impairment, and can include abnormal motion at joints unaffected by the primary impairment. Separating the primary cause from the secondary 'coping' mechanisms remains the main aim of gait analysis.

Loss of Dorsiflexion Strength

Study of the gait cycle reveals that the dorsiflexors play a key role at two critical points in the gait cycle. Firstly, immediately after initial ground contact, they control the plantarflexion of the foot induced by the ground reaction force (GRF); secondly, during swing phase they produce the small dorsiflexion moment necessary to lift the foot, which contributes to adequate ground clearance as the swing limb is advanced.

If the dorsiflexors are weak we can predict that the foot may be lowered abruptly following initial ground contact. Sometimes this can be an audible slap, known as 'foot slap'. It is possible to diagnose this type of patient by ear, as they approach the physiotherapy department, before coming into view!

Failure to adequately lift the foot during the swing phase may cause the toes to catch the ground, known as 'toe drag'. Coping mechanisms are often employed by the patient to enable adequate ground clearance to occur. Some of these mechanisms are detailed below. This list is not exhaustive, and neither are the mechanisms exclusive: a patient may adopt one of these coping mechanisms or a combination of many.

CIRCUMDUCTION

The swing limb can obtain ground clearance if it is swung outwards in an arc motion known as circumduction (Figure 8.10). This deviation is best viewed in the frontal plane.

VAULTING

Ground clearance for the swing limb can be attained if the patient rises into ankle plantarflexion on the contralateral stance limb during the mid-stance phase. This causes an exaggerated ver-

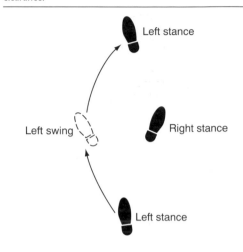

Figure 8.10   Circumduction. The swing limb moves in an arc, rather than straight forwards, to obtain adequate ground clearance.

tical rise during the gait cycle, which is very energy inefficient. Vaulting gait deviation is best viewed in the sagittal plane, although noticeable in the frontal plane.

HIGH STEPPAGE GAIT

A high steppage gait is, as the name suggests, one in which there is exaggerated flexion at both the hip and knee of the swing limb. These deviations lift the foot higher than usual, and therefore adequate ground clearance is obtained by the swing limb. This gait deviation is best viewed in the sagittal plane.

HIP HITCHING / HIKING

Hip hiking is elevation of the pelvis and swing limb, on the swing side, during the swing phase. This is achieved by contraction of the spinal lateral flexors. By tilting the pelvis up, often combined with increased pelvic rotation, limb advancement is achieved (see Figure 8.11). Observation is easiest in the frontal plane.

Figure 8.11 Hip hiking. The pelvis is lifted on the swing limb during the swing phase.

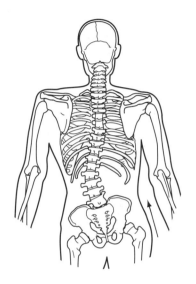

Knee Extensor Weakness

The knee extensors are active during early stance and late swing (rectus femoris is also active during early swing as a hip flexor). Their role in early stance phase is to control the rate of knee flexion induced by the GRF during loading response (weight acceptance). If the knee extensors are weak the patient may try to avoid uncontrolled knee flexion during loading response by increased anterior tilt of the trunk. If one limb is affected the trunk is straightened again during the second period of double support (as the contralateral limb starts to weight bear). If both limbs are affected the anterior trunk tilt will remain throughout the gait cycle. The purpose of the deviation is to displace the centre of gravity of the body anteriorly, which results in the line of force passing anteriorly to the knee (see Figure 8.12). In the long term damage can occur to the knee joint which becomes inherently unstable due

Figure 8.12 Anterior trunk bending brings line of force anterior to the knee, to compensate for knee extensor weakness. (Reproduced from Whittle, 1991, *Gait Analysis, An Introduction*, Butterworth-Heinemann, Oxford, with permission.)

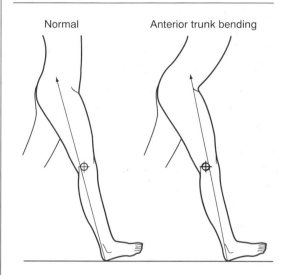

to continued thrusting of the knee into hyperextension.

Normal stair-climbing is impossible in the presence of knee extensor weakness. If there is one sound limb the patient will adopt a pattern of leading upstairs and following downstairs with the sound limb, which may allow the unstable knee to remain in full extension throughout the stair climb.

Excessive Knee Flexion

The knee is near full extension during terminal swing to initial ground contact, and during the mid-stance phase. Excessive knee flexion may occur at either of these phases of the gait cycle, or both. A fixed flexion contracture at the knee will obviously prevent full extension being obtained, and a flexion contracture at the hip may also prevent knee extension (thigh segment

Figure 8.13   (a) Antalgic gait and (b) Trendelenburg gait. Note pelvic obliquity during swing in the Trendelenburg gait. (Adapted from Jones and Baker, 1996, *Human Movement Explained*, Butterworth-Heinemann, Oxford, with permission.)

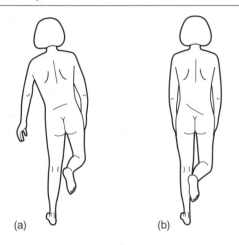

(a)   (b)

does not reach a vertical position during the stance phase of the gait cycle). Continual flexion at the knee has the effect of shortening the leg length, and coping mechanisms for leg length discrepancy may be adopted.

If there is spasticity of the knee flexors, which are able to overpower the knee extensors, a gait pattern of continual knee flexion may result. Other coping mechanisms may also be adopted such as anterior trunk lean to compensate for the relative weakness of the knee extensors.

Trendelenburg Gait

The main role of the abductors is to control the position of the pelvis in the frontal plane during the stance phase. If the abductors are weak, the pelvis will dip on the side of the foot which is off the ground. The patient often attempts to counteract this by lateral trunk bending towards the supporting limb. This has the mechanical effect of displacing the ground reaction force towards the supporting hip joint, and thereby reduces the hip adduction moment, and the counter hip abduction moment needed to control it (Figure 8.13).

Antalgic Gait

Antalgic gait is often adopted due to unilateral joint pain. The patient adopts a lateral displacement of the trunk towards the involved weight-bearing limb. If, for example, due to osteoarthritis the hip joint is painful, the amount of pain experienced depends largely on the force transmitted through the joint and the patient may adopt this lateral trunk displacement of the trunk in an attempt to reduce the total joint force through the painful hip. By reducing the horizontal lever arm between the painful hip and the body's centre of gravity there is less loading through the impaired joint.

Increased Lumbar Lordosis

Many people have an increased lumbar lordosis as part of their posture. Only when it is used as part of the gait cycle is it of interest in gait analysis. The most common cause of increased lordosis is flexion contracture at the hip. If hip joint range of motion is limited, there is a functional effect of a reduced stride length. Often to compensate for the failure of the thigh to reach a vertical position, there is an increase in extension of the lumbar spine, and therefore an increased lumbar lordosis. Muscle imbalance around the pelvis may also cause an increased lumbar lordosis, weakness of the anterior abdominal muscles or hip extensors may allow an increase in anterior pelvic tilt, with a consequent increase in lumbar lordosis.

Walking Aids

Walking aids such as sticks, crutches or frames are often recommended for patients and when correctly prescribed favourably modify the patient's gait pattern. Whichever type of aid is used, all support some of the body weight through the upper limb rather than the lower limb. Walking aids thus reduce the weight through a painful or unstable lower limb joint, plus increase balance and patient confidence. There are several types of aid available and choice will depend upon the individual patient and the level of independence that the patient is able to achieve.

Sticks

The simplest form of walking aid is the stick, held in the hand, which transmits force through the forearm and hand to the ground. Grip strength and the shape of the stick handle limit the amount of torque that can be applied to the stick. A variety of handle types are available, some of which are more suitable for an arthritic hand with impaired function. Sticks are only suitable for partial weight bearing, and are not able to safely transmit the entire body weight during gait.

One of the main reasons sticks are issued is to improve stability by increasing the size of the area of support; for maximum security two sticks are used. If a single stick is used it is advanced during the stance phase of the stable limb. If two sticks are used, these are individually advanced during the two periods of double limb support to ensure maximum stability throughout the gait cycle.

Another reason a stick is issued is to reduce loading of a painful limb. There remains much discussion regarding ipsilateral and contralateral stick usage to unload a painful limb. Many patients opt to use the stick ipsilaterally, especially those with painful arthritic hips and knees. The stick follows the motion of the affected limb, being advanced during the swing phase of that limb. Note the patient often has a rather ungainly gait with the stick being placed close to the foot, the patient leans over the stick in a lateral lurch to increase the loading on the stick and thus reduce the loading on the limb. When the stick is held in the contralateral hand, the lateral lurch is avoided, but the degree of vertical loading through the stick is reduced. Contralateral stick usage remains the first technique of choice for many therapists, as there is less disruption to the reciprocal gait cycle.

Tripod / Tetrapod

This variant on the walking stick has three (tripod) or four feet (quadripod). The feet provide extra stability, and each stick will stand up by itself. They are issued for a patient who has poor balance, and can be used during a gait re-education programme. The increased stability gained is at the expense of weight and size, which causes difficulties in doorways. They remain unsafe for use on stairs due to their large base size in respect to stair step dimensions.

Crutches

The main difference between a crutch and a walking stick is that a crutch can transmit significant forces in the horizontal plane. This is because the crutch has two points of attachment, one at the hand and the other higher on the upper limb, providing a lever arm for the transmission of force. The three main categories of crutch are (Figure 8.14):

- Axillary crutch (underarm);

- Elbow crutch (forearm);
- Gutter crutch (forearm).

AXILLARY CRUTCHES

As the name suggests they fit under the axilla. The top of the crutch should lean on the chest wall, and remain 50 mm below the axillary fold. If the crutches are too long or the patient uses them incorrectly, leaning on the top axillary bar there is serious risk of neurovascular damage. Correctly used with the axillary bar leaning on the chest wall, and the weight of the patient being predominantly transmitted through the hands they are suitable for non-weight-bearing gait. They provide good lateral stability, although they are rather energy cost inefficient.

ELBOW CRUTCHES

The upper point of body contact is the upper arm above the elbow, and thus the lever arm is shorter than the axillary crutch. This is seldom a problem and elbow crutches are suitable for both non-weight-bearing and partial weight-bearing gait. The advantages over axillary crutches are that they are lighter, suitable for long-term use, and the patient is still able to use their hand for functional activities such as opening a door, due to the retaining elbow cuff which prevents the crutch falling from the arm. Elbow crutches are suitable for use on stairs, and are often cosmetically more acceptable to the patient. Long-term use can create stress at the wrist, and as such are not suitable for patients with flexion contractures at the wrist and/or elbow.

GUTTER CRUTCHES

For patients with loss of functional handgrip due to pain, deformity or flexion contractures of the upper limb, gutter crutches are particularly useful. They enable more of the vertical force to be transmitted through the forearm itself rather than the hand. Most types of gutter crutch are adjustable in height, length of forearm support and angulation. If used incorrectly stress may be placed on the shoulder joints.

Walking Frame

The most stable walking aid is the walking frame. They have a very large base which enables the patient to walk within this area of support. Commonly used for the elderly when high levels of support are required, they are also used for children with neurological impairment. Differing types and weight frames are available, some fixed height, others adjustable. As with all types of walking aid, correct height adjustment is crucial for safe usage, the condition of the ferrules and/or wheels if a rollator frame need noting, and the frame should be carefully inspected for loose screws before it is issued. Jones and Baker (1996) provide a good review of the types of frame available.

Figure 8.14 Types of crutch: axillary (left), gutter (centre), elbow (right).

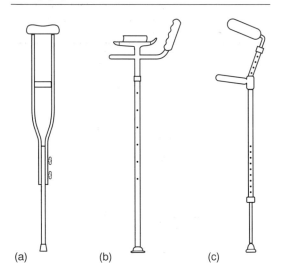

(a)   (b)   (c)

Walking with a standard walking frame disrupts the normal gait pattern, with only a 'walk-to' gait permissible. The usual method is to first move the frame forwards, and walk in to the frame with each foot, move the frame again etc. Walking is slow with a stop–start pattern. The patient needs to ensure that all four legs of the frame are firmly on the ground, a common fault being elevation of the front two legs, with a tendency for the patient to lean backwards.

The rollator is a variant on the walking frame, where the front two legs are replaced with wheels. Whilst the advancement of the frame is easier there is some loss of stability in the direction of forward progression.

Selection of Walking Aid

The correct selection of walking aid from the huge range available can assist the patient with impaired mobility to remain as independent as possible for as long as possible. Choice of walking aid is best based on the individual's home environment, lifestyle, and level of independence. All walking aids have to be correctly adjusted, with good ferrules and the patient needs to be competent in their use.

Gait Patterns With Walking Aids

Ipsilateral Two-Point Gait With One Stick
A single stick is used in the ipsilateral hand. The stick is advanced with the affected limb, during the stance phase of the non-affected limb.

Contralateral Two-Point Gait With One Stick
A single stick is used in the contralateral hand, to increase stability or reduce the loading on a single limb. The stick is advanced with the affected limb, allowing weight to be transferred through both the stick and the affected limb during advancement of the non-affected limb.

Three-Point Gait
Two walking sticks or crutches are used. Both aids are advanced together, followed by the affected limb, then the unaffected limb (Figure 8.15). Often used when partial weight-bearing is required, care must be taken to ensure the aids are in contact with the ground before the affected limb is advanced. Gait velocity is an important consideration: generally the faster the velocity the more weight is transferred through the affected limb. Sometimes a patient is permitted only to weight-bear a certain amount (e.g. 10 kg) and can be taught how to judge the correct weight transferred through the lower limb by standing on weighing scales.

Four-Point Gait
The four-point gait pattern is often used late in gait re-education training as a final step to learning

Figure 8.15   Three-point gait. (Reproduced from Jones and Baker, 1996, *Human Movement Explained*, Butterworth-Heinemann, Oxford, with permission.)

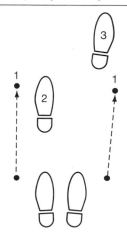

Figure 8.16   Four-point gait. (Reproduced from Jones and Baker, 1996, *Human Movement Explained*, Butterworth-Heinemann, Oxford, with permission.)

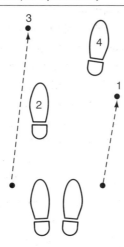

Figure 8.17   (a) Swing-through gait. (b) Swing-to-gait patterns. (Reproduced from Jones and Baker, 1996, *Human Movement Explained*, Butterworth-Heinemann, Oxford, with permission.)

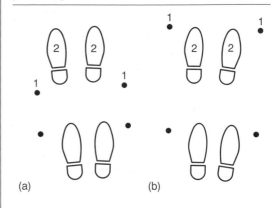

normal reciprocal gait. This pattern is not suitable for non-weight-bearing gait. The right stick is advanced, followed by the left lower limb; the left walking stick is advanced followed by the right lower limb (Figure 8.16). Therefore a single stick is moved forward only when the other stick and both limbs are in contact with the ground, thus producing a slower walking velocity.

Reciprocal Two-Point Gait

Using two sticks, the right limb and the left stick are advanced together, followed by the left limb and the right stick being advanced together. This is essentially the normal walking action, and appropriate for late stage gait re-education for patients with good balance and stability. Fast walking velocity can be achieved.

Swing-Through Gait

Both crutches are advanced forwards, both lower limbs are lifted and swung past the crutches. The crutches are quickly brought forwards again before balance is lost. Often adopted by spinal cord injury patients, with fast velocity achieved.

Only suitable for patients with good upper limb strength and control (Figure 8.17a).

Swing-To Gait

Similar to the swing-through gait, with both crutches being advanced together. However, the lower limbs are only lifted and advanced as far as the level of the crutches (Figure 8.17b).

Gait Re-education

Many of our patients will begin gait re-education within the full support of parallel bars in the physiotherapy department, and progress to walking aids, each with less support. Each walking aid encourages the patient to find a solution to being gait independent. Motor learning requires active problem-solving (see Bassille and Bock, 1996) which we encourage by teaching the patient to be independent of the therapist.

The literature identifies practice as the best predictor of learning. Therapists should decide which subtasks the patient needs to practise, and develop some gait activities for the patient to master emphasizing these subtasks. Winstein *et al.* (1989) studied an experimental group who were taught weight-shifting activities in addition to their daily therapy, and this group did not improve certain gait parameters any better than the control group. It is important to remember that practice of a subtask outside of the gait cycle may not automatically transfer into the gait cycle.

When practising gait training remember environment has an effect upon the patient. Walking in a protected environment on a smooth floor, in a well lit room without obstacles is not very representative of the more complex environment encountered outside. Encourage the patient to meet obstacles and other people walking along, and practise gait in the hospital corridor where the environment is less contrived. Consider the need for changes in gait velocity encountered in the urban environment. Crossing the road may require an increase in velocity and should be practised within gait re-education.

Gait re-education has the same fundamental aim as gait analysis: to identify the causal factors of the faulty gait pattern and offer a solution. Patients should be encouraged to be active problem-solvers themselves with the therapist encouraging various strategies to achieve a successful solution.

Summary

There is no single method of measurement that provides a complete analysis of gait. Although much of the expensive complex quantitative equipment remains unsuitable for routine clinical use, some of the qualitative methods (e.g. video) may be sufficient. It is not necessary for every patient to undergo a full gait analysis, which may be costly, extremely time consuming and intolerable to many patients. There need to be some criteria to determine which patients undergo which type of gait analysis. Firstly, the goal of the gait analysis must be defined. This must be based on the patient's problem and not driven by the possession of a piece of equipment. The treatment objectives should be clear, and the standard or measure by which you are to evaluate the intervention should be established. Consider the reliability, validity and appropriateness of the measurements undertaken (see Chapter 7).

Gait analysis has helped increase our depth and understanding of both normal and pathological gait, and supplies objective measures as to the efficacy of our treatments. With changing professional demands and finite resources available we need to organize further studies to provide evidence as to the effectiveness of our treatments. I would encourage therapists with access to gait analysis equipment to utilize it, and offer their skills in the interpretation of the data. Gait analysis has traditionally been one of our key clinical skills, and we must remain involved in moving gait analysis forward on a scientific basis.

References

Abuzzahab, FS, Harris, GF, Kidder, SM, Johnson, JE, Nery, J (1996) Foot and ankle motion analysis system instrumentation, Calibration and Validation, in Harris, GF (ed.) *Human Motion Analysis, Current Applications and Future Directions.* IEEE Press, New Jersey.

Astrand, PO, Rodhal, K (1970) *Textbook of Work Physiology.* McGraw, New York.

Bassille, CC, Bock, C (1996) Gait training, in Craik, RL, Oatis, CA (eds) *Gait Analysis – Theory and Application.* Mosby, Missouri.

Butler, P, Engelbrecht, M, Major, RE, Tait, JH, Stallard, J, Patrick, JH (1984) Physiological cost index for walking children and its use as an indicator of physical handicap. *Developmental Medicine and Child Neurology* 26: 607–612.

Cavanagh, PR (1987) The biomechanics of lower limb extremity action in distance running. *Foot and Ankle.* 7: 197–215.

Cavanagh, PR (1990) *Biomechanics of Distance Running.* Human Kinetics series. Champaign, Illinois.

Craik, RL, Oatis, CA (1985) Gait assessment in the clinic, in *Issues and*

Approaches in Measurement in Physical Therapy, Rothstein, JM (ed). Churchill Livingstone, MI.

Davis, R (1995) *Clinical Gait Analysis Instructional Course Handbook*. Enschede, The Netherlands.

Dec, JB, Saunders, JBDM, Inman, VT, Ebberhart, HS (1958) The major determinants in normal and pathological gait. *Journal of Bone and Joint Surgery.* **35**A, 543–558.

Finley, F, Cody, K (1970) Locomotive characteristics of urban pedestrians. *Archives of Physical and Medical Rehabilitation.* **51**: 423.

Finley, F, Cody, K, Finizie, R (1969) Locomotion patterns in elderly women. *Archives of Physical Medicine and Rehabilitation.* **70**: 140.

Gage, JR, (1991) *Gait Analysis in Cerebral Palsy.* MacKeith Press, London.

Gage, JR (1994) Editorial. The role of gait analysis in the treatment of cerebral palsy. *Journal of Paediatric Orthopaedics.* **14**: 701–702.

Gage, JR, Deluca, PA, Renshaw, TS (1995) Gait analysis: Principles and applications. *Journal of Bone and Joint Surgery.* **77**A (10): 1607–1623.

Goodwin, R, Diller, L (1973) Reliability among physical therapists in diagnosis and treatment of gait deviations in hemiplegics. *Perceptual and Motor Skills.* **37**: 727–734.

Hamil, J, Knutzen, K (1995) *Biomechanical Basis of Human Movement.* Williams & Wilkins, Baltimore.

Inman, VT, Ralston, HJ, Todd, F (1981) *Human Walking.* Williams & Wilkins, Baltimore.

Jones, K, Baker, R (1996) Walking aids and orthotics, in Baker, R, Jones, K (eds) *Human Movement Explained*, pp. 325–353. Butterworth-Heinemann, Oxford.

Kadaba, MP, Wootten, MG, Gainey, J et al. (1985) Repeatability of phasic muscle activity, performance of surface and intramuscular wire electrodes in gait analysis. *Journal of Orthopaedic Research.* **3**: 330.

Krebbs, DE, Edelstein, JE, Fishman, S (1985) Reliability of observational kinematic gait analysis. *Physical Therapy* **65**: 1027–1033.

Mario, GW, McDonald, M (1986) A biomechanical analysis of children's running patterns, in Watkins, J et al. (eds) *Sports Science.* London.

McGregor, J (1981) The evaluation of patient performance using long term ambulatory monitoring technique in domiciliary environment. *Physiotherapy* **67**: 30–33.

Miyazaki, S, Kubota, T (1984) Quantification of gait abnormalities on the basis of continuous foot-force measurement. Correlation between qualitative indices and visual rating. *Med. Biol. Eng. Comput* **22**: 70–76.

Moulin, F (1995) Observational gait analysis, in Craik, R and Oatis, C (eds) *Gait Analysis – Theory and Application.* Mosby, New York.

Murray, MP, Korg, RC, Clarkson, BH et al. (1969) Walking patterns in healthy old men. *Journal of Gerontology* **24**(2) 169–178.

Patrick, J (1991) Gait laboratory investigations to assist decision making. *British Journal of Hospital Medicine* **45**: 35–37.

Perry, J (1992) *Gait Analysis, Normal and Pathological Function.* Slack Inc, Thorofare, NJ.

Rose, J, Gamble, JG, Burgos, A, Mederos, J, Haskell, WL (1990) Energy expenditure index of walking for normal children and for children with cerebral palsy. *Developmental Medicine and Child Neurology* **32**: 333–340.

Rose, SA, Ounpuu, S, Deluca, PA (1991) Strategies for the assessment of paediatric gait in the clinical setting. *Physical Therapy* **71**(12) 961–980.

Salch, M, Murdoch, G (1985) In defence of gait analysis. *Journal of Bone and Joint Surgery* **67**B: 237–241.

Saunders, JB, Inman, VT, Eberhart, HD (1953) The major determinants in normal and pathological gait. *Journal of Bone and Joint Surgery* **35**A: 543.

Stallard, J, Tait, JH, Davies, JR (1978) Assessment of orthoses by means of speed and heart rate. *Journal of Medical Engineering and Technology* **2**: 22–24.

Sutherland, DH (1978) Gait analysis in cerebral palsy. *Developmental Medicine and Child Neurology* **20**: 807.

Sutherland, DH, Olshen, R, Cooper, R, Woo, L (1980) The development of mature gait. *Journal of Bone and Joint Surgery* **62**A: 336–353.

Sutherland, DH, Oishen, RA, Biden, EN, Wyatt, MP (1988) The development of mature walking. MacKeith Press, London.

Watts, HG (1994) Editorial. Gait laboratory analysis for preoperative decision making in spastic cerebral palsy: is it all it's cracked up to be? *Journal of Paediatric Orthopaedics* **14**: 703–704.

Weinstein, CJ, Gardner, ER, McNeal, DR, Barto, PS, Nicholson, DE (1989) Standing balance training: Effect on balance and locomotion in hemiparetic adults. *Archives of Physical and Medical Rehabilitation* **70**: 755.

Whittle, M (1991) *Gait Analysis, An Introduction.* Butterworth-Heinemann, Oxford.

Young, CC, Rose, SE, Biden, EN, *et al.* (1989) The effect of surface and internal electrodes on the gait of children with cerebral palsy, spastic diplegic type. *Journal of Orthopaedic Research.* **7**: 732.

C

Contemporary Therapeutic Approaches to Clinical Practice

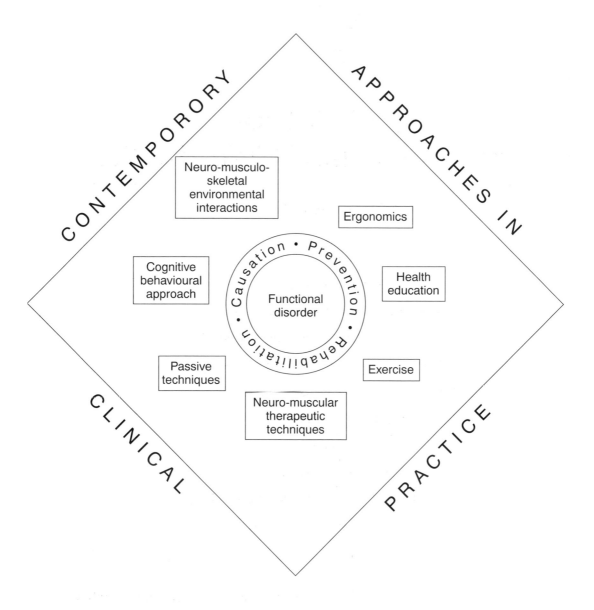

9

Passive Techniques:
A Review of their Use in Clinical Practice

KEVIN BANKS

Introduction

This chapter is approached from a clinical basis using case examples to highlight the content. Specific techniques of passive movement will not be included. Instead passive techniques will be approached from a functional, biomechanical, physiological and clinical point of view. This will help you to put passive movement into the functional context (whether passive movement of joint, muscle, nerve, or other soft tissue) and encourage you to think about tailoring techniques to the functional disorder encountered. The content will be reinforced by the research which is currently available on the subject and areas where further investigation is needed will be highlighted, along with possible ways of doing this.

Passive movement and soft tissue manipulation techniques and the reasons for selecting them have been described in detail in several different ways (Stoddard, 1983; Cyriax, 1983; Grieve, 1981; Paris, 1992; Maitland, 1991; Edwards, 1992; Kaltenborn, 1989; Mulligan, 1993; McKenzie, 1981; Butler and Gifford, 1989; Janda, 1983; Palastanga, 1986; etc). All of these approaches are based on relevant clinical models. All have been widely used in assessment examination and treatment of neuromusculoskeletal disorders. In this sense it is evident that no single approach to manipulative physiotherapy should be followed religiously. The prime goal of any approach should be to achieve its desired effect, ridding the patient of the symptoms and functional loss for which help has been sought.

The choice of passive technique or approach should be based on sound clinical reasoning (Chapter 6). Skilled handling is essential to perform techniques in a valid way, and an appropriate means of evaluation is necessary to gauge the effectiveness of what has been done. Passive techniques in themselves are only one tool in the toolbox for solving clinical problems.

Primarily, it is the intention, in this chapter, to deal with the principles and application of *treatment* by passive techniques.

Chapter Objectives

At the end of this chapter the student should be able to:

1 Define manipulation and mobilization;

2 List the structures influenced by passive techniques;

3 Understand what is meant by 'tissue biasing' of passive techniques;

4 Explain how passive techniques might be refined to make them clinically and structurally relevant;

5 Review the main criteria for the selection of a particular passive technique;

6 Discuss the criteria for progressing passive techniques to the point of patient discharge;

7 Discuss what would be the ultimate aim of the passive treatment technique and what would influence the decision to stop treatment;

8 Describe the effects of passive techniques;

9 Discuss how passive techniques can be evaluated scientifically;

10 Extrapolate the future considerations for the use of passive techniques in clinical practice.

Definitions of Passive Manual Techniques

Passive movement: A movement is passive when it is performed on a person by an outside force, that is, by another person or a piece of equipment.

Manipulation (general definition): A term used loosely to describe passive techniques of any kind. From the latin verb *manipulare* meaning *to handle*. The use of the hands in a skilled manner: skilled treatment by the hand.

Mobilization–manipulation (specific definitions): These two terms for passive movement techniques are usually described in the passive movement direction in which they are performed. Often a supplement is added to emphasize the purpose or purported desired effect, e.g. a transverse thrust at C4/5, a straight leg raise stretch, an anteroposterior glide of the tibia on the femur, long transverse strokes of the thoracic connective tissue.

Mobilization: A passive movement performed in such a manner or speed that it is at all times within the ability of the patient to prevent the movement if he so wishes. Mobilization can be oscillatory (varying speed and rhythm), small or large amplitude, in any part of the range into which it is being performed and with or without compression or distraction (for joints). Alternatively mobilization can be sustained stretching (with or without tiny oscillations) at the limit of the range. Continuous passive motion (CPM) by a mechanical device may also be described as mobilization.

Manipulation (thrust): A sudden movement or high velocity thrust performed at a speed that renders the patient powerless to prevent it. A manipulative thrust should always be carried out within the physiological limits of the the range into which it is being performed, but not necessarily at the limit of the range.

Manipulation under anaesthetic (MUA): The stretching of a joint and its associated structures to restore a full range of movement by breaking adhesions. Done as a steady controlled stretch, this procedure can also be done on a conscious patient under a local anaesthetic.

Connective tissue manipulation: A soft tissue manipulation technique directed at the fascial interfaces (Holey, 1995).

Transverse frictions: A specific manipulative procedure at right angles to the fibres of soft tissue (lesions) in order to achieve a localized effect (Cyriax, 1983).

Structures Influenced by Passive Movements

Generally speaking, passive techniques influence the inert structures of the neuromusculo/skeletal system. Most of the structures influenced are the connective and supporting tissue of joints, muscles, nerves and other soft tissues involved in movement. Passive movements may have mechanical and physiological effects on these structures. The clinical effects of passive techniques greatly concern the clinician, in that the presenting signs and symptoms may change as a result of an appropriately applied technique.

The following structures are influenced by passive movement techniques.

Joints

Maitland (1991) defined a joint for the purpose of considering mobilization, as follows: 'All of the intra-articular structures, the capsule, and all of the non-contractile tissue which moves during every passive and active movement'. Additionally a joint can be clinically and structurally subdivided into intra-articular and peri-articular components:

• Intra-articular structures include:

subchondral bone, which is innervated by type IV free nerve endings and thus a potential source of joint surface pain (LaRocca, 1992);

articular cartilage and synovial fluid. These structures are 'agitated' by passive motion and they play a key role in the health of the less vascularized parts of the joint. In addition they contribute to the reduced friction which facilitates efficient function of synovial joints (Lowther, 1988; Maroudas *et al.,* 1968).

synovial membrane, menisci, and fat pads are also intra-articular structures.

Clinical Example

A glenohumeral intra-articular disorder may be suspected if, for example, a patient presents with a deep ache within the joint whilst the joint surfaces are under compression (e.g. lying on it at night). There also may be a loss of the friction-free feel to passive movement of the joint when the joint surfaces are held under compression.

● Peri-articular structures include:

the highly innervated outer 2/3 of the joint capsule; supporting ligaments and related tendons.

The structure and function of the peri-articular tissues suggest a role in guiding and restraining movement (Evans, 1988). When mechanically and pathologically compromised they will contribute to the clinical phenomena of hypomobility, hypermobility and instability (Figure 9.1) (Chapter 6).

Clinical Example

Biasing of passive movements towards intra-articular or peri-articular structures of a joint may be a useful way of differentiating the source of a patient's symptoms and thereby help in the selection of a more effective treatment technique. For example, a 26-year-old hockey player is 80% recovered from a 'twisted knee' injury. He now only has mild pain on the medial side

Figure 9.1 Clinical representation of a typical synovial joint (Adapted from Barnett *et al.*, 1961, *Synovial Joints: Their Structure and Mechanics*, Longman, London, with permission).

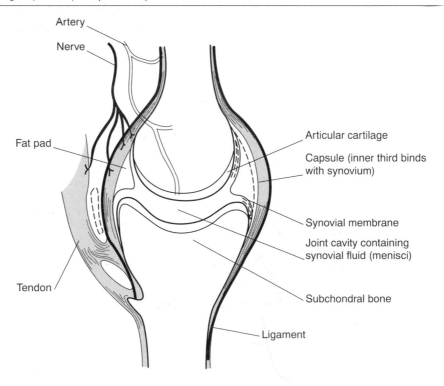

of the knee. On examination, in prone lying with the knee flexed to 90°, he has discomfort when the tibiofemoral joint is laterally rotated. If the same movement is performed with compression of the joint surfaces there is no discomfort (the intra-articular structures are suspected less). If the same movement is performed with the joint surfaces distracted his pain is reproduced (more stress on the peri-articular structures). A hypothesis of peri-articular damage is made. Therefore the knee is laterally rotated with distraction, as described above, to target the peri-articular tissue involved. The peri-articular tissues have been subjected to an inflammatory process and therefore need stretching to prevent the tendency for the tissues to contract in the later stages of repair.

A three-dimensional co-ordinates system (Gilmore, 1986; Kapandji, 1987) provides a useful model for describing planes and axes of passive movement. This highlights the large variety of physiological, accessory, or combined passive movements available (Figures 9.2 and 9.3).

Nerves

The nervous system (central nervous system, peripheral nervous system, and autonomic nervous system) should be considered as an anatomical, electrical, chemical and pathological continuum. It consists of highly metabolic specialized tissue (axons) and highly innervated connective tissue of various forms (Figure 9.4). These connective tissues provide protection and allow movement whilst the working functional environment of

Figure 9.2   A three-dimensional coordinates system representing the spectrum of passive movement directions available at a motion segment. ZZ, sagittal plane, coronal frontal axis; YY, transverse axis, longitudinal plane; XX, coronal plane, sagittal axis. (Adapted from Gilmore, 1986, Biomechanics of the lumbar motion segment, in Grieve, G (ed.) *Modern Manual Therapy of the Vertebral Column*. Churchill Livingstone, Edinburgh, with permission.)

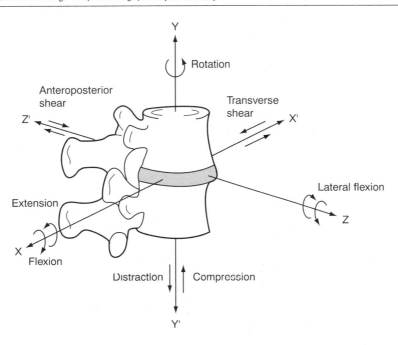

Figure 9.3 Three-dimensional coordinates system of the knee showing the potential spectrum of passive movement directions available along and about the axes. (Adapted from Kapandji, 1987, *The Physiology of the Joints. Vol. 2 Lower Limbs*, Churchill Livingstone, Edinburgh, with permission.)

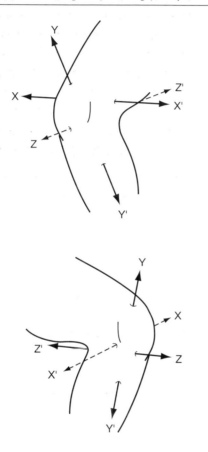

Figure 9.4 Cross-section of a peripheral nerve trunk showing the innervation of connective tissue by the nervi nervorum.

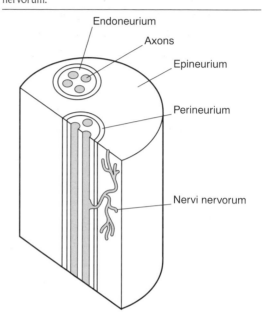

structures to move (slide) or to adapt to changes in tension (see Chapter 4).

the nerve is maintained during everyday activities. Consequently the whole of the nervous system, and its infrastructure, can be influenced by passive movements.

In recent years there has been a shift in emphasis towards 'biasing' passive movement techniques towards the structures of the nervous system. Neurodynamic tests and the models on which they are based, help to identify alterations in tissue compliance that are thought to be due to changes in the ability of the nervous system

Clinical Example

A 38-year-old woman suffered an inversion injury to the ankle two months ago. She is still experiencing a sharp pain on the outside of the ankle radiating into the top of the foot with foot inversion. This persists despite doing active stretching exercises. On further questioning she remembers experiencing a few minutes of 'tingling' in the outside of the foot immediately after the injury. Palpation examination of the superficial peroneal nerve reveals allodynia. Passive inversion of the foot reproduces her sharp pain. However, with her in supine lying and her foot held still in inversion, the addition of straight leg raise (SLR) and hip adduction causes an increase in the sharp pain and some tingling. These sensitizing additions show that the peroneal nerve was also damaged during the injury. The full mobility of the peroneal nerve can be restored by mobilizing ankle inversion in straight leg raise and hip adduction.

Muscles

Passive movement techniques will influence the connective tissue of muscles, their fascia, and their tendons. Common sites of mechanical vulnerability are the musculotendonous junction and the tenoperiostial junction. Synovial sheaths, bursae and the muscle fibre filaments (actin and myosin) may also be influenced. Skeletal muscle is richly innervated by A and C fibres (nociceptors) throughout, but more so in the regions of the tendon and fascia (LaRoca, 1992) (Figure 9.5). This

Figure 9.5   Sensory (and motor) innervation of muscle.

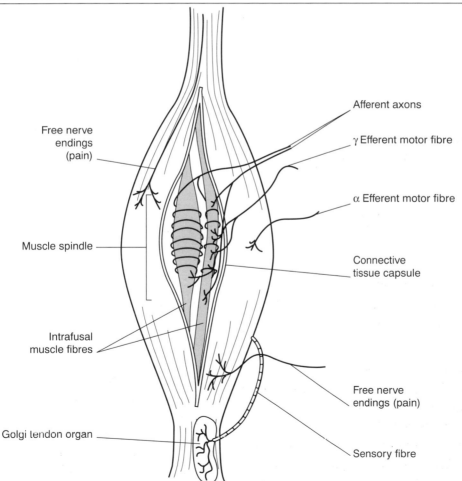

makes muscle a potential source of musculoskeletal pain. Muscle can be shortened or lengthened for various pathomechanical and pathophysiological reasons. Dysfunction of movement, strength and coordination will often result in muscle pain. Muscle length testing will reveal the need for passive stretching techniques of shortened muscle. Fascilitation methods can also be employed to influence muscle balance and length. Also examination of the soft tissues through palpation may reveal the need for local soft tissue manipulation techniques (e.g. transverse frictions or connective tissue massage).

Clinical Example

A 25-year-old body builder has developed a painful arc of shoulder abduction on the right due to an inflamed subacromial bursa. This occurred after weight training to build up his pectoral muscles. On examination no restriction in articular or neurodynamic mobility is evident. However, examination of the right sided pectoral muscles reveals they have become tight. Also the lower fibres of the trapezius muscle on the right has become lengthened. The result of this is a change in position of the right scapula. It has adopted a forward and downwardly rotated position. Consequently the subacromial bursa is being repeatedly compressed when the weights are lifted. By passively stretching the pectoral muscles and actively stabilizing the scapula the painful arc and subacromial compression quickly resolves (Figure 9.6).

Other Structures (e.g. skin, fascia, tendon sheath, lymphatics etc.)

Skilled palpation has been one of the key techniques which has set manipulative physiotherapists apart from the rest of the recognized medical professions. Through careful palpation the clinician may develop the ability to detect relevant clinical changes in: (1) skin temperature

Figure 9.6 Direction of fibres of pectoralis major and minor and lower trapezius indicating the direction for stretching of pectoralis minor and stabilization of the scapula by lower fibres of trapezius.

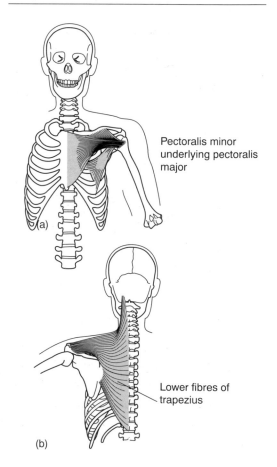

Pectoralis minor underlying pectoralis major

(a)

Lower fibres of trapezius

(b)

and sweating; (2) soft tissue near the surface and deep; (3) bony structure; and (4) tissue compliance to passive movement (Jull *et al.*, 1994). By means of passive techniques such as connective tissue manipulation, massage, and deep frictions the manipulative therapist has the ability to treat palpable soft tissue lesions in the skin, fascia, myofascia, muscle, ligament, nerve, lymph glands etc. (Palastanga, 1986; Holey, 1995) (Figure 9.7).

Clinical Example

'Tennis elbow' is a good example of how knowledge about structures can help the clinician to find the source of the patient's symptoms. A 66-year-old man presented with right 'tennis elbow' of three weeks duration, the onset of which corresponded to a 4-hour session of pruning the roses in his large garden. His main complaint was lateral elbow pain (Figure 9.8). This pain was brought on by activities that involved the use of the right hand for gripping and lifting. Pouring water from a kettle, and lifting a shopping bag were two such examples. On examination, the elbow was not painful to move actively. The right wrist and shoulder had minimal restrictions of movement. His neck was a little stiff and uncomfortable to move actively. There was a local area of palpable tenderness on and around the lateral epicondyle of the elbow.

His elbow joint movements were full and pain-free when tested passively. This included the special tests of elbow extension/abduction, extension/adduction, flexion/abduction, flexion/adduction (Maitland, 1991a).

The radial nerve supplies the lateral epicondyle of the elbow. The upper limb neural test biased towards the radial nerve (Chapter 4) was performed in this case. The neural tissue mobility was found to be full and symptom free.

The elbow pain was reproduced by isometric testing of the wrist and finger extensor. Local palpation of the common extensor origin at the lateral epicondyle of the elbow also reproduced the pain. It was concluded that the common extensor origin had become inflamed by the repeated action of pruning the roses and some of the fibres had become detatched from the periostium. Treatment therefore consisted of local transverse frictions to the common extensor origin with the aim of promoting local soft tissue healing and repair.

The local soft tissue manipulation techniques relieved the lateral elbow pain by 80%. A dull ache remained. On reflection the patient remembered having the same ache in the past when also suffering from a stiff neck.

As his elbow pain settled he had noticed his neck stiffness more, on the same side as the 'tennis elbow'. Palpation of his neck revealed stiffness and local discomfort at C5/6 on the same side as the remaining elbow ache. Mobilization of the neck improved his range of neck movement, improved the shoulder restriction and improved the elbow dull ache.

Some wrist restriction remained. Mobilization of the wrist joint improved the quality of gripping activities and therefore reduced the risk of further episodes of 'tennis elbow'.

Figure 9.7   Diagram of the layers and interfaces of the skin and its connective tissue. (Adapted from Holey, 1995, Connective tissue manipulation: towards a scientific rationale. *Physiotherapy.* 8I (I2): 730–739.)

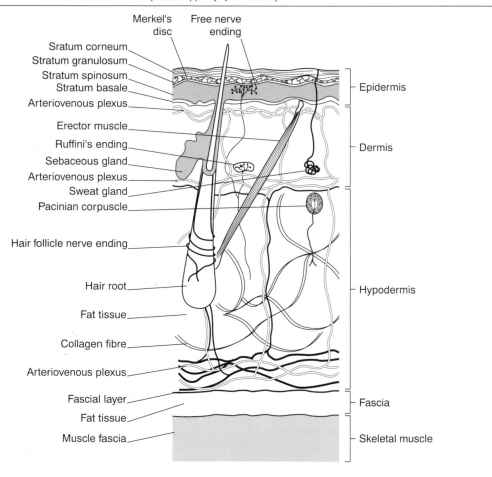

Figure 9.8   Symptom areas of a patient with 'tennis elbow'.

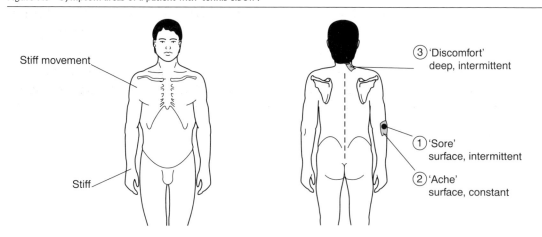

Principles of Passive Movement Techniques

For successful application of passive techniques it is important to consider the structures which are to be influenced. However it is also important to realise that the technique can rarely be entirely structure specific. For example, a technique often used to mobilize a stiff and painful hip joint is hip flexion/adduction. It should be realized, though, that the sciatic nerve, the various layers of buttock muscles, the sacro-iliac joint and the lumbar spine will also be mobilized. Therefore additional straight leg raise testing, muscle length testing, sacro-iliac stress testing, lumbar palpation and further testing of the hip joint will reveal the degree of involvement of each structure.

The stage of the pathological healing process and the extent of the patient's signs and symptoms also needs careful consideration. In this way an appropriate dosage of the technique will be applied (Figure 9.13).

It is clear that common principles of technique application exist between the different manipulative physiotherapy schools of thought. These principles apply no matter what structure is being targeted. In fact all connective tissues have similar compositions based on a glycoprotein matrix, collagen and elastin. They also have similar mechanical and physiological properties (Figure 9.23). Therefore passive movement techniques are likely to have similar effects on them.

In general passive techniques can be delivered to the appropriate site either through the skin or via limb and vertebral joint movement.

Passive Movement Direction

Once the proposed target structure and the method of delivery has been established, the most relevant movement direction, or range of movement, can be chosen. This will be in accordance with the desired effect of the technique. For example, stiffness at L4/5 may be treated with a posteroanterior technique if this is the stiffest direction; acute chondromalacia patellae may be treated by gently distracting the patella because this is the direction that is most pain relieving. The movement direction or range can be described in any appropriate way with symbols or diagrams (Maitland, 1991a,b; Kaltenborn, 1989) (Table 9.1). One example of visually depicting a passive movement direction is a linear model with A depicting any starting position and B depicting the end of an average normal range. B is thickened to account for the natural variability of the average normal end of range. This AB line can be shown in one or two dimensions with reference to any perceptable resistance to the movement. That is, resistance due to normal soft tissue compliance (Figures 9.9a, b and 9.10a, b) or due to stiffness (spasm-free resistance) (Figures 9.11a, b and 9.12a, b). Involuntary protective muscle spasm may also be considered as abnormal resistance to movement (Figure 9.16).

Table 9.1
Symbols. Symbols and abbreviations are used to denote the direction of movement of the technique or the test being used during examination or treatment. They help to make recording quick, brief, but understandable. (Reproduced, with permission, from Maitland, 1991, *Neuromusculoskeletal Examination and Recording Guide*, 5th edn, Lauderdale Press, Australia.)

↓ ↗	Central posteroanterior pressure (PAs) with a (L) inclination
↕	Central anteroposterior pressure (APs)
⌐•	Unilateral PAs on (L), ↘ with a medial inclination
↳•	Unilateral APs on the (L)
←•—	Transverse pressures towards (L) (+ ceph, + caud inclinations)
↻	Rotation of head, thorax, or pelvis to (L)
⟩	Lateral flexion towards (L)
←•→	Longitudinal movement (state ceph, caud)
—↓	Unilateral PAs at angle of (R) 2nd rib (or other rib)
•—↓	Further laterally on (R) 2nd rib
•—↑	Unilateral APs on (R)
CT ↗	Cervical traction in flexion for lower Cx and upper Tx joints
CT ↕	Cervical traction in neutral (sitting)
IVCT ↕	Intermittent variable CT neutral (sit or ly)
IVCT ↗	Intermittent variable CT in some F
IVCT ↗ 10 3/0 15	IVCT in flexion, 10 kg, 3 s hold/0 rest, for 15 min
LT	Lumbar traction
LT 30/15	Lt 30 kg, for 15 min
LT 50 0/0 10	Intermittent variable LT 50 kg, no hold/no rest, for 10 min

F	Flexion	Q	Quadrant
E	Extension	Lock	Locking position
AB	Abduction	F/AB	Flexion abduction
AD	Adduction	F/AD	Flexion adduction

Table 9.1
continued

↻	Medial rotation	E/AB	Extension abduction
↺	Lateral rotation	E/AD	Extension adduction
HF	Horizontal flexion	DISTR	Distraction
HE	Horizontal extension	COMPR	Compression
HBB	Hand behind back		
INV	Inversion	↓	Posteroanterior movement
EV	Eversion	↑	Anteroposterior movement
DF	Dorsiflexion	←→	Longitudinal movement
PF	Plantarflexion		Cephalad (ceph)
SUP	Supination		Caudad (caud)
PRON	Pronation		Body line/or other
EL	Elevation		e.g. femoral
DE	Depression		Forearm
PROTR	Protraction		
RETR	Retraction	←→	Transverse movement
MED	Medial		(R) or (L)
LAT	Lateral		
OP	Overpressure		Gliding adjacent joint
PPIVM	Passive physiological Intervertebral movements	↕	Surfaces
PAIVM	Passive accessory		
ULNT	Intervertebral movements Upper limb neural tests		
LLNT	Lower limb neural tests		

Joint abbreviations — see other texts.

Further Refinements of Passive Movement Techniques

GRADES

Passive oscillatory movements can be graded to indicate the amplitude and the position in the available range where the technique is being performed. This applies to movements that are within normal limits or movements that are pathologically limited (Figures 9.9–9.12). Classifying the technique in this way helps the clinician to think in finer detail about the techniques being used.

Kevin Banks

Figure 9.9   A range of movement and grades of passive mobilization (Maitland, 1991) – soft end feel. A, any starting position of the range. B, the end of average normal range. C, D, maximum quantity of resistance in this case. R_1, the start of resistance (normal average tissue compliance) soft end feel. R_2, the maximum quantity of resistance (normal average tissue compliance) soft end feel.

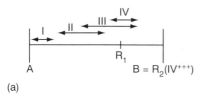

(a)

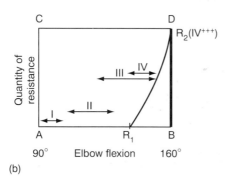

(b)

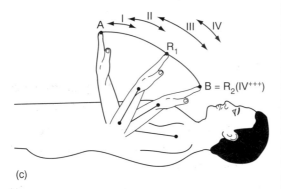

(c)

Also a grading system will form the best basis for communication with colleagues and for abbreviated recording.

Three examples of how grades may be described are as follows:

Figure 9.10   A range of movement and grades of passive mobilization (Maitland, 1991a) – hard end feel. A, any starting position of the range. B, the end of average normal range. C, D, maximum quantity of resistance in this case. R_1, the start of resistance (normal average tissue compliance) for a hard end feel. R_2, the maximum quantity of resistance/normal average tissue compliance) for a hard end feel.

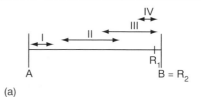

(a)

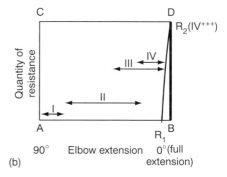

(b)

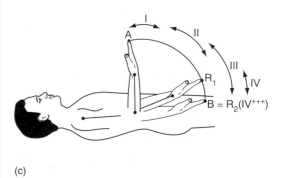

(c)

(Adapted from Maitland, 1991a)

I   A small amplitude movement performed at the beginning of the range, within the resistance-free part of the range;

II   A large amplitude movement performed within a resistance-free part of the range;

Figure 9.11 A movement diagram and grades of passive mobilization for a range of elbow extension limited by resistance (stiffness). A, any starting position of the range. B, the end of average normal range. C, D, the maximum quantity, or quality of the factors being plotted. R_1, the start of perceptible spasm-free resistance (stiffness). R_2, the maximum quantity of resistance. P_1, the point of onset of pain. P′ the quantity/quality of pain at the limit (not the maximum). L, pathological limit of range.

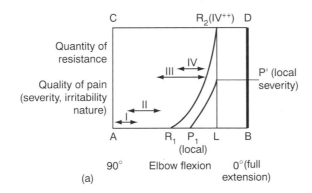

(a)

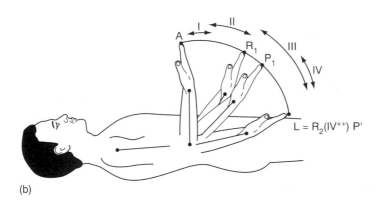

(b)

III A large amplitude movement performed into resistance or up to the limit of resistance;

IV A small amplitude movement performed into resistance or up to the limit of resistance;

V A high velocity, short amplitude thrust often near or at the limit of abnormal movement, at a speed outside of the patient's control (Figures 9.9–9.12).

Pluses or minuses can be used to refine the position in the available range further.

(Cyriax, 1983)

A Passive movement within the pain-free range (usually oscillatory, for acute conditions);

B Passive movement to the end of range (sustained stretching for increasing range in chronic stage);

C Passive movement to the end of range with overpressure of minimal amplitude (true manipulation to rupture small adhesions).

(Kaltenborn, 1989)

Translatory movements, traction, glide. Grades determined by the amount of slack the therapist feels when performing passive movements.

Figure 9.12   A range of passive movement and grades of passive mobilization for (a) an average normal posteroanterior lumbar spinous process with average normal tissue compliance (R₁ to R₂) and (b) a stiff (spasm-free resistance R₁ to R₂) painful posteroanterior lumbar spinous process. Note that in (b) a grade II is in the resistance-free part of the range but may still carry on into pain.

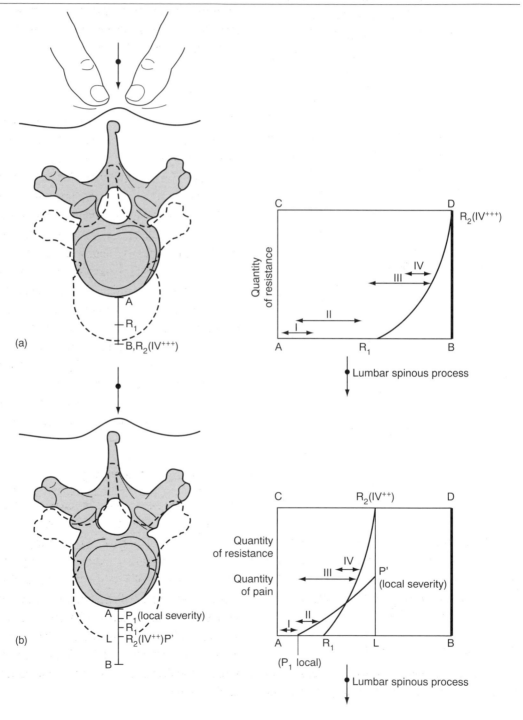

I Small amplitude of movement applied at the beginning of the range to loosen the joint;

II Large amplitude of movement applied up to the end of range which takes up the slack in the surrounding tissue tightening the joint;

III A greater force applied after the slack is tacken up, to stretch the tissue across the joint.

The three examples of classifying grades of passive techniques show several similarities. In each case the grades show graduation in position in range. The earlier grades have a gentleness about them, being performed at the start of the range or within the pain-free range. The later grades show a desire to improve the range of movement by stretching into resistance or tightness. Maitland and Kaltenborn refer to the amplitude of movement as well as the position in range. Cyriax and Kaltenborn refer to specific tissue effects. In contrast, the grades adapted from Maitland show more attention to detail and refinement. Also they are classified in terms of the clinician's perception of resistance to movement rather than tissue or joint effects. This is in keeping with Maitland's 'primacy of clinical evidence' model of technique selection. The Cyriax grades have a relationship to the stage of the soft tissue disorder. This corresponds to Cyriax's principles of accurate diagnosis of soft tissue lesions and his requirement that 'all treatment must reach the lesion'. The Kaltenborn grades relate to the biomechanical considerations of joint motion, and Kaltenborn's principles of selecting mobilization techniques which restore normal gliding in the joint. It is evident that the clinician can use the grading systems selectively, depending on each patient's particular clinical requirements.

RHYTHM, SPEED AND DURATION

Variations in the rhythm, speed and duration of the techniques (Figure 9.13) may affect the response the technique has during and after its performance. For example, a technique performed too quickly and with a jerky rhythm in the presence of protective muscle spasm, will only serve to enhance the protective response and the technique will be ineffective.

DOSAGE

Generally, guidelines on the selection of appropriate grade, rhythm, speed and duration of passive techniques (i.e. the 'dosage') have developed empirically through the years. 'Dosage' of passive techniques is an area that requires scientific evaluation so that fact can be added to clinical experience. A low dosage technique may be chosen initially if a patient has symptoms and signs which are functionally severe and pathologically active. On the other hand a disorder of minimal functional loss and pathological stability will be best dealt with using high dosage techniques. The clinical response during and after treatment will tell the clinician whether the technique has worked or not, i.e. does the patient feel better. Figure 9.13 details some clinical reasoning options when deciding upon the dosage of the technique.

Movement Diagrams

Passive techniques, whether biased towards joints, muscles, nerves or other soft tissues need to be modified according to the presenting history, symptoms, signs and pathological nature. Figures 9.9–9.11 give examples of how you can modify the grade of techniques when a range of elbow extension is normal and when it is limited by pain and stiffness following a fractured olecranon for instance. A further example (Figure 9.12) shows similar modifications for a normal and abnormal lumbar spine.

Figure 9.13   Technique dosage chart — clinically reasoned selection.

	Low dosage (when the severity, irritability or nature of the symptoms or disorder indicate caution) often pathophysiology.	High dosage (pathomechanics or maintained symptoms (pain)) often stiffness or pain related to stiffness.
Patient starting position	Most comfortable. As symptom free/discomfort free as possible.	Best position for access to apply forces in the appropriate direction.
Therapist starting position and application of forces	Light contact of hands/thumbs. Adapt to patient comfort whilst maintaining therapists body position in required direction and for accessibility of structure.	Firm but comfortable contact of hands/thumbs. Therapists body positioned in direction of technique with leverage giving optimal efficiency.
Passive movement direction (range)	Pain free or into slight/minimal pain or discomfort.	Into the restricted/painful direction at its limit (often in combined movements).
Grade (Maitland 1991) Amplitude and position in range	Reflex/neurophysiological effects I II	Mechanical related effects III IV V
Rhythm	Smooth oscillatory 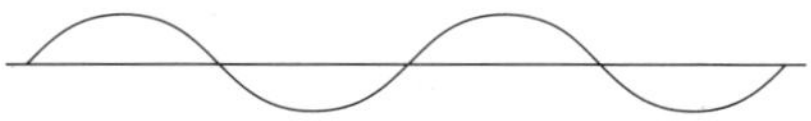	Staccato, sustained. Smooth alternated. 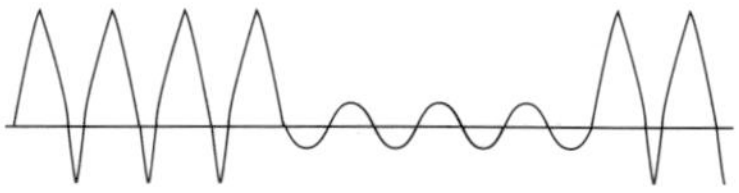
Speed	Slow e.g. 1 cycle/2 seconds	Fast e.g. 2–3 cycles/second
Duration	Short 30 seconds — 2 minutes	Long 2 mins — 5 mins × (n)
Advice/home programme	• Comfortable rest positions • Relieving positions/movements • Anti-inflammatory modalities if necessary • Gentle pain free movement	• Automobilizations • Prophylaxis

Movement diagrams (Figures 9.11a and 9.12b) are one method by which the clinician can express the extent of abnormal physical findings and the extent of symptoms (pain) the patient perceives when any passive movement direction is examined. Abnormal findings usually present are pain, stiffness (spasm-free resistance), or protective involuntary muscle spasm. Increased compliance to passive movement may also occur when instability is present. The detection of these clinically relevant signs by using the fingers and hands is learnt and refined over years of practice. There is evidence that skills such as the detection of resistance to movement by palpation improves with practice and feedback (Lee *et al.*, 1990).

A movement diagram is a dynamic, two-dimensional map which can be put to paper or visualized mentally. When a passive movement direction is found to be abnormal (e.g. elbow extension, or posteroanterior movement of the lumbar spinous process) and relevant to the patient's disorder a movement diagram can be constructed. The abnormal physical findings can be mapped out as you feel them with your fingers and hands (Figures 9.11 and 9.12). For example, when in the range does the patient start to feel his pain? (Detailed communication with the patient is needed for this.) What is limiting the movement and how much is limited compared with the ideal range? If stiffness is limiting the range, when in the range can you feel it starting? How much pain does the patient experience at the limit of the resistance? (A visual analogue scale is useful here sometimes.) And, finally, how do the pain and resistance to movement behave from where they start to where you can go no further? Is there, for instance, a gradual increasing of pain and resistance together?

Movement diagrams, therefore, represent passive movements which have become abnormal due to pathological processes. The factors limiting the passive movement usually correspond to the severity of the patient's symptoms and functional limitations. Thus the movement diagram may be useful in helping to select an appropriate dosage for a treatment technique (Figures 9.16–9.19). The movement diagram may also be useful as an evaluative tool to chart any progression made during treatment as the abnormal physical findings become less limiting (e.g. full elbow extension is being regained). Movement diagrams also serve as a valuable teaching and communication medium both with the patient and with colleagues. You should refer to Maitland (1991) and Magarey (1986) for more in depth descriptions of movement diagrams.

Method of Application

Passive techniques are skills that need to be learnt and practised extensively. Basic principles of leverage, line of gravity, and direction of forces should be applied. Thinking this way will help the clinician to apply passive movement forces efficiently and also achieve the desired effect of the technique. At the same time the clinician can learn to sense and 'feel' movement better. General principles should include thoughts about the following.

THE STARTING POSITION OF THE PATIENT

Wherever possible the patient should be positioned so as to reduce postural muscle activity and reduce the forces acting against the passive movement. For example, passive accessory movements of the glenohumeral joint are usually performed better in supported supine lying rather than in sitting. Positioning of the patient should also be considered in relation to the accessibility of the structures and direction of the selected technique. For example, it is much easier to apply forces to the lumbar spinous processes in prone lying or side lying than it is in supine lying. However, the patient's position may need to be modified if they have a very painful disorder. *Their* comfort then becomes a priority. For example, a patient with a very painful left hip joint may be most comfortable in supported right side lying. In this case the hip is still accessible for the clinician to perform accessory movement techniques.

Also some techniques may need to be performed in functional positions. For example, if a marathon runner can only reproduce his ankle pain when his weight is on it, the clinician may need to mobilize the accessory movements of the ankle with the patient standing.

THE STARTING POSITION OF THE THERAPIST (DIRECTION OF THE TECHNIQUE)

The mechanical advantage and efficiency of the technique will be determined by the therapist's starting position. The therapist's body should be positioned in the direction into which the technique will be performed so that the work is carried out with the minimum of effort. Wherever possible the principles of third-order levers should be applied to reduce the force required to produce the movement; for example, using the leg as leverage to mobilize the hip joint. Attention should be drawn to the ergonomics of the technique, i.e. the height of the plinth and the stresses and strains on the therapist's own body. Figure 9.14 show contrasting examples of this when treating the spine. One tip is to attempt to 'hug' the part being moved whenever possible.

THE MEANS OF APPLICATION

The highly sensitive organ of the fingers and hands best serves as the medium through which the passive technique can be directed, felt and controlled. There should be considerable attention given to where the hands are placed and the desired point of contact. The fingers and hands should not be the prime mover as this dilutes the perceived 'feel' of the movement. The arms and the body should be the main source of force production. Every therapist should feel the discomfort of someone pushing on their spine using

Figure 9.14 Examples of bad and good positioning when considering the therapist's starting position for a posteroanterior lumbar technique.

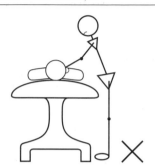

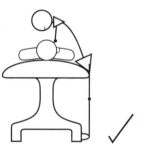

the thumbs as prime movers. In contrast they should also feel the softness of well placed hand contact and controlled body movement as the prime mover.

REFINEMENTS OF TECHNIQUE

Through training, the fingers and hands can become sensitive to the feel of the passive movement and can establish whether it falls into normal healthy parameters or whether it is related to dysfunction. Likewise the arms and body can be trained to refine the passive technique in order to modify the force applied, the depth or grade (position in range and amplitude) and the rhythm and speed, so helping it to achieve its desired effect.

These principles apply also to connective tissue

manipulation and other soft tissue techniques. They also have direction, depth, in some cases amplitude, and speed (Palastanga, 1986; Holey, 1995).

The Basis for Selection of Passive Techniques

The techniques you select and progress throughout an episode of care should not be based on one, but a series of reasoned factors. These should include the presenting history, symptoms and signs, the movement directions involved, the structures involved, the diagnosis, the pathology, the mechanism of pain production, and the nature of the person. All the factors involved should be considered in such a way as to make a strong case for the use of a particular technique. Considered decisions should be made about the structure to be treated, and the direction, position in range, depth and amplitude of the technique. It should also be considered whether the technique should be oscillatory or sustained, slow or quick, smooth or staccato, into pain or short of pain, with or without loading, for a short or long duration (Figure 9.13). You are referred to other texts for the techniques available (Maitland, 1986; Butler, 1991; Janda, 1983; Cyriax, 1983; Holey, 1995; Exelby, 1995).

The criteria for the selection and progression of techniques can be considered in terms of the clinical evidence and the theoretical basis.

The Clinical Evidence

QUESTION 1

The first question the patient is to be asked should be along the lines of 'As far as *you* are concerned, what do *you* feel is *your main problem?*' That is to say what does the patient consider to be his main problem in terms of symptoms (pain) and functional loss and how, therefore, by using the body's inherent capacity to give information, can this be used to help choose the best treatment technique?

Clinical Example

If a 79-year-old man experiences pain and stiffness deep in his left groin whilst releasing his crown green bowl and feels the same pain and stiffness when crossing his legs to put on his socks, it is likely that the pain and stiffness will also be reproduced in hip flexion/adduction. This direction may then be appropriate for a treatment technique.

CLUES FROM THE SYMPTOM BEHAVIOUR

Ask yourself whether the subjective information gives you clues to the source of the symptoms, the mechanism of their production and the treatment technique that may be used.

Clinical Examples

If a 44-year-old builder cannot work overhead because he experiences intense pain in the middle of his low back, he is likely to have problems in spinal extension. Examination and treatment are likely to be progressed gradually into spinal extension so that his functional loss is overcome.

If a 34-year-old salesman has pain down the back of his right leg when he is driving, and the pain increases when he looks down to change his CD (i.e. with neck flexion), a neurodynamic test such as the canal slump may be relevant to use in examination and treatment (Chapter 4). For example, a technique in the slump position (neck flexion or knee extension) is likely to mobilze the nervous system. This will then restore the neural structures to normal pain-free mobility.

If a 66-year-old secretary gets relief from her headache (Figure 9.15) by rubbing the base of her skull, transverse frictions of the suboccipital structures may well be a basis for treatment. This technique should aim to improve the mechanical and physiological properties of the suboccipital tissues and therefore relieve the woman's headache.

THE INJURING MOVEMENT

The mechanism and direction of an injury may be a clue to the structures involved, the amount of damage sustained, and the strength and direction of treatment techniques required.

Clinical Example

You have assessed a man who has twisted his back whilst shovelling concrete. His right-sided low back pain is intense initially, so you choose a low dosage technique into spinal rotation to start with. When he is 80% recovered you may well choose to clear the remaining symptoms and signs by using a combined movement technique in side lying at the limit of rotation and in spinal flexion (i.e. into the injuring movement direction).

THE ACTIVITY CAUSING THE SYMPTOMS AS DEMONSTRATED BY THE PATIENT (FUNCTIONAL DEMONSTRATION)

Analysis of the volunteered functional demonstration which reproduces the patient's symptoms will reveal both the likely source of the symptoms and the direction in which to treat them. Structurally biased differentiation may also be attempted to help specify the technique more.

Figure 9.15   Headache.

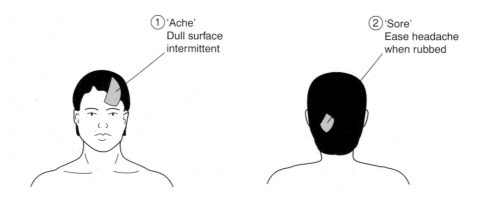

① 'Ache' Dull surface intermittent

② 'Sore' Ease headache when rubbed

A 26-year-old badminton player indicates that overhead smashing reproduces his mild right anterior shoulder pain. Asking him to adopt this position reveals that the right shoulder is in full elevation and lateral rotation, the neck is in extension, right lateral flexion and right rotation, the thoracic spine is in right rotation and extension, the elbow is almost fully flexed and the wrist is extended whilst the racket is gripped. Selectively altering any of these components and discovering which alters the pain will reveal where to direct treatment. With the patient in the functional position, if the anterior shoulder pain changes when the neck is taken further into extension, cervical techniques should be considered. If, however, the pain changes more when the shoulder is stressed more into elevation, the shoulder quadrant may be the technique to employ. If greater thoracic extension gives more pain, the use of thoracic techniques is indicated, whereas if further wrist extension causes more pain, a neurodynamic technique may need to be deployed.

CLINICAL GROUPINGS (CHASING THE PAIN)

Disordered neuromusculoskeletal structures will present you with clinically relevant abnormal physical signs when they are moved passively. They will also be painful. The pain and other signs — stiffness (spasm-free resistance), spasm, instability etc. — can be depicted on a movement diagram as discussed earlier. The extent of the signs and their relationship to each other can be classified into clinical groups which will give you a general basis for treatment selection as well as a means of communication with colleagues.

Pain (Often with Protective Spasm)
When a patient has pain that is severe or irritable, or where the nature of it requires caution (e.g. nerve root pain), and where only a small percentage of movement is possible, low dosage techniques (grades I and II pain-free, slow, smooth rhythm, for a short duration) will be most

Clinical Example

A patient with severe neck pain a few days after a whiplash injury fits into this clinical group. When you palpate the neck you find most pain and tenderness at C45. On passive accessory movement testing, pain increases immediately, is unbearable, and is accompanied by protective spasm. When passive mid-cervical rotation is tested, a few degrees each way are available before pain starts to increase and become unbearable (Figures 9.16 and 9.17). You therefore choose cervical rotation as a treatment technique as a small amount of pain-free passive oscillatory movement is available at the start of the range (grade I). If you perform the technique slowly (1 oscillation per 2 seconds), with a smooth rhythm and for a short duration (30 s–2 min), you are more likely to have mechanical and physiological effects on tissue healing and pain mechanisms without aggravating the patient's symptoms. Moreover, the patient is more likely to come back and see you again.

Figure 9.16 Movement diagram for selection of technique. S₁ S′, protective involuntary spasm.

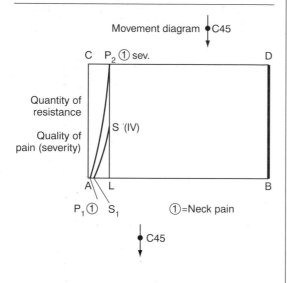

Figure 9.17 Movement diagram showing grade I (Maitland, 1991a) to be possible as a treatment technique.

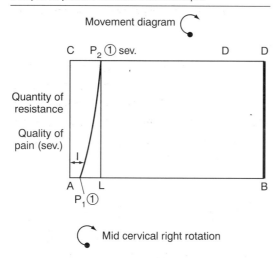

appropriate in most cases. Generally speaking, the structures responsible for the pain should be positioned and moved in the most pain-free manner possible. The intention of the technique should be to influence the pain mechanisms independent of any resistance.

Figure 9.18 Movement diagram of (for example) hip medial rotation showing through-range pain and spasm-free resistance (stiffness). Grade III (Maitland, 1991a) is the most appropriate grade, i.e. a large amplitude into the limiting resistance.

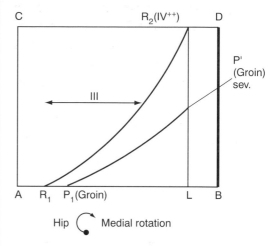

Pain and Stiffness (Spasm-Free Resistance) Together

By far the largest clinical grouping found in everyday practice is that in which the patient has both pain and stiffness together. In most cases the pain and stiffness are related to one another. If pain is dominant with little resistance, pain-free techniques may be chosen initially, but otherwise treatment techniques are more effective if carried into resistance. The amount of resistance the technique can move into will be dependent on the amount of pain accompanying it.

Pain and resistance generally occur together through a range or movement (ROM) or at the end of range (EOR). Occasionally, however, you may encounter stiffness on its own.

Through-range pain and resistance may respond better to techniques with larger amplitude (Figure 9.18). Often through-range pain and resistance are related to a hypothesis of joint surface pathology. In such cases compression of the joint surfaces may be of value to test the hypothesis further. Joint compression may help to reproduce the patient's pain and highlight the loss of friction-free movement associated with joint surface pathology. Selective, intermittent compression may be of value when treating joint surface disorders, as this may improve the distribution of synovial fluid on the articular cartilage and therefore improve its nutrition and healing capacity (Maitland, 1991a). End of range pain and resistance or stiffness alone will respond better to end of range oscillatory or sustained techniques (Figure

Clinical Examples

A 68-year-old women with a bunion on her right foot also experiences pain and stiffness in the big toe during the push-off phase of walking, but not enough to stop her. On examination, through-range pain and stiffness is reproduced with passive extension of the first metatarsophalangeal joint. When the joint is compressed the pain and stiffness feeling is the same as when she is walking. The selection of a technique into this direction (e.g. in lying, first metatarsophalangeal extension, with compression, grade III) will be justified if the pain and stiffness becomes less during and after the technique.

A 74-year-old man cannot tuck his shirt in because of stiffness and discomfort in his shoulder when he puts his hand up his back. On examination, he is found to have stiffness and pain at the end of passive medial rotation of the shoulder. By using a technique which stretches out medial rotation (e.g. grade IV) he can then perform his daily task.

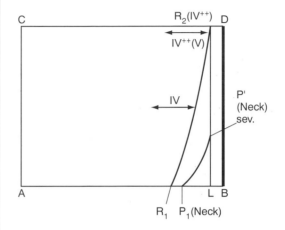

Figure 9.19 An end of range movement diagram (for example) of cervical lateral flexion showing end of range stiffness (R_1 to R_2) with some pain. Grades IV or V (Maitland, 1991a) are most appropriate in this case.

Cervical lateral flexion

9.19). Manipulation (e.g. grade V) rather than mobilization may also be a strong consideration.

Momentary Pain

Occasionally a clinical presentation is encountered whereby a patient experiences pain for a fleeting moment with certain activities and with little consistency, i.e. momentary pain. Usually combinations of movement will be required to find and treat the pain.

Clinical Example

A 19-year-old fast bowler experiences a fleeting sharp pain in the right side of his low back, during his delivery stride, on average once every two or three overs. The pain is reproduced and treated by a technique of unilateral posteroanterior pressure on L4 on the right whilst he is in spinal extension, right rotation and right lateral flexion.

343

Theoretical Basis

DIAGNOSIS/PATHOLOGY

Nachemson (1992) says of low back pain, 'Rarely are diagnoses scientifically valid'. Magarey (1986) says, 'A presumptive diagnosis is an important consideration when selecting treatment but in most instances the selection of a technique is made in response to the signs and symptoms'. Knowledge of the diagnosis and pathology on the other hand will often guide the dosage of the treatment technique, provided that this fits in clinically with the working hypothesis.

Clinical Examples

If a patient has a diagnosis of disc/nerve root lesion and clinically neurological changes are present, the emphasis on the treatment technique will be to perform it in a way that does not worsen the neurological signs.

If a patient has osteoarthritis of the hip, examination of the lumbar spine, sacroiliac joint and neurodynamics should still be carried out to exclude or implicate other components of the symptomology. Never assume anything!

STRUCTURES INVOLVED

Although an emphasis is placed on the clinical analysis of movement directions when selecting passive treatment techniques, knowledge of anatomy will give you a basis for biasing techniques towards one structure over another. Passive physiological and accessory movements, or combinations of these, will give you biasing towards joint tissue (with compression and distraction forces to influence more the intra- or peri-articular tissue). Derivatives of neurodynamic tests will give you an emphasis towards the nervous system structures. Knowledge about origins and insertions of muscles will help to bias length testing to the appropriate direction and also help interpretation of palpation findings. Knowledge of fascial interfaces will help interpret the effects of connective tissue massage and transverse frictions.

Clinical Example

A clinical example of tissue biasing may relate to the analysis of cervical lateral flexion. If a patient has right-sided neck pain and restriction of cervical lateral flexion to the left, think which structures could be responsible and which tests you have available to implicate structures and therefore direct your techniques appropriately. If you can work this out then you will have the ability to analyse any passive movement direction using the same principles.

Lateral flexion to the left reproducing right-sided pain will stress, for example, the intervertebral joints, the nerve roots and trucks, the scaleni muscles, sternomastioid and trapezius, and the subclavian artery in the thoracic outlet (Figure 9.20). To differentiate, you can passively laterally flex the neck to the left until the right-sided neck pain is felt. Next elevate the right shoulder girdle only. This will take the stress off the right-sided nerve, artery and muscles mainly. If the pain remains the same, and a hard articular end feel is felt, then the intervertebral joints on the right

Figure 9.20   A representation of structures related to the 'thoracic outlet'.

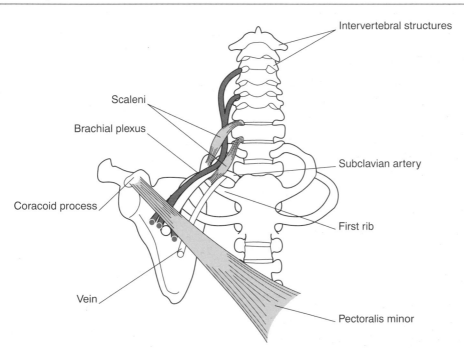

are likely to be the source of the pain. (Passive physiological and accessory movements of the cervical spine will confirm this hypothesis.)

If the pain goes with elevating the right shoulder girdle, and the neck can be taken further and pain-free to the left, the muscle or nerve or artery on the right is a more likely source. In this case, if left lateral flexion to the pain is performed with the right arm in a ULNT position, and the pain and range changes with right wrist sensitization, a neural bias is implicated. If there are no neurodynamic restrictions or signs, the muscles may be the source of the right-sided neck pain, in which case the right scaleni length can be tested, for example, by fixing the insertion at the right first rib using the heel of the left hand and side flexing the neck to the left using the left hand to cradle the head and neck. If this test is more comparable, then muscle bias treatment techniques (e.g. myofascial release, stretching, muscle balance exercises etc.) may be employed. The right subclavian artery may best be implicated by the presence of vascular changes (e.g. colour, temperature changes in the limb or lack of peripheral pulses).

BIOMECHANICS

Techniques may be selected on the grounds of biomechanical consideration. This is acceptable as long as the biomechanical restrictions fit in with the clinical picture and the desired effect is

Clinical Examples

Joints may become stuck or 'locked' due to loose bodies, meniscal tears or synovial impingement. The biomechanical function of the joint is lost (i.e. the roll, spin, slide mechanism). In the case of cervical 'facet-locking wry neck' the joint biomechanics are thought to be affected in this way. The neck becomes stuck with a contralateral side flexion and rotation deformity, often after a sudden movement. This condition often responds well to grade V manipulative thrust techniques with the intention of 'gapping' the offending joint to unlock it and therefore restore its ideal mechanical function. 'Facet-locking wry neck' should not be confused with 'discogenic wry neck' which comes on more gradually, has a deformity more into flexion, and takes longer to resolve, responding best to mobilization techniques rather than manipulative thrust techniques.

Passive techniques performed along the plane of a joint may be a biomechanical consideration in restoring pain-free movement. Such techniques may be performed with or without active movement (Exelby, 1995). For example, if thoracic flexion is locally painful and restricted, it may be appropriate to use a unilateral technique on the relevant facet joints in the plane of the joint, inclined towards the head (Figure 9.21), with the intention of restoring pain-free movement. This can be performed passively with the patient in prone lying, or in a sitting position, during active thoracic rotation.

The roll, spin and slide mechanism of joints surfaces may need to be considered as a way of improving pain-free joint range. In this respect, the quality of physiological movement is only as good as the quality of the accompanying accessory or joint play movement. For example, shoulder abduction is accompanied by roll upwards and slide downwards of the head of the humerus in relation to the glenoid. In the case of 'frozen shoulder', capsular thickening prevents this. On examination accessory movements of the glenohumeral joint to allow the head of the humerus to drop down during abduction are lost or reduced. Accessory movement techniques in different arm positions, depending on pain tolerance, should be used to mobilize the joint and restore the lost movement.

Often, however, the painful restricted joint movement does not correspond to biomechanical principles. For example, when open chain knee extension is painful and restricted (e.g. extending the knee whilst sitting on a plinth) the concave/convex rule suggests that to restore this movement direction the tibia needs to slide forwards on the femur. A posteroanterior technique of the tibia on the femur is suggested. If, however, this accessory movement direction is full range and pain-free but the anteroposterior direction of the tibia on the fumur in knee extension is stiff and painful, it may be more appropriate clinically to use the 'non-biomechanical' direction in treatment. What is known biomechanically does not always translate into what we expect to find clinically with patients. Therefore, on the one hand, clinicians should be reappraising their biomechanical knowledge continually. On the other hand, clinicians should be prepared to search clinically for techniques that are more effective if a biomechanical model is not being helpful.

Figure 9.21   Plane of the vertebral articular facets.

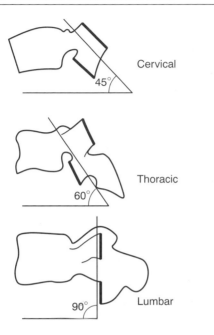

Cervical
45°

Thoracic
60°

Lumbar
90°

achieved. That is to say, the patient's pain and restrictions are relieved.

THE NATURE OF THE SYMPTOMS

Great care in selection of technique should be taken if symptoms arise that indicate the need for caution; for example, where there are symptoms and signs of nerve root compression or vertebral artery insufficiency. In such cases treatment techniques should be chosen carefully in order to avoid exacerbation of such symptoms. Always think whether the technique you have chosen could be harmful.

THE NATURE OF THE PERSON

The dosage of the selected technique may be influenced by your judgement about the way your patient responds to ill health. Therefore, be aware of the pain acceptance and pain tolerance of the patient, given such factors as his cultural background, his social and economic frame of reference, his reaction to a 'medical' environment and so on. For example, a stoical person may not reveal the true extent of his problem because they do not like to complain, and in such cases overtreatment may be harmful. At the other extreme, a patient with a low pain acceptance may require you to reduce the dosage of the technique because of his reaction to painful stimuli rather than because of the pathological nature of his disorder.

CREATIVITY OF PASSIVE TECHNIQUE SELECTION

At times you will find it appropriate to invent a technique for a particular patient's clinical presentation. You should, in fact, be prepared to try new things within the framework of clinical safety, and indeed if you avoid using set routines of selection of techniques, you will solve clinical problems that do not respond to standard practice. Choose each technique on its merit and make it functionally relevant. (An example of weak reasoning would be to choose, for example, a posteroanterior technique for glenohumeral pain because that usually does the trick.) Above all be self-critical if the desired effect of the technique is not achieved. The clinical examples below show how the clinician can 'invent' techniques.   A logical approach will ensure the techniques still have a relevant clinical basis.

Clinical Examples

A 28-year-old builder has a history of gradually increasing anterior shoulder pain, especially with horizontal extension movements. An anteroposterior (AP) movement on his coracoid process reproduces some of the pain and pins and needles in his index finger. When the arm is then placed in ULNT1 position with horizontal extension the AP on the coracoid is more painful. This position and movement is then adopted as a treatment technique. This clinical example shows how techniques can be invented. A logical approach is required so that techniques still have a clinically relevant basis to them, but at the same time go beyond documented, textbook techniques.

The only way the deep ankle pain of a 33-year-old marathon runner can be reproduced is by an AP direction of the tibia and fibular on the talus in standing with the ankle dorsiflexed. This is used as a treatment technique.

A 42-year-old builder who experienced a deep ache in the left side of his low back after bending over laying bricks for a few hours is treated with a transverse pressure on L4 on the left with him standing and in a half flexed position. This is the only way his pain could be reproduced and treated successfully.

Progression of Techniques

Progression of techniques may initially involve changing a component of the technique already being used, either as the technique is being performed or as a response to its effects during subsequent visits.

Clinical Example

A patient with strong neurogenic pain in the wrist (e.g. carpal tunnel syndrome) is being treated using a grade II shoulder depression technique, short of pain, to influence the neurodynamic component of the pain mechanism. The technique may be progressed by increasing the grade to a II+ or by performing the technique for longer.

Another consideration for progression may be to treat the structures in a different movement direction.

Clinical Example

A patient with anterior knee pain may improve only slightly with patellofemoral longitudinal passive mobilization but improve considerably more quickly with a transverse technique.

At some stage in the progression of treatment, recovery may have slowed down. In such cases it is probably relevant to treat a different structure contributing to the patient's symptoms or to add on treatment techniques.

Clinical Example

A 24-year-old man was having difficulty bending because of right-sided back pain following a rear impact car accident two weeks before. On examination, a hypothesis was made that three components were responsible for the symptoms and functional loss. These were: the intervertebral joints T10–S1, identifiable because joint signs were found on passive intervertebral testing; the right erector spinae, suggested by soft tissue swelling and thickening within the muscle found on palpation; and thirdly altered neurodynamics, indicated by reduction in SLR and increasing back pain with ankle dorsiflexion in SLR. Initially, the pain and restricted bending did not improve with passive accessory techniques on T10–S1. However, soft tissue manipulation (kneading) of the erector spinae improved the pain and bending by 50%. A passive SLR technique gave another 10% improvement, and a further 30% improvement only came when going back to mobilizing the intervertebral joints into a rotation direction (the spine was twisted at the point of impact). The last 10% recovery was attributed to natural history and a home exercise programme.

In some cases where recovery has slowed with treatment, or where the symptoms seem to be improving on their own, it may be relevant to advise a period of time without treatment to establish whether the intervention has been effective or of only temporary relief, or whether the natural progression of the disorder is causing recovery.

The effects of the previous technique on the patient's symptoms and functional restrictions will determine the rate of progression and final outcome. It is often useful to estimate the rate of progression and prognosis given the diagnosis and clinical evidence. In this way the decision to carry on using a technique or whether to change technique may be helped. The ultimate aim of the technique is to relieve the patient of his signs and symptoms and by prophylaxis to influence the future history or recurrence of the problem (Figure 9.22).

Prognosis

The decision to stop treatment should be made by balancing factors that may lead to a favourable or unfavourable prognosis. Factors to consider are:

- The natural history of the disorder: Has the disorder run its natural course? What is the stage and stability of the disorder, the state of the structures and the known pathology?
- The response to treatment. Has the disorder progressed at an acceptable rate? If not, are further medical investigations required or is there an element of the patient becoming dependent on therapy?
- What is acceptable for the patient. Can they accept a level of discomfort and restriction or not? Do they consider that their original main problems have been solved?
- Prophylactic measures required. Is a specifically tailored home programme required to add to the rate of recovery or to maintain the recovery?
- Above all prognosis should be realistic!

Figure 9.22 Considerations when planning technique progression.

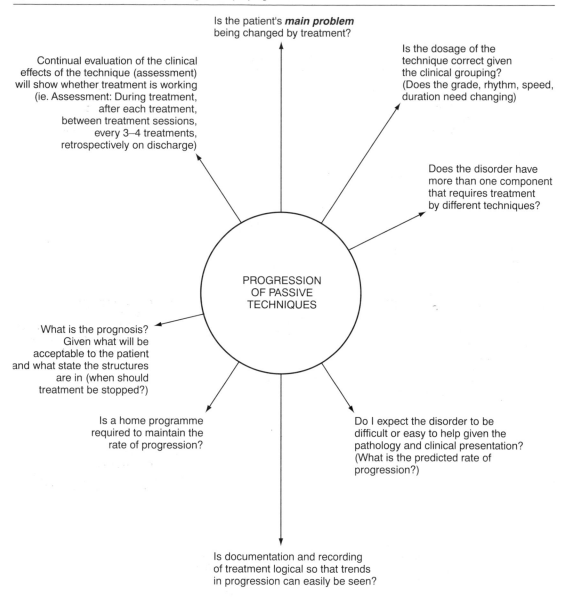

Is the patient's **main problem** being changed by treatment?

Continual evaluation of the clinical effects of the technique (assessment) will show whether treatment is working (ie. Assessment: During treatment, after each treatment, between treatment sessions, every 3–4 treatments, retrospectively on discharge)

Is the dosage of the technique correct given the clinical grouping? (Does the grade, rhythm, speed, duration need changing)

Does the disorder have more than one component that requires treatment by different techniques?

PROGRESSION OF PASSIVE TECHNIQUES

What is the prognosis? Given what will be acceptable to the patient and what state the structures are in (when should treatment be stopped?)

Is a home programme required to maintain the rate of progression?

Do I expect the disorder to be difficult or easy to help given the pathology and clinical presentation? (What is the predicted rate of progression?)

Is documentation and recording of treatment logical so that trends in progression can easily be seen?

Effects of Passive Techniques

Passive techniques impart kinetic energy to the tissues and cells being moved. The author postulates that passive movements should adhere to the general rules of energy conservation and energy transfer. That is, energy cannot be created, it can only be transferred from one form to another (Figure 9.23). The clinical and therapeutic effects of passive movements are well known (Frank *et al.,* 1984). Interest is now being directed at their metabolic, physiological and neurophysiological effects. The reductionist path of scientific enquiry

Figure 9.23   Proposed effects of passive movement techniques according to the laws of energy conservation and transfer.

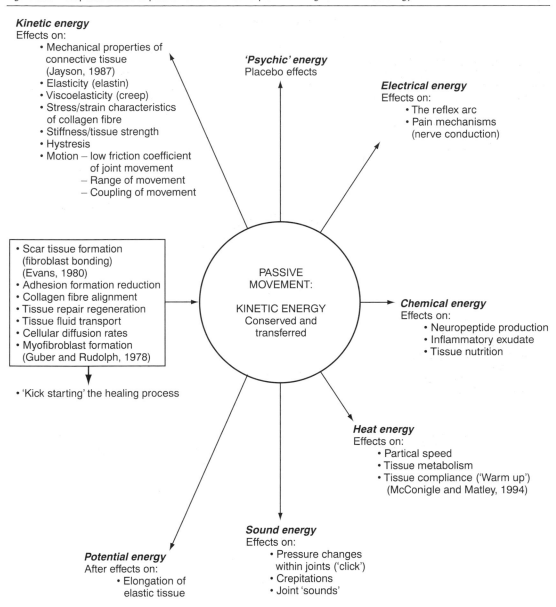

helps to classify at which macroscopic or microscopic level passive movement techniques might be having an effect.

Clinical Level

When compared with other therapeutic modalities, passive mobilization and manipulation has been shown to be more effective in most valid studies (Di Fabio, 1992). However, most studies have been concerned with the effects on spinal disorders, and at present there are few studies relating to peripheral structures. The lack of evidence highlights the difficulties of using prospective group comparison studies when researching the effectiveness of manipulative physiotherapy. The ethical question arises when a non-treatment control group is needed. It is impossible to carry out a double blind study as a trained clinician is required to perform treatment. Large numbers of subjects are required to obtain statistically significant results. And showing that the results are representative of the population as a whole is difficult with a patient group in a specific geographical location. Therefore the logistics of valid clinical research in this field are extensive. The single case study approach (Riddoch and Lennon, 1991) has been suggested as a means of overcoming some of these difficulties and at the same time obtaining results that can be scrutinized statistically. However, the main clinical effects of passive techniques that are evident are: a reduction in pain of neuromusculoskeletal origin, increase in ranges of movement and return to functional normality. For example, Saal et al. (1996) showed that most of a group of patients with cervical disc herniation responded well to nonsurgical management, including manual techniques. They returned to their pre-injury activity levels with little limitation. Another clinical consideration should be the placebo effect of 'having something done' and the psychological benefits of manual therapies.

Tissue Level

Frank et al. (1984) have shown that passive movement applied to ligament will affect tissue compliance, collagen alignment and the strength and stiffness of the ligament. Salter (1989) hypothesized that continuous passive motion (CPM)

should enhance the nutrition and metabolic activity of articular cartilage and other joint tissue. He found that, in the knee joints of rabbits, CPM stimulates the pluripotential undifferentiated mesenchymal cells to differentiate into articular cartilage (as opposed to either fibrous tissue or bone) and therefore lead to regeneration of articular cartilage. He also found, again in rabbits, that CPM accelerates the healing of articular cartilage and peri-articular tissue such as tendon and ligament. This is backed up by Lundborg (1988) in respect of nerve repair. Twomey and Taylor (1995) also suggest that the health of spinal joints depends on repeated low stress movement.

Metabolic Level

Caterson and Lowther (1977) showed that mechanical stress is important to normal metabolism of articular cartilage and to its ability to resist deformation under load. In their experiment using a population of sheep they found that the sheep who had their legs immobilized and non-weightbearing had a significantly reduced proteoglycan content of their articular cartilage (proteoglycan is a normal metabolic constituent of articular cartilage). Lundborg and Rydevik (1973) have shown that elongation of a nerve by 11% will produce ischaemia and therefore affect the normal metabolic demands of the nerve. This may occur if the normal mobility or stretch capacity of neural tissue is compromised by pathology. Therefore mobilizing neural tissue has the potential of improving the mechanical proporties of the nervous system and at the same time restoring an ideal metabolic environment. Holey (1995) suggests that connective tissue massage has metabolic effects on soft tissues via the local reflex effects on circulation.

Neurophysiological / Chemical Level

LaRoca (1992) describes C fibres, which are abundant in connective tissue, as containing neuropeptides including substance P. These neuropeptides play an important part in the production of tissue and neurogenic inflammation, nociception and neurogenic pain. C fibres are also thought to be involved in the monitoring of the metabolic state of the tissue and therefore processes such as protein synthesis. Passive movement of the tissue will affect these processes in some way. Wright (1995) argues that the endogenous control system in the periaquiductal grey matter of the dorsal horn is stimulated by spinal manipulation and is therefore a reason for postmanipulation analgesia. In chronic pain states (e.g. osteoarthritis of the knee) pain-free passive movement may, by plasticity, make the wide dynamic range (WDR) neurones in the dorsal horn revert to a role in movement and touch rather than in pain perception. Wright (1995) also refers to the trend in recent studies to relate to the effects of manipulation on the sympathetic nervous system – i.e. the effects of mobilization on temperature and skin conductance (sweating) and the effects of spinal posteroanterior mobilization on mechanical and thermal pain thresholds.

Cellular and Subcellular Levels

Studies on nerves have shown that axoplasmic flow within nerves is improved by movement (Butler, 1989). The transport mechanism and consequently the metabolic activity are thus improved. Guyton (1979) states that if a cell is to live and survive and grow it must obtain nutrients and other substances from the surrounding fluid. This will be done in part by active transport mechanisms, pinocytosis, and in part by diffusion. Passive movement will impart kinetic energy to the tissues, some of which will be transferred to cellular level (Frank et al., 1984). Kinetic energy will increase local temperature, which means there will be an increase in the speed of the randomly moving particles. As a result, the rate of diffusion will increase and this will help the cell to live, survive and grow.

Passive movements have plenty of beneficial effects, as you can see. However, be aware that overjudicious or inappropriate use may also have detrimental effects at all these reductionist levels. Among the possible consequences to consider are tissue trauma, vascular embarrassment, nerve damage, prolonged inflammatory response, nociceptive reinforcement and sympathetic disturbance.

The Validity and Reliability of Passive Movement Techniques

Passive movement techniques, especially manipulative thrust techniques, have been shown in a number of controlled trials to effectively relieve acute spinal neuromusculoskeletal pain and restore voluntary movement (Keir and Goats, 1991; Nachemson, 1992; Di Fabio, 1992) (Table 9.2). Despite this evidence for the efficacy of manual therapy it is currently unclear how these treatments may achieve their effects (Zusman, 1986).

With this in mind Jull (1987) challenged manual therapists to 'PROVE IT OR LOSE IT – MANUAL DIAGNOSIS'. She highlighted the need for manual diagnosis and treatment techniques to be accepted by recognized medical practice and to stand up to the rigours of scientific investigation.

Table 9.2
Valid efficacy studies of manual therapy. (From DiFabio, 1992, Efficacy of manual therapy. *Physical Therapy* **72**(12): 853–863, with kind permission of the american Physical Therapy Association.)

Author(s)	Citation	Primary comparison	Results statistically supporting the primary intervention[a]
Meade *et al.*	*BMJ* (1990) **300**: 1431–1437	Lumber manipulation versus mobilization	Y
Hadler *et al.*[b]	*Spine* (1987) **12**: 703–706	Lumbar manipulation versus mobilization	Y
Ongley *et al.*[c]	*Lancet* (1987) **18**: 143–146	Lumbar manipulation versus mobilization	Y
Sanders *et al.*[b]	*J Manipulative Physiol Ther* (1990) **13**: 391–395	Lumbar manipulation versus control	Y
Hoehler *et al.*[b]	*JAMA* (1981) **245**: 1835–1838	Lumbar manipulation versus control	Y
Glover *et al.*[b]	*Br J Ind Med* (1974) **31**: 59–64	Lumbar manipulation versus control	Y
Fisk	*NZ Med J* (1979) **90**: 288–291	Lumbar manipulation versus control	Y
Evans *et al.*	*Rheumatol Rehabil* (1978) **17**: 46–53	Lumbar manipulation versus control	Y
Nwuga	*Am J Phys Med* (1982) **61**: 273–278	Lumbar mobilization versus control	Y
Farrell and Twomey[b]	*Med J Aust* (1982) **1**: 160–164	Lumbar mobilization and manipulation versus control	Y
Mathews *et al.*	*Br J Rheumatol* (1987) **26**: 416–423	Lumbar mobilization and manipulation versus control	Y
Parker *et al.*	*Aust NZ J Med* (1978) **8**: 589–593	Cervical manipulation versus mobilization	N
Howe *et al.*	*JR Coll Gen Pract* (Occas Pap). (1983) **33**: 574–579	Cervical manipulation versus control	Y
Cibulka *et al.*	*Phys Ther* (1988) **68**: 1359–1363	Sacral manipulation versus control	Y

[a]Y = yes, N = no.
[b]Immediate or short-term symptomatic reduction found for manipulated groups. Long-term effects were comparable for all groups or not analysed.
[c]Treatment combined with proliferant injections, analgesics, and exercise.

There was and still is a need to leap from empirical clinical practice to valid, reliable and consistently effective methods of dealing with disorders of neuromusculoskeletal pain and movement.

- *The people who need to be convinced are:* manual therapists themselves (are they doing what they believe they are doing?); the general public at large (the biggest market);

medical practitioners and health sevice providers (demanding scientific fact).

- *the direction for research suggested by Jull:*

  investigating the sensitivity of manual diagnosis in identifying symptomatic levels in spinal pain patients;

  quantifying intertherapist and intratherapist reliability in detecting pathological states accurately;

  using animal research to convert empirical description of manual examination and treatment techniques into sound scientific fact.

- *The focus of manual therapy research should be relevant to the following definitions:*

  Validity: the degree to which the results of a measurement correspond to the true state of the phenomenon being measured (Valkari-Juntura *et al.*, 1989). Validity is measured by sensitivity and specificity. For instance, Goddard and Reid (1965) suggested that the straight leg raise test can be used to measure abnormal neural mobility in lumbosacral nerve root lesions. Therefore is a limited SLR a true reflection of the presence of an L5/S1 nerve root lesion?

Sensitivity: the proportion of people with a disease (disorder) who have a positive test for the disease (disorder). For instance, do all people with an L5/S1 nerve root lesion have a reduced SLR?

Specificity: the proportion of people without the disease (disorder) who have a negative test for the disease (disorder). For instance, do all people who do not have an L5/S1 nerve root lesion have an ideal SLR?

Reliability: the extent to which repeated measurements of a relatively stable phenomenon fall closely to each other. Thus if 20 therapists measured the SLR of a patient with an acute L5/S1 nerve root lesion (intertherapist reliability) or, if one therapist measured it 20 times (intratherapist reliability), would all the measurements be the same?

Predictive value: the probability of disease, given the results of a test. For instance, if a patient has a painful restricted SLR, what is the probability of his having an L5/S1 nerve root lesion?

Has your opinion of the SLR test changed?

From this you can see that using scientific enquiry (observation, experimentation, measurement, interpretation of results, discussion and conclusions drawn) gives you a means by which you can provide scientific fact for the clinical phenomena that you encounter. For example, small amplitude pain-free passive movements (grade I) are often used clinically to treat movement severely restricted by pain. If executed appropriately and skilfully these techniques contribute to the reduction in pain with movement. This is a recurring clinical observation but at present there is debate about the mechanisms by which it occurs. Therefore research is required to explore the mechanism of a grade I passive movement technique, its validity, its reliability, its predictive value and ultimately its mechanical, physiological, biomechanical and pathological effects.

Modern manual therapists (Grieve, Maitland, McKenzie, Kaltenborn, Paris etc) have set us on the road to scientific acceptability by emphasizing clinical problem-solving and the continual evaluation and self-criticism of manipulative physiotherapy. The task of the next generations is consolidation and further scientific study coupled with acceptable marketing strategies to promote our product. The approaches in research over the last generation can be charted in the following way.

Testing Segmental Mobility

Evans *et al.* (1988) reviewed previous studies on intervertebral palpation of the resistance to passive movement, given that, if the manual therapists could detect the onset of resistance to movement and relate this to the normal mechanical compliance of tissue, then abnormal passive mobility related to pathological states could be detected. Kaltenborn and Lindahl (1969), Gonella *et al.* (1982) and Johnson (1976) used several therapists to examine passive physiological movement of selected joints and grade them into: ankylosed, considerable restriction, slightly restricted, normal, slightly increased mobility and unstable. They found that intratherapist reliability in testing was good but intertherapist reliability was poor. Quin (1986) and Bain (1987) also found that assessment of passive accessory intervertebral movement failed to indicate good intertherapist reliability.

Other studies looked at the validity of techniques used in the manual examination and treatment of peripheral joint movement. Bastian (1988) aimed to determine the intratester reliability of examination of accessory movements of the knee (tibiofemoral) joint and the accuracy of performing grades II and IV as described by Maitland (1986). Ten experienced therapists tested six healthy knees. The Genucom knee analyser was used to measure and record displacement forces produced. The study found that there was a fair ability to reproduce a grade IV and a poor ability consistently to reproduce grade II. Chesworth *et al* (1991) studied the clinical evaluation of passive ankle joint stiffness in patients with ankle fractures, using movement diagrams against the values generated by a computerized torque measurement system. Results of this study showed a large discrepancy between the individual movement diagrams and the torque measurements, and

considerable variation between therapists was also evident.

Good intratherapist reliability had been established in these tests. However, it became clear from studies of intertherapist evaluation of passive movement and grading of passive movement that levels of reliability being attained were low. Among the reasons for this may be variables of measurement and experimental design, the biological variability of what is normal and abnormal movement and the inter/intra therapist variables — namely, training, education and clinical experience. With this in mind, Lee *et al.* (1990) found that concurrent feedback was associated with a significant improvement in accuracy and consistency in the application of a mobilizing force. The conclusion is that 'practice makes perfect'.

Exploring the Value of the Pain Response During Passive Testing

In 1985 Matyas and Bach suggested that knowledge of pain response was a more accurate and reliable way of determining symptomatic spinal levels than assessment of spinal stiffness and changes in tissue compliance. They suggested that the pain provoked on palpation was enough to localize treatment techniques to the most relevant symptomatic level and the most relevant passive movement direction. This approach has limitations when it is considered that several segments of the spine may be innervated by the same branch of the sinuvertebral nerve. Therefore a tender spinal level is not necessarily the level that is the real source of the tenderness.

Lee and Evans (1994) related the force displacement curve of the spinal posteroanterior (PA) mobilization technique, as visualized on a movement diagram, to the normal tissue compliance for soft tissue. However, they challenged the reliability of palpation of PA mobility alone and suggested that pain response during PA movement may be useful in diagnosing spinal levels of lesions. As an aside, they also suggested that the PA produces an extension force in the spine more than a pure shear force, and that, from cadaver studies, the restraint to the PA force is mainly from the intervertebral disc. However, evidence for this assertion is lacking.

Testing Segmental Mobility and the Pain Response

Jull et al. (1994) challenged the 'pain response is the major cue' school of thought. As part of a larger study (using manual diagnosis to identify patients with headaches of cervical origin), they found their manual testing of cervical joints to be highly sensitive and specific. The manual testing included soft tissue palpation, passive accessory intervertebral movement testing and passive physiological intervertebral movement testing. There was a high correlation between their own judgement (without verbal cues from the patient) and those of the patients as to whether the joints were painful, slightly painful or non-painful. This suggests that pain is not the only reliable cue in such circumstances.

As a development from this, Jull et al. (1988) and Philips and Twomey (1993) evaluated the sensitivity and specificity of manual assessment skills (mobility testing and pain response) in the cervical and lumbar spines respectively. These skills are clearly seen as comparing well with what is regarded as the most widely used medical diagnostic method currently available, namely spinal anaesthetic block. However, conclusions drawn suggest that both segmental mobility testing and verbal pain response make the detection of symptomatic segmental levels more sensitive and specific, rendering more effective treatment possible. Further studies on correlating the detection of symptomatic levels with the effectiveness of treatment techniques are needed.

Additionally Magarey et al. (1993) found, in a study comparing commonly used passive restraint tests for the shoulder (e.g. quadrant, lock, instability tests, and differentiation tests) with arthroscopic diagnosis, that by themselves the tests were not reliable as predictors of specific disorder. Reliability and predictive value was improved when an overall examination process was used, including subjective features, pain patterns, palpation and more extensive movement testing.

The Pain Sciences Approach

Zusman (1994) suggested that provocative mechanical stimulation may not be an infallible means of accurate localization of the pathological source of pain. If, for example, a patient's shoulder movement is painful this does not necessarily mean that there is anything pathologically wrong with the shoulder. Subsequently, if you treat the patient's cervical spine, and the shoulder movements become full and pain-free, then you have influenced pain mechanisms affecting the shoulder rather than any pathological process within it. Related to this is an awareness of the need for a wider understanding of pain mechanisms, i.e. nociception, neurogenic pain, secondary hyperalgesia, central pain mechanisms and chronic pain, together with the role of the autonomic nervous system and maintained pain states, non-organic elements to pain and the role of the cortex.

Although these approaches relate more to joint disorders, within a relatively distinct field, it is important to note that similar findings are evident in the evaluation of manual diagnosis and techniques biased towards muscles, nerves and other soft tissue. That is, clinically observed phenomena, mechanical effects of testing and techniques, diagnostic value, and clinical effects.

Future Achievement and Potential

After decades of specific manual therapy approaches being taught and used, there is a need to highlight the development of multistructural approaches to the manual therapy management of neuromusculoskeletal disorders, with the patient at the centre of the model.

Consideration should be given to the requirement for research to confirm clinical observations, notably the dosage of passive techniques, the hypothesis of tissue biasing and the predictive value of passive testing.

Clinicians should embrace the philosophy of open-mindedness and a self-critical approach to practice. This will contribute to a healthy evolution of skills and knowledge.

An extract from prominent researchers signals the direction for future clinicians Frank *et al.* (1984) say of passive joint motion

> Clinical and experimental evidence supports the probable effectiveness of passive joint motion at joint and tissue levels, but without a better quantitative understanding of the mechanisms of action, dose-responsiveness, and specific tissue effects, passive motion will continue to be used suboptimally with inconsistent results. When these clinical and research deficiencies are corrected, passive motion will attain its proper place as a powerful and reliable orthopedic tool.

Summary

- There are several different manipulative physiotherapy approaches to the assessment, examination and treatment of neuromusculoskeletal disorders. No one approach should be followed religiously. The prime aim of any approach should be to achieve its desired effect, thus ridding the patient of the symptoms and functional loss for which help has been sought.
- Passive techniques are usually the primary means by which manipulative physiotherapists treat neuromusculoskeletal disorders. Generally speaking, passive techniques influence the mobility and the biological functional environment of connective tissues. The connective tissues influenced most by passive techniques are those of joints, nerves, muscles and other soft tissues including skin and fascia.
- Passive techniques performed skillfully can be biased towards specific structures (i.e. joints, nerves, muscles and other soft tissues) in order to target tissues at fault.
- Common principles apply to the clinical application of passive techniques. Passive techniques may be classified in terms of the movement direction being performed, grades of passive movement, dosage refinements (i.e. speed, rhythm, and duration) and method of delivery to the appropriate tissues. This gives the clinician a relevant clinical model on which to base the selection of the most appropriate treatment technique.
- The selection of passive techniques for treatment should be based on sound clinical reasoning related to the presenting clinical evidence (history, symptoms and signs), the diagnosis and pathological nature of the disorder, the requirements of specific structures,

biomechanical knowledge and the nature and expectations of the patient.

- Progression of treatment should be based on the effects of the passive techniques selected. That is, are they working? Are they relieving the patient of his symptoms? In this way relevant adjustments to the techniques can be made to improve the chances of the patient getting better at a desirable rate.

- Clinical research has given manipulative physiotherapists some mechanical and biological basis to the effects of passive movement techniques at clinical, tissue, metabolic, neurophysiological, chemical, cellular and subcellular levels.

- Clinical research into the validity of passive techniques has established consistency in the predictive value of some manual therapy approaches.

- Future achievements in the universal acceptance of manual therapies should be helped by the need for a multistructural, multifactorial approach to the mangement of neuromusculoskeletal disorders. Also there is evidently a need for more basic research into the validity and reliability of the passive techniques used by clinicians. These achievements are possible if there is an open-minded, self-critical approach to manipulative physiotherapy.

Further Reading and References

Bain, D (1987) 'The assessment of passive accessory intervertebral motion and physiotherapist reliability' Thesis, South Australian Institute of Technology.

Bastian, S, Harris, B, Dyrek, D (1988) Performance of extremity joint mobilisation: consistency and accuracy. *Physical Therapy*, 68 (5): 781–782

Barnett, CH, Davies, DV, MacConaill, MA (1961) *Synovial Joints: Their Structure and Mechanics.* Longman, London.

Butler, DS (1989) Adverse mechanical tension in the nervous system: A model for assessment and treatment. *Australian Journal of Physiotherapy* 35 (4): 227–229.

Butler, DS (1991) *Mobilisation of the Nervous System.* Churchill Livingstone, Edinburgh.

Butler, DS, Gifford, L (1989) The concept of adverse mechanical tension in the nervous system. *Physiotherapy* 75 (11): 622–636.

Caterson, B, Lowther, D (1978) Changes in the metabolism of the proteoglycans from sheep articular cartilage in response to mechanical stress. *Biochimica et Biophysica Acta*, 540: 412–422.

Chesworth, B, Vandervoort , A, Koval, J A pilot study to compare the subjective and objective evaluation of passive ankle joint stiffness. *Physiotherapy Canada*, 43 (4): 13–18.

Cyriax, J (1983) *Textbook of Orthopaedic Medicine*, vol. 2 (Treatment by Manipulation, Massage and Injection). WB Saunders, London.

Di Fabio, R (1992) Efficacy of manual therapy, *Physical Therapy*, 72 (12): 853–864.

Edwards, BC (1992) *Manual of Combined Movements.* Churchill Livingstone, Edinburgh.

Evans, D, Trott , P, Pugatschen , A, Baghurst, P (1988) Manual palpation of resistance to movement, parts 1 and 2, in *IFOMT Proceedings*, Cambridge.

Evans, P (1980) The healing process at cellular level: a review, *Physiotherapy* 65 (8): 257–259.

Evans, P (1988) Ligaments, joint surfaces, conjunct rotation and close-pack, *Physiotherapy*, March 105–114.

Exelby, L (1995) Mobilisation with movement: a personal view, *Physiotherapy*, 81 (12): 724–729.

Frank, C, Akeson, WH, Woo, SL-Y, Amiel, D, Coutts, R (1984) Physiology and therapeutic value of passive joint motion, *Clinical Orthopaedics and Related Research*, 185: 113–125.

Gilmore, KL (1986) Biomechanics of the lumbar motion segment in Grieve, G (ed) *Modern Manual Therapy of the Vertebral Column*, pp. 103–111. Churchill Livingstone, Edinburgh.

Goddard, MD, Reid, JD (1965) Movements induced by straight leg raising in the lumbosacral roots, nerves and plexuses and in the intrapelvic section of the sciatic nerve. *Journal of Neurology, Neurosurgery and Psychiatry* 28 (12):.

Gonella, C, Paris, SV, Kutner, M (1982) Reliability in evaluating passive intervertebral motion, *Physical Therapy*, 62 (4): 436–444.

Grieve, GP (1981) *Common Vertebral Joint Problems.* Churchill Livingstone, Edinburgh.

Guber, S, Rudolph, P (1978) The myofibroblast. *Surgery, Gynaecology and Obstetrics*, 146: 641–644.

Guyton, A (1979) *Physiology of the Human Body*, 5th edition. WB Saunders, London.

Holey, L (1995) Connective tissue manipulation: towards a scientific rationale, *Physiotherapy*, 81 (12): 730–739.

Janda, V (1983) *Muscle Function Testing.* Butterworth, London.

Janda, V, Jull, G (1988) Muscles and cervical pain syndromes. In Grant. R. (ed.) *Physical Therapy of the Cervical and Thoracic Spine*, pp. 153–166. Churchill Livingstone, New York.

Jayson, M (ed.) (1987) *The Lumbar Spine and Back Pain* 3rd edn. Churchill Livingstone, Edinburgh.

Johnston, W (1976) Interexaminer reliability in palpation, *Journal of the American Osteopathic Association*, 81: pp. 298–313

Jull, G (1987) Manual examination – prove it or lose it, In *Proceedings, Manipulative Therapists Association of Australia*, fifth biennial conference, pp. 351–358. Melbourne.

Jull, G, Bogduk, N, Marsland, A (1988) The accuracy of manual diagnosis for cervical joint pain syndromes, *Medical Journal of Australia*, 148: 233–236.

Jull, G, Treleaven, J, Versace, G (1994) Manual examination: is pain provocation a major cue to spinal dysfunction *Australian Journal of Physiotherapy*, 40 (3): 159–165.

Kaltenborn, FM (1989) *Manual Mobilisation of the Extremity Joints.* Orthopaedic Physical Therapy Products, Minneapolis.

Kaltenborn, F, Lindahl, O (1969) Reproducerbarheten vid rorelsundersckning av enskilda kotor, *Lakertidningen*, vol. 66, pp. 962–965.

Kapandji, IA (1987) *The Physiology of the Joints. vol 2. Lower Limb.* Churchill Livingstone, Edinburgh.

Keir, KAI, Goats, GC (1991) Introduction to manipulation, *British Journal of Spinal Medicine* 25 (4): 221–226.

LaRocca, H (1992) A taxonomy of chronic pain syndromes, *Spine*, 17 (10S): 344–355.

Lee, M, Moseley, A, Refshauge, K (1990) Effect of feedback on learning a vertebral joint mobilisation skill, *Physical Therapy*, 70 (2): 97–102.

Lee, R, Evans, J (1994) Towards a better understanding of spinal postero-anterior mobilisation, *Physiotherapy*, 80 (2): 68–73.

Liebesman, JL, Cafarelli, E (1994) Physiology of range of motion in human joints: a critical review, *Critical Reviews in Physical and Rehabilitation Medicine*, 6 (2): 131–160.

Lowther, D (1988) The effect of compression and tension on the behaviour of connective tissue, In *Aspects of Manipulative Physiotherapy*, Lincoln Institute of Health Sciences, Melbourne, Australia, pp. 15–21.

Lundborg, G (1988) *Nerve Injury and Repair*, Churchill Livingstone, Edinburgh.

Lundborg, G, Rydevik, B (1973) Effects of stretching the tibial nerve of the rabbit, *Journal of Bone and Joint Surgery*, 55B pp. 390–401.

McConigle, T, Matley, KW (1994) Soft tissue treatment and muscle stretching, *Journal of Manual and Manipulative Therapy*, 2 (2): 55–62.

McKenzie, R (1981) *The Lumbar Spine Mechanical Diagnosis and Therapy*, Spinal Publications Ltd., New Zealand.

Magarey, ME (1986) The first treatment session, In Grieve, G (ed) *Modern Manual Therapy of the Vertebral Column.* Churchill Livingstone, Edinburgh. chap. 6, pp. 661–672.

Magarey, M, Hayes, M, Trott, P (1993) The shoulder complex: How useful are our differentiating procedures? A preliminary analysis of the predictive value of clinical differentiating procedures of the shoulder complex. In Singer, KP (ed) *Integrated Approaches – Proceedings of the 8th Biennial Conference of the Manipulative Therapists Association of Australia*, 24–27, Perth, W. Aust., pp. 43–45.

Maitland, GD (1986) *Vertebral Manipulation*, Butterworth, London

Maitland, GD (1991a) *Peripheral Manipulation*, Butterworth Heinemann, London.

Maitland, GD (1991b) *Neuromusculoskeletal Examination and Recording Guide*, 5th ed., Lauderdale Press, S. Aust.

Maroudas, A, Bullough, P, Swanson, SAV, Freeman, MAR (1968) The permeability of articular cartilage, *Journal of Bone and Joint Surgery*, 50B (1): 166.

Matyas, T, Bach, T (1985) The reliability of selected techniques in clinical arthrometrics', *Australian Journal of Physiotherapy*, 31 (5): 175–199.

Mulligan, BR (1993) Mobilisation with movement, *Journal of Manual and Manipulative Therapy*, 1 (4): 154–156

Nachemson, A (1992) Newest knowledge of low back pain: a critical look, *Clinical Orthopaedics and Related Research*, 279 pp. 8–20.

Palastanga, N (1986) Connective tissue massage, In Grieve, G. (ed.) *Modern Manual Therapy of the Vertebral Column*, Churchill Livingstone, Edinburgh, 80 pp. 827–833.

Paris, S (1992) The Paris approach. In *IFOMT Proceedings, Fifth International Conference, Vail, Colorado*, pp. 21–22.

Phillips, DR, Twomey, L (1993) Comparison of manual diagnosis with a diagnosis established by a unilevel lumbar spinal block procedure, In Singer, KP (ed), *Integrated Approaches – Proceedings of the 8th Biennial Conference of the Manipulative Therapists Association of Australia*, Perth, W. Aust., pp. 55–61.

Quin, S (1987) *Reliability of passive accessory intervertebral movements*, Thesis, South Australian Institute of Technology.

Riddoch, J, Lennon, S (1991) Evaluation of practice. The single case study approach. *Physiotherapy Theory and Practice*, 7 pp 3–11.

Saal, JS, Saal, JA, Yurth, EF (1993) Non-operative management of herniated cervical intervertebral disc with radiculopathy. *Spine*, 21 (16): 1877–1883.

Salter, R (1989) The biological concept of continuous passive motion in synovial joints; The first 18 years of basic research and its clinical application, *Clinical Orthopaedics and Related Research*, 242, 12–25.

Stoddard, A (1983) *Manual of Osteopathic Practice*, Hutchinson, London.

Sunderland, S (1978) *Nerve and Nerve Injury*, 2nd edn Churchill Livingstone, Edinburgh.

Twomey, L, Taylor, J (1995) Exercise and spinal manipulation in the treatment of low back pain, *Spine*, 20 (5): 615–619.

Valkari-Juntura, E, Parras, M, Laasonen, EM (1989) Validity of clinical tests in the diagnosis of root compression in cervical disc disease, *Spine*, 14 (3): 253–257.

Wright, A (1995) Hypoalgesia post-manipulative therapy: a review of potential neurophysiological mechanisms, *Manual Therapy*, 1 (5): 11–16.

Zusman, M (1986) Spinal manipulative therapy: a review of some proposed mechanisms and a new hypothesis, *Australian Journal of Physiotherapy*, 32 (2): 89–99

Zusman, M (1994) The meaning of mechanically produced responses, *Australian Journal of Physiotherapy*, 40 (1): 35–39.

10

Neuromuscular Therapeutic Techniques and Approaches

JUDITH PITT-BROOKE

Introduction

It has been shown in previous chapters that the nature of most clinical problems is complex. This requires clinical physiotherapists to possess a broad repertoire of skills to enable them to both assess and treat patients whose problems may arise from dysfunction of one or more of many different structures or tissues.

This chapter aims to introduce the reader to a range of approaches and techniques which have primarily been developed to deal with problems of the neuromuscular system. The aim is set in the context of problems primarily of the musculoskeletal system and excluding problems associated with upper motor neurone damage to the central nervous system. Assessment and treatment of problems of muscle length, strength and coordination and the assessment of static and dynamic posture are covered including different approaches to relaxation therapy. The scope of each of these areas is purposely limited to that of contemporary practice. As with all areas of clinical practice, new concepts are continually emerging and being developed and students need to be aware that there is a need to broaden and deepen the extent of their basic knowledge and understanding of the foundations of practice. The approaches and techniques described in this chapter will provide the student with a sound introduction to the theoretical background which underpins the treatment of muscle related problems. As the reader progresses through the chapter, the links and influences between the musculoskeletal system and central nervous system will emerge. As new approaches to physiotherapeutic treatment develop, the most striking feature is that it is becoming more and more obvious that to exclude the influence of one system on another is to disregard reality. Developments in the field of neurodynamics have demonstrated this more clearly than ever (see Chapter 4).

Chapter Objectives

After reading this chapter you should be able to:

1 Understand the importance of acquiring a knowledge of a broad range of approaches and techniques applicable to muscle dysfunction;

2 Appreciate the range of factors which require consideration in the assessment of muscle dysfunction;

3 Understand the value of specific contemporary approaches to assessment and treatment of muscle dysfunction;

4 Demonstrate an awareness of the theoretical and scientific bases of neuromuscular techniques commonly used in contemporary physiotherapy practice;

5 Discuss the effects of prevention and treatment strategies which utilize neuromuscular techniques in the light of the limitations of current scientific knowledge;

6 Discuss future directions for scientific research to facilitate the extension of knowledge of the value of the approaches and techniques presented.

Where do I Start in the Assessment of Movement Problems?

The successful analysis of human movement dysfunction requires the recognition of four basic factors.

1 *Visual observational skills* Firstly there is the need to develop reliable observational skills. This is perhaps a contradiction in terms, although much clinical practice relies on visual observation!

2 *Tactile skills* It is also important to develop confidence in the skills of palpation. Information which emerges from the palpation of different structures often reinforces visual information and supports or negates it.

3 *What is normal movement?* Thirdly, it is important to develop a knowledge and understanding of the variations of human movement which fall within the bounds of 'normal'. This takes time. For undergraduate students, observation of each other's movement will show you that there is considerable variety in the way individuals perform a set movement with a stated objective, e.g. getting down onto the floor from a standing position. All are likely to be considered normal. If one extends this idea outwards to the population at large, it immediately becomes evident that there is a

huge variety of what we might call 'normal movement'.

4 *Impact of movement on the body's structures*
The fourth factor important to the understanding and successful analysis of movement dysfunction is that every movement involves a degree of structural change in the body's tissues. It is important therefore to recognize the immediate, short-term and long-term reactions to movements in terms of both structural reactions and possible modifications of sensory and motor patterns. It is important to recognize the impact of day-to-day movement requirements on the body in terms of active movement and postural control. There is often a recognizable association between day-to-day movement habits and the development of certain dysfunctions which affect different tissues. This is particularly evident in the fields of occupational injury and sports injury, but these may just be areas in which extreme demands are placed on certain anatomical structures. An assessment of the impact of posture and movement on the body's structure should always be part of the analysis of movement problems.

The development of manual and visual skills must not be mutually exclusive. In order to acquire sophisticated assessment and treatment skills it is necessary to adopt a 'cognitive-visuo-tactile' approach in which each element is important. What you see and what you feel provide information which enable thought processes to be triggered and hypotheses developed regarding the presentation of painful problems associated with movement or muscle dysfunction. As you see more and feel more, the thought processes can be developed.

The Neuromusculoskeletal Environment Interactions Concept (NMEI)

As has been stated, analysis of movement is fundamental in attempting to prevent injury, determining the cause of injury and to the rehabilitation of musculoskeletal disorders. The degree to which you develop skills in the analysis of movement will depend on the level of understanding of basic scientific concepts which relate to human movement. An approach to the analysis of human movement problems, based on a synthesis of knowledge about biomechanical and physiological factors, was developed several decades ago by a Scottish physiotherapist, Tom McClurg Anderson (McClurg Anderson, 1951). The approach was termed 'human kinectics'. The essence of the ideas were further developed, particularly in the field of patient handling, by Vasey and Crozier (1982) who have published their views under the title 'A neuromuscular approach to human movement'. This section draws on some of the original ideas put forward by McClurg Anderson which have been extended in the light of more recent scientific findings as a concept of 'neuromusculoskeletal environmental interactions' (NMEI) to explain the possible causation of some musculoskeletal disorders and also to suggest an approach to their prevention treatment and rehabilitation (Pitt-Brooke, 1997). A preliminary account of the NMEI in the context of the development of muscle imbalance was suggested earlier (Pitt-Brooke, 1995).

McClurg Anderson (1971) identified the need to recognize the basic requirements of normal day-to-day movement habits on muscle function from the perspective of both mobility and postural control and suggested that such function may materially influence the condition of certain body tissues and therefore the manner in which they fulfil their function. He suggested for the same reason, that day-to-day movement habits may determine to a considerable extent the injuries or dysfunctions likely to affect those tissues.

The approach to the analysis of movement advocated consideration be given to the following features of each movement:

1 The initial stimulus; and
2 The fundamental character of the movement, which entails certain actions:

(a) *lock actions* – defined as 'putting a (body) part into a position which will automatically stabilize other parts of the body and lead to more efficient action with the minimum of effort'. An example of this would be the lock action of the neck, lower cervical extension with slight upper cervical flexion, i.e. tucking in the chin, which tends to draw the rest of the spine into extension, as well as stimulating retraction of the shoulder girdle. This provides a stable and balanced position from which to move the upper limbs.

(b) *check actions* – defined as 'the proper placing of the feet or body to prevent possible overbalancing while performing a particular movement'. For example, ensuring that the feet are placed and adjusted so that the base of support is widened in the direction of movement.

(c) *evasive actions* – defined as 'protective limitation of action in a part which leads to alteration in the character of a movement, and to compensatory actions'. These actions most commonly arise as a result of protective inhibition in response to discomfort. An example here is that of someone with shoulder weakness or pain, who tries to reach out to grasp something. Instead of flexing/elevating the arm, the individual tilts the body forward and to the opposite side as well as using shoulder girdle elevation excessively. Inhibition of gleno-humeral joint movement is the evasive action whilst all other movements are compensatory.

If movement is to be harmonious in terms of minimizing stresses to the body's structures, there must be a regard for this basic framework. When any part of a movement is altered without regard to its basic framework, compensatory actions are established. This disturbs the harmony of a movement and produces unnecessary muscular tension.

Movement Defined in Terms of Efficiency of Muscular Effort

In this context, McClurg Anderson defined movement in terms of efficiency and his views led him to believe that some patterns of movement were efficient and some were not. Those that were not were the movements which were most likely to cause unnecessary strain to the musculoskeletal system. A definition of good movement according to McClurg Anderson (1971) is:

> A movement which fulfils its function with the minimum of effort and the minimum of strain.

Minimum effort refers to the type of muscle work involved in producing and regulating movements. This muscle work relies on coordination of muscular action. Remember that muscles always work together in groups and that different muscles perform different roles within the group. The type of muscle work will depend upon the role of the muscle or muscle group. (Refer back to

Chapter 2, if you are not sure about this. It is very important.) Coordination of muscular action relies upon reciprocation between:

1 Agonistic and antagonistic muscles / groups;
2 Muscles concerned with adjusting and maintaining balance throughout movement;
3 Muscles which stabilze the spinal joints and the limb girdles during movement.

In order for a specific objective movement to occur, e.g. lifting a book from a shelf at eye level, there is coordination of many different muscles, all performing these different roles.

1 There will be isotonic action of the agonists to grasp and lift the book off the shelf.
2 This action will be allowed by the reciprocal relaxed lengthening of the antagonists (assuming they have normal muscle length).
3 The bones to which the origins of the agonists are attached will be stabilized by muscles also to attached to those bones, but also with attachments to bones not required as part of the primary movement. These muscles work isometrically. It is this stabilization work which is responsible for the majority of energy expenditure due to muscle contraction during the course of a day.

Building on this understanding it is possible to develop a model to explain the development of some nonspecific painful musculoskeletal conditions.

1 When muscles are subjected to excessive tension in resting, postural or active functions, their natural extensibility (contractile element) and elasticity (tendinous element) will be reduced. This is probably due to changes in the structure of fascia and connective tissue within the muscles (McClurg Anderson, 1951; Goldspink et al., 1974; Goldspink and Williams,

1981) in respone to microtraumas that initiate the inflammatory response (Pecina and Bojanic, 1993). In addition, sensitivity may be altered as well as blood and lymphatic circulation.

2 Over a period of time deterioration of anatomical structures (e.g. connective tissues — muscle, fascia, ligament) results from excessive tension in different parts of the body. This frequently occurs in a cumulative subliminal fashion leading to cumulative strain in certain structures and tissues. Unfortunately, as already mentioned, cumulative strain is difficult to demonstrate in clinical and laboratory experiments. There is, however, growing evidence that structural deterioration of body tissues can result from progressive injury as a result of excessive tension being experienced in different parts of the body (Goldspink et al., 1974; Goldspink and Williams, 1981; Adams and Hutton, 1985; Adams et al., 1987; Pecina and Bojanic 1993). Such deterioration results in progressive adaptive shortening of structures in response to repeated small-scale inflammatory responses within the tissues, in response to repetitive subliminal strains. Muscle and fascia adapt to their function both in terms of length and structure.

3 In the context of cumulative strain, the most costly form of muscle work is that which involves sustained contraction, i.e. isometric or static muscle work. It is inefficient in terms of the utilization of energy because sustained contraction leads to a reduction in blood flow through the muscle. This is the characteristic muscle work of postural control and is predominant in the trunk and around the limb girdles in most activities of daily living. Pause to analyse tasks such as brushing one's teeth, filling a kettle, reaching to a cupboard, ironing, pushing a shopping trolley around corners! Some of

these muscles may be adapted for their function, i.e. they have a high proportion of slow-twitch fibres, and these probably become subjected to overuse injury. In other cases, muscles more commonly associated with mobility functions may be required to act as stabilizers, as a result of poor posture or movement patterns. This may particularly be so in the case of 'top heavy' movements.

Figure 10.1

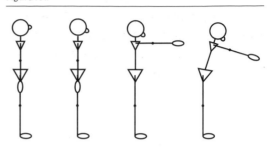

Practical Task

To give you an idea of which areas of the body typically sustain the abuse which human movement can inflict on some muscle groups, stand up in a space, with your feet comfortably apart and your arms down by your sides [Figure 10.1]. Drop your chin to your chest and keep it there. After approximately half a minute and keeping your head down, lift your arms up straight in front of you to the horizontal position and maintain them there. Maintain this position for approximately half a minute. Start to become aware of the areas in your body which are becoming uncomfortable, or where you are conscious of tension. Maintain this position and then bend forward at the hips by about 30°. Again, maintain this position for about half a minute. You will experience a feeling of discomfort or tension in any of the following areas: lower leg — gastrocnemii, thighs — quadriceps, thighs — hamstrings, low back — erector spinae and quadratus lumborum, shoulders — trapezii and deltoids.

4 It seems likely that many problems associated with pain in the musculoskeletal system could be associated with movement patterns which cause cumulative strain on body structures. Painful disorders of the musculoskeletal system which develop insidiously, often with no memorable incident of injury may be resulting from the gradual deterioration of structures, in particular muscular, ligamentous and connective tissues which have been subjected to insidious subliminal strain, but which over a period of time, reach a threshold of intolerance and give rise to pain.

5 One of the most predominant movement patterns which is likely to be associated with the development of cumulative strain is the 'top heavy bending' movement in which movements begin with the hands, head and upper trunk moving forward. This forward movement of the upper part of the body requires the trunk and leg muscles to stabilize the lower part of the body, rather like an anchor and chain take the strain of a boat when moored. This 'top heavy' movement pattern dominates many human actions at work, in recreational activities as well as everyday movements in the home.

6 To treat the source of many musculoskeletal problems it may be necessary to change the physical movement habits of those who suffer the painful consequences of strain on soft tissues.

It therefore becomes necessary to consider the basic principles of what may be described as 'good movement' (hereafter termed efficient movements) in terms of minimizing the cumulative strain which results from excessive postural stabilization.

Characteristics of Efficient Movements

The essential feature of a good movement may be considered to be its segmental nature, in which the various parts of the body come into action progressively in the proper sequence. In addition, an efficient movement will facilitate the recruitment of all available forces and reduce the need for reflex postural activity to a minimum. Efficient movements are based on the following principles:

1 The lower the centre of gravity of an object, the greater its stability. In terms of human movement, if the centre of gravity of the body is lowered, reflex postural activity is reduced. Moreover, the nearer the line of gravity falls to the centre of the base of support, the more balanced the movement will be. The lower the centre of gravity and the wider the base of support, the greater is the chance that the line of gravity will fall near the centre of the base. This principle can be applied to movement of all body parts. In the trunk for example, to lower the body from standing, this principle can be effected by relaxing the knees, hips and low back into flexion.

2 The greater the area of the base of an object, the greater the stability. Again, in terms of human movement, the base from which movement occurs needs to be wide to ensure maximum stability. This is difficult as the base is likely to be part of that movement. If a foot is moved in the direction of intended movement, or in the direction to which the body is tending to fall, reflex postural activity will be reduced. Turning of a foot in this manner is associated with rotation at the hips and this is likely to reduce or prevent unwanted rotation in the spine. Principles 1 and 2 combined allow the development of a dynamically stable efficient movement. In other words, a moving body requires a mobile base in order to maintain stability. This is essential. It is the inability to adjust the base as part of a movement which leads to evasive actions elsewhere in the body. Evasive actions are likely to lead to strain or injury.

3 In terms of leverage the closer a load is applied to the fulcrum of the lever, the less the effort is required to balance it. In human movement, any part of the body or limb part which is above, in front or behind its centre of gravity, constitutes a load. In addition, external loads, however large or small, are usually taken by the hands. The fulcrum may be at the wrist or elbow. In either case, if the load is kept as near to the centre of gravity as possible the less will be the effort to balance displacement of the load. In the case of loads taken in a hand, if they are kept in the hand or forearm as near to the fulcrum as possible it is likely that the use of gripping actions will be minimized. Intense gripping actions require substantial stabilizing muscle work and should be avoided where possible. Reaching beyond the object to be moved with outstretched fingers, applies a stretch to the palmar fascia, which then recoils. The combination of these actions tends to discourage overgripping and encourage the load to fall nearer the palm of the hand rather than the fingers.

A further example of this point lies in analysis

of reaching actions. Following these principles, in any reaching action, movement should begin at the shoulder girdle with an initial elevation. This should be followed segmentally, by extension of the elbow and flexion of the shoulder joint, then relaxation of the shoulder girdle. The muscles which would otherwise fix the shoulder girdle become part of the movement and the action progresses segmentally in a distal direction. Theoretically, this should minimize the need for stabilizing muscle activity in the upper trunk and shoulder girdle.

4 All basic actions in human movement which require a change in body posture involve an element of lowering and raising the mass of the body. In order to effect an efficient lowering of the body's mass within its base of support it should be lowered segmentally starting with the body parts closest to the base. The lowering phase should therefore be initiated by a 'relaxation' of the knees and hips. In continu-

ing this relaxation, gravity would tend to effect a 'relaxation' in the trunk, i.e. flexion in the lumbar spine and increased flexion in the thoracic spine, whilst the cervical spine increases its lordosis. One only needs to look at the effect of gravity in producing a kyphosis over 70–80 years in many elderly people to see that this is true. This position of 'collapse' is also compatible with fulfilling the requirements of maintained balance on the basis of the principles outlined above.

The 'effort' phase, or raising of the body's mass, should be initiated by gentle cephalad movement of the head, so that the cervical, thoracic and lumbar segments become elongated in that order (10.2b), restoring themselves to their neutral position within the base of support. Raising and lowering the body in this way enhances balance in movement and may help to maintain mobility in the spine (see Figure 10.2).

Figure 10.2   The influence of head position in relation to trunk movement reactions.

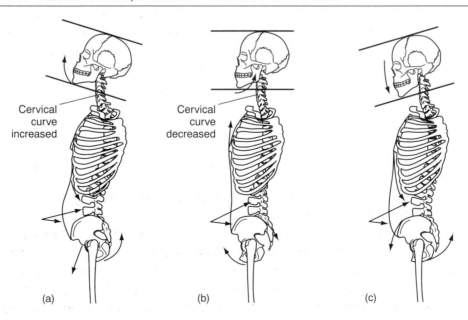

Cervical curve increased

Cervical curve decreased

(a)   (b)   (c)

Practical Task

It may be useful to the reader to consider at this point, the application of these principles in basic movement actions such as pushing, pulling, lifting, reaching and turning. In particular, next time you visit a supermarket, consider the movements involved in moving a shopping trolley. Pushing and pulling? Do you do this by moving your base or by moving the upper body forward with a fixed base? How do you hold the bar? Do you grip it or do you handle it at the edges of the bar taking hold in the palms of the hands? How do you reach to the top shelf? How do you manoeuvre the trolley around those nasty corners?

Requirement for Conditioned Change in Movement Habits

Inherent in this approach to movement rehabilitation is that there is usually a need to initiate change in the habitual movement patterns of individuals. In order to do this, thorough assessment of movement habits is required. Subsequent to the analysis of problems, there will be a need to prepare the individual for a change in movement habits by preparing areas of the body for change. This can be done through specific preparatory exercises or 'conditioning' movements which should be designed both to gain physiological relaxation in target muscle groups and also to increase sensory awareness of areas of tension in the body. Failure to recognize the need to prepare the individual for movement pattern rehabilitation in this way may merely contribute further

to their problems. It's rather like encouraging a baby to walk before it has mastered control of its reflexes, resulting in a stiff, inefficient and unbalanced walking pattern.

The role of muscles in the genesis of neuromusculoskeletal disorders has received increasing attention in recent years. This signifies a healthy return to a more balanced assessment of the origin of pain in the neuromusculoskeletal system after a decade in which many physiotherapists have paid excessive attention to an arthrogenic and discogenic view.

Having highlighted the need to consider movement pattern re-education in the context of 'normal' and 'efficient' movement as a primary objective in the rehabilitation of patients it becomes necessary to consider in more detail how to assess the effects of poor or inefficient patterns in individuals experiencing pain. Over the past 20 years, a concept of 'muscle imbalance' has gained both popularity and credibility. It draws attention to the problems which may be created by muscle shortening. Contemporary physiotherapy practice has embraced the concept and both anecdotal and research evidence has helped to develop a range of assessment and treatment techniques to identify and rectify problems of muscle imbalance.

Posture and the Concept of Muscle Imbalance

Posture is concerned with the alignment of different body segments and the interrelationship between them. Movement of one body segment will influence that to which it is adjacent. It is important for students of physiotherapy to

Figure 10.3   Normal postural alignment. (Adapted, with permission, from Kendall *et al.*, 1993, *Posture and Pain*. 4th edn, published by Williams & Wilkins, Baltimore.)

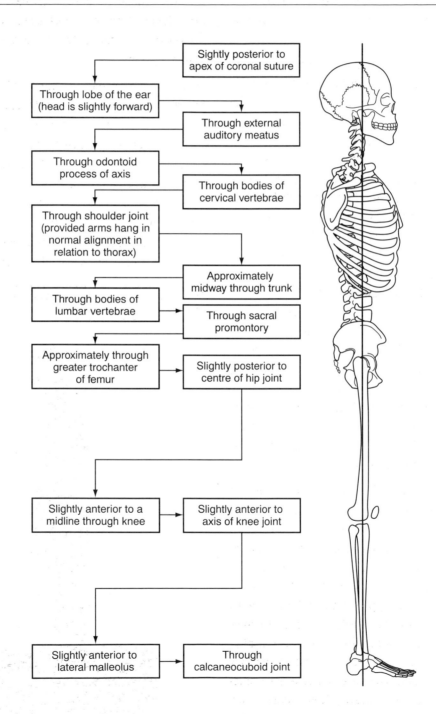

consider the effect of movement of one body segment on another, both in static and dynamic postures and its effect on the musculoskeletal system.

Some of the most influential extrinsic factors affecting posture are the muscles of the body (Lowman and Young, 1960). Reflection on the roles of different muscles in the production and control of movement enables a case to be made for a therapeutic approach to musculoskeletal disorders which considers muscle function a causative factor. A concept of muscle imbalance has developed over the past two or three decades as a result of clinical studies in the fields of physical medicine, neurology and physiotherapy. Many of the ideas have developed from those first attributed to Janda and Schmid (1980). These studies have suggested that muscle imbalance, i.e. movement dysfunction caused by length associated changes in muscles, can contribute to the development of musculoskeletal pain (Gossman et al., 1982; Caillet, 1981; Janda, 1983). Indeed, some authors, such as Janda (1983) and Kendall et al. (1993) have placed the role of muscles in musculoskeletal dysfunction at the forefront of therapeutic assessment and treatment.

The literature in the field of posture and muscle imbalance is based to a large extent on anecdotal observation although recently there have been a small number of studies which are attempting to analyse the theory underpinning the concept more scientifically (Gossman et al., 1982; Wohlfahrt et al., 1993; Toppenberg and Bullock, 1990; White and Sahrmann, 1994). Anatomical definitions of 'good posture' have abounded in physiotherapy for many years. These definitions suggest a relationship between the skeletal framework and the line of gravity. It is important for students of physiotherapy and practising clini-

cians to consider the effect of postural alignment and malalignments on the musculoskeletal system. Observation of normal alignment posture demonstrates balance between agonistic and antagonistic groups.

In Figure 10.3, the erector spinae and hip flexors are balanced with the abdominal muscles and the hip extensors. Alterations in normal alignment are likely to be associated with imbalance between these muscles. For example, a kyphotic–lordotic posture as described by Kendall and Kendall (1994) is associated with adaptive shortening of the lumbar erector spinae and the hip flexors with relative lengthening of the abdominals (see Figure 10.4). A comprehensive and detailed description of

Figure 10.4 Subject demonstrating a kyphotic–lordotic posture.

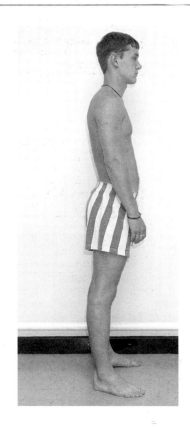

postural malalignments is offered by Kendall and Kendall (1993).

More dynamically, analysis of muscle work involved in a typical posture associated with handling objects or lifting, involving flexion at the hips, reveals postural fixation in the gastrocnemii, hamstrings and quadriceps, erector spinae and quadratus lumborum, in order to counteract forward displacement of the centre of mass of the body. This is a predominant functional posture involved in many everyday activities, such as lifting, push-

ing and pulling with and without loads (see e.g. Figure 10.5). It is also a posture which has been associated with the development of cumulative trauma disorders in the trunk. The muscles identified here are also included in a group of muscles identified by Janda (1983) which are commonly found to be shortened. These are listed in Table 10.1. Perhaps there is an indication here of a reason why adaptations in muscle length occur in what seem to be selected muscle groups.

The reader is referred to the papers by Janda and Schmid (1980), Toppenburg and Bullock (1990), Sahrmann (1992) and Norris (1995) for a more detailed account of patterns of muscle imbalance.

The muscle shortening here is described as a detectable shortening of a muscle–tendon unit or muscle group which prevents full range of movement in the joint(s) over which it passes either through contraction of the antagonist muscle or through passive stretching. Shortened muscles do not show spontaneous electrical activity and therefore are not actively contracting in order to prevent full lengthening (Janda, 1983).

However, we still don't know to what extent the connective tissues and muscle fibres are involved in this type of muscle shortening. (Muscle shortening associated with upper motor neurone damage, i.e. spasticity, has a different type of contracture as a result of the release of excessive reflex activity.)

Clinico–anatomical tests have been developed to assess the length of most muscles in the body (Janda, 1983; Kendall et al., 1993). Their use is becoming widespread and a common feature of many physiotherapeutic assessment procedures in many areas of practice. There is no doubt that some of these tests are very valuable in detecting muscle shortening and its inevitable impact on active and passive movement. However, it is always

Figure 10.5   Typical posture associated with handling objects.

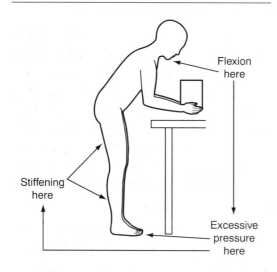

Table 10.1
Muscles most commonly found to be shortened (Janda, 1983)

Anteriorly	Posteriorly
Pectoralis major	Levator scapulae
Finger flexors of the hand	Trapezius (upper part)
Iliopsoas	Erector spinae
Adductors of the thigh	Quadratus lumborum
Rectus femoris	Piriformis
Tensor fascia lata	Hamstrings
	Gastrocnemius and soleus

important to remember that muscle shortening may be readily detectable by virtue of a limited range of passive movement at a joint, but it may not be *responsible* for that limitation. Other structures associated with or crossing the joint may be contracted. For example, it would be reasonable to suspect that tibialis posterior muscle shortening is responsible for a loss of range of motion of eversion and dorsiflexion if the patient feels a stretch deep in the calf as the ankle is dorsiflexed and everted. However, it may not be possible to be confident of this conclusion because it is possible that the limitation is being caused by other muscles or peri-articular structures. Assessment of muscle length in itself, then, does not necessarily yield enough information about range of motion. Yet if it is not assessed adequately, it is very likely that inaccurate conclusions about a patient's problem will be drawn.

Some examples are offered here to help understanding. As the reader considers these examples it is suggested that he/she considers the points raised above.

In the upper limb, observation anteriorly of subjects in supine with both arms elevated gives an indication of the likely length of muscles between the trunk and the humerus.

The subject in Figure 10.6 below, demonstrates good muscle length, with both arms resting in the horizontal plane, close to the ears. Good length in the pectoralis major and latissimus dorsi allow this resting position. The subject in Figure 10.7 is unable to rest in this position demonstrating a particular difficulty with the right upper limb. This subject has near normal active range of motion but not full range of motion. On this basis, consider the factors which might cause limitation of full range of motion. What appears to have been lost is passive range of motion. This may be due to joint structures, nerve structures or muscle shortening. The pectoralis major and latissimus dorsi were shortened in this subject.

More specific assessment can reveal adaptive length changes in particular muscles. The subject in Figure 10.8, demonstrates good length in the pectoralis major, with the upper limb resting in the horizontal plane. The subject in Figure 10.9, demonstrates some shortening of the pectoralis major muscle with the upper limb failing to rest in the horizontal plane. Rotation of the trunk away from the upper limb in this subject gives further evidence of the findings.

The same starting position is adopted in the assessment of length of the latissimus dorsi muscle. Additional adduction and external rotation of

Figure 10.6   Good muscle length between the trunk and the humerus.

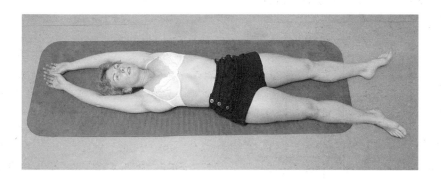

Figure 10.7   Evidence of shortening of muscles between the trunk and humerus.

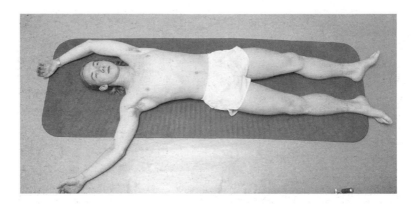

Figure 10.8   Subject demonstrating good length in pectoralis major.

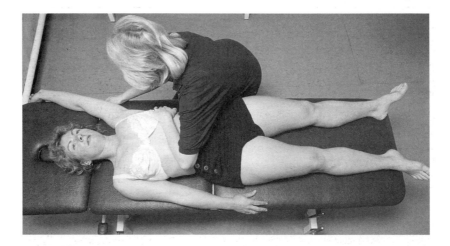

the gleno-humeral joint is applied with passive hip and lumbar flexion in order to stretch the lower fibres of the muscle. The subject in Figure 10.10 demonstrates good length whilst the subject in Figure 10.11 tested with resistance to lumbar flexion and discomfort in the shoulder region limiting the full movement. This suggests a shortened latissimus dorsi.

Simple visual observation of standing posture in the sagittal plane gives an indication of muscle length around the low back and pelvic girdle

(see Figure 10.12a). This subject has a particularly flat back. Assessment of the hamstrings in this subject reveals a severely shortened hamstring group with resistance being met at 50° (Figure 10.12b). The subject in Figure 10.13 demonstrates a more normal length in the hamstring group, with 80° of passive hip flexion before resistance caused knee flexion.

The test position for iliopsoas and rectus femoris is the same. Fixation of posterior rotation of the pelvis is achieved by the subject holding the oppo-

Figure 10.9   Subject demonstrating shortening of the pectoralis major.

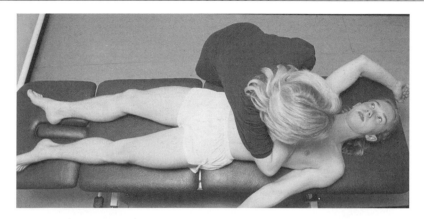

Figure 10.10   Subject demonstrating good length in latissimus dorsi.

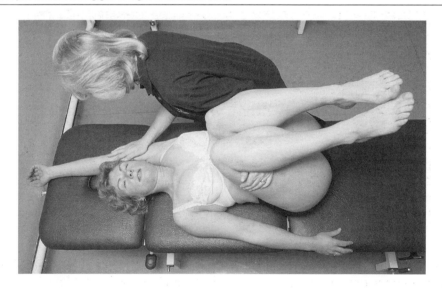

site leg in full hip flexion. In Figure 10.14, the subject demonstrates good length of iliopsoas where the posterior aspect of the thigh falls to the horizontal indicating normality (Janda, 1983). The subject in Figure 10.15 demonstrates slight shortening in this muscle with the posterior thigh just resting above the horizontal. Pressure applied to the top of the thigh here resulted in discomfort in the groin and low back. The subject in Figure

10.14 also has good length in the rectus femoris with the lower leg falling vertically from a horizontal thigh. The subject in Figure 10.15 has a shortened rectus femoris, with the lower leg clearly failing to rest in a vertical position.

The subject in Figure 10.16 demonstrates both a shortened iliopsoas and rectus femoris with the thigh failing to rest in a horizontal position and

Figure 10.11 Subject demonstrating shortening of latissimus dorsi.

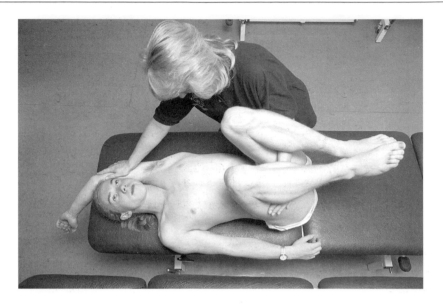

Figure 10.12a Subject demonstrating a flat back.

Figure 10.12b The same subject demonstrating short hamstrings.

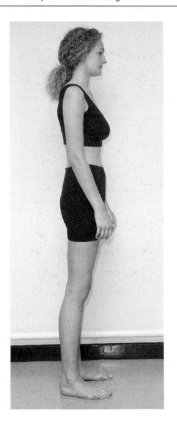

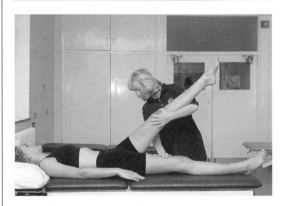

the lower leg unable to fall vertically. External pressure is applied to the lower leg showing that the subject is still unable to allow the leg to reach the expected position indicating severe shortening.

Various methods have been described for the assessment of length of tensor fascia latae and the reader is referred to Janda (1983), Kendall *et*

Figure 10.13 Subject demonstrating normal hamstring length.

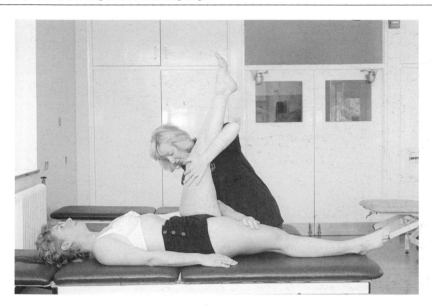

Figure 10.14 Subject demonstrating good length in iliopsoas and rectus femoris.

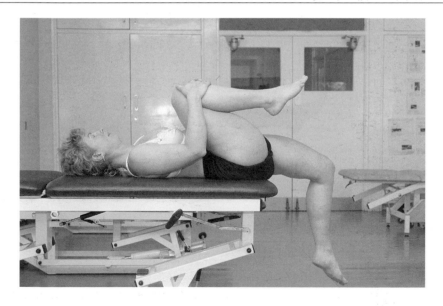

al. (1993) and Melchoine and Sullivan (1993). Fixation of the pelvis creates difficulties in all these tests.

Length of spinal muscles is more difficult to assess as the clinico-anatomical tests require the use of two or three operators to get an accurate result. However, observation of the sequence of movement in subjects under specific instruction to

Figure 10.15   Subject demonstrating slightly short iliopsoas and short rectus femoris.

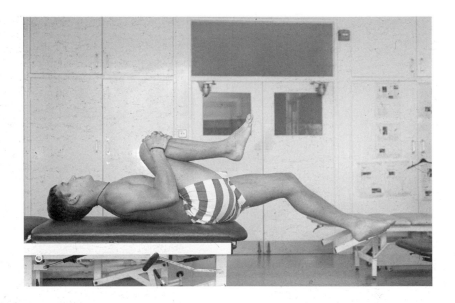

Figure 10.16   Subject demonstrating more severe shortening of rectus femoris.

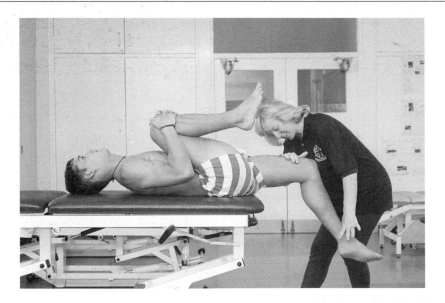

lower themselves to the ground can reveal information about the likely length of the lumbar erector spinae and quadratus lumborum muscles. The subjects in Figure 10.17a and 10.17b were instructed to reach to the ground using the term 'collapse' to encourage a movement which includes posterior rotation of the pelvis. This maybe termed the 'drop' test. Anecdotal evidence suggests that in subjects with good length, rotation of the pelvis can be observed near the begin-

Figure 10.17a,b   Subjects demonstrating differences in the 'drop test'.

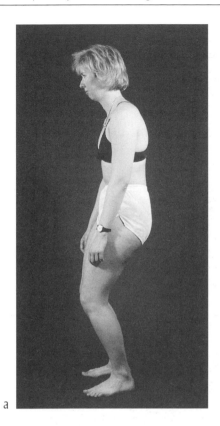

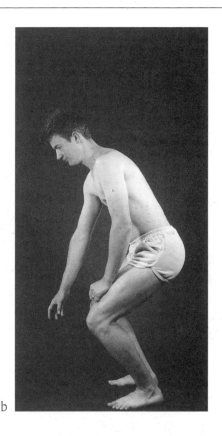

a

b

ning of the sequence of movement. In subjects with shortening of the lumbar dorsal musculature, rotation of the pelvis occurs at the end of the sequence of movement and sometimes not at all.

Painful conditions of the neuromusculoskeletal system often present with patterns of muscle shortening and imbalance. Some of these may be associated with occupational or recreational activities. Such muscle imbalances may distort alignments which may then lead to undue tension and stress on joints, ligaments and muscles. This may be an important factor in the causation of subsequent painful postural conditions (Sahrmann, 1992; Kendall *et al.*, 1993; Pitt-Brooke, 1995).

It is essential, therefore, that physiotherapists are able to identify and correct faulty posture and movement patterns. This necessarily involves the assessment of both length and strength although as Sahrmann (1992) suggests, 'muscle imbalance syndromes are more a function of faulty length than of faulty strength'.

The concept of muscle imbalance is characterized by two main elements:

1 adaptive length changes in muscle (shortening and lengthening);
2 recruitment changes with respect to both inhibition and overstimulation.

Adaptive Length Changes in Muscle

Kendall *et al.* (1952) observed length-associated changes in patients with faulty postural alignment. They described patients who had muscles in a lengthened position as a result of postural alignment. They went on to define stretch, stretch weakness, and shortness as follows (Kendall *et al.*, 1993).

> **Stretch** means to elongate or extend in length.
> **Stretch weakness** is the effect on muscles of remaining in an elongated position beyond the physiological rest position, but not beyond the normal range of muscle length.
> **Shortness or tightness** are terms which are used interchangeably to indicate a slight or moderate decrease in muscle length; movement in the direction of elongating the muscle is limited.

Recent studies on animals have investigated the effects of length-associated changes in muscles. Although we should be cautious in extrapolating the results to humans, these studies give us an indication as to how muscle tissue may adapt under certain circumstances.

Animal studies carried out by Tabary *et al.* (1972) suggest that muscle adapts to a lengthened position by increasing its number of sarcomeres and by reducing their length. These studies were conducted on immobilized limbs. The adaptation began within 24 hours of immobilization. When immobilization was discontinued, the muscles regained their 'normal' sarcomere number and length. Age may be a factor in determining the nature of the adaptive response. In young animals the length of the muscle belly decreases and the tendons elongate (Tabary *et al.*, 1972) whilst in the

adult there is no change in tendon length and the muscle adapts by increasing the number of sarcomeres.

In muscles which have been lengthened, the length–tension curve is similar to that of controls and the amplitude of the peak active tension generated by the lengthened muscle may be up to 35% greater than that of controls (Crawford, 1973). The peak occurs at approximately the position where the muscle has been immobilized, as it will develop its strength relationships depending on its new length.

Possibly in the light of these findings, Sahrmann (1987) defined the term 'positional weakness' which is a more helpful and understandable term to the clinical therapist and indicates the importance of testing a muscle's strength in different positions, based on an understanding of alterations in the length–tension curve described above.

The clinical importance of the alteration in a muscle's length–tension curve is that it may be unable to develop the required tension in the position imposed by the joint or body posture and may therefore necessitate the use of synergistic muscles in order to control the action otherwise carried out by the prime mover. This in turn may lead to abnormal movement patterns (White and Sahrmann, 1994). It is important to realize that a muscle which has been continually stretched as a result of postural malalignment may test stronger in its new extreme length and weaker in a standard muscle test, leading to a false diagnosis and therefore a possible error in therapeutic intervention.

Adaptive shortening occurs when a muscle is immobilized in a shortened position, the adaptation occurring through a loss of sarcomeres. Gossman *et al.* (1982) described how the active tension developed by shortened muscles is less than in controls and how the peak of the tension occurs at the point of immobilization. It has been suggested by some that this may be due to a slower rate of adaptation of connective tissue which leads to an increase in the proportion of connective tissue relative to sarcomeres and consequent reduced extensibility (Gossman *et al.*, 1982).

Tightness weakness is a phenomenon which was identified by Janda (1993) in which a shortening in a muscle is associated with weakness. This may be due to increased overlap between actin and myosin filaments, a relative increase in connective tissue and a remodelling of the endomysium and perimysium causing an increase in thickness. This results in an increase in compression of the fascial bag, compression of small arteries and consequent ischaemia of the muscle. Nutritional conditions of the muscle deteriorate resulting in weakness of the muscle.

Recruitment Changes in Muscle

It has been well documented that muscles which are prone to tightness are recruited more easily within a movement pattern than their elongated synergists (Jull and Janda, 1987; Sahrmann, 1992; Norris, 1995). However, most of this documentation refers back to the early work of Sahrmann and Janda, whose theories are based primarily on their own preliminary studies of movement patterns. Janda (1978) described electromyographic studies suggesting that the excitability threshold of a tight muscle is lowered and that this can result in overactivation of a tight muscle during a movement. This may explain variations in recruitment patterns and the timing of synergists. If these variations are extreme, imbalance may develop between agonistic and antagonistic muscles resulting in a faulty movement pattern through the predominance of a tight overactive muscle during activity, or recruitment of such a muscle when it should be inactive.

The reader is referred to the papers by Williams and Goldspink (1971), Gossman *et al.* (1982), Norris (1995) for a more detailed account of biased recruitment.

Consequences of Muscle Imbalance

If the musculoskeletal system and the central nervous system are part of a single functional unit, then there may be a number of consequences of muscle imbalance. These may not be confined to a local muscle dysfunction (see Figure 10.18).

In addition, it is inevitable that there will be impaired reciprocal innervation, a situation in which the tight or shortened muscle is inhibiting its antagonist, again, producing altered proprioception, impacting on motor control and the programming of movement patterns.

Muscle imbalances are likely to influence joint biomechanics → altered distribution of pressure on joint structures → overstress on joint structures → painful conditions of peri-articular structures.

Whilst the shape of joint surfaces is a structural element which physiotherapy cannot directly change, bony change may occur in immature bone as a result of load transmission (White and Sahrmann, 1994). Balance between muscles is therefore of paramount importance in the development and maintenance of correct postural alignment and hence avoidance of faulty

Figure 10.18   The consequences of muscle imbalance.

Local effect of a shortened muscle is mainly limited range

Compensation for the localized dysfunction

May lead to compensatory hypermobility in surrounding structures

May lead to an alteration in proprioceptive input

Further impaired movement control

force transmission through the musculoskeletal system. Correction of kinetics at an early stage may contribute to the normal development of bones and joints and restrict later postural problems.

Therapeutic Intervention to Normalize Muscle Balance

Having identified an abnormal movement pattern and analysed the length and strength of the muscles involved in a particular pattern, therapeutic intervention should be aimed at facilitating the appropriate recruitment of muscles within that pattern.

Jull and Richardson (1994) offer the approach shown in Figure 10.19 to the assessment and treatment of painful musculoskeletal conditions. Our attention here is to the section in bold type. The evidence from clinical observation and experimental studies clearly indicates that muscle is a tissue which is prone to change. This change is more pronounced in a muscle which becomes shortened than a muscle which

becomes lengthened. Although the changes may be detrimental to efficient movement, they are often reversible and this enables the correction of movement dysfunction.

Proprioceptive Neuromuscular Facilitation Techniques

Muscular dysfunction resulting from acute, chronic, segmental or multiple injury is common among patients referred to physiotherapy. Restoring normal function requires the therapist to consider muscle function, balance and coordination in the context of the morphological and physiological features which are associated with different forms of dysfunction.

Stimulation of the proprioceptive system as a basis for re-education of muscle has been the focus of attention of many physiotherapists for several decades. Many of these ideas have been based on the original work of Herman Kabat (1965).

Figure 10.19   The assessment and treatment of painful musculoskeletal conditions. (Adapted from Jull and Richardson, 1994).

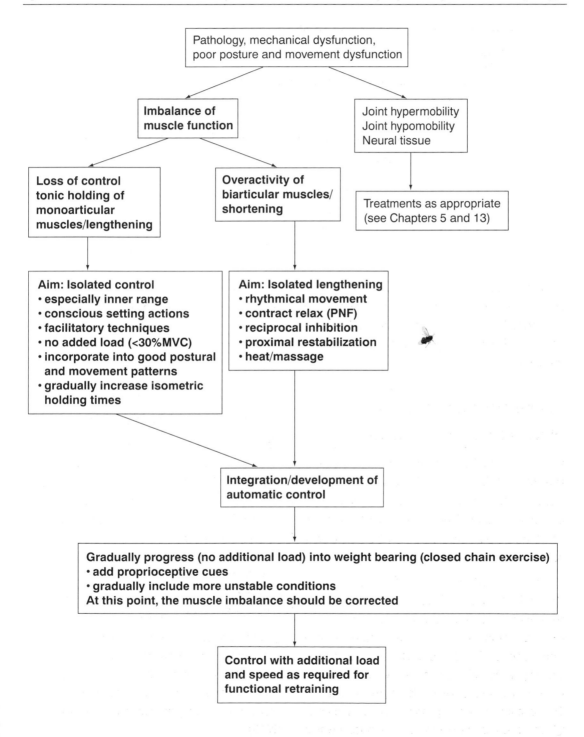

Kabat's Theories

Kabat reported that a greater motor response can be attained when employing facilitation techniques in addition to resistance when compared to resistance alone. His findings suggested that this facilitation resulted from a number of factors:

1 Application of stretch;
2 The use of particular movement patterns;
3 The use of maximal resistance in order to induce 'irradiation'.

In order to understand fully the basis of proprioceptive neuromuscular facilitation (PNF) techniques certain terms need to be clearly defined:

Proprioceptive: Anything to do with the sensory receptors which give information concerning body position and movement.

Neuromuscular: Involving nerves and muscles.

Facilitation: Making easier.

Proprioceptive neuromuscular facilitation is an approach to treatment of muscular dysfunction which encompasses a positive and reinforcing integration of physical and psychological facets to help patients achieve their highest level of function. This is in keeping with Kabat's philosophy that all human beings, including those with disability, have untapped existing potential.

The work of Charles Sherrington was influential in the development of the techniques of PNF. References to his original work are difficult to locate and for this reason some important terms are defined below. They are all taken from his early work (Sherrington, 1947).

Reciprocal innervation: (Reciprocal inhibition) The contraction of agonistic muscles is accompanied by simultaneous inhibition of their antagonists. This is a reflex response and is a necessary condition of coordinated movement.

As we shall see later in this section, relaxation techniques make use of this principle.

Temporal summation: A succession of weak, subliminal stimuli which occur within a short period of time can combine to cause excitation.

Spatial summation: Similarly, several weak stimuli, applied simultaneously to different parts of the body, can reinforce each other and cause excitation. In practice, temporal and spatial summation occur simultaneously to produce greater activity.

Successive induction: Contraction of the antagonistic muscle immediately prior to the stimulation of the agonist, increases (induces) excitation of the agonist.

Irradiation: This occurs when either the strength or the number of stimuli is increased. It is a spreading and increased strength of response to other indirect muscles.

Afterdischarge: The effect of a stimulus continues after the stimulus has stopped. Afterdischarge is proportional to the strength and duration of the stimulus. This principle explains the perception of increased power that follows a maintained static contraction.

Essentially, PNF techniques can be used to achieve the following objectives:

- Increase or facilitate range of movement;
- Increase muscle strength;
- Increase endurance;
- Increase or facilitate muscular coordination;
- Reduce pain.

PNF employs a range of manual techniques all of which adhere to the same basic principles. These principles are outlined below.

Principles Underpinning PNF Techniques

MAXIMAL RESISTANCE

All techniques involve the use of maximal resistance. The term 'maximal' indicates that sufficient resistance must be applied such that the patient uses maximum effort, but which is not deleterious to the quality of the muscular response. In practice, this is difficult to judge and takes some experience. Often, student physiotherapists and inexperienced practitioners of PNF techniques, tend to be a little heavy-handed. This point is made to encourage the inexperienced to persevere and to feel the quality of movement throughout muscular contraction. However, the great advantage with manual resistance here, is that once you begin to develop skill levels, you are able to accommodate resistance and adapt to the patient's needs sensitively throughout the range of movement. In this regard, manual resistance is akin to 'isokinetics' (see Chapters 6, 8 and 12) and can be more useful than 'dead weight' resistance.

MANUAL CONTACT

All techniques are dependent upon manual contact. There are particular handholds associated with different patterns of movement (see below). The main principles to consider when applying the manual contact is that their purpose is to guide the movement by stimulating movement of the body part into the hands. In addition, the hands are the vehicle for the provision of resistance. Grip and pressure are used to provide this resistance. For example, if one wishes to resist adduction, the hand(s) would be placed on the adductor surface on the limb and a pressure applied in the direction of abduction. This principle holds for all PNF techniques.

PATTERNS OF MOVEMENT

Kabat identified patterns of movement in which muscles seemed to produce better responses. The concept of patterning has also gained support in other therapeutic approaches (i.e. Bobath, Rood, Brunnstrom). The patterns identified by Kabat all have a diagonal end spiral component, thereby taking exercise out of the cardinal planes and introducing composite movements as a more appropriate way of re-educating muscles (Figures 10.20 and 10.21). Many therapists are convinced that the use of mass movement patterns yields better therapeutic results. There is, however, little scientific evidence that this is actually the case. It is not recommended that the concept of these movement patterns be disregarded, merely that their true value in therapeutic exercise requires further scientific substantiation. Many experienced therapists, including the author, would suggest that subjectively it is possible to detect better responses from muscles when they are worked in pattern than out of pattern. It may be that this is more perceptible in some patterns than others, possibly because of the functional nature of the patterns and/or because of the proprioceptive input.

(For a detailed description of the patterns, see Voss, Ionta and Meyers, 1985.)

Practical Task

Try reaching over the top of your head and down the back of you spinous processes. Note the movement. External rotation of the shoulder, supination and radial deviation?

Try putting your hands to the back of your seat and push off using your finger tips. Note the movement. Internal rotation, pronation and ulnar deviation?

Put your arm out in front of you with the elbow straight. Externally rotate your shoulder and keep going. What happens in the forearm, Supination? Keep going.

What happens at the wrist. Radial deviation? Probably!

Go through the same procedure starting with internal rotation and note the opposite associated movements. Interesting isn't it?

Clearly, there is something in these patterns which merits proper scientific investigation.

The PNF patterns seem to be very difficult to remember. You will find it easier if you remember and understand the associated movements as suggested above.

Note that there are *four* patterns associated with each limb and that these patterns represent *two* diagonals of movement. So that, the flexion/adduction/external rotation pattern in the lower limb is directly opposite to the extension/abduction/internal rotation pattern. In order to induce stretch, the extreme of the extension pattern is the starting position if one is working the muscle in the flexion pattern. This may become clearer when the techniques are described.

STRETCH

Stretch is used to elongate the muscle and also to facilitate contraction through the stretch reflex. The stretch stimulus occurs when a muscle is elongated. This facilitatory effect is augmented when all the synergistic muscles of a limb or the trunk are elongated. In addition, the stretch reflex can be elicited from muscles which are under tension or subject to contraction and this may help to produce a more powerful functional contraction. Therefore, all PNF techniques begin with an initial elongation of the pattern to be worked and an extra 'tweak' to elicit a stretch reflex.

Figure 10.20 Upper limb patterns. Note that in the upper limb patterns, external rotation always goes with flexion and internal rotation always goes with extension. Also, pronation and ulnar deviation always go with internal rotation and supination and radial deviation always go with external rotation. These are natural composite movements i.e. elements of movement which are associated in function.

Shoulder Forearm Wrist Fingers	Flexion/abduction/external rotation Supination Extension/radial deviation Extension/abduction		Flexion/adduction/external rotation Supination Flexion/radial deviation Flexion/adduction
		Upper limb	
Shoulder Forearm Wrist Fingers	Extension/abduction/internal rotation Pronation Extension/ulnar deviation Extension/abduction		Extension/adduction/internal rotation Pronation Flexion/ulnar deviation Flexion/adduction

Figure 10.21   Lower limb patterns. Again, note that in the lower limb patterns, adduction always goes with external rotation. Remember this by remembering ADDER. Further to this, inversion always goes with external rotation. This seems to follow a functional movement pattern. Consider the movements involved in the swing phase of walking?

Hip Ankle/Subtalar Toes	Flexion/abduction/internal rotation Dorsiflexion/eversion Extension/abduction			Flexion/adduction/external rotation Dorsiflexion/inversion Extension/abduction
			Lower limb	
Hip Ankle/Subtalar Toes	Extension/abduction/internal rotation Plantarflexion/eversion Flexion/adduction			Extension/adduction/external rotation Plantarflexion/inversion Flexion/adduction

TRACTION AND APPROXIMATION

The application of traction and approximation by elongation or compression of the limbs helps to facilitate movement or stability, probably by stimulating the joint receptors (Voss et al., 1985).

Traction also elongates the muscles thereby acting as a stretch stimulus. Traction is used to facilitate movement, especially pulling movements (flexion in the lower limb), whilst approximation is used to facilitate compression or pushing movements (extension in the lower limb). Approximation will also facilitate stabilization.

TIMING

Timing is a term which refers to the sequencing of movements. Normal movement requires a smooth sequence of activity and coordinated movement requires precise timing of that sequence. The normal sequence of many movements is from distal to proximal (though perhaps we should question whether this is efficient — remember the principles of efficient movement outlined by McClurg Anderson above). PNF techniques use this so-called 'normal' timing sequence with movement beginning distally.

BODY POSITION AND THE DIAGONAL OF MOVEMENT

It is generally accepted that the diagonal of movement within the patterns should be narrow. In accordance with this, a more efficient resistance can be applied if the therapist's body is in line with the required movement. The therapist should therefore attempt to line up their hips and shoulders perpendicular to the line of movement, with the hands and arms kept in alignment (Adler et al., 1993). The resistance should come from the therapist's body to ensure efficient body mechanics. This enables the therapist to retain relaxed hands which can then detect patient responses.

VERBAL COMMANDS

Verbal commands tell the patient what to do. It is important that these are given clearly and that they are brief and well timed with the initiation and sequence of movement.

VISUAL STIMULUS

If the patient is able to see the movement it may help them to control it better. Moving the eyes influences the position of the head and neck and this may be beneficial. Certainly, the eyes are an important part of the sensory system and feedback from them may help to provide a more powerful contraction.

Techniques

Proprioceptive neuromuscular facilitation techniques have been used by physiotherapists for many years in the re-education of muscles, for increasing range of movement in certain circumstances and for pain relief. The aim of these techniques is to promote functional movement through facilitation, strengthening, inhibition and relaxation of muscles or muscle groups. The facilitatory procedures outlined above are a feature of all techniques and are graded and combined to suit the needs of each patient.

RHYTHMIC INITIATION

This technique can be used to improve coordination in movement and to facilitate a normal speed of movement. It can also be used to help patients relax and to assist in initiating movements.

Indications
- Uncoordinated movement
- Movement which is too slow or too fast
- General tension or agitation
- Difficulty in initiating movement

Description The therapist moves the patient or limb part through the range of movement passively at an appropriate speed. This is reinforced by verbal commands.

The patient is then encouraged to work actively, the movement therefore becoming active-assisted. The return movement remains passive, conducted by the therapist.

When the patient has gained active control of the movement, together with appropriate coordina-

tion at an appropriate speed, the therapist introduces resistance, whilst maintaining the rhythm with verbal commands.

The technique is usually done with active motion in one direction of the diagonal, but may be modified to work both patterns actively.

Practical Tips

In the passive phase, use the term, 'Let me move you . . . now, let me move you back'.

In the active assisted phase, use the term, 'Now help me move you . . . now relax and let me move you back'.
In the active and resisted phases, use the terms, 'Now move into my hands, push into my hands . . . let me move you back'.

*In this way, your commands are reassuring and can be used to induce an appropriate rhythm. Emphasis on the word 'now' in each command enhances this instruction particularly in the active phase, e.g., **now** move, **now** push.*

RHYTHMIC STABILIZATIONS

This technique is an isometric technique which is used to facilitate contraction in muscles around a joint in order to encourage stabilization. It is also based on the neurophysiological principle of successive induction as well as temporal and spatial summation. It is particularly useful as a warm-up activity and also in conditions in which there is a painful joint.

Indications
- Pain, particularly when the joint is moved
- Limited range of joint motion
- Joint instability
- Poor muscle coordination

Description

The therapist places the joint in the required position, which must be pain-free. She then resists contraction of the stronger muscle group first, giving the instruction to the patient, 'Don't let me move you'. This will induce a strong isometric contraction. The resistance is increased gradually until the patient has responded fully. The therapist then moves the distal hand to resist the opposite pattern, repeating the command, 'Don't let me move you'. As the patient changes his reaction, the therapist moves the second hand to reinforce resistance of this pattern. The resistance is built up slowly and once the patient has responded, the therapist again moves the distal hand to resist the opposite pattern, and so on.

Practical Tips

Beginners with this technique should not attempt to alternate between all four patterns. Start with two and then change to the two patterns in the opposite diagonal.

It is essential not to build up the resistance too quickly. The patient must not be able to move the joint. It is important to convey to the patient that they are not attempting to move the joint, merely to maintain the joint's position. This may be important in gaining the patient's confidence if he has a painful joint.

Do try to position yourself so that you have a physical advantage, i.e. so that you are stabilized properly. Otherwise you may find this a tiring procedure to perform.

Once the therapist has become skilled, she may alternate between all four patterns for the limb,

therefore inducing a rhythmical contraction of all muscle groups around the joint. Alternatively, the therapist may choose to work in one diagonal and then move to the other diagonal, moving rhythmically from one pattern to the other within each diagonal separately. This process is repeated rhythmically until the patient fails to respond effectively, indicating early fatigue. After some rest, it may be repeated or another technique may be used.

HOLD–RELAX, CONTRACT–RELAX AND AGONIST CONTRACT

These techniques can be used to facilitate and increase range of motion when muscle is thought to be a cause of limitation. It involves an isometric or limited isotonic contraction of the limiting muscles.

Indication

- Limited range of motion, especially where there is limitation of passive movement.

Description

The therapist, with or without the patient's assistance, moves the joint or body part to the end of pain-free passive range of motion. The therapist then asks the patient to produce a strong contraction of the restricting muscle / muscle group (i.e. the antagonists). The therapist, whilst resisting most of the motion, allows enough to be sure that all muscles, particularly the rotators to be contracting (contract–relax). This contraction should be maintained for 3–6 seconds (Balnave et al., 1987).

The therapist then tells the patient to relax. It has been suggested that both the patient and therapist relax for a period up to 2 minutes (Balnave et al., 1987) after which the patient's limb part or joint is repositioned, usually passively, by the therapist, to the new limit of passive range. However, Enoka (1994) suggested that the stretch should be applied during the 10 seconds immediately following contraction when the excitability of the muscle spindle and the motor neurone pool is reduced. The author's experience suggests the latter is probably more effective.

This can be modified by asking the patient to actively move into the new range (contract–relax–contract) after the initial contract and relax period.

The technique is repeated until no further range is achieved.

In the technique of hold–relax, the same procedure is followed except that the patient produces a strong contraction which is resisted by the therapist, restricting it to an isometric technique. In practice, few therapists are able to fully control such a strong contraction and some movement inevitably occurs, usually through lack of therapist skill. Therefore, even in cases of an attempted hold–relax technique, frequently the result is a contract–relax technique.

Practical Tips

It is really important to stretch the rotational component to facilitate the best contraction of the resisting muscle group. This is probably why the contract–relax technique is more used in contemporary practice.

Use the term, 'Don't let me move you', even though your intention may be to allow a little rotary movement. You will probably find that unless your body mechanics are absolutely first rate, or that as the therapist, you are considerably bigger and stronger than the patient, you will find it difficult to 'hold' the patient once they have built up the strong contraction. The command 'Don't let me move you' is, however an excellent motivator for the patient to provide a strong contraction.

Build the resistance to the patient's movement up slowly. In this way you will gain far more control. Until one becomes quite skilled, the tendency is to be heavy-handed with manual resistance. It is important to enable the patient to gain control of the contraction before you increase the resistance.

AGONIST CONTRACT

The agonist contract technique is based on the principle of reciprocal relaxation and requires the patient to contract the agonistic muscle whilst the therapist stretches the antagonist.

Indications
- Limited range of motion, especially where there is passive limitation.

Description
The therapist takes the limb to the point of limitation of range of motion and then instructs the patient to contract the agonistic muscle. The patient is allowed to develop the contraction adequately before the therapist applies pressure in a direction to assist the contraction and stretch the antagonistic muscle which is limiting the movement. Pressure should be applied very gradually.

REPEATED CONTRACTIONS

Repeated contractions make use of isotonic contractions to increase active range of motion, facilitate the initiation of a motion and increase muscle strength. They are based on the neurophysiological principles of temporal and spatial summation.

Indications
- Muscle weakness including an inability to initiate movement
- Decreased awareness of movement

Description
Basic repeated contractions: The therapist takes the limb or body part into the elongated position, ensuring that the rotational component in particular is stretched. A gentle extra 'squeeze', is given together with the preparatory command 'Now' on top of the elongation in order to initiate the stretch reflex.

The patient is instructed to 'move' in the direction indicated with the command 'Now push' or 'Now pull' so that the patient's response coordinates with the induction of the stretch reflex.

The resulting contraction is resisted, isotonic and through full range. The limb part is then returned to the starting position and the process is repeated.

Advanced repeated contractions: The therapist conducts the above. Further to this, if there is a detectable weakness at a specific point in the active range, an isometric hold can be incorporated.

The therapist facilitates an isotonic contraction to the weak point in the range and then instructs the patient to 'Hold it there, don't let me move you'. Having built up a strong isometric contraction, the therapist then stretches the rotational component in the pattern and together with the command 'Now pull up/push up', allows the limb to complete the pattern. This can be repeated at several points in the range in order to allow the facilitation of overflow from a strong part of the pattern to a weak part.

Timing for emphasis: A further modification to the basic repeated contraction can be made in order to facilitate overflow from stronger proximal muscle groups to distal ones. In this modification, the repeated contraction is restricted to a point in the range at which the proximal joints are held isometrically, usually near the middle of their range, whilst the distal joints continue with isotonic repeated contractions. In this way, the normal timing of the pattern, in which movement is from distal to proximal, is altered to emphasize movement at a distal joint by facilitating overflow as indicated above.

Practical Tips

Simple repeated contractions are often the first technique encountered by students of PNF, as they are the means by which one learns the patterns.

The most important element of skill to develop is the ability to time the elongation, extra squeeze or stretch and the command 'Now pull, or now push' in order to coordinate the effects of these different forms of stimulus. This coordination is the key to the development of skills in all other techniques and it is well worth practice. It is also important to practice on different subjects as the tension in the musculotendinous structures will feel different from subject to subject.

SLOW REVERSALS

This is an isotonic technique in which the stronger muscles of the antagonistic pattern in a diagonal are facilitated and active motion is continued from this direction to the opposite without relaxation. It is based on Sherrington's neurophysiological principle of successive induction, the theory being that excitation in the antagonistic group can help to increase excitation in the weaker agonists as long as relaxation between the patterns is prevented. This technique is used to increase strength and coordination, prevent fatigue and increase active range of motion where muscle weakness or incoordination is identified.

Indications
- Weakness of agonistic muscles
- Poor coordination with inability to alter direction of motion

Description
The starting position is the position of elongation and stretch for the antagonistic pattern. The therapist offers resistance through the range of motion in this pattern and at the end of the range, alters the manual grips to facilitate the opposite pattern without allowing relaxation. Again at the end of range of motion of the agonistic pattern, the process is repeated, again without relaxation. In this way, the reversals are developed. It is thought that successive contraction of muscles in each pattern also induces a reflex relaxation in the opposing group as a result of reciprocal relaxation and that this helps to prevent fatigue.

Practical Tips

It is important not to attempt to complete the reversal too quickly. The changeover from one pattern to the other must be smooth. It is facilitated by maintaining the distal hand hold in the upper limb and the proximal hand hold in the lower limb. In this way the hands are able to maintain the traction or approximation component of the pattern and this helps to maintain the contraction in each direction.

It is important to coordinate the timing of the changeover with an emphasis in the verbal command, 'now pull back, now push back' etc.

The use of traction and approximation are also particularly useful in facilitating the smooth changeover from one pattern to the other.

On the whole, if the therapist is careful not to over-resist the patient particularly at end of range, the changeover will be more smooth. Remember that patients are generally weaker in outer range and inner range, so resistance needs to be modified accordingly. If this is not done the patient will be inhibited by over-resistance.

Clinical Use of PNF Techniques

Considerable practice is required to develop the complex psychomotor skills required to implement all the principles associated with this approach to the re-education of muscles. In some areas PNF techniques are widely used and in others they are underused. The reason for this is usually that they have been poorly taught in undergraduate or pre-registration training and therapists feel that unless they can perform the techniques perfectly, they are of little value. In fact the opposite may be true. There is little scientific evidence to suggest that techniques are only effective if used in the proper patterns and with all components of the skills adequately executed.

The use of the patterns advocated by Voss *et al.*, (1985) has been the subject of some debate (Basmajian, 1967; Stern *et al.*, 1970) and there is considerable anecdotal evidence to suggest that use of the principles of PNF techniques can be valuable even if the full patterns are not used. This is, however, only anecdotal and there is a need for more extensive research in this area.

However, the techniques associated with the PNF approach are currently showing increasing favour particularly in the treatment of muscle imbalance problems, probably because of their versatility in terms of objectives. The techniques have been outlined independently above but in practice, they are all very much used together. A therapy

Clinical Example

Miss P was a 17-year-old amateur sportswoman. She suffered a rotator cuff injury and glenohumeral ligament strain after an awkward twist whilst doing handsprings. She presented with pain anteriorly, superiorly and posteriorly around the glenohumeral joint which could be localized on palpation and testing to be arising from injury to the supraspinatus and infraspinatus muscles and the glenohumeral ligaments. (There was an underlying coracohumeral ligament and acromioclavicular joint sprain.)

Following management of the immediate inflammatory response and pain over a period of a few days, PNF techniques were used to further relieve pain, restore length, strength and coordination to the rotator cuff muscles.

Sessions started by warming the muscles up and aiming to reduce pain arising from stiffness and reduced circulation. Rhythmic stabilizations were progressed from patterns in one diagonal to both diagonals. Following the warm-up period, a hold–relax technique was used to stretch the extensor muscles which *had become a little tight, inhibiting flexion. With each gain in range of flexion, two or three repeated contractions of the flexors into the new range were introduced, with intermittent hold–relax stretches to maximize the gain in range. Following several interchanges between these two techniques, some slow reversals were introduced to facilitate coordination between the flexor and extensor muscle groups, with particular attention to the newly facilitated range. A last stretch to the extensor muscles was applied using the agonist contract method and following two or three repeats of the technique a rhythmic stabilization was performed near to the facilitated range.*

New range was gained but, as important, the quality of the whole range was improved substantially. Pain from stiffness was reduced.

Subsequent treatments focused increasingly on the strengthening techniques to prevent the development of instability at the shoulder complex.

session may start with rhythmic stabilizations to warm the problem area up, then techniques with either a strengthening or mobilizing objective may be used. These may be used in succession with each other, so that a treatment session may include an interplay of several techniques dependent upon the responses of the patient. An example of this is given below.

The aim of PNF is to facilitate and promote functional movement through the excitation and inhibition of appropriate muscle groups. The techniques outlined above form the basis upon which the assessment and treatment of patients with movement dysfunction may be evaluated and determined using the philosophy and principles formulated by Kabat and developed by Voss *et al.* (1985).

Relaxation

Many patients entering physiotherapy departments have painful problems associated with dysfunction of the neuromusculoskeletal system. These problems are often multifactorial and one component may be an element of stress. Stress is a physiological adaptation response to environmental agents or stimuli recognized as 'stressors'. The body's initial reaction to a stressor is a complex of reactions initiated by hypothalamic stimulation of the sympathetic division of the autonomic nervous system and the adrenal medulla (Tortora and Agnostakos, 1990). Heart rate and strength of cardiac muscle contraction increase, along with the level of vasoconstriction, thereby increasing cardiac output and blood pressure. Respiratory rate is elevated, gastric motility is decreased and perspiration increases. The response may be prolonged by sympathetic stimulation of the adrenal medulla which increases adrenaline and noradrenaline secretion. A degree

of stress, however, may be beneficial to the stimulation of the nervous system to enable the individual to respond to the environment in which we live. It is the prolonged response which may give rise to impairment of performance. This is demonstrated in the inverted U hypothesis of arousal shown in Figure 10.22.

It has been suggested that emotional stimuli can be the most common stressors and that the endocrine, autonomic and musculoskeletal systems may all be involved in the body's response. Although all systems are exposed equally to stress, it is believed that the weakest area is most vulnerable to diseases or dysfunctions of adaptation. It therefore follows that if a patient complains of a musculoskeletal dysfunction and the subjective assessment uncovers a source of stress for that patient, there may be a requirement for the therapist to consider means by which physical stress relief may benefit the patient.

Stress Reduction and Approaches to Relaxation

The concept of relaxation has a long and varied history. However, the current interest in forms of relaxation therapy stems from an increase in self-

Figure 10.22   The inverted U hypothesis of arousal.

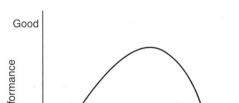

awareness which accompanied the 'body boom' of the 1960s and 1970s.

Relaxation techniques broadly fall into two main categories:

1 Meditative, in which the meditative element is the major component, e.g. Benson's controlled breathing which includes the use of a mantra (Benson, 1972),
transcendental meditation;
2 Physical, in which physical activity is the major component, e.g. Jacobson's progressive relaxation, Mitchell's physiological relaxation.

In some techniques, both elements are equally important, e.g. the Alexander technique and yoga.

There has been considerable research into relaxation techniques and there seems little question that all these techniques have been able to show alleviation of responses to stress (Alexander and Michlich, 1972; Benson, 1972; Patel, 1973; Stone and De Leo, 1976; Leggat et al., 1981) though there is little evidence that any one procedure is more effective than another or indeed if any of them produce a larger effect than placebos. A meta-analysis conducted by Abrams et al. (1989) concluded that transcendental meditation had the greatest effect on trait anxiety.

Relaxation Approaches Commonly Used by Physiotherapists

THE CONCEPT OF PROGRESSIVE RELAXATION

The concept of progressive relaxation therapy was pioneered by Jacobson in 1938 (Jacobson, 1939). It is now a universally accepted technique used by many physiotherapists and has come to be known as Jacobson's progressive relaxation.

The progressive relaxation approach encourages patients to tense, then relax sequentially, groups of muscles while also attending to the somatic components of tension and relaxation which are being experienced. Jacobson (1939) suggested that by teaching the patient to contract a muscle and develop recognition of the tension signals, recognition of tension in daily life would be possible. Following contraction, the muscle fibres lengthen and relaxation occurs. (Remember the PNF principle of maximal contraction is followed by maximal relaxation. Jacobson's work preceded Sherrington's, but Sherrington's findings which were applied to muscle re-education techniques, also underpin Jacobson's concept.) As the patient progressed in the technique it was assumed that physiological progression would occur. There are several studies which support Jacobson's claims. It appears to be of clinical value, particularly with respect to hypertension, reduction of seizures in epileptics and the reduction of respiratory distress (Dahl et al., 1987; Bindemann et al., 1991).

However, recent studies have indicated that isometric contraction of small muscle groups may be associated with increased sympathetic activity, resulting in increased heart rate and contractility and increased arterial pressure, particularly with regard to systolic blood pressure (Federici et al., 1993; Costa and Baggioni, 1994). This has led to numerous hospitals withdrawing progressive relaxation from cardiac rehabilitation regimes in fear of eliciting adverse effects (Harvey cited Salt, 1995). However, this was not found to occur in normotensive patients by Salt (1995) in a study of the effects of this method. Indeed a significant reduction in both systolic and diastolic blood pressure was reported.

MITCHELL'S SIMPLE PHYSIOLOGICAL RELAXATION

In 1963, Laura Mitchell, a physiotherapist, introduced a method of simple physiological relaxation to the World Confederation for Physical Therapy. In this presentation, she claimed that patients suffering from stress were in the grip of the flight–fight response. She placed particular emphasis on muscular tension and expressed her observations that stressed patients appeared to present with the same posture in a recognizable pattern.

The aim of simple physiological relaxation was to eliminate the state of muscle tension in the body whilst simultaneously preserving the patient's awareness of this posture (Mitchell, 1963).

The method is based on three simple physiological factors:

1 The all or none law of muscle fibre contraction states that each fibre contracts fully or not at all, and consequently tone can be increased or decreased at will or by reflex from the mid brain.
2 Information arising from the joint, muscles and tendons is signalled to the cerebral cortex to assist in constructing the plastic image of the body.
3 In the group action of muscles there is reciprocal innervation of opposing groups, whereby contraction in agonistic muscles is accompanied by reflex relaxation of antagonists.

The rationale of Mitchell's method is therefore that it is possible for the patient, if aware of increased tension, to gain reflex relaxation in tense muscle groups by contracting their antagonists. Based on this hypothesis, Mitchell developed a complete scheme of ordered movements designed to work through the tense muscles of the body, replacing increased muscle tension with relaxation (see Table 10.2). Essentially, this involves moving the body away from the fear/stress positions of flexion, adduction, medial rotation and elevation and encouraging the patient's awareness of this posture.

Respiration control is also encouraged with instruction directed towards diaphragmatic and lateral costal deep breathing.

Note the muscle groups in the right-hand column of Table 10.2 and compare the overlap with the muscles identified by Janda as muscles prone to shortening in the section on muscle imbalance.

Table 10.2
Muscle groups targeted in Mitchell's simple physiological relaxation

Shoulder depressors	to induce relaxation in	Shoulder elevators
Elbow extensors	to induce relaxation in	Elbow flexors
Shoulder abductors	to induce relaxation in	Shoulder adductors
Finger and thumb extensors	to induce relaxation in	Finger and thumb flexors
Hip lateral rotators	to induce relaxation in	Hip medial rotators
Ankle dorsiflexors	to induce relaxation in	Ankle plantarflexors
Trunk flexors	to induce relaxation in	Trunk extensors
Neck extensors	to induce relaxation in	Neck flexors

WHAT DO WE LEARN FROM THE LITERATURE?

Mitchell's method has become the more popular technique in clinical usage over recent years, yet there is little scientific evidence that it is more or less effective than Jacobson's method. A study carried out by Jackson (1991) concluded that Mitchell's method appeared to be of value with respect to tension reduction in patients with rheumatoid arthritis. In a robust controlled study of both Jacobson's method and Mitchell's method Salt (1995; Salt and Kerr, 1997) found that both methods elicited reductions in the physiological parameters systolic and diastolic blood pressure, heart rate and respiration rate, but that there was no significant difference between the methods, suggesting that both methods could be of value in the treatment of stress-related disorders. It seems that as there is no evidence to date that one method is more effective than the other, the choice of relaxation therapy should be a decision made by the patient. The freedom to choose a technique which conforms to the patient's requirements is also likely to enhance compliance (Benson, 1972).

Conclusions

Contemporary physiotherapy practice is emerging from a prolonged period in which excessive attention has been paid to an arthrogenic view of many painful musculoskeletal disorders. The role of muscles in the genesis of these disorders has received increasing attention in recent years signifying a healthy return to a wider assessment of the origin of pain in the musculoskeletal system.

This chapter has outlined specific neuromuscular approaches which are used by physiotherapists in the prevention and rehabilitation of disorders of the musculoskeletal system. The knowledge base which is common to these approaches has been suggested demonstrating a need on the part of the clinician to integrate and synthesize this knowledge. Each approach has something to offer and it is important that a fully competent physiotherapist attempts to broaden their knowledge adequately in order to provide a range of clinical skills necessary to fulfil the demands of complex clinical reasoning. What is presented here is only one area of practice for physiotherapists and must be augmented with the valuable information and knowledge provided elsewhere in this text and other specialist texts.

Key Points

1 Most clinical problems are complex, requiring clinical physiotherapists to develop a broad repertoire of skills. There are a range of neuromuscular approaches and techniques in contemporary practice which deserve the attention of students of physiotherapy.

2 In order to treat painful disorders of movement and muscle function it is important to develop a 'cognitive-visuo-tactile' approach to the assessment of such disorders in order to ensure that a comprehensive picture of the problem is gained. Of particular importance in this equation is a detailed analysis of movement patterns.

3 Many painful disorders of the musculoskeletal system are associated with adaptations in muscle length and abnormal muscle strength and coordination. The role of static and dynamic posture in the genesis, treatment and rehabilitation of these problems is significant.

4 There are a range of clinico-anatomical tests which have been developed to assess muscle

length and a range of stretching techniques which are designed to prevent and treat short muscles. These are widely used in clinical practice and although their reliability is questionable in part, if executed rigorously and with attention to detail, they form a valuable set of procedures.

5 Manual techniques are often criticized because of subjectivity in their execution. However, manual techniques which are used in the assessment and treatment of muscle length and strength have many advantages. These include: the ability to acquire knowledge through palpation which would otherwise not be discovered; facilitatory and inhibitory effects on muscle function through the proprioceptive system; the ability to adapt assistance / resistance to movement dependent on objectives and individual ability; and the reassurance offered to the patient by careful application of manual contact.

6 The underpinning knowledge for all neuromuscular approaches and techniques is similar. This allows biomechanical, environmental and physiological principles to be applied to each treatment approach, whether it be considerations about how best to induce relaxation in a patient demonstrating signs of stress, decisions about how to assess muscle length or facilitate an increase in the strength of a weak muscle group, or how to re-educate a more efficient movement pattern.

7 Painful disorders of the musculoskeletal system usually manifest themselves in movement dysfunction and thereby muscular dysfunction. A sound understanding of the interaction between body mechanics, muscular factors, nervous system factors and the environment will enable a successful approach to the analysis, diagnosis, treatment and re-education of many painful musculoskeletal disorders.

8 Many of the ideas contained within the approaches considered in this chapter need more scientific appraisal in relation to musculoskeletal disorders. Further scrutiny of these ideas will result in better rehabilitation strategies.

References and Further Reading

Abrams, AI, Eppley, KR, Shear, J (1989) Differential effects of relation techniques on trait anxiety: a meta-analysis. *Journal of Clinical Psychology*, **45** (6): 957–973.

Adams, M, Hutton, W (1985) Gradual disc prolapse. *Spine* 10 (6).

Adams, M, Dolan, P, Hutton, W (1987) Diurnal variations in the stresses on the lumbar spine. *Spine* 12 (2).

Adler, SA, Beckers, D, Buck, M (1993) *PNF in Practice: An Illustrated Guide*. Springer Verlag, New York.

Alexander, AB, Michlich, PH (1972) The immediate effects of systematic relaxation training on peak expiratory flow rates in asthmatic children. *Psychosomatic Medicine* **35** (5): 388–393.

Balnave, RJ, Cilless, JE, Goonan, R, Mansfield, J, Sanderson, DE, Smith, DR, Trollor, S, Waniganayake, A, Wilson, S, Wu, H (1987) Physiological mechanisms underlying the techniques increasing hip flexion range of movement. World Congress of Physiotherapists, Sydney, Australia.

Basmajian, JV (1967) *Muscles Alive: Their Functions Revealed by Electromyography*. Baltimore, Williams & Wilkins Co.

Benson, H (1972) Systematic hypertension and the relaxation response. *New England Journal*, **296**: 1152–1156.

Bindemann, S, Soukoup, M, Kaye, SB (1991) Randomised control study of relaxation training. *European Journal of Cancer* **27** (2): 170–174.

Costa, F, Biaggioni, I (1994) Role of adenosine in the sympathetic activation produced by isometric exercise in humans. *Journal of Clinical Investigation* **93** (4): 1645–1660.

Crawford, GNC (1972) The growth of striated muscle immobilised in extension. *Journal of Anatomy* **114**: 165–183

Dahl, J, Melin, L, Lund, L (1987) Effects of a contingent relaxation treatment programme on adults with refractory epileptic seizures. *Epilepsia* **28**: 125–132.

Enoka, RM (1994) *Neuromechanical Basis of Kinesiology*, 2nd edn. Human Kinetics, Champaign, Illinois.

Federici, A, Ciccone, M, Noia, D, Selvaggi, G, Antenolli, G, Rizzon, P (1993) The non-invasive assessment of coronary flow during isometric exercise by Doppler ultrasonography of the internal mammary artery anastomosed to the left coronary. *Cardiologia* **38** (9): 555–559.

Goldspink, G, Williams, PE (1981) *Mechanisms of Muscle Adaptation to Functional Requirements*, vol 24. Gubba, F, Marechall, G, Takais, O (eds). Perganon Press, Oxford.

Goldspink, G, Tabary, JC, Tabary, C, Tardian, G (1974) Effect of denervation on the adaptation of sarcomere number and extensibility to the functional length of the muscle. *Journal of Physiology* 236: 733–742.

Gossman, MR, Sahrmann, SA, Rose, SJ (1982) Review of length associated changes in muscle. *Physical Therapy* 62 (12): 1799–1808.

Harvey, J (1995) personal communication, cited Salt, V (1995) Mitchell's simple physiological and Jacobson's progressive relaxation techniques: a comparison. Undergraduate thesis. School of Physiotherapy, University of Nottingham.

Jacobson, E (1939) *Progressive Relaxation.* University of Chicago Press, Chicago.

Jackson, M (1991) An evaluation of the Mitchell method of simple physiological relaxation in women with rheumatoid arthritis. *British Journal of Occupational Therapy* 54 (3): 105–107.

Janda, V (1983) *Muscle Function Testing.* Butterworths, London.

Janda, V (1993) Muscle strength in relation to muscle length, pain and muscle imbalance. In Harms-Ringdahl, K (ed.) *Muscle Strength.* International Perspectives in Physical Therapy, vol. 8. Churchill Livingstone, London.

Janda, V, Schmid, HJA (1980) Muscles as a pathogenic factor in back pain. In *Proceedings of I.F.O.M.T. Conference,* New Zealand, 2–23.

Jull, GA, Janda, V (1987) Muscles and motor control in low back pain: Assessment and management. In Twomey, LT and Taylor, JR (eds), *Physical Therapy of the Low Back,* Clinics in Physical Therapy. Churchill Livingstone, New York.

Jull, G, Richardson, C (1994) Active stabilisation of the trunk. Seminar notes. United Kingdom Nov/Dec.

Kabat, H (1965) Proprioceptive facilitation in therapeutic exercise. In Licht, S (ed.) *Therapeutic Exercise.* Waverly Press, New Haven.

Kendall, HO, Kendall, FP, Boynton, DA (1952) *Posture and Pain* volume ii, pp. 103–124. Williams & Wilkins, Baltimore.

Kendall, FP, McCreary, EK, Provance, PG (1993) *Muscle Testing and Function,* 4th edn. Williams and Wilkins, Baltimore.

Leggat, EA, Mandel, AR, Shein, GF, Milner, M (1981) Effects of relaxed breathing on circulatory and respiratory parameters in severely asthmatic children. *Physiotherapy Canada* 33 (6): 366–370.

Lowman, C, Young, C (1960) *Postural Fitness. Significance and Variances,* pp. 112–134. Lea & Febiger, Philadelphia.

McClurg Anderson, T (1951) *Human Kinetics and Analysing Body Movements.* Heinemann, London.

McClurg Anderson, T (1971) Human kinetics and good movement. *Physiotherapy* 57: 169–176.

Melchione, WE, Sullivan, MS (1993) Reliability of measurements obtained by use of an instrument designed to indirectly measure iliotibial band length. *JOSPT* 18 (3).

Mitchell, L (1963) A Mitchell method of physiological relaxation. *Physiotherapy* 49: 249–256.

Norris, C (1995) Spinal stabilisation. Muscle Imbalance and the low back. *Physiotherapy* 81 (3): 127–138.

Patel, CH (1973) Yoga and biofeedback in the management of hypertension. *The Lancet,* 1053–1055.

Pecina, M, Bojanic, I (1993) *Overuse Injuries of the Musculoskeletal System.* CRC Press Inc., USA.

Pitt-Brooke, J (1995) The relation of movement patterns to muscle length and strength in health and dysfunction: The case for a wider approach to musculoskeletal disorders. *Clinical Anatomy* 8 (2).

Pitt-Brooke, JCL (1997) Neuromusculoskeletal environmental interactions concept (NMEI): an approach to the causation, prevention and rehabilitation of some musculoskeletal disorders, in Tidswell, M (ed), *Cash's Textbook of Orthopaedics for Physiotherapists.* Mosby, St Louis.

Sahrmann, SA (1992) Posture and muscle imbalance: Faulty lumbar-pelvic alignment and associated musculoskeletal pain syndromes. Orthopaedic Division Review. Canadian Physiotherapy Association, Orthopaedic Division, pp. 13–20.

Sahrmann, SA, Rose, SJ, (1982) Review of length associated changes in muscle. *Physical Therapy* 62 (12).

Salt, V (1995) Mitchell's simple physiological and Jacobson's progressive relaxation techniques: a comparison. Undergraduate thesis. School of Physiotherapy, University of Nottingham.

Salt, VL, Kerr, KM (1997) Mitchell's Simple Physiological Relaxation and Jacobson's Progressive Relaxation Techniques: A comparison. *Physiotherapy* 83 (4).

Sherrington, C (1947) *The Integrative Action of the Nervous System.* Cambridge University Press, New Haven.

Stern, PH, McDowell, F, Miller, JM, et al. (1970) Effects of facilitation exercise techniques in stroke rehabilitation. *Archives of Physical and Medical Rehabilitation* 51: 526–531.

Stone, RA, De Leo, J (1976) Psychotherapeutic control of hypertension. *New England Journal of Medicine* 294: 81–86.

Tabary, JC, Tabary, C, Tardieu, C et al. (1972) Physiological and structural changes in the cat's soleus muscle due to immobilisation at different lengths in plaster casts. *Journal of Physiology* 224: 231–244.

Toppenberg, R, Bullock, M (1986) The interrelationship of spinal curves, pelvic tilt and muscle lengths in the adolescent female. *Australian Physiotherapy* 32 (1).

Toppenberg ,R, Bullock, M (1990) Normal lumbo-pelvic muscle lengths and their relationship in adolescent females. *Australian Physiotherapy* 36 (2).

Tortora, GJ, Agnostakos, NP (1990) *Principles of Anatomy and Physiology,* 6th edn. Harper Collins Publishers, USA.

Vasey, J, Crozier, L (1982a) A move in the right direction. *Nursing Mirror,* 28 April.

Vasey, J, Crozier, L (1982b) Get into condition. *Nursing Mirror,* 5 May.

Vasey, J, Crozier, L (1982c) At ease. *Nursing Mirror,* 12 May.

Voss, DE, Ionta, M, Meyers, B (1985) Proprioceptive neuromuscular facilitation: patterns and techniques, 3rd edn. Harper and Row, New York.

White, SG, Sahrmann, SA (1994) A movement system balance approach to management of musculoskeletal pain. In: Grant, R (ed.), *Physical Therapy of the Cervical and Thoracic Spine.* Churchill Livingstone, London.

Williams, PE, Goldspink, G (1971) Longitudinal growth of striated muscle fibres. *Journal of Cell Science* 9: 751–767.

Wohlfahrt, D, Jull, G, Richardson, C (1993) The relationship between dynamic and static function of abdominal muscles *Australian Physiotherapy* 39 (1).

11

Exercise in Health

KATE KERR

Introduction

. . . it is evident from the structure of the body, that exercise is not less necessary than food for the preservation of health (William Buchan, 1792)

'Exercise is synonymous with physical effort, physical activity and exertion' (Knuttgen, 1976), and may vary both in the extent of total body involve-ment and in the degree of intensity. It appears that Buchan may have viewed the increased use of carriages and sedans to be dictated 'more by fashion than by necessity' and regarded it strange that 'men should be such fools as to be laughed out of the use of their limbs, or to throw away their health, in order to gratify a piece of vanity', identifying himself as one of the early protago-nists of the role of exercise in health.

In recent years more and more studies have been published highlighting the importance of exercise in physical health (Anthony, 1991). A report by the Royal College of Physicians (1991) on the medical aspects of exercise noted that, in spite of evidence from both clinical and epidemiological studies that exercise in early and middle life may be beneficial by delaying the onset or progression of a variety of diseases, regular physical activity has been greatly reduced in everyday life, both among adults and children.

It is well known that the body and individual body systems react and develop in response to the forces and stresses placed upon them; thus exercise may be used as a positive measure to improve health and prevent dysfunction, and also in the development, improvement, restoration or maintenance of normal function.

Chapter Objectives

At the end of this chapter, the student should be able to:

- Review the general health benefits of exercise;
- Consider the potential effects of exercise on disease processes affecting the various systems of the body:
  - cardiovascular disorders,
  - respiratory disorders,
  - the skeletal system,
  - the reproductive system;
- Investigate the links between exercise, health and obesity;
- Consider the role of health-related exercise in the elderly;
- Review the psychological benefits of exercise.

Physical Activity and Health

'Exercise can be of considerable benefit to everyone' (Morris et al., 1987). It contributes to a reduction in mortality and morbidity, and adds to the enjoyment of life. It is of value not only to young healthy individuals, but also to the elderly in prolonging an active and independent life, and to those with chronic diseases and disabilities. Much of the evidence for the benefits of exercise has been known for a long time, but it is only recently that the public, the medical profession and the government have recognized it (Morris et al., 1987).

Health-related exercise can take many forms and, at least until recently, has been most commonly associated with the prevention of coronary heart disease. However, with the accumulative evidence for the therapeutic and preventive benefit in many other conditions, exercise is emerging as a key element in most national health promotion recommendations and strategies. For example, the physical activity category is the first priority area of the Healthy People 2000 initiative (Cooper, 1991), aimed at improving a number of health issues for Americans. Cooper (1991) summarized the aim of the initiative as 'to improve the general health of all Americans through emphasis on prevention of illness and disability', and noted that one of the primary goals is to encourage regular exercise for everyone.

The ability to perform physical activity is intrinsic to most aspects of human life. When normal individuals who have been sedentary for some time participate in vigorous exercise, they immediately become aware of their limited capacity for physical activity, and of the discomfort it produces (Fentem et al., 1988). However, after a few weeks of regular exercise there is a training effect, and the capacity for physical activity improves. After training, an individual of any age can work harder, longer and with less effort than previously, and there is a reduced sense of effort for any given task.

Exercise is of general benefit at all ages because it is necessary for the preservation of optimal function and structure of muscles, bones, joints and the cardiovascular system. This ensures that the range of activities an individual can perform with confidence and ease is maintained, and the constraints of a low physical working capacity or fatigue are avoided. This also contributes to an improvement in well being. Fentem *et al.*, (1988) provide an excellent paper on the case for exercise.

In spite of the overwhelming evidence to support the health benefits of exercise (Fentem *et al.*, 1988), and its high priority in relation to health goals, it seems that little progress has been achieved in reaching national targets to increase participation in regular activity (McGinnis, 1992). Of particular concern are the shortfalls in the areas of physical activity in children, and in women (Anderson *et al.*, 1987; Welsh Heart Programme Directorate, 1987; Allied Dunbar Fitness Survey, 1992; McGinnis, 1992; Roberts *et al.*, 1994).

In recognition of the increasing encouragement for individuals to become involved in various forms of physical activity aimed at developing and maintaining cardiorespiratory and muscular fitness in healthy adults, the American College of Sports Medicine has produced a number of 'position statements' regarding the quantity and quality of exercise (ACSM, 1978, 1990). The statements of 1978 and 1990 were very similar in content, and put forward the following guidelines:

- Frequency of training: 3–5 days per week;
- Intensity of training: 60–90% of maximum heart rate (HR_{max}) or 50–85% of maximum oxygen uptake (VO_{2max});
- Duration of training: 20–60 minutes of continuous aerobic activity. Duration is dependent on the intensity of the activity, so that lower intensity activity should be performed over a longer period of time. Higher intensity activity (85–90% HR_{max}) over a shorter period of time (15–20 minutes) may be more appropriate to the younger more active person, whereas lower intensity (60%) over a longer period of time (60 minutes) might suit the older, less athletic individual.
- Mode of activity: any activity which uses large muscle groups, that can be maintained continuously, and is rhythmical and aerobic in nature. These include running/jogging, walking/hiking, swimming, skating, cycling, cross-country skiing.

The 1990 statement added a recommendation for resistance training, to develop and maintain fat-free weight.

- One set of 8–10 repetitions of eight to ten exercises that condition the major muscle groups, at least two days per week.

The combination of frequency, intensity and duration of chronic exercise has been found to be effective in producing a training effect. The interaction of these factors provide the *overload stimulus*. In general, the lower the stimulus, the lower the training effect, and the greater the stimulus the greater the training effect. Endurance training of fewer than two days per week, at less than 50% of maximum oxygen uptake, and for less than 10 minutes per day, is insufficient for developing and maintaining fitness for healthy adults (ACSM, 1990).

Physical Fitness Versus Physical Activity and Health

A more recent statement extended the *physical fitness model* to a *physical activity and health paradigm* (Pate *et al.*, 1995). This advised that 'every US adult should accumulate 30 minutes or more of moderate intensity physical activity on most, preferably all, days of the week'.

Regular physical activity has been shown to reduce the risk of mortality from all causes by more than 25% (Paffenbarger *et al.*, 1990). Furthermore, a study by Pekkannen *et al.* (1987) indicated that regular physical activity can increase life expectancy by more than 2 years over the population average, and this was supported by Heydon and Fodor (1988) who suggested that a 1- to 2-year increase in life expectancy can be expected for men who are physically active in their lifestyle compared with inactive men.

The National Children and Youth Fitness Survey, carried out in America by Ross and Gilbert (1985) and Ross and Pate (1987), indicated that at least half of today's youth do not participate in physical activity appropriate to long-term health promotion, and that less than half of elementary and secondary schools offer daily physical education classes; of those hours of physical activity offered, less than half were considered as designed to 'shape and nurture lifelong physical activity and fitness patterns' (McGinnis, 1992).There is growing scientific evidence to suggest that activity patterns influence fitness levels (Pate *et al.*, 1990), but the nature of the activity patterns, and the social and environmental factors most likely to encourage these patterns of activity have not yet been identified.

Benefits of Exercise in Relation to Health

The benefits of regular physical activity have been identified with regard to the prophylactic management of a wide variety of pathological conditions. It is increasingly accepted that exercise should form an integral part of many disease management programmes, both as a primary or secondary preventive measure. The benefits accrued from regular physical activity may also provide a means of reducing the impact of chronic disease processes by improving physical work capacity and thereby reducing handicap and helping to avoid or delay the necessity for institutional care (Fentem *et al.*, 1988). The health benefits of exercise include the following:

- Reduction in the likelihood of developing coronary heart disease (Berlin and Colditz, 1990);
- Reduction of systolic and diastolic blood pressure (Nelson *et al.*, 1988);
- Reduction of required insulin in late-onset diabetes (Trovati *et al.*, 1984);
- Weight reduction and control (Miles, 1991);
- Maintenance or increase of bone density, and thus protection against osteoporosis (Marcus *et al.*, 1992);
- Improved exercise tolerance in chronic respiratory problems (Lertzman and Cherniack, 1976).

Having established the key benefits of exercise in health, it may be useful to consider the role of regular physical activity in specific situations.

Exercise and Cardiovascular Disorders

There is an increasing body of evidence to support the potential role of exercise in both the prevention and treatment of cardiovascular disease. Changes in lipid circulation brought about by regular aerobic exercise and an accompanying reduction of arterial pressure appear to inhibit the formation of atheromatous plaques. Population studies have shown that physical inactivity is associated with an increased incidence of coronary heart disease, and that there is an association between physical activity and relatively lower blood pressure.

Coronary Heart Disease

A sedentary lifestyle is a recognized risk factor for major diseases such as coronary heart disease (CHD) (Sopko et al., 1992). Two meta-analyses of data from more than 40 studies have reviewed the evidence which associated high levels of habitual physical effort with low incidence of coronary heart disease. Powell et al. (1987) affirmed that the association is causal, at least in men, and quoted nine well designed studies on male subjects which supported a causal link. Berlin and Colditz (1990) concluded that physically inactive individuals are 1.9 times more likely to develop CHD than active persons, independent of other risk factors (hypertension, hypercholesterolemia and smoking). The mechanism through which exercise might be preventive in coronary heart disease could be by its effects on the main coronary risk factors. Aerobic exercise reduces blood pressure (Duncan et al., 1985), increases high density lipoprotein concentration which in turn reduces hypercholesterolemia (Mankowitz et al., 1992), facilitates smoking cessation (Marcus et al., 1991) and reduces obesity (Bray, 1988). Exercise also has a part to play in secondary prevention. O'Connor et al. (1989) in an overview of exercise rehabilitation programmes following myocardial infarction, found a reduction of about

25% in recurrent infarction and sudden death from heart failure.

Strong evidence for the beneficial effects of exercise on either longevity or coronary artery disease in women is lacking, possibly because fewer women develop the disease before old age. However, of those studies which reported separate data for women, the trend for greater risk of coronary events (CHD, myocardial infarction, angina) with decreased levels of physical activity were similar to male subjects, but in many cases more pronounced (Brunner et al., 1974; Brownell and Stunkard, 1981; Campos et al., 1988; Blair et al., 1989; Burke et al., 1991). This suggests that the relationship between fitness and health may be stronger in women than in men. However, only limited data exist to suggest the efficacy of the clinical treatment of women with exercise rehabilitation following the diagnosis of coronary heart disease (Douglas et al., 1992).

Exercise appears to have a similar protective/preventive effect regarding obesity and CHD in children as in adults. Among children as young as 4–8 years, the fattest were found to be the least active (Berkowitz et al., 1985), and this can lead to further decrease of activity levels and obesity (Dietz and Gortmaker, 1985). Obese children show significantly increased levels of cholesterol, triglycerides and blood pressure, compared to their lighter weight and more physically active peers (Fripp et al., 1985). As in adults, exercise has also been shown to have a beneficial effect on the coronary heart disease risk factors in children and adolescents, especially on blood pressure (Hofmann et al., 1987; Hagberg et al., 1983). So the same message comes across for both children and adults — there is clear evidence of a link between activity levels and CHD risk factors.

Paffenbarger and Hyde (1984) described the type of exercise necessary to reduce the risk of suffering a heart attack as 'vigorous, regular and current'. Vigorous activity in turn was defined by Morris et al. (1987) as activity which requires an energy expenditure of 7.5 kcal per minute, and is maintained for at least three periods of 20 minutes each week. This concurs with the American College of Sports Medicine position statements of 1978 and 1990. In practical terms, it is probably easier to judge the intensity of exercise required by increasing the rate of activity (for example brisk walking, jogging, swimming) until heart rate has increased to 60–90% of age-related maximum heart rate (calculated as 220 minus age in years), and maintaining that rate for 20 minutes. The lower end of the scale (60% of age-related maximal heart rate) may be more appropriate for the older, less fit individual, while the upper end (90%) should be the target for active, athletic individuals.

Hypertension

Hypertension can be controlled to some extent by exercise. Nelson et al. (1988) demonstrated a graded hypotensive response among mild to moderate hypertensives (baseline blood pressures in the region of 149/99 mmHg), with a fall in pressure of 11/9 recorded following a programme of regular exercise, for 45 minutes, three times a week, at an intensity of 70% maximum working capacity. Sincolfi et al. (1984) demonstrated significant decreases in systolic blood pressure in hypertensive subjects on beta-blocking medication following a single exercise protocol involving supine cycling on a cycle ergometer for 30 minutes. These studies suggest that exercise may be used to augment the effect of medication in subjects with mild to moderate hypertension, and consequently reduce the dosage required.

Exercise taken at regular intervals may also have a protective role by inhibiting the age-dependent rise in blood pressure observed in middle-age in western societies, thus reducing the frequency with which arterial hypertension develops. This may in turn have a 'knock-on' protective role in the development of coronary heart disease and stroke.

A study by Roman et al. (1981) demonstrated a significant reduction in resting blood pressure in women with established hypertension following a 3-month dynamic exercise programme, and a return to baseline after 3 months without training; when training was reintroduced, resting

Clinical Application

Physiotherapists are in an excellent position to encourage patients to increase their general activity levels. Too often exercise programmes are directed specifically at a part of the body (back, knee, shoulder) without considering the overall pattern of physical activity in the patient. We should incorporate our specific exercise programmes into a more general 'physical activity' package, in which we provide the patient with a physical activity plan, appropriate to the patient's age, level of fitness, limitations associated with their individual disability and access to amenities. This would send out a much more positive 'health message' to our patients, rather than the rather narrowly focused home exercise programmes aimed at increasing specific joint range, or strengthening specific muscle groups.

blood pressure was again found to be reduced when compared with pre-training levels.

Exercise and Respiratory Disorders

The benefits of exercise training for special populations are becoming increasingly recognized. Included in these special populations are several types of chronic disease patients, including those with respiratory diseases. Although the degree to which these patients can exercise may be limited by their pathology, exercise is usually beneficial for these patients.

Most asthmatics benefit from exercise, and should therefore be encouraged to participate. However, a minority of severe asthmatics are distressed by physical activity, so it is important to identify them to avoid potential danger. Exercise-induced asthma appears to be caused by a cooling and drying of the sensitive airways which triggers an inflammatory response (Royal College of Physicians, 1991).

Asthmatic children can take exercise safely, even vigorous outdoor activity, provided their medication is adequate. Swimming in indoor heated pools is of particular benefit as the warm moist air does not cause airway constriction. Endurance training can help to reduce the symptoms of asthma, and a good physical capacity permits participation in normal everyday physical activities; similarly, with cystic fibrosis, moderate to vigorous aerobic activity has produced improvements in respiratory function and reduced dependence on treatment (Andreasson et al., 1987).

In patients with chronic obstructive airways disease (COPD), exercise training, independent of comprehensive rehabilitation, has demonstrated significant improvements in work tolerance and

reduction in dyspnoea. Carter et al. (1992) reviewed the use of exercise training aimed at reducing dyspnoea and restoring functional capacity in patients with COPD. They found that most patients demonstrated positive responses to exercise conditioning, with reductions in dyspnoea and extended work tolerance, with little or no change in pulmonary function. Possible explanations for the response, with no concomitant improvement in pulmonary function, include psychological encouragement, improvements in mechanical efficiency, improved cardiovascular conditioning, improved muscle function, biochemical adaptations responsible for reducing glucose utilization, desensitization to dyspnoea and contributions from better self-care. The fact that some patients did not respond positively to exercise conditioning suggests that careful selection of patients and / or conditioning programme is required to achieve the best results. Further investigation is required to attempt to define the characteristics of those patients most likely to benefit from conditioning programmes, and also to identify the nature of the programmes most appropriate to different patient groups.

Clinical Application

Patients with respiratory problems are often very anxious about participating in physical activity, as it makes them breathless. However, by avoiding physical activity, the patients become involved in a vicious cycle of events in which their ever-decreasing activity levels result in decreased exercise tolerance. As part of their physiotherapy management, it is important that these patients are encouraged to recognize that although their exer-

cise tolerance is limited by their respiratory status, other factors (such as avoiding physical activity) can compound the problem. To break the cycle of lack of physical activity and decreasing exercise tolerance, these patients need to learn how to cope with their breathlessness, and consequently reduce their anxiety about participating in physical activity. Once they feel they have a degree of control over their breathing, they should embark on a progressive general activity programme aimed at improving cardiovascular and muscular endurance and efficiency. Objective markers (distance walked, number of repetitions, duration of activity before breathlessness causes the patient to stop) can be used to monitor progress and to provide indicators for progression, and to provide motivating feedback for the patient. A pulmonary rehabilitation class might create a nonthreatening, supportive environment to initiate such programmes, from which the patients would be encouraged to continue on their own.

Exercise in the Control of Obesity and Diabetes Mellitis

Exercise promotes the secretion of a number of hormones, particularly those of the gonads and the pituitary. Insulin sensitivity increases, demonstrated by the body's ability to take up and utilize glucose in response to a smaller amount of insulin. Control of general metabolism alters in response to vigorous rhythmic exercise, resulting in an increase in aerobic metabolism (oxygen consumption) above the resting metabolic rate both during and after exercise.

Obesity

Obesity can be broadly defined as an excessive enlargement of the body's fat stores. The total amount of body fat exists in two sites as either essential or storage fat. Essential fat is necessary for normal physiological functions, and is found in differing quantities in all organs and throughout the central nervous system. Storage fat is deposited in adipose tissue, is largely subcutaneous, and can be mobilized as a source of energy; it is the storage fat which can be affected by diet or exercise, with the quantity of essential fat remaining relatively constant.

A simple measure of 'fatness' can be obtained by calculating the body mass index (BMI) or Quetelet's Index which is calculated by dividing the body weight (W) in kilograms by the height squared (H) in metres ($BMI = W/H^2$). The health risks associated with obesity increase as the BMI exceeds 30. Associated with obesity is the increased prevalence of health problems such as coronary heart disease, hypertension, diabetes mellitus, abnormal lipid and lipoprotein concentrations, impaired heat tolerance, osteoarthritis and gout, renal disease and pulmonary diseases (Miles, 1991). The presence of a high waist-to-hip circumference ratio (exceeding 0.90) is highly correlated with the presence of cardiovascular disease (Pacy et al., 1986).

It has been demonstrated that the most effective way to lose weight and maintain a desirable body weight long term is through a combination of mild caloric restriction and increase in caloric expenditure through regular endurance exercise.

Figure 11.1 Weight loss in (a) caloric restriction alone and (b) caloric restriction and exercise. (From Lamb, *Physiology of Exercise: Responses and Adaptations* 2nd edn. Copyright © 1984 by Allyn and Bacon. Adapted by permission.)

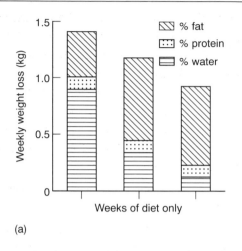

(a)

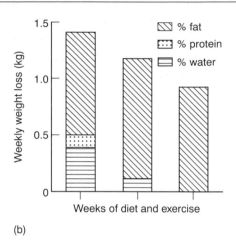

(b)

Incorporating exercise into a weight-reduction programme prevents the undesirable loss of lean body mass which is frequently associated with reduction programmes based solely on caloric restriction (Hagan *et al.*, 1986; Lampman *et al.*, 1986; Dargie and Grant, 1991; Miles, 1991). Weight loss through caloric restriction alone often includes a large loss of water, and some lean tissue, especially early in a dietary programme. This is illustrated in Figure 11.1.

A programme of regular aerobic physical activity, such as walking, jogging, cycling or swimming (Sheldahl, 1986) is particularly appropriate for obese subjects, and will increase energy consumption not only during the period of exercise, but for several hours afterwards (Wilson, 1990).

McGinnis (1992) expressed concern over the profile of physical activity patterns for women, and supported this with evidence from a National Health and Nutrition Examination Survey, which indicated that 27% of American women between the ages of 20 and 74 were classified as being overweight. Most of the studies on the response to exercise have been performed in male subjects,

so that when the small number of studies carried out with female subjects are considered, the overall results are often inconclusive. However, the addition of regular aerobic exercise into a dietary weight-reduction programme in a group of moderately obese women accelerated weight loss, when compared with a control group on dietary restriction alone (Hill *et al.*, 1989). Similarly, compliance with a weight reduction programme was found to be better when aerobic exercise was introduced into the programme in a group of moderately obese children and adolescents, when compared to a control group treated with dietary restrictions alone (Reybrouck *et al.*, 1990).

Diabetes Mellitis

Diabetes mellitis is a disease associated with problems in controlling blood glucose, resulting primarily in *hyperglycemia*. There are two types of diabetes mellitis: type I (insulin dependent or juvenile-onset diabetes), resulting from a deficiency in insulin production in the pancreas; and type II (non-insulin dependent or adult-onset diabetes), usually associated with decreased cellular insulin sensitivity. Type I diabetics are dependent on regular injections of insulin, whereas type II diabetics are often obese, and can control hyperglycemia through dietary restrictions and weight loss, although they may also require oral medication to reduce blood glucose levels.

Insulin increases the rate of glucose transport into muscle, and also increases glycogen synthesis. Exercise also speeds up these processes, and additionally has the effect of improving insulin sensitivity. Consequently, less insulin is required to regulate blood glucose after training than before. The improved insulin sensitivity is probably related to the binding capacity of insulin to receptor sites of the individual muscle cells (McArdle et al., 1986). There is little evidence to suggest that the control of blood glucose levels among type I diabetics is improved with exercise, but it has been suggested that with regular exercise, the dosage of required insulin can be reduced. A beneficial effect in the control of blood sugar by exercise in type II diabetics has been seen (Trovati et al., 1984), and Taylor et al. (1984) showed that type II diabetes is less common among physically active men, although this has not been supported by other studies.

In general, diabetics can participate in the same types of exercise as non-diabetics. Daily exercise is recommended for both types I and II diabetics, for the purposes of regulation of insulin doses and weight management respectively (ACSM, 1991). Although exercise may contribute to the management of diabetes, there are certain risks which must be taken into consideration. In diabetics with a high level of insulin (perhaps following injection) exercise may result in an excessive lowering of blood glucose levels, causing *exercise-induced hypoglycemia*, characterized by feelings

of hunger, nervousness, profuse sweating, alternate pallor and flushing of the face, and faintness. In diabetics with low levels of insulin, exercise may result in *hyperglycemia* (with decreased glucose uptake by the cells) *and ketosis* (production of *ketone bodies* by the incomplete metabolism of fat) which is caused by the mobilization of fat to a greater extent than the body can use in response to insufficient carbohydrate metabolism (McArdle et al., 1986). This can in severe cases cause unconsciousness, and is accompanied by a characteristic 'pear drop' odour on the breath.

The risk of hypoglycemic events occurring may be reduced by taking the following precautions:

1 Monitoring blood glucose frequently when initiating an exercise programme;
2 Decreasing the insulin dose or increase carbohydrate intake prior to the exercise bout;
3 Injecting insulin into an area such as the abdomen that is not active during exercise;
4 Avoiding exercise during periods of peak insulin activity;
5 Eating carbohydrate snacks before and during prolonged exercise bouts;
6 Being knowledgeable about the signs and symptoms of hypoglycemia;
7 Not exercising alone.

Clincial Application

Many elderly patients, while having physiotherapy for other problems, present with both obesity and type II diabetes. With the knowledge that daily exercise can regulate insulin dosage and help in weight management, physiotherapists should encourage these patients to develop a regular exercise habit. As in the case of lack of physical activity and decreased exercise tolerance in respiratory disorders, obesity and sedentary lifestyle can develop into a vicious cycle in which excessive weight makes exercising difficult, and lack of exercise contributes to weight gain. As part of their ongoing patient management, physiotherapists can provide expert guidance on exercise prescription for these patients, again identifying objective markers to monitor progress both in exercise tolerance and weight regulation. Referral to a dietician for advice on dietary intake should also be considered for both obese patients and those with type II diabetes. A possible knock-on effect of exercise-induced improvements in insulin and blood glucose regulation in diabetic patients might be a reduction in the circulatory changes which can ultimately lead to amputation. With younger type I diabetic patients, physiotherapists should feel confident to advise these patients on the possible effects of exercise, on sensible precautions to be taken, and on the importance of living a 'regular' lifestyle. Above all, these patients should not feel the need to restrict either the intensity or duration of their physical activity — merely to keep it on a fairly consistent level.

Effect of Exercise on Bone Density and the Reproductive System

The general area of women's health has attracted increasing interest in recent years, with the establishment of clinics and hospitals dealing with a variety of disorders found primarily in women. Osteoporosis, generally defined as a decrease in bone mineral density, affects both males and females, but occurs earlier and consequently has a greater impact in females. An increasing body of research has investigated the relationship between exercise and bone density, in an attempt to determine whether exercise has a protective or remediative role in osteoporosis. The other major area of interest in women's health is the effect of exercise on reproductive function. Although menstrual disorders have been observed in large numbers and proportions of women participating in athletic pursuits, the prevalence of reproductive disturbances in women of varying gynaecological age and differing degrees of participation is poorly documented.

Osteoporosis

The World Health Authority define osteoporosis as 'a disease characterized by low bone mass and microarchitectural deterioration of bony tissue, leading to enhanced bone fragility and a consequent increase in fracture risk'. The condition usually develops gradually and without symptoms, the pre-fracture state being referred to as osteopenia. Most patients are initially diagnosed with the condition following a fracture. There is a slow loss of bone density in both sexes as they age, but there is an accelerated phase in women during the decade following the menopause (Cooper and Aihie, 1994).

Hip fractures, which are a common manifestation of osteoporosis, are an important cause of morbidity, with patients requiring expensive institutional care (Dargie and Grant, 1991). The risk of fracture is directly related to bone mineral content which falls progressively with time from its peak in early adulthood. The higher the initial bone mineral content, the longer it takes to reach the 'fracture threshold', so there is a strong case for pre-menopausal women to take active measures to minimize osteoporosis. During puberty, considerable increases in bone mineral content occur in the axial and appendicular skeleton. Physical activity can influence bone formation (and breakdown) positively through the physical stresses placed on the skeleton by the appropriate muscles and external forces. Thus it would seem to be appropriate to encourage young females to participate in physical activity to increase bone mineral content to a high level to protect against osteoporosis in later life. Bone density can be maintained by moderate weight-bearing exercises; physical activity and its attendant stresses stimulate bone metabolism (Krolner et al., 1983), and can have the effect of increasing bone mass even after the menopause (Chow et al., 1987). Exercise intervention trials generally support the conclusion that exercise promotes bone mass (Marcus et al., 1992), and cross-sectional studies have shown that a positive correlation exists between activity level and bone mineral density, with athletes having higher bone mineral density than non-athletes (Marcus et al., 1985; Lane et al., 1986; Smith and Gilgan, 1987). With the recognition of the link between physical activity and bone mineral density, it is of considerable concern that major surveys (Allied Dunbar Fitness Survey, 1992; Roberts et al., 1994) have indicated low levels of activity in young women, at the very time when they should be building up their bone mineral content.

The type and extent of exercise recommended to protect against osteoporosis has yet to be established, although it is generally agreed that it should involve anti-gravitational load or weight-bearing activities. Chow et al. (1987) advocated 5 to 10 minutes of stretching and warm-up exercises followed by 30 minutes of walking, jogging and dance routines on a daily basis, whereas Krolner et al. (1983) have suggested that 1 hour walking plus aerobic exercise twice weekly will increase bone mineral density in the spine. It appears that physical activity in the elderly, both men and women, protects against hip fracture (Wickham et al., 1989).

Due to the increased risk of osteoporosis in postmenopausal women, this is an area in which the effects of exercise in female populations has been relatively extensively researched. Marcus et al. (1992) reviewed a number of cross-sectional studies and intervention trials using a variety of weight-bearing physical activities including walking, jogging and dancing, and concluded that physically active women had higher bone mineral density than inactive women, and that exercise intervention increased levels of bone mineral density. The relationship between the nature of the activity and the site of increased bone mineral density has not been clarified.

Reproductive System

Exercise-related menstrual dysfunction is a well recognized syndrome which occurs in women who participate in endurance sports and professional dance. The problem is particularly frequent in elite athletes with low weight (Warren, 1991), and may be manifest by delayed menarche, amenorrhoea or inadequate luteal phases (Schwartz et al., 1981; Shangold and Levine, 1982; Bullen et al., 1985). However, a causal link between exercise and menstrual disorders has not been established (Warren, 1991; Loucks et al., 1992), and physical activity alone without some other predisposing cause is unlikely to be the cause of reproductive dysfunction. Possible predisposing factors include low body weight, changes in nutrition, eating disorders, weight loss and a history of late menarche or previous menstrual irregularity (Bullen et al., 1895).

Pregnancy

Pregnant women present a unique problem with respect to exercise because of the possible competition between exercising maternal muscle and the foetus for blood flow, oxygen delivery, glucose availability and heat dissipation. The American College of Sports Medicine (1991) suggest that it is not advisable for pregnant women to begin a *new* strenuous exercise programme during the first or third trimesters of pregnancy, when the risks to mother and foetus are greatest. During the second trimester, gradual increases of activity are appropriate, but should not be further increased into the third trimester. However, maintaining a physical activity programme of moderate exercise of 15–30 minutes duration, 3–5 times per week will help to maintain physical work capacity; other benefits thought to accrue from exercise during pregnancy are improved aerobic and muscular fitness, facilitation of labour and recovery from labour, enhanced maternal psychological well-being and establishment of permanent healthy lifestyles (ACSM, 1991). The best modes of exercise during pregnancy are walking and non-weight-bearing activities such as stationary cycling or exercise in water. The intensity of activity cannot be based on heart rate, as this alters during pregnancy; it is suggested that the intensity is excessive if the individual cannot carry on a conversation during exercise (the 'talk test!').

Clinical Applications

Physiotherapists work regularly with women of all ages, and we should use our sound understanding of the benefits derived from participating in physical activity, to encourage and advise our female patients on the role of exercise in women's health. With knowledge that the risk of fractures associated with osteoporosis may be decreased if individuals develop a high bone mineral density between puberty and the menopause, we should be encouraging our female patients to participate in physical activity. Although the precise nature of the activity has not been defined, it appears that weight-bearing exercises, of a nature and intensity similar to those suggested to reduce risk of CHD would be appropriate. For female patients who present with overuse injuries associated with endurance sports (running, walking) and professional dance, and are also suffering from menstrual dysfunction, the physiotherapist should suggest that they investigate nutritional factors and menstrual history, as physical activity is unlikely to be the sole cause. Finally, we should also encourage pregnant women to maintain physical activity throughout their pregnancies, with the precaution of avoiding increasing activity during the first and final three months.

The Elderly

Ageing is a term which has been used to describe the biological, physiological and sociological changes which occur in individuals over time (Elia, 1991), and has been associated with a gradual decline in the body's functional capacity and a reduction in the system's resistance stress and disease. Shephard (1987) stated that 'physical activity has more potential for promoting healthy ageing than anything else science or medicine has to offer'.

Physiological Changes Associated With Ageing

The changes which occur with ageing can affect the cardiovascular system, the respiratory system, the nervous system and the musculoskeletal system (Figure 11.2). Furthermore, basal metabolic rate and maximal oxygen uptake gradually decrease with age, as does glucose tolerance which is associated with late onset (non-insulin dependent) diabetes. Relative body fat increases as lean body mass decreases with age. Total cholesterol and low density lipoprotein levels increase, while high density lipoprotein levels remain constant, which change in balance places the elderly individual at increased risk of coronary heart disease.

CARDIAC CHANGES

Ageing can result in a decline in resting stroke volume, maximal heart rate and cardiac output, and because of a reduction in the elasticity of the blood vessels, an increase in blood pressure. Maximum cardiac output in elderly subjects is 20%–30% less than that of a young adult, and the return to pre-exertion levels of heart rate, blood

Figure 11.2 Influence of ageing on functional capacity. From Lamb, *Physiology of Exercise: Responses and Adaptations.* 2nd edn. Copyright © 1984 by Allyn and Bacon. Adapted by permission.)

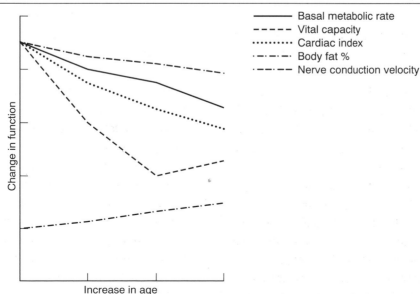

——— Basal metabolic rate
- - - - Vital capacity
·········· Cardiac index
·—·—· Body fat %
·—··—· Nerve conduction velocity

pressure, oxygen consumption and carbon dioxide elimination is slower in elderly subjects.

PULMONARY CHANGES

Lung compliance increases with age, while thoracic mobility decreases. This results in an increase in residual volume (by 30%–50%) and a similar (30%–50%) reduction in vital capacity. In response to exercise, the elderly subject increases the rate of respiration, but the tidal volume remains constant, which creates an increased workload on the respiratory muscles to overcome the added elastic resistance (De Vries and Adams, 1972).

CHANGES IN THE NERVOUS SYSTEM

The response of the nervous system to ageing involves a reduction in conduction velocity by 10%–15%, with a resultant increase in reaction time. This affects both sensory and motor responses, and almost certainly are related to the 35%–40% increase in falls in subjects over the age of 60 years (Shephard, 1987).

MUSCULOSKELETAL CHANGES

Ageing causes decrease in both the size and number of muscle fibres (particularly fast-twitch fibres), which can result in muscle strength decrements of up to 20%–40% (Kach et al., 1990), and this is demonstrated in decreased speed and strength of contraction and early onset of fatigue. Fascia, ligaments and tendons become less extensible with aging, resulting in decreased range of motion at joints, both active and passive. Loss of bone with ageing has already been mentioned.

Benefits of Exercise for the Elderly

Although it is accepted that some reduction of physical capabilities is an inevitable consequence of ageing, it is also suspected that this reduction is greater than is warranted by the loss in capacity (Fentem et al., 1988). Improvements in physical capacity and control of chronic disease resulting from exercise have been found in the elderly, similar to younger people (Seals et al., 1984; Bassey, 1987). While the consequences of ageing cannot be completely reversed, appropriate exercise can increase muscle bulk and strength by 10%–20% in men in their early seventies (Aniansson et al., 1980), and other research has shown that stamina can improve with training even after 65 years (Haber et al., 1984; Seals et al., 1984). Regular stretching exercises either at home (Fentem et al., 1988) or in a class (Frekany and Leslie, 1975) can maintain range of motion in major joints, and the lubrication of joints through such movements can maintain function and limit the effects of degenerative disease.

As in all exercise programmes, those aimed at the elderly population should take into account the health status and needs of the individual. Walking, chair and floor exercises, and modified strength/flexibility exercises are well tolerated by most elderly individuals. Water exercise, swimming or cycling may be more appropriate for those with joint problems affecting the lower limb (ACSM, 1991).

It is vital that older people are encouraged to maintain their physical activities, as reduced activity in itself can lead to further reductions in capacity. Goals for physical activity for the elderly include maintaining functional capacity for independent living, reduction in the risk of cardiovascular disease, deceleration of the progression of chronic degenerative disease processes, promotion of psychological well-being and the opportunity for social interaction (ACSM, 1991). Once again, physiotherapists should see themselves as having a vital role in encouraging regular physical activity in the elderly, and in offering specific advice as to the nature and intensity of that activity. Physiotherapists working with the elderly in both hospital and community settings can do much to dispel the notion that ageing is automatically associated with inactivity. On a wider remit, we might use our specific knowledge of exercise and of the effects of degenerative disease processes to encourage setting up activity sessions suitable for older individuals in community and leisure centres.

Psychological Benefits of Exercise

Most people who participate in regular exercise claim to feel better in more than a purely physical sense. Psychological assessment suggests that those who exercise regularly feel less depression, tension, fatigue, and aggression, and have better sleep patterns. A sense of achievement, improved physical appearance, distraction from worries and the presence of companionship and pleasant surroundings may all contribute to a sense of 'well-being' (Royal College of Physicians, 1991). Recently, interest has increased in the possible benefits of exercise in the psychological parameters of depression, anxiety, stress, self-concept and intellectual functioning (Anthony, 1991).

Regular aerobic training has been found to be of benefit in the treatment of mild depression and anxiety, equal to other therapeutic interventions including psychotherapy (Martensen, 1990). North et al. (1990) concluded from a meta-analysis of studies on exercise and depression that all modes of exercise, both aerobic and anaerobic, were effective in decreasing depression, with the longest programmes having the greatest effect, and exercise being more effective at reducing depression than relaxation or other enjoyable activities. It is thought that a biochemical mechanism may be responsible for the antidepressant effect of exercise; two suggestions are the increased release of endorphines, but there is little evidence to support their increased levels in the brain (Markoff et al., 1982), and increased production and metabolism of central monoamines (Chaoulof, 1989). Similar mechanisms may explain the 'runner's high' experienced by long distance runners, and the feeling of 'withdrawal' in a few athletes when forced to stop exercise. They may also explain why in the USA, running programmes have in the past been regarded as an acceptable alternative to drug abuse (Schuster, 1989).

Although music therapy in itself has become more recognized in recent years as a means of managing certain psychological states, Sinyor and Seraganian (1983) found that aerobic exercise was more successful at reducing the effects of stressful activities than either a course of music appreciation or meditation; the authors suggest that as both exercise and stress have similar effects on heart rate, blood pressure, release of adrenaline and other biochemical responses, improving the body's ability to cope with exercise stress will have a similar effect on its ability to cope with mental stress. Similarly, regular participation in physical activity can moderate the effects of stressful life events on health (Howard et al., 1984). Some research has also suggested that regular aerobic physical activity can decrease the elements of type-A personality characteristics (hostile, aggressive, competitive, rushed, driven) (Blumenthal et al., 1980) which make these personalities twice as likely to suffer a heart attack before the age of 65 as more easy-going personalities (Case et al., 1985).

Exercise has also been shown to help individuals with low self-concept to improve their views of themselves (Eichoff *et al.*, 1983) particularly if supported by counselling (Hilyer and Mitchell, 1979), and several studies have demonstrated that participation in regular exercise can improve intellectual functioning, memory and imagination (Anthony, 1991); this is the case even in psychogeriatric patients, where improved mental function has been demonstrated (Diesfeldt, 1977).

How to Motivate Patients to Exercise

In addition to providing the information, we must also consider how we can motivate our patients to exercise. Anthony (1991) provides eight suggestions.

Establishing a Baseline

The three major areas which physical activity programmes encompass are cardiovascular fitness, muscular strength and flexibility. In an ideal situation a maximum exercise stress test would be administered to determine cardiovascular fitness, and specific strength and flexibility measures taken to establish a baseline from which improvement can be monitored. However, it is probably more realistic, and indeed appropriate, to identify functional objective markers which are meaningful for the patients, and which the patients can measure themselves. These might include distance walked / run / swam, distance walked / run / swam in a specific time, number of repetitions of an activity, pre- and post-exercise heart rate, weight lifted, distance stretched.

The Exercise Prescription

The exercise prescription should be based not only on the patient's physiological and physical baseline measures, but also on the ability to fit the exercise programme into an existing lifestyle without unacceptable disruption. Thus the patient should understand that the exercise prescription establishes a range of exercise in terms of mode, intensity, frequency and duration, and that benefits can still be derived from the lower end of the range. A lower level prescription might fit better into the patient's lifestyle, and the patient will not feel that unreasonable demands are being made. Once the exercise programme has been established, and patient compliance is assured, it may be possible to increase the prescription at a later stage.

Goal Setting

Realistic goal setting can also create motivation for compliance with exercise programmes. If the goals are unrealistically high, the patients will lose heart and give up! If they are too low, they become meaningless and do not stimulate the patients to fulfil their potential. Thus, attainable and challenging short-term goals should be set in consultation with the patients, so that they understand what is realistic and what is not.

Educating the Patient

With increased knowledge comes a greater chance of compliance. The physiotherapist should educate the patient in terms of the rationale behind the mode, intensity, frequency and duration of the exercise programme. This should be done in language appropriate to the level of understanding of the patient.

Individualizing the Prescription

Helping the patient to find forms of exercise which suit his or her lifestyle and temperament, and which are accessible, can often lead to greater motivation and compliance.

Supervision, Positive Reinforcement and Feedback

Supervision, reinforcement and feedback are particularly important in the early stages of implementation of an exercise programme, before the patient develops the 'exercise habit' and it becomes self-enforcing. Often it is not until 2–3 weeks into an exercise programme that the patient begins to feel benefits, so it is important to encourage continuance of the programme at this stage. Once the programme is established, and the patient feels the benefits, the ability to use objective markers to monitor their own progress becomes a powerful feedback tool.

Convenience, Fun and Variety

Physiotherapists can be helpful in encouraging their patients to make exercise as convenient, fun, novel and 'painless' as possible. Encouraging the participation of family and friends can make exercise more fun, and the recognition of how much daily activities (such as walking, gardening and climbing stairs) can contribute to an exercise programme means that exercise can be incorporated into a patient's daily lifestyle with minimum inconvenience.

Role Modeling

If physiotherapists are to encourage exercise and the benefits of an active lifestyle, they should themselves be prepared to provide a positive role model by participating in such a lifestyle themselves. To remain a 'couch potato' while encouraging others to exercise is to send contradictory messages to the patients, which can demotivate them.

Weighing Up the Benefits and Risks

This chapter has summarized some of the health benefits of exercise. There is substantial evidence to support the view that regular exercise of an aerobic nature (such as walking, jogging, cycling, swimming, dancing) is beneficial to general physical and psychological health. Regular aerobic exercise has been found to be effective particularly in the prevention of coronary heart disease, and is increasingly seen as a means of maintaining bone density, and thus preventing osteoporosis. Exercise is also accepted as having a contribution to the management of diabetes and obesity, and as an important means of maintaining or improving physical working capacity in a wide range of chronic disease processes, thus improving quality of life.

However, those involved in the promotion of exercise should be aware of the potential risks. Exercise obviously places increased demands on the heart; in normal healthy individuals, regular exercise of appropriate intensity will provide a training effect which the cardiorespiratory system will accept without undue stress. For those with existing cardiac disease, and for those who decide to embark upon a course of vigorous exercise after a prolonged sedentary period, an inappropriate exercise programme can lead to cardiovascular symptoms. Other risks associated with exercise include:

1 Exercise-induced asthma;
2 Sudden death (usually associated with exercising in the presence of a viral myocarditis);

3 Menstrual dysfunction and haemoglobinuria (blood in the urine) — (associated with strenuous endurance training);

4 Musculoskeletal injuries associated with repetitive loading (stress fractures, tendinitis).

Generally speaking, a sensible approach to the frequency, duration and intensity of exercise will avoid these risks. People who have been sedentary, who have a history of cardiovascular problems, or who have other disorders which may be affected by exercise, should seek advice before embarking on an exercise programme. Usually, starting at a low level of activity, and gradually building up to the required level is the best approach, with a gentle warm-up and warm-down procedure integrated into the programme. Patients should be advised on possible symptoms, such as chest pain, awareness of cardiac irregularity, faintness or excessive dyspnoea, and told to report them immediately.

The benefits of exercise must ultimately be set against the potential hazards. Patients with cardiorespiratory pathology can usually be introduced to cardiac and pulmonary rehabilitation programmes in a safe environment, and encouraged to maintain their activity following the programme. For those with other specific risks, individually tailored programmes can be devised to minimize the potential hazards of exercise and maximize the benefits. For the vast majority of the population, sensible exercise offers many more benefits than risks. The Royal College of Physicians concluded their report on the 'Medical aspects of exercise' (1991) with the following recommendations:

1 There is now good evidence of the many physical and psychological benefits available to the population from regular exercise, which should be recognized by all those in health care.

2 The habit of taking regular exercise is best started in childhood and should be continued into middle age and where possible old age, because exercise helps to make the most of diminishing capacity.

3 Doctors should ask about exercise when they see patients, particularly when they come for routine health checks, and should be aware of and advise on suitable exercise programmes (this should apply to physiotherapists too).

4 The value of exercise for patients with a wide range of disorders should be considered and advice given on the type and extent of activity to be undertaken.

5 Doctors (and physiotherapists) should be aware of the relevant risks that exercise might pose for individual patients. In particular, they should warn against unaccustomed, severe or inappropriate activity. When exercise is of a suitable intensity for the individual, is taken regularly and with sensible precautions, the benefits far outweigh the risks.

Summary

- Physical activity has been shown to impart benefits in a number of disease processes including cardiovascular disorders, respiratory disorders, and disorders of the musculoskeletal and reproductive systems, and to have a positive effect on diabetes and obesity.

- Exercise is of general benefit at all ages because it is necessary for the preservation of optimal function and structure of muscles, bones, joints and the cardiovascular system. It is thought that physical activity has more potential for promoting healthy ageing than anything science or medicine has to offer!

- Although there is substantial evidence to support the health benefits of exercise, there are considerable shortfalls in the amount of physical activity taken by women and children.

- The combination of frequency, intensity and duration of chronic exercise has been found to be effective in producing a training effect. For a training effect, frequency of training should be 3–5 times per week, intensity should be 60–90% maximum heart rate or 50–85% VO_{2max} and duration should be 20–60 minutes of continuous aerobic activity.

- An alternative exercise prescription, related to the *physical activity and health paradigm*, suggests an accumulation of at least 30 minutes of moderate physical activity every day.

- In addition to physical and physiological benefits, it has been shown that those who exercise regularly feel less depression, tension, fatigue, and aggression, and have better sleep patterns.

- Physiotherapists can motivate their patients to exercise by establishing objective markers to monitor progress, devising an appropriate and individualized exercise programme which maintains interest and fits easily into the existing lifestyle, educating the patient, setting realistic goals, providing reinforcement and feedback, and finally by acting as a role model.

- The benefits of exercise must ultimately be set against the potential hazards, but individually tailored programmes can minimize the risks and maximize the benefits.

- Physiotherapists are in daily contact with patients presenting with a wide range of physical problems. In addition to managing these specific problems, the physiotherapist is in a unique position to consider the general physical capacity of the patient, and to advise and promote health-related exercise programmes to improve physical and psychological well-being. Too often it appears that we are concerned only with the specific problems which have necessitated physiotherapy intervention, and ignore the total health picture. Perhaps we do not see ourselves as having a role in promoting health-related activity. But who is in a better position, and indeed better qualified to do this than physiotherapists, with their extensive knowledge of exercise and of the physical and physiological effects of pathological processes? There is no reason why, as part of our physiotherapy intervention, we should not promote health-related activity by devising exercise / activity programmes for the young and old, fit and unfit, able-bodied and disabled.

References

Allied Dunbar / Health Education Authority / Sports Council (1992) Allied Dunbar National Fitness Survey: a report on activity patterns and fitness levels. Main findings and summary document. Sports Council / Health Education Authority, London.

American College of Sports Medicine (1978) The recommended quantity and quality of exercise for developing and maintaining fitness in healthy adults. *ACSM Position Stands and Position Statements (1975–1985)*. ACSM, Indianapolis.

American College of Sports Medicine (1990) The recommended quantity and quality of exercise for developing and maintaining cardio-respiratory and muscle fitness in healthy adults. *Medicine and Science in Sport and Exercise* 22(2): 265–274.

American College of Sports Medicine (1991) Exercise prescription for special populations, in *Exercise Testing and Prescription*. Lea & Febiger, Philadelphia.

Anderson, LB, Henckel, P, Saltin, B (1987) Maximal oxygen uptake in Danish adolescents 16–19 years of age. *European Journal of Applied Physiology* 56: 74–82.

Andreasson, B, Jonson, B, Kornfalt, R, Nordmark, E, Sanstrom, S (1987) Long-term effects of physical exercise on working capacity and pulmonary function in cystic fibrosis. *Acta Paediatrica Scandinavica* 76: 70–75.

Aniansson, A, Grimby, B, Rundgren, A (1980) Isometric and isotonic quadriceps strength in 70 year-old men and women. *Scandinavian Journal of Clinical and Laboratory Investigation* 24: 315–322.

Anthony, J (1991) Psychologic aspects of exercise. *Clinics in Sports Medicine* 10(1): 171–180.

Bassey, EJ (1987) Benefits of exercise in the elderly, in Isaacs, B (ed) *Recent Advances in Geriatric Medicine*. Churchill Livingstone, London.

Berkowitz, RI, Agras, WS, Korner, AF, Kraemer, HC, Zeanah, CH (1985) Physical activity and adiposity: a longitudinal study from birth to childhood. *Journal of Paediatrics* **106**: 734–738.

Berlin, JA, Colditz, GA (1990) A meta-analysis of physical activity in the prevention of coronary heart disease. *American Journal of Epidemiology* **132**: 612–628.

Blair, SN, Goodyear, NN, Gibbons, LW, Cooper, KH (1984) Physical fitness and incidence of hypertension in healthy normotensive men and women. *Journal American Medical Association* **252**: 487–490.

Blair, SN, Kohl, HW, Paffenbarger, RS, Clark, DG, Cooper, KH, Gibbons LW (1989) Physical fitness and all-cause mortality: prospective study of healthy men and women. *JAMA* **262**: 2395–2401.

Blumenthal, JA, Williams, RB, Williams, RS (1980) Effects of exercise on type-A (coronary prone) bahaviour pattern. *Psychosomatic Medicine* **42**: 289–296.

Bray, GA (1988) Exercise and obesity, in Bouchard, C, Shephard, RA, Stephens, T, Sutton, JR, McPherson, BD (eds) *Exercise, Fitness and Health*. Human Kinetic Books, Champaign, Il.

Brownell, KD, Stunkard, AJ (1981) Differential changes in plasma high-density lipoprotein-cholesterol levels in obese men and women during weight reduction. *Archives of Intern Medicine* **141**: 1142–1146.

Brunner, D, Manelis, G, Modam, M, Levin, S (1974) Physical activity at work and the incidence of myocardial infarction, angina pectoris and death due to ischaemic heart disease. An epidemiological study in Israeli collective settlements (kibbutzim) *Journal of Chronic Disease* **27**: 217–233.

Bullen, BA, Skrinar, GS, Beitins, IZ, von Mering, G, Turnbull, BA, McArthur, JW (1985) Induction of menstrual disorders by strenuous exercise in untrained women. *New England Journal of Medicine* **312**: 1349–1353.

Burke, AP, Farb, A, Virman, R, Goodin, J, Smialek, JE (1991) Sports-related and nonsports-related sudden cardiac death in young adults. *American Heart Journal* **121**: 568–575.

Campos, H, McNamara, JR, Wilson, PWF, Ordovas, JM, Schaefer, EJ (1988) Differences in low density lipoprotein subfractions and apolipo-proteins in premenopausal and postmenopausal women. *Journal of Clinical Endocrinology and Metabolism* **67**: 30–35.

Carter, R, Coast, JR, Idell, S (1992) Exercise training in patients with chronic obstructive pulmonary disease. *Medicine and Science in Sport and Exercise* **24**(3): 281–291.

Case, RB, Heller, SS, Case, NB (1985) Type A behaviour and survival after acute myocardial infarction. *New England Journal of Medicine* **312**: 737–741.

Chaoulof, A (1989) | Physical exercise and brain monoamines: a review. *Acta Physiologica Scandinavica* **137**: 1–13.

Chow, R, Harrison, JE, Notarius, C (1987) Effect of two randomised exercise programmes on bone mass of healthy menopausal women. *British Medical Journal* **295**: 1441–1444.

Clapp, JF, Rokey, R, Treadway, JL, Carpenter, MW, Artal, RM, Warrnes, C (1992) Exercise in pregnancy. *Medicine and Science in Sport and Exercise* **24**(6): S294–S300.

Cooper, DL (1991) Year 2000 fitness objectives for the Nation. *Clinics in Sports Medicine* **10**(1): 223–226.

Cooper, C, Aihie, A (1 994) Osteoporosis: recent advances in patho-genesis and treatment. *Quarterly Journal of Medicine* **87**: 203–209.

Dargie, HJ, Grant, S (1991) Exercise. *British Medical Journal* **303**: 910–912.

De Vries, HA, Adams, GM (1972) Comparison of exercise responses in old and young men. *Journal of Gerontology* **27**: 344.

Diesfeldt, HFA (1977) Improving cognitive performance in psychogeri-atric patients: the influence of physical exercise. *Age Ageing* **6**: 58–64.

Dietz, WH, Gortmaker, SL (1985) Do we fatten our children at the television set? Obesity and television viewing in children and adolescents. *Paediatrics* **75**: 807–811.

Douglas, PS, Clarkson, TB, Flowers, NC, Hajjar, KA, Horton, E, Klocke, FJ, LaRosa, J, Shively, C (1992) Exercise and atherosclerotic heart disease in women. *Medicine and Science in Sport and Exercise* **24**(6): S266–S276.

Duncan, JJ, Farr, JE, Upton, SJ, Hagan, RD, Oglesby, ME, Blair, SN (1985) The effects of aerobic exercise on plasma catecholamines and blood pressure in patients with mild essential hypertension. *Journal of the American Medical Association* **254**: 2609–2613.

Eichoff, J, Thorland, W, Ansorge, C (1983) Selected physiological and psychological effects of aerobic dancing among adult young women. *Sports Medicine Physical Fitness* **23**: 278.

Elia, EA (1991) Exercise and the elderly. *Clinics in Sports Medicine* **10**(1): 141–155.

Fentem, PH, Bassey, JE, Turnbull, NB (1988) The new case for exercise. *Sports Council/Health Education Authority.*

Frekany, GA, Leslie, DK (1975) Effects of an exercise programme on selected flexibility measurements of senior citizens. *Gerontologist* April: 182–183.

Fripp, RR, Hodgson, JL, Kwiterovitch, PO, Werner, JC, Schuler, HG, Whitman, V (1985) Aerobic capacity, obesity, and atherosclerotic risk factors in male adolescents. *Paediatrics* **75**: 813–818.

Haber, P, Honiger, B, Klicpera, M, Niederberger, M (1984) Effects in elderly people 67–76 years of age of three-month endurance training on a bicycle ergometer. *European Heart Journal* **5**(suppl. E): 37–39.

Hagan, RD, Upton, SJ, Wong, L, Whittam, J (1986) The effects of aerobic conditioning and/or caloric restriction in overweight men and women. *Medicine and Science in Sport and Exercise* **18**(1): 87–94.

Hagberg, JM, Goldring, D, Ehsani, AA, Heath, GW, Hernandez, A, Schechtman, K, Holloszy, JO (1983) Effect of exercise training on the blood pressure and haemodynamic features of hypertensive adolescents. *American Journal of Cardiology* **52**: 763–768.

Heydon, S, Fodor, GJ (1988) Does regular exercise prolong life expec-tancy? *Sports Medicine* **6**: 63–71.

Hill, JO, Schlundt, DG, Sbrocco, T, Shaorp, T, Pope Cordle, J (1989) Evaluation of an alternating calorie diet with and without exercise in the treatment of obesity. *American Journal of Clinical Nutrition* **50**: 248–254.

Hilyer, JC, Mitchell, W (1979) Effect of systematic physical training combined with counselling on the self concept of college students. *Counselling and Psychology* **26**: 427–436.

Hofmann, A, Walter, HJ, Connely, PA, Vaughan, RD (1987) Blood pressure and physical fitness in children. *Hypertension* **9**: 188–189.

Howard, JH, Cunningham, DA, Rechnitzer, PA (1984) Physical activity as a moderator of life events and somatic complaints. *Canadian Journal of Applied Sports Science* 9: 194–200.

Kach, FW, Boyer, JL, VanCamp, SP (1990) The effect of physical activity and inactivity in aerobic power in older men. *Physician and Sports Medicine* 18: 73.

Knuttgen, HG (1976) *Neuromuscular Mechanisms for Therapeutic and Conditioning Exercise*, 2nd edn. University Park Press, Baltimore.

Krolner, B, Toft, B, Nielson, SP, Tondevold, E (1983) Physical exercise as prophylaxis against involutional vertebral bone loss: a controlled trial. *Clinical Science* 64: 541–546.

Lampman, RM, Schteingart, DE, Foss, ML (1986) Exercise as a partial therapy for obesity. *Medicine and Science in Sport and Exercise* 18(1): 19–24

Lane, NE, Bloch, DA, Jones, HH, Marshall, WH, Jr, Wood, PD, Fries, JF (1986) Long distance running, bone density and osteoarthritis. *Journal American Medical Association* 255: 1147–1151.

Lertzman, MM, Cherniack, RM (1976) Rehabilitation of patients with chronic obstructive pulmonary disease. *American Review of Respiratory Disease* 114: 1145–1165.

Loucks, AB, Vaitukaitis, J, Cameron, JL, Rogol, AD, Skrinar, G, Warrem, MP, Kendrick, J, Limacher, MC (1992) The reproductive system and exercise in women. *Medicine and Science in Sport and Exercise* 24(6): S288–S293.

McArdle, WD, Katch, FI, Katch, VL (1986) *Exercise Physiology: Energy, Nutrition and Human Performance*, 2nd edn. Lea & Febiger, Philadelphia.

McGinnis, MJ (1992) The public health burden of a sedentary lifestyle. *Medicine and Science in Sport and Exercise* 24(6): S196–S200.

Mankowitz, K, Seip, R, Semenkovitch, CF, Daugherty, A, Schonfeld, G (1992) Short-term interruption of training affects both fasting and post-prandial lipoproteins. *Atherosclerosis* 75: 181–189.

Marcus, BH, Albrecht, AE, Niaura, RS, Abrams, DB, Thompson, PD (1991) Usefulness of physical exercise for maintaining smoking cessation in women. *American Journal of Cardiology* 68: 406–407.

Marcus, R, Drinkwater, B, Dalsky, G, Dufek, J, Raab, D, Slemenda, C, Snow-Harter, C (1992) Osteoporosis and exercise in women. *Medicine and Science in Sport and Exercise* 24(6): S301–S307.

Markoff, RA, Ryan, P, Young, T (1982) Endorphins and mood changes in long-distance runners. *Medicine and Science in Sport and Exercise* 14: 11–15.

Martensen, EW (1990) Physical fitness, anxiety and depression. *British Journal of Hospital Medicine* 43: 194–199.

Miles, DS (1991) Weight control and exercise. *Clinics in Sports Medicine* 10(1): 157–169.

Morris, JN, Everitt, MG, Semmence, AM (1987) Exercise and coronary heart disease. In Macleod D, Maughm R, Nommo M, Reilly T, Williams C (eds), *Exercise Benefits, Limits and Adaptations*. E and FN Spon.

Nelson, L, Esler, MD, Jennings, GL, Korner, P (1988) Effects of changing levels of physical activity on blood pressure and haemodynamic in essential hypertension. *Lancet* II: 473–489.

North, TC, McCullagh, P, Tran, ZY (1990) Effect of exercise on depression. In Pandolf, KB, Holloszt, JO (eds), *Exercise and Sports Science Review* 18: 379–415.

O'Connor, GT, Buring, JE, Yusuf, S, Goldhaber, SZ, Olmstead, EM, Paffenbarger, RS Jr (1989) An overview of randomised trials of rehabilitation with exercise after myocardial infarction. *Circulation* 80: 234–244.

Pacy, PJ, Webster, J, Garrow, JS (1986) Exercise and obesity. *Sports Medicine* 3: 89.

Paffenbarger, RS, Hyde, RT (1984) Exercise in the prevention of coronary heart disease. *Preventive Medicine* 13: 3–22.

Paffenbarger, RS, Hyde, RT, Wing, AL (1990) Physical activity and physical fitness as determinants of health and longevity. In Bouchard, C, Shephard, RJ, Stephens, T, Sutton, JR, McPherson, BD (eds), *Exercise, Fitness and Health*. Human Kinetic Books, Champaign, Illinois.

Pate, RR, Dowda, M, Ross, JG (1990) Association between physical activity and physical fitness in American children. *American Journal of Diseases in Childhood* 144: 1123–1129.

Pate, RR, Pratt, M, Blair, SH (1995) Physical activity and publoc helath: a recommendation from the Centres for Disease Control and the American College of Sports Medicine. *Journal of the American Medical Association* 273: 402–407.

Pekkannen, J, Marti, B, Nissinen, A, Tuomilehto, J, Punsar, S, Karvonen, MJ (1987) Reduction of premature mortality by high physical activity: a 20 year follow-up of middle-aged Finnish men. *Lancet* I: 1473–1477.

Powell, KE, Thompson, PD, Casperson, CJ, Kendrick, JS (1987) Physical activity and the incidence of coronary heart disease. *Annual Review of Public Health* 8: 253–287.

Reybrouck, T, Vinckx, J, Van den Berghe, G, Vanderschueren-Lodeweyckx, M (1990) Exercise therapy and hypocaloric diet in the treatment of obese children and adolescents. *Acta Paediatricie Scandinavica* 79(1): 84–89.

Roberts, H, Dengler, R, Zamorski, A (1994) Trent Lifestyle Fitness Survey: technical report to Trent Regional Health Authority.

Roman, O, Camuzzi, AL, Villalon, E (1981) Physical training program in arterial hypertension: a long-term prospective follow-up. *Cardiology* 67: 230–243.

Ross, JG, Gilbert, GG (1985) The National children and youth study: a summary of findings. *JOPERD* 56: 44–51.

Ross, JG, Pate, RR (1987) The National children and youth study II: a summary of findings. *JOPERD* 58: 51–56.

Royal College of Physicians (1991) *Medical Aspects of Exercise: Benefits and Risks*. The Royal College of Physicians, London.

Seals, DR, Hagberg, JM, Allen, WK, Hurley, BF, Dalsky, GP, Ehsani, AA, Holloszy, JO (1984) Glucose tolerance in young and older athletes and sedentary men. *Journal of Applied Physiology* 56: 1521–1525.

Schuster, J (1989) Running injuries. Presentation at the Northern Ireland Institute Conference, Coleraine.

Schwartz, B, Cumming, DC, Riordan, E (1981) Exercise associated amenorrhoea: a distinct entity? *American Journal of Obstetrics and Gynaecology* 141: 662.

Shangold, MM, Levine, HS (1982) The effect of marathon training upon menstrual function. *American Journal of Obstetrics and Gynaecology* 143: 862.

Sheldahl, LM (1986) Special ergometric techniques and weight reduction. *Medicine and Science in Sport and Exercise* 18(1): 25–30.

Shephard, RJ (1987) *Physical Activity and Ageing* 2nd edn. Aspen, Rockville, MD.

Sincolfi, SF, Carleton, RA, Elder, JP, Bouchard, PA (1984) Hypotension after exercise and relaxation. In Cantu, RC (ed.) *Clinical Sports Medicine.* The Colamore Press.

Sinyor, D, Seraganian, P (1983) Aerobic fitness level and reactivity to psychosocial stress: psychological, biochemical and subjective measures. *Psychosomatic Medicine* **45**: 205–216.

Smith, EL, Gilgan, C (1987) Effects of inactivity and exercise on bone. *Physician and Sports Medicine* **15**: 91–102.

Sopko, G, Obarzanek, E, Stone, E (1992) Overview of the National Heart, Lung, and Blood Institute workshop on physical activity and cardiovascular health. *Medicine and Science in Sport and Exercise* **24**(6): S192–S195.

Taylor, R, Ram, P, Zimmet, P, Raper, LR, Ringrose, H (1984) Physical activity and the prevalance of diabetes in Melanesian and Indian men in Fiji. *Diabetologica* **27**: 578–582.

Trovati, M, Carta, Q, Cavalot, F, Vitali, S, Banaudi, C, Lucchina, PG, Fiocchi, F, Emannuelli, G, Lenti, G (1984) Influence of physical training on blood glucose control, glucose tolerance, insulin secretion and insulin action in non-insulin dependent diabetic patients. *Diabetes Care* **7**: 416–420.

Welsh Heart Programme Directorate (1987) Exercise for health: health related fitness in Wales. *Heartbeat report no 23.*

Warren, MP (1991) Exercise in women. *Clinics in Sports Medicine* **10**(1): 131–139.

Wickham, CAC, Walsh, K, Cooper, C, Barker, DJP, Margetts, BM, Morris, J, Bruce, SA (1989) Dietary calcium, physical activity and the risk of hip fracture. *British Medical Journal* **299**: 889–892.

Wilson, MA (1990) Treatment of obesity. *American Journal of the Medical Sciences* **299**(1): 62–68.

12

Exercise in Rehabilitation

KATE KERR

Introduction

We are constantly reminded by the media of the desirability of being 'fit' in the sense of physical fitness. The term 'fit' or 'fitness' is used in many contexts: in relation to health (as discussed in the previous chapter), in conjunction with the general activity levels of the population, and, perhaps most prominently, as a prerequisite to success in sport. De Vries (1980) recognized the problems associated with attempting to provide a definition of physical fitness, and suggested that concepts of *motor fitness* and *physical working capacity* (PWC) should be incorporated into any working definition of physical fitness.

Elements of motor fitness

- Strength
- Speed

- Agility
- Endurance
- Power
- Coordination
- Balance
- Flexibility
- Body control

Elements of physical working capacity (PWC)

- Cardiovascular function
- Respiratory function
- Muscular efficiency
- Strength
- Muscular endurance

The elements of motor fitness have traditionally formed the basis of 'physical education' and training. The elements associated with physical working capacity suggest a more extensive view of physical fitness, and have been widely accepted by members of the medical profession (particularly cardiologists) and physiologists. Perhaps it is appropriate that physiotherapists, as members of a profession with knowledge of exercise and of pathological processes associated with injury and disease, should develop a unified concept of physical fitness in the context of the rehabilitation of patients following injury and disease.

Chapter Objectives

After reading this chapter, the student should be able to:

- Identify the elements of physical fitness in the context of rehabilitation;
- Define the concept of rehabilitation;
- Identify the effects of immobilization;
- Identify the role of exercise in rehabilitation;

- Consider the factors influencing muscle performance;
- Investigate various approaches to the restoration/improvement of muscle performance:
  - specific programmes,
  - rationale,
  - effects,
  - evidence;
- Consider cardiovascular fitness;
- Identify other factors to be considered in exercise programmes:
  - fatigue,
  - closed versus open kinetic chain exercises,
  - isokinetic exercise,
  - eccentric exercise,
  - manual v. mechanical techniques,
  - combined programmes.

The *Concise Oxford English Dictionary* defines 'fit' as: well adapted or suited (for some purpose or status); qualified, competent, worthy (to do . . .); in good athletic condition or health.

After reading these two chapters on exercise in health and rehabilitation, can you create a definition of fitness as it might pertain to **health** and to **rehabilitation**? Do you think it is possible to provide a definition to encompass all aspects of fitness, or are specific definitions necessary?

Therapeutic Exercise in the Rehabilitation of Muscle Performance

The ultimate goal of any therapeutic exercise programme is to regain symptom-free movement and function (Kisner and Colby, 1996), and may take the form of a dynamic programme of prescribed exercise for preventing, limiting or reversing the deleterious effects of inactivity, injury or disease processes, while returning individuals to a level of activity as close as possible to their former pre-injury/pre-pathology level. The scope of therapeutic exercise in its widest sense is vast, and may encompass the rehabilitation of patients with neurological dysfunction, patients with respiratory dysfunction, and patients with neuromuscular and musculoskeletal disorders. This chapter will concentrate primarily on the rehabilitation of muscle performance, although the concept of cardiovascular fitness will also be addressed; neural pathodynamics and neuromus-

cular therapeutic techniques are addressed elsewhere in this book (Chapters 5 and 10).

The importance of exercise and movement in rehabilitation programmes following injury or disease is emphasized when we consider the effects of immobilization on soft tissues. Harrelson (1991) provided a comprehensive summary of these effects (see Figures 12.1–12.3 and Tables 12.1–12.3).

Hertling and Kessler (1996) recognized five types of therapeutic exercise which are necessary to prevent the effects of immobilization, to restore or to maintain a healthy musculoskeletal system,

Figure 12.1 Transverse section of frog sartorius muscle, showing thick myosin filaments, surrounded by thin actin filaments, and dark glycogen particles. (Adapted from Leeson, TS, Leeson, CR, Papero, AA (1988) *Text/Atlas of Histology*, p. 243. WB Saunders, Philadelphia.)

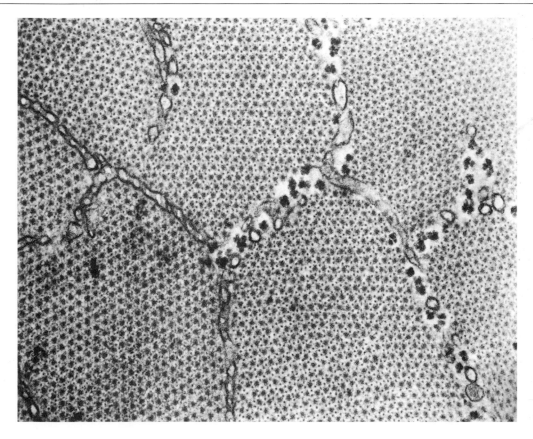

Figure 12.2   Dense regular connective tissue. The fibres tend to follow a wavy course, with fibroblasts arranged in rows between the collaganous fibres. (Adapted from Leeson, TS, Leeson, CR, Papero, AA (1988) *Text/Atlas of Histology*, p. 155. WB Saunders, Philadelphia.)

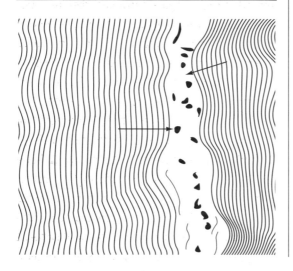

namely strength training, flexibility training, endurance training, neuromuscular control training, and aerobic training. These aspects of exercise link closely with the elements of *motor fitness* and *physical working capacity* as proposed by De Vries (1980); a reasonable conclusion might be that any comprehensive rehabilitation programme should consider the components of *strength*, *muscle endurance*, *power*, *flexibility*, attributes of neuromuscular control, which might include *proprioception* and *skill*, and *cardiovascular endurance*. These elements will form the basis of this chapter, with the inclusion of some additional related elements.

Figure 12.3   Hyaline (left), elastic (centre) and fibrocartilage (right), showing intercellular elastic and collagenous fibres. (Adapted from Leeson, TS, Leeson, CR, Papero, AA (1988) *Text/Atlas of Histology*, p. 161. WB Saunders, Philadelphia.)

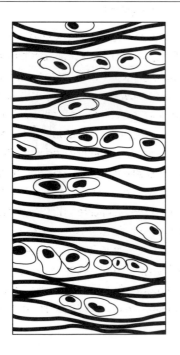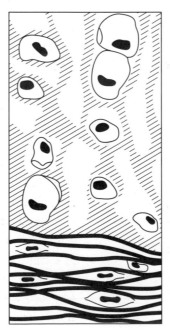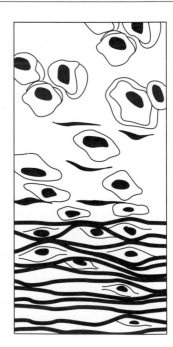

Table 12.1
The effects of immobilization on muscle histopathology

Effects of immobilization on muscle

Decrease in muscle fibre size
Decrease in size and number of mitochondria
Decrease in total muscle weight
Increase in muscle contraction time
Decrease in muscle tension produced
Decrease in levels of glycogen and ATP
More rapid decrease in level of ATP during exercise
Greater increase in lactate concentration during exercise
Decrease in protein synthesis

Table 12.2
The effects of immobilization on cartilage histopathology

Effects of immobilization on articular cartilage

Decrease in proteoglycan synthesis
Softening of articular cartilage
Decrease in articular cartilage thickness
Adherence of fibrofatty connective tissue to cartilage surfaces
Pressure necrosis at points of cartilage–cartilage contact
Chondrocyte death

Table 12.3
Effects of immobilization on ligament histopathology

Effects of immobilization on ligament

Significant decrease in linear stress, maximum stress and stiffness
Decrease in ligament fibril cross-sectional area, resulting in a decrease in fibril size and density
Decrease in synthesis and degradation of collagen
Haphazard arrangement of new collagen fibres
Reduction in load and energy-absorbing capabilities of the bone-ligament complex
Decrease in glycoaminoglycan level reducing water content and extensibility
Increase in osteoclastic activity at the bone–ligament junction, causing an increase in bone resorption in that area

Strength

The American College of Sports Medicine (1990) expanded their original recommendations, published in 1978, for exercise in healthy adults to include exercise prescription for muscular strength and endurance. They described physical fitness as being 'composed of a variety of characteristics included in the broad categories of cardiorespiratory fitness, body composition, muscular strength and endurance and flexibility'. DiNubile (1991) concluded that strength training can therefore be regarded as one of the cornerstones of a comprehensive fitness programme. Harms-Ringdahl (1993) observed that 25 years ago, muscle strength was a rather 'easy' concept in physiotherapy; it was evaluated by physiotherapists with their hands, and usually rated as *normal*, *reduced* or *none (paralysed)*. However, since then the complexity of the relationship between muscular strength and performance and function has been increasingly recognized.

The concept of muscle strength has been defined in a number of ways, from the simple definition proposed by McArdle *et al.* (1986) 'the maximum force generated by a muscle or muscle group' to a more extended and functional definition: 'the ability of skeletal muscle to develop force for the purpose of providing stability and mobility within the musculoskeletal system, so that functional movement can take place' (Harris and Watkins, 1993). Enoka (1994) suggested that the term *strength* should apply only to those situations of isometric contraction, that is for all contractions in which the velocity of shortening is zero, and that for all contractions in which the velocity of contraction is greater than zero, the term *power* should be used.

However, this might be regarded as a rather narrow definition of strength, and not one which can be easily applied to functional performance. Thus, for the purposes of this chapter, the term *strength* will encompass the force developed in both static and dynamic contractions, as suggested in the definitions by Galley and Forster (1987) ('the maximum effective force that can be actively exerted by a muscle in a specific movement'), Kisner and Colby (1996) ('the ability of a muscle or muscle group to produce tension and a resulting force in one maximal effort, either dynamically or statically, in relation to the demands placed upon it') and the previously quoted definitions by Harris and Watkins (1993) and McArdle *et al.* (1986). Similarly, the term *power* is defined the rate at which a muscle can do mechanical work (Galley and Forster, 1987), or as the maximum strength producing capability of an individual relative to time (DiNubile, 1991), and takes into consideration the force, distance and time taken to perform the task. Power is usually associated with explosive strength.

Factors Influencing the Development of Muscle Strength

In designing therapeutic exercise programmes to develop strength, the factors influencing muscle performance must be taken into consideration. Although these have been considered in detail in Chapter 2, a brief summary in the context of application of exercise programmes may be useful here.

THE NATURE AND RECRUITMENT OF MOTOR UNITS

Muscle strength depends on the number of motor units activated, the fibre-type composition of the motor units, and the frequency of their rate of contraction. With increasing load, recruitment of more motor units is most important, but as the load becomes heavy, increase in the rate of firing becomes the most important mechanism to develop greater force (Sale, 1987). Slow motor units (composed of slow-twitch fibres) are recruited earlier and at lower thresholds of activation than fast twitch fibres, which are recruited in interval training activities with more intensive contractions, and consequently contribute more to strength and power (Lamb, 1984).

CENTRAL INFLUENCES

Astrand and Rodahl (1977) have emphasized the role of central inhibitory mechanisms in the manifestation of muscle strength: effective inhibitory mechanisms reduce the number of motor neurones activated in a voluntary maximal contraction in untrained individuals, resulting in reduced force output.

This may have important implications in clinical practice. Training in technique, and the use of other facilitatory tools (such as repetition, manual contact, verbal encouragement) can reduce the influence of inhibitory mechanisms, resulting in increased overall facilitation, and increased recruitment of motor units. The suggestion that central factors are decisive in the development of strength is also supported by the observation that in the early stages of strength training, increases in strength can be achieved without concomitant muscle hypertrophy, which would indicate an increase in the number and/or size of muscle fibres. When training for muscle strength for a specific activity, the best training is *that* activity; the gain in strength when one is engaged in 'unfamiliar' procedures is comparatively modest even when they activate the muscles which are being trained (Astrand and Rodahl, 1977). This is an example of *specificity of training* which will be discussed in more detail later.

FORCE–VELOCITY RELATIONSHIPS

The dynamic capabilities of any single joint system is determined by the force–velocity characteristics of muscle contraction (Enoka, 1994) (see Figure 12.4). Basically, *as the velocity of shortening increases, the amount of force a muscle can exert decreases.* When a muscle contracts and shortens, it produces movement and performs a *concentric contraction*; when a muscle contracts and remains the same length (that is, it produces no movement), it performs an *isometric contraction*. The force exerted by a concentric contraction is less than the force exerted by an isometric contraction. This can be explained by the fact that during an isometric contraction the velocity of shortening is regarded as zero, whereas during concentric contractions the velocity of shortening is always greater than zero, and consequently the force exerted is less.

(a) velocity > 0; isotonic eccentric (lengthening) contraction — *greatest force*

(b) velocity = 0; isometric contraction — ↓ ↓ ↓ ↓ ↓ ↓

(c) velocity > 0; isotonic concentric (shortening) contraction — *least force*

When a muscle contracts and lengthens, it also produces movement, and in this case performs what we describe as an *eccentric contraction*. This occurs when the force opposing the action of the muscle (the external force) is *greater* than the force produced by the muscle, for example in lowering a weight (the force produced by the weight is greater than the force exerted by the

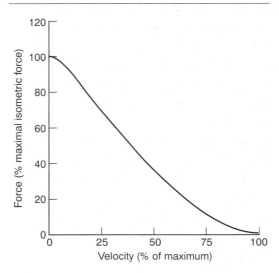

Figure 12.4 Relationship between force and speed of contraction. (Adapted from Lamb, DR *Physiology of Exercise. Responses and Adaptations*, 2nd edn, p. 265. Copyright © 1984 by Allyn and Bacon. Adapted by permission.)

muscles controlling its descent). In concentric contractions, the external force is *less* than the muscle force, and in isometric contractions, the external force is *equal* to the muscle force.

Of all types of muscle contraction, perhaps *eccentric contraction* is the most difficult to understand. Most simply, it may be regarded as producing a *controlling force* over a movement which is produced by another opposing force. The opposing force may be produced by mechanical means (for example, a weight), by gravity, or by muscular contraction. Let us look at examples of all three.

Practical Task

1. If you wish to lower a full basin of water on to a table, it is obviously important that you don't just drop it onto the table, or the water will spill. You therefore lower the container slowly and carefully until it rests on the table. The weight of the container is tending to produce a downwards force which must be controlled by your arms, or the container will fall. Thus you hold the container with your arms flexed at the elbow, and gradually straighten them as you lower the container to the table. Your elbow flexors are working (you can feel them!), but your elbow is extending – your elbow flexors are working eccentrically to control the descent of the container.

Working with a partner, try lifting and lowering a weight on to a table. Palpate both the flexors and extensors of the elbow during both actions. You will find that the flexors are working during both actions. How are they working when you lift the weight?

2. Consider sitting down on a chair. Although we sometimes flop on to a chair, we usually lower ourselves gradually. As soon as you prepare to sit down, you bend forward at the hips, and start to flex your knees. This causes you to move out of the alignment which maintains stability in standing, and the force of gravity will tend to flex your hips and knees further in an uncontrolled manner, until you land either on the chair (if you are lucky!) or on the floor. To prevent this uncontrolled descent, your hip extensors work eccentrically to control the speed of hip flexion, and the knee extensors also work eccentrically to control knee flexion.

Working with a partner, observe what is happening at the hip and knee when you descend stairs. Palpate the hip extensors and knee extensors. Describe how they are working and why.

3. During walking, as you take a step forward, the hip and knee flex and the ankle dorsiflexes to lift the leg through during the swing phase. As the leg continues to swing forward, the hip continues to flex (due to action of the hip flexors) and the knee starts to extend to prepare for heel strike (partly by quadriceps action, and partly by pendular activity). If there was no controlling influence on the hip flexion and knee extension during this latter part of the swing phase, the leg would swing forward excessively (as though you had just kicked a ball) with each step. Thus the hip extensors work eccentrically to control the amount and rate of hip flexion, and the hamstrings work eccentrically to control knee extension. This means that there is no excessive lift of the leg in preparation for heel strike.

As it may be difficult to palpate muscle action during walking, carefully watch someone walking to observe hamstring activity just prior to heel strike. What happens to the foot following heel strike? What muscles are working, how and why?

Early research using isolated muscle preparations (Hill, 1938, cited in Harris and Watkins, 1993) demonstrated that during concentric contractions, the magnitude of force generated declines with increasing speed of contraction, and that during eccentric contraction, force production increases with increasing speed of contraction. Although the force–velocity relationship has been substantiated in human subjects for concentric contractions, the evidence in eccentric contractions is less convincing.

In physiological terms, the relationship between force and velocity has been explained by reference to the sliding filament theory; as the rate of shortening increases, the average force exerted by each cross-bridge decreases, and there may be fewer cross-bridge attachments as the muscle shortens more quickly. In lengthening contractions, it has been suggested that the force required to break a cross-bridge is greater than that required to hold in an isometric contraction, resulting in greater force exerted by the cross-bridge (Enoka, 1994).

LENGTH–TENSION RELATIONSHIPS

Length–tension relationships in human muscle demonstrate that muscle in a very lengthened or a very shortened state generates less force than in mid-ranges (Figure 12.5) (resting length, which is defined as half-way between fully lengthened and fully shortened (Enoka, 1994).

According to the sliding filament theory, force can be exerted only during the phase of attachment of cross-bridges, and the magnitude of the force depends on the number cross-bridge attachments occurring at the same time. As the

length of the muscle changes, and the actin and myosin filaments slide past one another, the number of binding sites available for cross-bridge formation changes. As the filaments slide towards one another, the sarcomere length decreases, and the possibility of cross-bridge formation decreases. Similarly, as the filaments are pulled away from one another (as in an excessive stretch), again the possibility of cross-bridge formation decreases. At a sarcomere length of 2 μm there is maximum potential for cross-bridge formation. This is illustrated in Figures 12.6 and 12.7.

Although these factors may appear theoretical in nature, they are important to consider in the development of treatment programmes for patients. Consider a patient who has had a temporary (neuropraxia) injury to the axillary nerve following anterior dislocation of the shoulder, with resultant severe weakness (grade 2) of deltoid.

- As eccentric force is greater than concentric force, you might start rehabilitation by asking the patient to try to control lowering of the arm from a partially abducted position, rather

Figure 12.6　Relationship between contractile force, sarcomere length and myofilament overlap. (Adapted with permission from Enoka, RM, 1994, *Neuromechanical Basis of Kinesiology*, 2nd edn, p. 201, Human Kinetics Publishers)

Figure 12.5　Relationship between muscle length and active tension. (Adapted from Lamb, DR *Physiology of Exercise. Responses and Adaptations*, 2nd edn, p. 262. Copyright © 1984 by Allyn and Bacon. Adapted by permission.)

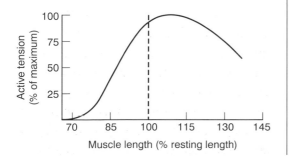

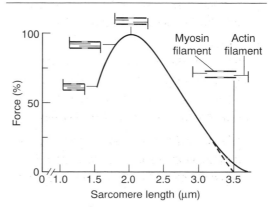

Figure 12.7 Effect of muscle length on the number of potentially active cross-bridges. (a) Optimal length, its effective cross-bridges, maximum strength. (b) Too much stretch, 12 effective cross-bridges, reduced strength. (c) Too much shortening, 14 effective and 2 antagonistic cross bridges for net of 12, reduced strength. [Adapted from Lamb, DR *Physiology of Exercise. Responses and Adaptations*, 2nd edn, p. 262. Copyright © 1984 by Allyn and Bacon. Adapted by permission.]

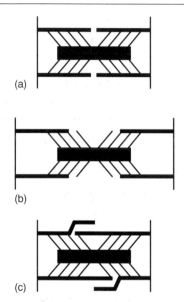

than asking the patient to attempt to lift the arm.

- Rehabilitation might also commence with strengthening in outer/middle range rather than inner range, as it is possible to exert greater force with the muscle in a lengthened rather than a shortened position.

- To attempt to influence central inhibitory mechanisms, you might use facilitatory techniques (such as tapping over the muscle, verbal encouragement) to increase overall facilitation and increase recruitment of motor units.

- repetitive low intensity activity will recruit slow-twitch fibres (which are recruited before fast-twitch fibres) with the added bonus of training in technique, which tends to increase motor unit recruitment.

- As the muscle gains in strength, isometric and concentric work may be incorporated, working the muscle into inner range, and high intensity/low repetition activity (to recruit fast-twitch fibres) may be introduced.

Practical Task

Following injury or surgery to the knee, patients often exhibit an 'extension lag' — that is when, for example, it might be possible to passively extend the knee fully, but the patient's active extension against gravity stops 20° short of full extension. Using the theoretical framework above, can you:

1 *provide an explanation why the patient cannot actively extend this last 20°;*
2 *devise a progressive treatment programme.*

Principles of Strength Training

Basic to any training, exercise or rehabilitation programme are the concepts of overload and specificity of training. These concepts relate to an organ's ability to adapt to imposed stress and include both structural and functional changes. Without adherence to these principles, gains in performance cannot be achieved.

OVERLOAD

As a general rule, a muscle working close to its maximum force-generating capacity will increase in strength (McArdle *et al.*, 1986). During everyday functional activities, this level of demand is rarely achieved, so extra stress or *overload is* required to achieve a strengthening effect. Overload is accomplished when an individual physically demands more of his or her muscles than are normally required or used (DiNubile, 1991). Although the absolute level of the overload will vary according to the individual, the principle of overload remains the same. It has been suggested that before adaptive responses will occur, a threshold point must be exceeded (Enoka, 1994). For example, the threshold for isometric training is thought to be about 40% of maximum; that is, adaptations will occur only if the load exceeds 40% of maximum. Similarly, Berger (1982) suggested that the threshold for isotonic training should be about 50% of maximum.

Furthermore, not only must overload be applied, but the magnitude of the overload must be progressively increased as the individual adapts to the training and increases in strength. This approach to the application of overload is known as *progressive resistance exercise* (PRE), a term which was first coined by DeLorme (1945), when he described a method of increasing muscular strength using a system of cables and pulleys with gradual increase in resistance. McQueen (1954) advanced this concept to incorporate specificity when he developed different PRE training programmes to develop muscle power on the one hand, and hypertrophy on the other. Both DeLorme and McQueen based their progressive resistance programmes on the concept of the 10 RM (Resistance Maximum), that is the maximum load which can be lifted ten times and ten times only. Thus, a training programme might consist of ten lifts of 10 RM, repeated three times, or in three *sets*. Examples of progressive resistance programmes based on the 10 RM concept are demonstrated in Figure 12.8.

Figure 12.8   Examples of progressive resistance programmes.

The DeLorme Programme

10 lifts of 50% 10 RM
rest
10 lifts of 75% 10 RM
rest
10 lifts of 10 RM

Performed 5 times weekly
1 RM tested weekly

The McQueen Programme

The 'Hypertrophy' programme

10 lifts of 10 RM
rest
10 lifts of 10 RM
rest
10 lifts of 10 RM

The 'Power' programme

10 lifts of 10 RM
rest
8 lifts of 6–8 RM
rest
and so on until 1 RM is reached

Berger (1962a, cited in Berger, 1982) compared different numbers of repetitions per set, and different numbers of sets to determine which were most effective for improving strength. The results showed that six repetitions and three sets achieved maximal strength gains. Furthermore, the same author (Berger, 1962b, cited in Berger, 1982) found that the optimal number of repetitions to execute when performing one set only is

Figure 12.9   The optimal programme as advocated by Berger (1962a,b cited Berger, 1982).

The Berger programme

6 lifts of 6 RM
rest
6 lifts of 6 RM
rest
6 lifts of 6 RM

---

closest to the 6 RM. The optimal programme as advocated by Berger (1962a, b, cited in Berger, 1982) is shown in Figure 12.9.

SPECIFICITY

Specificity relates to the nature of the changes (structural, functional, systemic, local) that occur in an individual as a result of training. Training adaptations are specific to the cells and their structural and functional elements that are overloaded, that is, a training effect will be achieved which is specific to the type of training imposed. Thus isometric exercises improve isometric strength, and concentric exercises improve concentric strength, most of all for the angular speed exercised (Harms-Ringdahl, 1993). This is referred to as the SAID principle (Specific Adaptation to Imposed Demands) (DiNubile, 1991), and is the basis underlying the design of training programmes. This can be seen in the different training programmes adopted by 'power' athletes (sprinters, jumpers, throwers) and 'endurance' athletes (marathon runners, race walkers). Although the specificity of general approaches to training is well established, there is still some disagreement as to the degree to which specificity can be applied to the more finite details of muscle performance. Jones *et al.* (1989) and Sale and McDougall (1981)

reported that adaptations specific to the task, muscle length and velocity of contraction occurred during strength training, but Peterson *et al.* (1990) found no specificity with respect to concentric and eccentric contractions, and Behm and Sale (1993) similarly found no specificity with respect to isometric and rapid contractions.

However, in spite of these areas of controversy, it is generally accepted that training programmes should be designed to meet the specific requirements of the individual – is the strength needed for isometric contractions, concentric contractions or eccentric contractions – and at what joint angles? Analysis of performance at work and in leisure must be used to set the goals of the training programme, and will almost inevitably reveal that all aspects of muscle perfomance are involved, to a greater or lesser degree!

Summary – Principles of Strength Training

1 Muscle strength depends on the nature (slow- or fast-twitch) and number of motor units activated.
2 Central inhibitary mechanisms can influence (reduce) force output by limiting or reducing the number of motor neurones activated in a voluntary contraction. Inhibition of these central factors will result in increased force output, in the absence of hypertrophy.
3 As the velocity of *shortening* increases in *concentric* contractions, the force output decreases. As the velocity of *lengthening* increases in *eccentric* contractions, the force output increases.
4 Muscle in a very lengthened or a very shortened state generates less force than in mid-ranges (115% of resting length).

5 Muscle strengthening programmes are based on the principles of *specificity* and *overload*.
6 Strength programmes are generally based on the concept of high resistance/low repetition. Loads of 80–100% of resistance maximum, with a repetition of 6–10 create a training effect.

Muscle Endurance

Muscular endurance refers to the ability of a muscle or group of muscles to sustain contractions over a period of time, and depends on:

- The strength of the muscle/s involved, localized muscle energy stores (Galley and Forster, 1987);
- The capacity of the circulatory system (heart, blood vessels and blood) and the respiratory system (lungs) to deliver oxygen to the working muscles, and to carry chemical waste products away from them (Lamb, 1984);
- The fibre-type composition of the muscles involved (DiNubile, 1991).

The degree to which circulation and respiration limit sustained activity depends on many factors, primarily the intensity of exercise, the duration of the activity, and the amount of static muscle contraction involved.

Short-term, high intensity exercise acquires the necessary energy from anaerobic metabolism; for sustained activity, aerobic metabolism is necessary to supply adequate oxygen to the working muscles, and to remove lactic acid from the blood. The exercise level or level of oxygen consumption at which the blood lactate begins to show a systematic increase (where lactic acid is formed at a rate which exceeds its removal from the blood) is termed the point of *onset of blood lactate accu-*

mulation (OBLA). Once blood lactate levels begin to rise above resting values, fatigue occurs with resulting impaired muscle performance (Lamb, 1984). The OBLA normally occurs between 55 and 65% of oxygen uptake (the maximum amount of oxygen taken up by the body as it exercises against increasing loads) in healthy untrained subjects, but may be at 80% in more highly trained endurance athletes (McArdle et al, 1988). This indicates that with specific training, an individual can sustain activity at a higher intensity, or maintain activity for a longer period, without experiencing fatigue related to lactic acid accumulation.

De Vries (1980) summarized the elements of endurance as a factor in human performance as shown in Table 12.4.

The development of muscular endurance is closely related to the development of muscle strength and power. If a muscle or muscle group increases in strength, it will be able to perform a given task at lower percentages of its resistance maximum, and consequently sustain the activity for a longer period without fatigue. However, to improve local muscle endurance, it is not enough to merely improve muscle strength, so the twin principles of training (specificity and overload) must be applied, as they are in strength training.

Whereas strength training relies on the application of high resistance with a low repetition rate, endurance training involves lower levels of resistance applied over a greater number of repetitions.

However the load, although not as high as in strength training, (where it is usually between 80 and 100% of resistance maximum), must still apply overload, or an endurance training effect will not be achieved. One approach to the training

Table 12.4
Elements of endurance

Physiological elements	Psychological elements
Local endurance (one or several localized muscle groups) • strength of the particular muscle group/s • energy stores • peripheral circulatory factor General endurance (whole body activity) • strength of general musculature • energy stores • systemic circulatory factor • heat regulatory mechanisms • neural factors Muscular efficiency	Willingness to take pain Motivation

of muscular endurance is to perform an activity repeatedly against a moderate load to the point of fatigue (Kisner and Colby, 1996); progress is demonstrated by increasing the number of repetitions before fatigue causes the subject to stop the exercise. The load must however be of a threshold level to impart a training effect. Kottke (1971, cited in Galley and Forster, 1987) suggested that using loads of less than 15% of maximal strength is inadequate to produce a training effect, and advocated loads of 30–50% of maximal strength in endurance training programmes. Berger (1982) suggested that loads which could be lifted more than 25 times should be regarded as having an endurance training effect rather than strength training, but did not quote an upper value. Although the literature on specific strength training programmes is extensive, this is not the case for muscle endurance — it appears that loads of 30–50% of resistance maximum, lifted 25–35 times will produce an endurance training effect.

As in strength training, neural factors may be utilized to improve endurance performance. If groups of muscles are exercised repetitively in specific patterns of movement, the subject's level *of skill* in performing the task will improve. Unnecessary movements are eliminated, thus reducing the energy requirements of the task, and allowing the subject to continue performing the task over a longer period of time (Galley and Forster, 1987).

When an activity performed over a prolonged period of time involves large percentages of the body's musculature, general *cardiovascular endurance* is required in addition to local muscular endurance. This will be covered in a separate section.

Summary: Principles of Endurance Training

1 Muscular endurance refers to the ability of a muscle or group of muscles to sustain contractions over a period of time.
2 The development of muscle endurance is closely related to the development of strength and power. A stronger muscle can perform a given task at lower percentages of its resistance maximum for a longer period without fatigue.
3 Resistance training relies on the application of

lower levels of resistance applied over a greater number of repetitions. It appears that 30–50% of resistance maximum, lifted 25–35 times will produce an endurance training effect.

4 As in strength training, the principles of overload and specificity apply to endurance training.

Power

When an explosive movement occurs, power is the physical component involved. Power may be defined as the amount of work performed in a unit of time (Berger, 1982). When a graph is plotted of load against speed of contraction, maximum isometric strength at any joint angle is always greater than dynamic concentric strength at the same angle. In eccentric contractions, maximum strength at a given joint angle is greater when the muscle is lengthening than when it is contracting either concentrically or isometrically. The relationship between load and speed of contraction suggests that there must be an optimal combination of speed and force to provide the greatest muscular power. A muscle is said to develop its greatest power when its velocity of shortening is approximately one third of the maximum possible, and the force produced is approximately one third of the isometric force that the muscle can generate (Astrand and Rodahl, 1977). This is illustrated in Figure 12.10.

If muscular power combines the components of force and speed, training either or both of these components should result in an increase in muscular power. Muscles differ in their ability to produce fast movement, in that those muscles with a high percentage of fast-twitch fibres can

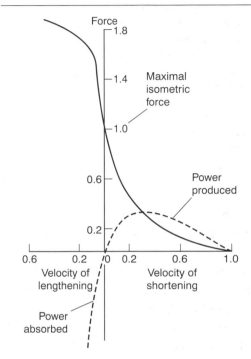

Figure 12.10 Force–velocity curve in shortening and lengthening contractions. (Adapted from Astrand and Rodahl, 1977, *Textbook of Work Physiology: Physiological Bases of Exercise*, p. 104, McGraw-Hill, New York. Copyright © Per-Olof Astrand.

contract more rapidly than the postural muscles which are composed predominantly of slow-twitch fibres. De Vries (1980) noted that although evidence is lacking, the ultimate maximal speed capacity is probably limited by the intrinsic speed of an individual's muscle tissue, and by the nicety of his/her neuromuscular coordination patterns. Neither factor is amenable to changes to the same extent as those possible in strength and endurance training.

It appears also that speed is both limb specific, and movement specific; thus an individual who can run fast will not automatically be able to throw a ball fast. Consequently, if one is to improve speed of action, specific speed training for that particular action is required. But if speed of movement is limited by the intrinsic speed of an individual's muscle tissue, how can this be enhanced? De Vries (1980) suggested that repeated practice of the specific activity at speeds as fast as those required by a specific target activity will improve speed of performance; this is supported by studies carried out on acquisition of skill and changes of performance during practice, which found that successive performances of the same task tended to become more uniform, that the rate of improvement with practice depended on potential variability within the task, and that the more subtasks within the overall task, the greater was the potential to improve and to continue improving (Welford, 1976). Thus improvements in skill acquisition and neuromuscular coordination can result in increased speed of performance

Furthermore, those factors which might provide resistance to movement should be addressed; flexibility should be improved until range of motion is such that no resistance is offered to the movement, and this may be enhanced by an adequate and appropriate warm-up to increase deep muscle temperature.

It can be seen that training of muscular power is rather more complex than strength or endurance training. However, an understanding of the components of power provides the basis for training programmes, and the application of overload in the strength training aspect, and specificity in both strength training and skill acquisition and practice, demonstrate that these same fundamental principles can be applied in a variety of situations.

Taking these basic principles on board, a power programme might be developed in the following way;

- Analyse the activity to break it down into its components;

- Analyse the muscle activity involved;
- Analyse the joint ranges of motion necessary;
- Strengthen muscles / muscle groups involved;
- Increase / maintain range of motion required by the activity;
- Improve speed / skill of performance of individual components of the activity by practice and repetition;
- Perform components of the activity against a resistance of 30% maximal isometric strength as fast as possible;
- Perform total activity against resistance of 30% maximal isometric strength as fast as possible.

Practical Task

Using the framework above, devise power programmes for sporting activities (throwing the javelin, long jump) and functional activities (rising from a chair, going upstairs).

Summary: Principles of Power Training

1 Muscular power combines the components of force and speed.
2 Training programmes which address either or both of these components should result in increases in power.
3 The speed at which muscles can contract depends on the fibre composition — muscles with a high percentage of fast-twitch fibres can contract more rapidly and produce more power than those whose fibre composition is predominately slow-twitch.
4 Speed of contraction also depends on neuromuscular coordination.
5 As fibre composition and the intrinsic speed of

neuromuscular firing patterns are not easily enhanced, repeated practice of a task will improve skill at that task, and result in improved speed of performance.

6 Increased flexibility will reduce resistance to movement at the extremes of ranges, and contribute to speed or movement.

Flexibility

In addition to strength and endurance, mobility of soft tissues is necessary for the performance of normal everyday functional activities. During normal activity, the soft tissues selectively lengthen and shorten to permit and produce movement, and this constant alteration in length maintains the appropriate length of the tissues involved. If normal movement is restricted in any way, selective adaptive shortening of the soft tissues occurs, resulting in limitation of range of motion of the joint/s involved. Fibrosis and shortening can occur within 4 days of the onset of immobilization/immobility (Stap and Wodfin, 1986).

Whereas flexibility can be defined at its simplest as 'the range of possible movement in a joint' (De Vries, 1980), more specifically, range of motion may be regarded as the available amount of movement about a joint, whereas flexibility is the ability of the soft tissue structures, such as muscle, tendon, and connective tissue to elongate through the available range of joint motion (Middleton, 1991). The aspect of neural tension is addressed elsewhere (Chapter 5). The concept of elongation of the soft tissues during movement is an important one, as possible range of motion in a joint, measured in a static position, does not necessarily provide an indication of the stiffness or looseness of that joint as it is required to move

quickly with minimal resistance to the movement. This introduces the notion of two different components of flexibility – *static flexibility*, which may be regarded as the range of motion in a joint, and *dynamic flexibility*, which gives an indication of the degree of stiffness, or the forces that resist throughout the range of motion of a joint (De Vries, 1980).

In keeping with the relatively simple concept of static flexibility, the measurement of this component is also relatively simple, and may involve direct measurement of joint angle by goniometry, or indirectly by measuring linear distance between reference points (usually bony points). Dynamic flexibility is more difficult to assess, and requires more complex equipment; isokinetic equipment with a passive mode (rather like a continuous passive motion machine) may be used to measure resistance to movement, and some of the opto-electric systems have the capability of measuring joint displacement over time, which may also provide an indirect measure of resistance to movement (see Chapters 6 and 8).

The basic factors influencing joint range of motion have already been discussed (Chapter 2). In considering the potential to lengthen soft tissues, and to reduce the resistance they offer to movement, Wright and Johns (1960, cited in De Vries, 1980), investigated the physical factors which contribute to joint stiffness, and therefore limit dynamic flexibility, in normal and diseased joints. They investigated the effects of *elasticity, viscosity, inertia, plasticity* and *friction,* and found that inertia and friction had a neglible effect, viscosity accounted for only one tenth of the torque used in moving the joint passively, and that elasticity and plasticity were the major factors.

Connective tissue is composed of collagen and other fibres within a ground substance, and has viscoelastic properties, defined as two components of stretch, which allow elongation of tissue. The viscous component allows for a plastic stretch, which results in permanent elongation of the tissue after the load has been removed. Conversely, the elastic component allows for elastic stretch, a temporary elongation, and the connective tissue returns to its original length when the stressing force is removed. Range of motion exercises should primarily be designed to produce plastic deformation (Middleton, 1991).

Muscle tissue has the ability to lengthen considerably under certain conditions (Anderson and Burke, 1991). The Golgi tendon organs (GTOs) are sensory receptors located at the musculotendinous junction, which respond to tension. Tension can be imparted to the tendon in two ways: firstly, active contraction of the muscle will create a pull on its tendon, and secondly, sustained passive stretch of the muscle will also provide tension in the tendon. The purpose of the GTOs is to protect the muscle and its tendon from excessive forces; when a sustained, significant force is applied to the musculotendinous unit (either by static stretch or isometric contraction), the GTOs are stimulated, and trigger an inhibiting response which causes the muscle to relax, and thus reduce the tension. This then creates a situation in which the relaxed muscle can be further lengthened, achieving a length greater than that it originally possessed.

There are a number of approaches designed to stretch muscle and other soft tissues which may limit flexibility. In general, flexibility exercises aim to increase the range of motion either with the limb muscles passive (static) or with one or more of the muscles attempting to assist the stretch (dynamic). Anderson (1981) supports the use of the *static stretch*, and provides the following instructions.

- When you stretch, spend 10–30 seconds in the *easy stretch*. No bouncing! Go to the point where you feel a *mild tension*, and relax as you hold the stretch. The feeling of tension should subside as you hold the position. If it does not, ease off slightly and find a degree of tension that is comfortable. The easy stretch reduces muscular tightness and readies the tissues for the *developmental stretch*.

- After the easy stretch, move slowly into the *developmental stretch*. Again, no bouncing. Move a fraction of an inch further (*from the limit of the easy stretch*) until you again feel a mild tension, and hold for 10–30 seconds. Be in control. Again, the tension should diminish; if not, ease off slightly. The developmental stretch fine-tunes the muscles and increases flexibility.

Anderson and Burke (1991) suggest that during the stretch, the Golgi tendon organs initiate sensory impulses, resulting in reduced resistance to stretched soft tissue by inhibiting muscle contraction in the stretched tissue. This relaxation phenomenon does not occur when a stretch is performed quickly (Guyton, 1981).

Ballistic (bouncing) stretching is a rapid, jerky movement in which a body part is put into motion, and momentum carries it throughout the range of motion until the muscles are stretched to the limit (Anderson and Burke, 1991). Thus the antagonists are stretched by the dynamic movement of the agonists (De Vries, 1980). However, Anderson and Burke (1991) suggest that as the individual bounces, the muscle responds by contracting, to protect itself from overstretch, probably through stimulation of the muscle spindle. Thus internal tension develops in the muscle, and prevents it from being fully stretched.

De Vries (1959, cited in De Vries, 1980) compared the outcome of static and ballistic methods of stretching in seven training periods of 30 minutes, and found that both methods resulted in significant gains in static flexibility of trunk flexion, trunk extension, and shoulder elevation. There was no significant difference between the two methods. However, De Vries (1980) concluded that the static method was the method of choice, citing three distinct advantages: there is less danger of exceeding the extensibility limits of the tissues involved and consequently potential damage, energy requirements are lower, and although ballistic stretching is apt to cause muscular soreness, static stretching will not; in fact, De Vries suggests, static stretching relieves soreness.

A further approach has been applied to gaining flexibility, namely proprioceptive neuromuscular facilitation (PNF), in which relaxation of muscle is achieved through spinal reflexes. Although the PNF approach to the rehabilitation of movement has been described in detail in Chapter 10, a brief description in the context of improving flexibility will be given here. Three applications of the approach have been described. The *hold–relax* (HR) stretch involves an initial maximal contraction of the muscle to be stretched, followed by relaxation and stretch of the muscle to the limit of the range of motion. The stretch should be applied during the 10 seconds immediately following the isometric contraction, when the excitability of the muscle spindle and the motor neurone pool is reduced (Enoka, 1994), and can be performed with the assistance of a partner or therapist.

Example

To stretch the hamstrings, with the knee maintained in extension, the hip is flexed as far as is possible. The hamstrings then perform a maximal isometric contraction at their most lengthened position, followed by relaxation and stretch.

The agonist contract stretch involves the therapist or partner moving the limb to the limit of antagonist range, the subject then contracts the agonist while the partner/therapist applies a stretch to the antagonist. This technique is based on activation of the agonist, and through reciprocal inhibition, relaxation of the antagonist.

Example

To stretch the quadriceps, with the hip maintained in extension, the knee is flexed as far as is possible. The hamstrings then contract maximally against resistance, while the quadriceps are stretched.

Finally, a combination of the two techniques may be used — *hold–relax, agonist contraction* — in which there is an initial isometric contraction of the antagonists, followed by relaxation and stretch of the antagonists, which is further facilitated by contraction of the agonists.

Example

To stretch the plantarflexors, with the knee maintained in extension, the ankle is dorsiflexed as far as is possible. The plantarflexors perform a maximal isometric contraction against resistance, followed by relaxation and stretch,

> augmented by subsequent maximal contraction of the dorsiflexors.

Research has also shown that temperature has an important influence on the mechanical behaviour of tissue under conditions of stretch (Sapega and Quendenfield, 1981). Increased connective tissue temperature increases extensibility, and higher therapeutic temperatures at prolonged low loads produce the greatest elongation with the least damage (Middleton, 1991). Muscular activity demands increased blood flow to muscle, and therefore increased intramuscular temperature. Stretching should not be performed at the beginning of a warm-up, as the tissue temperature is low. Cold muscles and tendons are less extensible, and thus more vulnerable to injury. Lehman *et al.* (1966, cited in Middleton, 1991) reported that the use of ultrasound prior to joint mobilization elevated deep tissue temperature, and improved extensibility. Furthermore, Middleton (1991) suggests that it is advantageous to stretch immediately following a rehabilitative exercise session, and then to apply ice to the involved part while stretching continues, which is probably based on desensitization of myofascial trigger points (Middleton, 1991).

In conclusion, there are several approaches to increasing flexibility, all of which have demonstrated effectiveness. The choice of technique should be based on the one most appropriate to the specific individual, and which can be performed most effectively by the individual.

Summary of Principles of Stretching

1 Both static and ballistic stretching achieve similar results, but ballistic stretches are more likely to produce muscle soreness.

2 Stretches using PNF techniques appear to produce greater improvements in flexibility, but there does not seem to be a consistent difference between the different techniques (Moore and Hutton, 1980).

3 There is general agreement that flexibility exercises should be directed at inducing plastic rather than elastic changes in connective tissue, because plastic changes produce more permanent changes in tissue length (Enoka, 1894).

4 It is thought that static stretching has its greatest effect on the noncontractile connective tissue elements, whereas PNF influences the length of the contractile elements by adding sarcomeres to its length.

Proprioception

Proprioception may be defined as the information received from sensory receptors which provides knowledge (conscious and unconscious) of the position and movement of the body and body parts in space, and the response to that information. Proprioceptors include muscle spindles, tendon organs and joint and skin receptors. These respond to the mechanical variables (position, movement) associated with muscles and joints which are due to actions generated by the system itself (Enoka, 1994) and by external forces. Hasan and Stuart (1988) suggest that proprioceptors have two roles — first to control movement to a form which is appropriate to the surroundings in which the movement occurs, and second, to produce movement which takes into account the musculoskeletal dynamics of the system as a whole.

Example

A relatively simple example is provided by the proprioceptive feedback loop mechanism which provides stability to the lateral compartment of the ankle. In normal circumstances, if the lateral ligament of the ankle is stretched, afferent discharge from the mechanoreceptors in the ligament travels to the dorsal horn of the spinal cord, synapses with the motor efferents to the peroneal muscles, which contract to relieve the stretch on the lateral ligament. If the stretching force is too rapid, too strong or is sustained, the muscular response may be inadequate, and the ligament will tear.

Damage to the ligament will damage the proprioceptors within the ligament, making it more susceptible to repeated injury – recurrent lateral ligament sprains are a common problem. It is therefore of paramount importance that rehabilitation programmes should include activities directed at restoring the effectiveness of the proprioceptive feedback mechanism. This may involve 'training' other proprioceptors to take over the role of the damaged receptors, and improving the effectiveness of the muscular response (see below for more detail).

An associated sense, *kinaesthesia*, provides information which enables the system to determine the position of its limbs, and to identify what has produced the movement (i.e. internal or external force). Like proprioceptive input, kinaesthetic input is derived from a variety of afferent sources – skin, muscles, tendons, joint capsules, ligaments – and from centrally generated motor commands, and the sensations include those concerning position and movement, effort and heaviness, and the perceived timing of movements (Enoka, 1994). In contrast to proprioceptive input which is more general, kinaesthetic sensations are perceived, and include vestibular sensations and input from muscles and joints which might not be consciously perceived (Goodwin *et al.*, 1972). Highboard and springboard divers, and gymnasts require a highly developed kinaesthetic awareness, as it is important that they are aware of exactly where their limbs are in space. Both senses are essential for coordinated movement, and the terms are often used interchangeably.

Although joint receptors were originally thought to provide the sensory information necessary to determine joint position and movement, it is now thought that the muscle spindle is more important (Goodwin *et al.*, 1972). It appears that appreciation of joint position or movement, and the sense of heaviness or effort, is the result of integration between *corollary discharges* which provide the sensory centres with information about outgoing motor commands, and the incoming information from the sensory receptors themselves. Correct balance between these two systems is necessary for appropriate coordinated muscular action during normal functional activity.

Normal functioning of joints during skilled actions is likely to be inadequate as a result of distortion of proprioceptive signals following injury (Glencross and Thornton, 1981). Damage to proprioceptive systems commonly occurs through trauma to a joint, either through acute injury, or as the result of chronic overuse. This can result in partial deafferentation of the joint, with subsequent impairment of normal reflex muscular stabilization, awareness of joint movement and position (Freeman, 1965; Beard, 1994; Borsa et al., 1994) and a decreased ability to detect large ranges of motion (Glencross and Thornton, 1981). This may be due to actual damage to the sensory receptors in the muscle or joint structures (Freeman, 1965; Wyke, 1972; Borsa et al., 1994), to a problem with the transmission and integration of afferent impulses (Revel et al., 1991), or to an inability to recruit sufficient numbers of receptors necessary to detect extremes of range of motion (Smith and Brunoli, 1989).

Lack of proprioceptive and kinaesthetic sense will result in impairment of the normal reflex muscular stabilization of joints, which may in turn lead to functional instability and risk of further injury, and possibly the development of early degenerative changes (Barrett et al., 1991). This is demonstrated in recurrent inversion sprains of the ankle (Ryan, 1994) and in shoulder instability following traumatic dislocation (Smith and Brunoli, 1989). Proprioceptive training should be regarded as an essential part of any rehabilitation programme, particularly in patients following injury to joint structures.

Summary: Principles of Proprioception Training

Specific exercise techniques can be applied to assist patients in regaining stability.

1 O'Sullivan and Schmitz (1994) describe *placing and holding* (positioning a limb or part of a limb, and asking the patient to maintain the position against the force of gravity), *alternating isometrics* (alternate isometric contraction of opposing muscle groups against resistance), and *rhythmic stabilizations* (similar to alternating isometrics, but resistance is applied to opposing muscle groups simultaneously at different locations). (Note that this terminology is used differently by Knott and Voss – see Chapter 10.)

2. Other resistive PNF techniques applied in patterns of movement (described in Chapter 10) may be used to promote coordinated activity of groups of muscles.

3. Weight-bearing exercises for both upper and lower limbs, based on the *closed kinetic chain* principle (described later in this chapter) should be introduced at the earliest opportunity, to redevelop proprioceptive and neuromuscular functions (Balduini et al., 1987; Vegso and Harmon, 1982).

4. Wobble boards (Derscheid and Brown, 1985) and gymnastic balls can be used during weight-bearing to challenge and re-educate proprioceptive reflexes.

Skill

'Skill is highly co-ordinated movement that allows for investigation and interaction with the physical and social environment' (O'Sullivan and Schmitz, 1994). Skilled movement relies on proximal joint / segment stability, which leaves the distal segments free for manipulation, locomotion and other functional activities. Skilled movements are consistent, intentional and with purpose, performed with economy of effort, and are regulated with precise timing and direction. Skill lies in the efficient and effective use of capacities as a result of experience and practice. Welford (1976) described the chain of events leading to the acquisition of skill as having three main divisions: first, perceptual coding of the incoming data which involves the selection and integration of sensory information; second, the translation from perception to response which involves decision-making; and third, the phasing and sequencing of action, all of which take place before the movement sequence is performed.

Galley and Forster (1987) describe a similar model of skill acquisition, referred to as an information processing model of perceptual–motor skills. Figure 12.11 summarizes the model.

Skilled motor performance is acquired through a process of learning (Welford, 1976). Experience, and therefore learning, are cumulative in that the way in which an individual deals with any new situation is inevitably influenced by previous experience, and each new experience modifies the manner of dealing with subsequent situations. In the development of skilled performance, two main elements are essential, namely understanding what is required of the task, and repetition and practice of the task.

Galley and Forster (1987) cite Fitts and Posner (1967) in identifying three stages in learning a new perceptual–motor skill. First is the *early* or *cognitive phase*, in which the learner/patient attempts to identify and understand what is required of the task. Full comprehension can be assured only if there is precise information about what has to be learned, and this in turn requires a careful and accurate analysis of the task. Feedback on the accuracy of performance is important at this stage to enable the patient to judge the appropriateness of his responses. Explanation and demonstration of the skill by the physiotherapist is useful at this stage, as is mental practice by the patient.

The second or *intermediate* or *associative phase* involves a move from understanding what to do, to how to do it. This phase involves practice to establish the movement pattern, to eliminate errors and improve efficiency and coordination.

Figure 12.11   Summary of information processing model of perceptual-motor skills.

Perpetual mechanism

Identifies and classifies information in **the light of past and present experience**

Decision mechanism

Receives information and decides on a plan of action. This is done by searching long-term memory, where information has been **stored in a more permanent form as a result of practice**, in order to make an appropriate response.
This takes time, especially if there are a number of possible responses. Time is reduced with practice.

Effector mechanism

Uses the plan of action selected by the decision mechanism to organize an appropriate response.
The necessary motor commands are sent to the muscles in **correct sequential and temporal** order to perform the desired task, taking into consideration the specific demands of the task.

Feedback mechanism

Feeds back information to the system about 'knowledge of performance' during performance of the task, and 'knowledge of results' after the task is completed.
This allows the individual to **compare the actual response with the desired response**, and forms the basis of decisions concerning the next move.

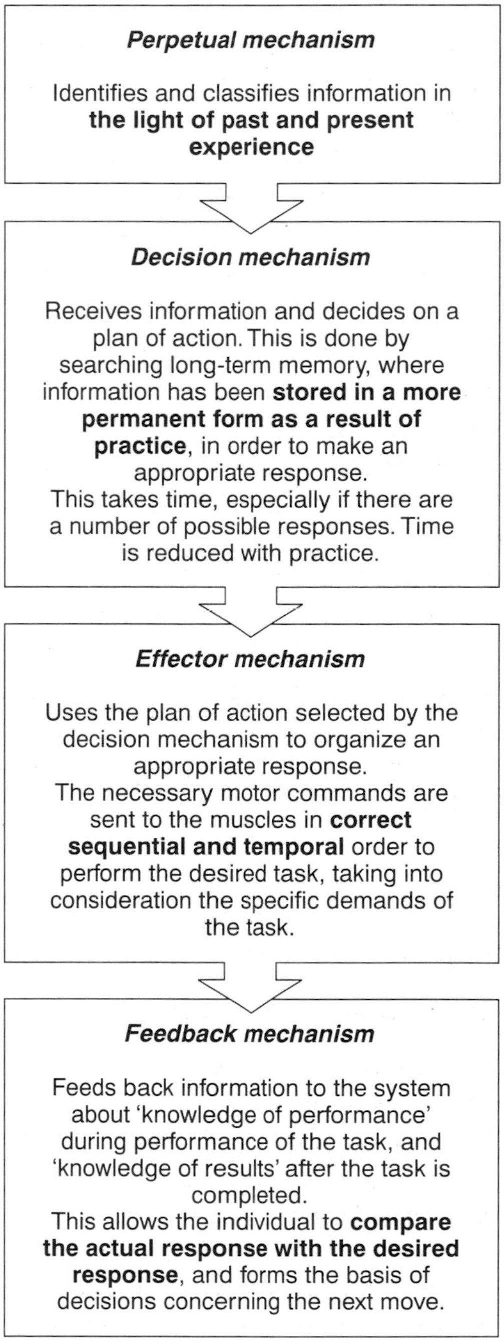

During this phase, the learner may change the cues used to promote accurate performance of the skill. For example, in the early stages of learning a skill, visual cues may be the primary source of information, but other sensory sources may take over later as greater proficiency is achieved. Although this may to a certain degree be desirable, in the long term the learner may become dependent on the 'new' cues instead of learning to observe those inherent in the task, and performance may ultimately deteriorate, particularly when the task has to be transferred to a new environment (Welford, 1976). With practice, the individual components of a task become increasingly subsumed within the task as a whole, and performance improves both in terms of uniformity and in performance time.

The final or *autonomous phase* is an extremely advanced phase, and one which not everyone will achieve (Galley and Forster, 1987). At this stage, the task has become so well learned that its performance is almost automatic. The learner no longer needs to think about the performance of the task, and can simultaneously devote attention to other events or thoughts. Think of the concentration required to learn to ride a bicycle, and how eventually it becomes so easy that you don't have to think about it!

Most research into the acquisition of skill has been directed at sport and industrial tasks, in which specific skills outside the sphere of everyday functional activities have to be learned. Following injury or disease, patients have to relearn what were originally normal functional activities as if they were new skilled tasks. It is important in the early stage that the patient understands the nature of the task, and this can be enhanced by careful identification of the individual elements of the task, and by clear explanations and demonstrations. Practice of elements of the task can gradually be combined to form the complete task, with appropriate feedback given at all times to improve the patient's 'knowledge of performance'. It is obvious that physiotherapists must have a sound understanding of the stages of learning a new (or relearning an old) skill so that they can facilitate patients' learning; they should also be aware that individuals may prefer and respond to different 'cues' (visual, auditory, kinaesthetic), and consequently modify their approach to achieve the best response.

As skill in the performance of the task is achieved, efficiency in processing incoming data and initiating action seems to increase, improving general efficiency in performance, and reducing fatigue due to unnecessary actions (Welford, 1976). It is important that repeated practice of a skill (or functional activity) does not endanger flexibility, or the ability to adapt the skill to other environments. For example, in re-educating gait, it is important that the patient is capable not only of walking forward in a straight line on a smooth level surface, but also of adapting the basic skill to walking backward, around obstacles, on inclines, on uneven ground, on carpets, and up and down kerbs and stairs.

Summary: Principles of Skill Training

1 Skilled movements are consistent, intentional, performed with purpose and with economy of effort, and are regulated with precise timing and direction.
2 Three main phases of skill development have been identified:

- cognitive phase: identification and understanding of the elements of the task;
- associative phase: moving from understanding what to do, to how to do it;
- advanced phase: the skill is so well developed that the performance is almost automatic.

3 In practice, relearning a 'lost' skill or learning a new one might be achieved by:
- identifying elements of the task;
- practicing individual elements;
- refining individual elements through feedback on performance;
- combining some of the elements, and practicing performance;
- refining combined elements through feedback on performance;
- combining all elements to practice the complete task;
- refining the complete task through feedback of performance.

4 Finally the re-acquired or newly learnt skill should be applied to different situations, so that the patient can adapt to different circumstances.

Cardiovascular Endurance

Total body endurance is necessary for performance of repetitive motor tasks in daily living, and carrying on a sustained level of functional activity, such as walking or climbing stairs (Kisner and Colby, 1996). Aerobic capacity, a measure of cardiovascular endurance, which is defined as the highest rate of aerobic metabolism during the performance of rhythmic dynamic muscle work which exhausts the subject in 5–10 minutes, is assessed through the measurement of the maximal oxygen uptake (VO_{2max}) which is the maximum volume of oxygen consumed per minute

(Galley and Forster, 1987). Following bedrest, resting heart rate increases, stroke volume is diminished and VO_{2max} is markedly lowered. Furthermore, muscle atrophy occurs and mitochondria are reduced in size and their capacity for aerobic metabolism is diminished, and the circulatory system is unable to maintain normal blood pressure when the patient assumes the upright position (Lamb, 1984).

Although *complete* bedrest is prescribed less commonly in modern medical practice, reduction in a patient's normal level of activity following injury or illness will result in a reduction of aerobic fitness. Therefore any rehabilitation programme following illness or injury should include general activities to improve the patient's cardiorespiratory fitness, as well as the more specific treatments aimed at his local condition (Galley and Forster, 1987).

Dynamic exercise that involves consistent contractions of the body's large muscle groups stimulates the cardiorespiratory system. To promote cardiorespiratory adaptations, these dynamic exercises should be performed over an adequate period with sufficient oxygen present — *aerobic exercise*. Cardiorespiratory adaptations occur centrally (heart) and peripherally (muscles), and it is thought that the changes incurred are probably due to interaction between these two systems, rather than one or the other (Cox, 1991).

Central Mechanisms

Aerobic exercise improves the efficiency of the cardiorespiratory system demonstrated by greater ventricular chamber size, with corresponding larger end-diastolic volumes at rest and during exercise, increase in stroke volume at rest and during exercise, and an increase in

Kate Kerr

maximal cardiac output. Blood volume also increases in response to aerobic training, enhancing the oxygen delivery capacity of the cardio-respiratory system.

Peripheral Mechanisms

An increase in the number and size of mitochondria occurs in response to aerobic training. This enables the muscle cells to extract and use oxygen more efficiently, thus improving the muscles' ability to oxidize both fat and carbohydrates. An increase in the concentration of myoglobin improves the muscles' oxygen-diffusing capacity and promotes efficient metabolic exchange.

The adaptations which occur in response to regular aerobic exercise involving progressively increasing workloads seem to improve the body's ability to respond to the challenges of increasing metabolic rates. De Vries (1980) summarized the physiological changes brought about by aerobic training:

- Lower resting heart rate;
- Lower heart rate for any submaximal workload;
- Greater maximal stroke volume;
- Lower ventilation equivalent (less ventilation required per unit of O_2 utilized);
- Greater maximal O_2 consumption;
- Less utilization of anaerobic energy sources for a given work load;
- Capacity for greater O_2 debt;
- Less displacement of physiological function by any given level of work load, and faster recovery to baseline after completion of exercise.

This basically means that with training, improved aerobic capacity will allow an individual to exercise longer, at higher workloads, with less distress to the system.

As in other types of training, the concept of overload is central to aerobic training. The American College of Sports Medicine (1990) put forward a position statement on the recommended quantity and quality of exercise for developing and maintaining cardiorespiratory fitness, body composition and muscular strength and endurance in healthy adults (see below).

Summary: Principles of Cardiovascular Endurance Training

1 *Frequency of training*: 3–5 days per week.
2 *Intensity of training*: 60–90% of maximum heart rate or 50–85% of maximum oxygen uptake (VO_{2max}).
3 *Duration of training*: 20–60 minutes of continuous aerobic activity. Duration is dependent on the intensity of the activity; thus, lower intensity activity should be conducted over a longer period of time. Because of the importance of 'total fitness' and the fact that it is more readily attained in longer duration programmes, and because of the potential hazards and compliance problems with high intensity activity, lower to moderate intensity activity of longer duration is recommended for the non-athletic adult.
4 *Mode of activity*: any activity which uses large muscle groups, and can be maintained continuously, and is rhythmic and aerobic in nature, e.g. walking, running/jogging, cycling, rowing, and swimming are appropriate activities.
5 *Resistance training*: strength training of a moderate intensity, sufficient to maintain fat-free weight should be an integral part of an adult fitness programme. One set of 8–12

repetitions of eight to ten exercises that condition the major muscle groups at least twice per week is the recommended minimum.

Further Considerations and Applications

Fatigue

Muscular fatigue is the inability to maintain or repeat the production of a given force by muscular contraction (Lamb, 1984). Fatigue of muscles during physical exercise has been experienced by everyone – its rate of onset often determines success in sport, productivity in industry/labour, and frustration in attempting to become physically fit following injury or disease.

The site of neuromuscular fatigue has been a focus for much research, and a number of possible sites have been suggested, namely the central nervous system, the final motor neurone, the neuromuscular junction and the muscle itself. Several arguments have been put forward to support each potential site, and it may well be that the source of neuromuscular fatigue is multifactorial.

Electromyographic evidence indicates that as a muscle exhibits fatigue, the amplitude of EMG output increases, indicating that more motor units are recruited in an attempt to sustain the same force of contraction. Following maximal contraction, when all the available motor units are recruited, the force of contraction declines, but the EMG remains constant, suggesting that the site of fatigue is in the muscle itself. Eventually, as the contraction continues, the contractile elements in the muscle will fail, and the EMG will decrease.

Sustained work can produce discomfort, possibly from the accumulation of lactic acid. Pain may cause the exerciser to cease working before there is any evidence that the muscles themselves can no longer sustain the contraction. Motivation and the ability to withstand pain/discomfort vary greatly among individuals, and consequently the manifestation of fatigue may vary accordingly.

The concept of fatigue must be taken into consideration when developing therapeutic exercise programmes; the level of activity must be appropriate to the individual, sufficiently intense to provide overload, but not excessive to the point of causing early onset of fatigue. Strategies for increasing motivation should be explored (setting short-term goals, improving understanding of the effects and purposes of the exercise programme), and careful planning of the exercise programme by involving different elements of muscle performance, and alternating high and low intensity work.

Closed Kinetic Chain Activities

The analysis and rehabilitation of multi-joint motion is becoming increasingly accepted as the focus of rehabilitation programmes, as a result of the growing awareness of the need to integrate motions and emphasize the whole rather than the part. This is another example of *specificity of training*, as we rarely use single joint systems in everyday functional activity. This approach relies on the concept that no single segmental movement can be performed in complete isolation, but depends on, and influences movement and/or muscle activity in other segments. This raises the concept of the *open kinetic chain* (OKC) and the *closed kinetic chain* (CKC).

The open kinetic chain can be described as a series

or chain of linked or articulated segments, the proximal of which is regarded as fixed, and the distal of which is free to move. Examples of OKCs in the body are the upper limb, in which the proximal segment is the thorax, and the distal segment is the hand, and the lower limb during non-weight-bearing activities, in which the proximal segment is the pelvis, and the distal segment is the foot when free to move through space. Examples of rehabilitation activities involving the OKC concept include free weight-lifting, in which a weight is attached to the hand or foot, and lifted freely through space (see Figure 12.12).

The closed kinetic chain is a series of articulated segments, in which the proximal and distal segments are linked, thus joining together the ends of the 'chain' and closing it. Dvir (1995) uses the example of hand-assisted rising from a chair to illustrate the CKC. As long as the hands grip the forearm rests, the chain consists of the 'articulation' between the floor and the feet, the articulated body segments leading to the hands, and back to the floor via the chair. Other examples of the CKC are prone kneeling, in which the floor

betweeen the hands and feet provides the final 'articulation' which links the ends of the chain, and double support standing, in which the floor between the feet again acts as the final linking 'articulation'.

In the closed kinetic chain, unlike the open, not only is the distal segment not free to move in an unconstrained manner, but all segments in the chain are constrained by the links they have to adjacent segments. Although not a CKC in the true sense, in that the distal and proximal segments are not necessarily linked by an 'articulation', once any distal segment is constrained in its movement, the system behaves like a CKC. Therefore, most weight-bearing activities, either of the upper or lower limbs, can be regarded as CKC activities.

Practical Task

To observe the influence of movement of one segment on other linked segments, in the upright standing position, supinate both feet; the tibia will externally rotate, as will the femurs, creating a tendency for valgus at the knee, the hips will extend, with backward tilting of the pelvis and flattening of the lumbar curve. Now observe what happens when you pronate your feet! Similarly, stretch your arm forward and grip a stable object (like a wallbar) with your palm facing downward; now laterally rotate your shoulder, and observe what happens in the upper limb as a whole.

In addition to providing a logical and functional approach to rehabilitation, CKC exercises can avoid undue stresses on structures due to excessive force production in a specific group of

Figure 12.12   Open kinetic chain exercise for the extensors of the knee. (Adapted, with permission, from Enoka, 1994, *Neuromechanical Basis of Kinesiology*, 2nd edn. Human Kinetics Publishers.)

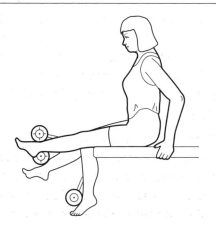

muscles. This has been extensively applied in rehabilitation following anterior cruciate ligament (ACL) reconstruction; the more traditional approach to quadriceps strengthening by lifting free weights places excess stress on the reconstructed ligament, whereas CKC activities reduces this stress by *coactivation* of hamstrings and the application of compression forces on the knee (Shelbourne and Nitz, 1990).

Coactivation refers to the concurrent activity in the muscles comprising an agonist/antagonist set. It has the mechanical effect of making a joint more stable (stiffer) and more resistant to displacement. With its function of increasing stability, coactivation would appear to be a useful feature to employ in the learning of novel tasks, tasks which require a high degree of accuracy, in tasks involving high forces, and in functional rehabilitation of muscle groups whose primary role is stability.

Enoka (1994) illustrates three types of situation in which an individual might use coactivation:

- In movements which require rapid changes in direction — it seems more economical to modulate the level of tonic activity in an agonist/antagonist group, than to turn them alternately on and off;
- In activities when individuals move heavy loads, or when high forces are applied to a joint system;
- In activities in which power may be transferred from one joint system to augment power in another. This relies on the capability of two-joint muscles to transfer power from one joint to another.

Inappropriate coactivation of opposing muscle groups can occur in pathological states involving the central nervous system, for example the rigidity experienced in Parkinson's disease.

Isokinetic Exercise

Exercise machines in which the load is controlled by gear or friction systems (e.g. Cybex, Kincom, Biodex) provide an accommodating resistance, which can generate a load which is equal in magnitude, but in an opposite direction to the force exerted by the subject. This can produce a movement in which the angular velocity of the moving segment is kept constant — *isokinetic* (Enoka, 1994).

All isokinetic systems are based on the principle that the lever arm moves at a pre-set angular velocity, however great the force applied by the user. If the user pushes harder, the muscle generated force is increased, and this tends to try to increase the speed of movement. However, the machine increases its resistance correspondingly and maintains the speed of movement within very narrow margins about the original pre-set angular velocity.

Because of the accommodating property, the resistance of the device varies in proportion to the capabilities of the user over the range of motion. Isokinetic dynamometry was introduced about 25 years ago, and has been used extensively in physiotherapy research to provide quantitative analysis of muscle performance. Dvir (1995) has quoted evidence to support the reliability of isokinetic devices when used within an accepted protocol, and to a lesser extent the validity of test findings for a number of specific dysfunctions (see also Chapter 8 for reliability and validity).

Isokinetic devices can be used with concentric and eccentric contractions, depending on the equipment available. For a concentric test, the individual pushes against the device, which controls the rate of movement of the segment, and positive work is performed. For an eccentric test, the individual must resist and control the load applied by the device, resulting in negative work. Although much of the early work done with isokinetic devices has involved laboratory-based research, isokinetic equipment is increasingly being used in training/rehabilitation settings.

Research has indicated that, as with other training methods, isokinetic training demonstrates the characteristic of specificity, with the greatest gains being achieved at the specific training speed. Speed selections in isokinetic devices range from 0° per second to 300° per second, which covers the speed of movement in a wide range of functional activities, but not some of the more sport-related activities such as jumping, running and throwing (Enoka, 1994). However, when you consider that in training programmes which use dead weights, angular velocities of 60° per second are common, and the angular velocity of the shank (lower leg) during normal speed walking reaches almost 350° per second (Winter et al., 1974, cited in Dvir, 1995), the potential value of isokinetic equipment becomes apparent.

Another significant advantage of isokinetic training is that a muscle group can be stressed differently throughout its range of motion, which means that the patient can reduce the effort at painful parts of the range, and the equipment accommodates to that effort. This is of obvious benefit in rehabilitation settings. Different characteristics of muscle performance can also be accommodated in isokinetic training, with strength training using low repetitions at low speeds, endurance training using high repetitions at high speeds, the application of diagonal patterns of movement to simulate those used in the PNF approach, and more recently the introduction of closed kinetic chain applications. The

major disadvantage of isokinetic devices in the clinical setting is their high cost!

Eccentric Exercise

Eccentric or lengthening contractions of muscle form an important aspect of everyday functional activity, and consequently should be included in any therapeutic exercise programme. It is accepted that when an active muscle is lengthened and an eccentric contraction is performed, forces are generated which are greater than those generated in either an isometric or a concentric contraction of the same muscle. Newham (1993) explained the differences in tension generation with respect to the sliding filament theory of Huxley (1974). During concentric contraction, the cross-bridge bonds are repeatedly broken as the myosin molecules move on to each new actin site, and while the bonds are broken, no active tension can be generated by the myosin molecules. This reduces the potential for total muscle force generation. Conversely, during eccentric contractions, the tension generated by the cross-bridges is increased by the force which is produced by the existing actin–myosin bonds being stretched; this force will increase until the actin–myosin bond is broken, whereupon the myosin will attach to another actin site, and further generation of tension will occur.

If eccentric contractions are capable of generating the greatest tension, it might be assumed that they would be the most effective mode of contraction to use in strengthening programmes. However, there is little evidence to support this, with no additional increase in strength found when using eccentric training, compared with concentric and isometric training (Jones and Rutherford, 1987). However, Enoka (1994) suggests that there are probably differences at submaximal levels of activation, such as the co-ordination and control of muscle activity.

However, the need for the controlling influence of eccentric contractions in functional activity is well recognized – during the gait cycle (Sutherland *et al.*, 1980), and during descending to the seated position (Kerr *et al.*, 1997) – and if the principle of specificity of training is applied, it is important within rehabilitation programmes to match the training activity to the desired functional activity. However, the particular role for eccentric exercise in rehabilitation is at present largely speculative, and little evaluation has been carried out (Newham, 1993).

The main drawback of using eccentric exercise in training, is the production of delayed onset muscle soreness (DOMS), long associated with unaccustomed eccentric muscle activity, and described as a localized soreness which appears 24–48 hours following activity (De Vries, 1980). While normal healthy subjects, and those with no specific muscle pathology recover rapidly and completely from DOMS, it is not known whether this is the case in individuals who already have some primary muscle disease (Newham, 1993).

Furthermore, precautions should be taken in the application of eccentric exercise in some patients, as there is potential for greater stress on the cardiovascular system (increased heart rate) when eccentric exercise is performed against heavy resistance. Therefore this type of exercise may not be suitable for some patients.

Manual v. Mechanical Techniques

Most forms of therapeutic exercise in rehabilitation programmes demand the application of load, which may be applied either *manually* or *mechanically.*

MANUAL TECHNIQUES

Manual resistance is a form of active resistance exercise in which the resisting force is applied by the therapist in either a static or a dynamic contraction. There are several advantages in the application of manual resistance:

- The therapist can modify the resistance in response to the patient's ability throughout the range of motion.
- The point of application of resistance can be varied in response to the desired lever arm, to avoid painful areas and to exclude areas of instability (e.g. fracture sites).
- Resistance can be applied in anatomic planes of motion, or in diagonal patterns with rotatory components as in PNF techniques (see Chapter 10)
- Both isometric and isotonic contractions can be resisted to provide emphasis.
- The patient–therapist relationship can be established, in which the patient can feel supported and encouraged by the therapist in attempting to achieve common goals.
- It is particularly useful during early stages of rehabilitation when muscle performance is poor, and when pain may be a significant element.

There are also some disadvantages:

- It is impossible to record objectively the amount of resistance applied.
- It is therapist intensive.
- It may encourage patient dependence on the therapist.
- With stronger patients, the therapist may not be able to apply sufficient resistance to constitute overload.

MECHANICAL TECHNIQUES

Mechanical techniques involve the application of force by some type of equipment, which may include free weights, weight and pulley systems, springs, extensible bands, multigyms, and isokinetic devices. As with the application of manual techniques, mechanical techniques have both advantages and disadvantages.

Advantages of mechanical techniques include the following:

- The resisting force can be recorded objectively, and consequently the overload principle applied in progressive resistance exercise.
- It is less therapist intensive.
- It allows the patient to become more independent and take more control of his treatment.
- It can be used during the more advanced stages of rehabilitation when greater resistance is necessary for overload.
- Patient motivation may be increased with knowledge of progression of loads.

Disadvantages of mechanical techniques include the following:

- The therapist no longer has the same degree of control over the patient's performance, and incorrect techniques may be used. Close supervision and attention to clear and accurate instructions may overcome this.
- Patient–therapist interaction may be reduced as the patient works more independently.
- There is less flexibility of application to adapt to the patient's response (for example, variation in strength throughout range).
- It is less easy to combine isometric and isotonic contractions to provide emphasis.

It may often be appropriate to combine both manual and mechanical techniques in a rehabilitation programme – specific manual techniques may be used to address individual identified problems of the injured part, while mechanical techniques may be used to improve the more general elements of muscle performance, both in the specific injured part, and more generally throughout the body. Thus the advantages of both approaches can be exploited, with individual problems being addressed in the one-to-one patient–therapist interaction, and patient independence and more general rehabilitation being promoted in the use of mechanical methods. Furthermore, variety and interest can be built into the programme by the integration of the two approaches.

Combined Programmes (Pyramid Training)

With the recognition that individuals often, indeed usually, require a combination of elements of muscle performance, *a pyramid training programme* has been developed to encompass a variety of aspects (see Figure 12.13). It involves exercising at different intensities (resistance) and different repetition rates. Exercising at a low number of repetitions (1–5) but at a high resistance (75–100% of resistance maximum) produces muscle strength by improving intramuscular coordination. Training at 8–10 repetitions and a resistance intensity of 40–60% resistance maximum improves strength by increasing muscle mass, and training at high repetitions (15 or more) and at a low resistance 20–40% resistance maximum will improve endurance (Gustavsen and Streeck, 1993)

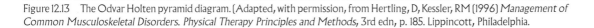
Figure 12.13   The Odvar Holten pyramid diagram. (Adapted, with permission, from Hertling, D, Kessler, RM (1996) *Management of Common Musculoskeletal Disorders. Physical Therapy Principles and Methods,* 3rd edn, p. 185. Lippincott, Philadelphia.

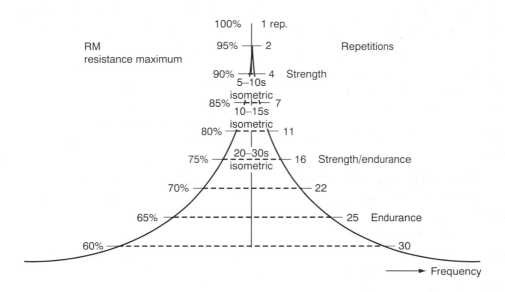

Summary

- Rehabilitation programmes should encompass a unified concept of physical fitness.
- There are five basic types of therapeutic exercise which should be included in rehabilitation programmes – strength training, flexibility training, endurance training, neuromuscular control training, and aerobic training. Strength training should include the related element of power, and attributes of neuromuscular control should include proprioception and skill.
- The twin principles of *overload* and *specificity* should be applied to all types of training. These principles relate to an organ's ability to adapt to imposed stress by creating both structural and functional changes.
- *Overload* implies the application of a demand to a structure or system, which is greater than that normally experienced by that structure or system. As the structure/system responds by adaptively changing, the magnitude of the demand must be progressively increased to maintain the overload.
- *Specificity* refers to training adaptations that are specific to the type of training imposed. Thus, for example, different training programmes are adopted by different athletes – consider the different programmes for 'power' athletes (sprinters, jumpers, throwers) and 'endurance' athletes (marathon runners, race walkers).
- *Repetition* can be built into rehabilitation programmes to improve strength and power (high resistance/low repetition), endurance (low resistance/high repetition) and skill.
- The concept of fatigue must be taken into consideration in the development of training programmes – the level of activity must provide an appropriate level of overload, but should avoid causing early fatigue.
- *Closed kinetic chain* exercises, in which the distal segment of a series of joints is not free

to move, can be used extensively in functional rehabilitation.

- *Isokinetic* dynamometers are specialized devices which can control the speed and type of muscle contraction. They can be used to train and measure different types of muscle performance (isometric, concentric, eccentric).

- Physiotherapists should make use of both manual and mechanical resistance in rehabilitation programmes. Manual resistance is particularly (but not exclusively) useful in the early stages of rehabilitation programmes, but it is time consuming, and lacks objectivity.

- As shown in this chapter, the physiotherapist has a wide range of approaches which may be incorporated into rehabilitation programmes. A sound knowledge of the principles upon which these approaches are based, and comprehensive understanding of the needs and demands of individual patients, should equip the physiotherapist with the essential information to develop specific and effective rehabilitation programmes to ensure return to maximal function.

References

American College of Sports Medicine (1990) The recommended quantity and quality of exercise for developing and maintaining cardiorespiratory and muscle fitness in healthy adults. *Medicine and Science in Sport and Exercise* **22** (2): 265–274.

Anderson, RA (1981) *Stretching*. Pelham Books, London.

Anderson, B, Burke, ER (1991) Scientific, medical and practical aspects of stretching. *Clinics in Sports Medicine* **10** (1): 63–86.

Anthony, J (1991) Psychologic aspects of exercise. *Clinics in Sports Medicine* **10** (1): 171–180.

Astrand, PO, Rodahl, K (1977) *Textbook of Work Physiology: Physiological Bases of Exercise*. McGraw Hill, New York.

Balduini, FC, Vegso, JJ, Torg, JS, Torg, E (1987) Management and rehabilitation of ligamentous injuries of the ankle. *Sports Medicine* **4** (3): 63–64, 80.

Barrett, DS, Cobb, AG, Bentley, G (1991) Joint proprioception in normal, osteoarthritic and replaced knees. *Journal of Bone and Joint Surgery (Br)* **73–B**: 53–56.

Beard, DJ, Dodd, CAF, Trundle, HR, Hamish, A, Simpson, RW (1994)

Proprioception enhancement for anterior cruciate ligament deficiency: a prospective randomised trial of two physiotherapy regimes. *Journal of Bone and Joint Surgery* **76–B** (4): 654–657.

Behm, DG, Sale, DG (1993) Intended rather than actual movement velocity determines velocity-specific training response. *Journal of Applied Physiology* **74**: 359–368.

Berger, RA (1982) *Applied Exercise Physiology*. Lea and Febiger, Philadelphiaa.

Borsa, PA, Lephart, SM, Kocker, MS, Lephart, SP (1994) Functional assessment and rehabilitation of shoulder proprioception for glenohumeral instability. *Journal of Sport Rehabilitation* **3**: 84–104.

Cox, MH (1991) Exercise training programmes and cardiorespiratory adaptation. *Clinics in Sports Medicine* **10** (1): 19–32.

DeLorme, TL (1945) Restoration of muscle power by heavy resistance exercise. *Journal of Bone and Joint Surgery* **27**: 645–667.

Derscheid, GL, Brown WC (1985) Rehabilitation of the ankle. *Clinics in Sports Medicine* **4** (3): 527–544.

De Vries, HA (1980) Physiology of exercise for physical education and athletics, 2nd edition. William Brown.

Diesfeldt, A (1977) Improving cognitive performance in psychogeriatric patients: the influence of physical exercise. *Age Ageing* **6**: 58–64.

DiNubile, NA (1991) Strength training. *Clinics in Sports Medicine* **10** (1): 33–61.

Dvir, Z (1995) *Isokinetics. Muscle Testing, Interpretation and Clinical Applications*. Churchill Livingstone, Edinburgh.

Enoka, RM (1994) Neuromechanical basis of kinesiology, 2nd edition, Human Kinetics, Champaign, IL.

Freeman, MA (1965) Co-ordination exercises in the treatment of functional instability of the foot. *Physiotherapy* **51** (12): 393–395.

Galley, PM, Forster, AL (1987) Human movement: an introductory text for physiotherapy students. Churchill Livingstone, Edinburgh.

Glencross, D, Thornton, E (1981) Position sense following joint injury. *Journal of Sports Medicine* **21**: 23–27.

Goodwin, GM, McCloskey, DI, Matthews, PBC (1972) The contribution of muscle afferents to kinaesthesia shown by vibratiion induced illusions of movement and by the effects of paralysing joint afferents. *Journal of Neurophysiology* **95**: 705–748.

Gustavsen, R, Streeck, R (1993) Training therapy; prophylaxis and rehabilitation. Thieme Medical Publishers, New York.

Guyton, AC (1981) *Textbook of Medical Physiology*, 6th edition. WB Saunders, Philadelphia.

Harms-Ringdahl, K (ed) (1993) *International Perspectives in Physical Therapy – Muscle Strength*. Churchill Livingstone, Edinburgh.

Harrelson, GL (1991) Physiologic factors of rehabilitation, in Andrews, JR, Harrelson, GL (eds) *Physical Rehabilitation of the Injured Athlete*. WB Saunders, Philadelphia.

Harris, MP, Watkins, BA (1993) Evaluation of muscle performance, in Harms-Ringdahl, K (ed) *Muscle Strength*. Churchill Livingstone, Edinburgh.

Hasan, Z, Stuart, DG (1988) Animal solutions to problems of movement control: the role of proprioceptors. *Annual Review of Neurosciences* **11**: 199–223.

Hertling, D, Kessler, RM (1996) *Management of Common Musculo-skeletal Disorders. Physical Therapy Principles and Methods*, 3rd edn, Lippincott, Philadelphia.

Huxley, HE (1974) Review lecture: muscular contraction. *Journal of Physiology (London)* **243**: 1–43.

Jones, DA, Rutherford, OM (1987) Human muscle strength training: the effects of three different regimes and the nature of resultant changes. *Journal of Physiology* **391**: 1–11.

Jones, DA, Rutherford, OM, Parker, DF (1989) Physiological changes in skeletal muscle as a result of strength training. *Quarterly Journal of Experimental Physiology* **74**: 233–256.

Kerr, KM, White, JA, Barr, DA, Mollan, RAB (1997) Analysis of the sit-stand-sit movement cycle in normal subjects. *Clinical Biomechanics* **12** (4): 236–245.

Kisner, C, Colby, LA (1996) Therapeutic exercise; foundations and techniques. 3rd ed. FA Davis, Philadelphia.

Lamb, DR (1984) *Physiology of Exercise: Responses and Adaptations.* 2nd ed. Allyn and Bacon, MA.

McArdle, WD, Katch, FI, Katch, VL (1986) Exercise physiology, energy, nutrition and human performance, 2nd ed. Lea and Febiger, Philadelphia.

McQueen, I (1954) Recent advances in the technique of progressive resistance exercise. *British Medical Journal* **2**: 328–338.

Middleton, K (1991) Range of motion and flexibility, in Andrews, JR, Harrelson, GL (eds) *Physical Rehabilitation of the Injured Athlete.* WB Saunders, Philadelphia.

Moore, MA, Hutton, RS (1980) Electromyographic investigation of muscle stretching techniques. *Medicine and Science in Sport and Exercise* **12** (5): 322–329.

Newham, DJ (1993) Eccentric muscle activity in theory and practice, in Harms-Ringdahl (ed) *Muscle Strength.* Churchill Livingstone, Edinburgh.

O'Sullivan, SB, Schmitz, TJ (1994) *Physical Rehabilitation: Assessment and Treatment.* 3rd ed. FA Davis, Philadelphia.

Peterson, SR, Bell, GJ, Bagnall, KM, Quinney, HA (1990) The effects of concentric resistance training on eccentric peak torque and muscle cross-section area. *Journal of Orthopaedic and Sports Physical Therapy* **13**: 132–137.

Revel, M, Ander-Deshays, Minquet, M (1991) Cervicocephalic kinaesthesia sessibility in patients with cervical pain. *Archives of Physical Medicine and Rehabilitation* **72** (5): 288–291.

Ryan, L (1994) Mechanical stability, muscle strength and proprioception in the functionally unstable ankle. *Australian Journal of Physiotherapy* **40** (1): 41–47.

Sale, DG (1987) Influence of exercise and training on motor unit activation, in Pandolf, KB (ed) *Exercise and Sports Science Reviews*, vol 15. McMillan, New York.

Sale, D, McDougall, D (1981) Specificity in strength training: a review for the coach and athlete. *Science Periodical on Research and Technology in Sport*, Ottawa. The Coaching Association of Canada.

Sapega, AA, Quendenfield TC (1981) Biophysical factors in range-of-motion exercise. *Physician in Sportsmedicine* **9** (12): 57–63.

Shelbourne, KD, Nitz, P (1990) Accelerated rehabilitation after anterior cruciate ligament reconstruction. *American Journal of Sports Medicine* **18**: 292–299.

Smith, RL, Brunoli, J (1989) Shoulder kinaesthesia after anterior glenohumeral joint dislocation. *Physical Therapy* **69** (2): 106–112.

Stap, LJ, Wodfin, PM (1986) Continuous passive motion in the treatment of knee flexion contracture. *Physical Therapy* **66**: 1720–1722.

Stevenson, JC, Lees, B, Davenport It Cust, NW, Granger, KF (1989) Determinants of bone density in normal women: risk factors for future osteoporosis. *British Medical Journal* **298**: 924–928.

Sutherland, DH, Cooper, L, Daniel, D (1980) The role of the ankle plantarflexors in normal walking. *Journal of Bone and Joint Surgery* **62** (3): 3 54–3 63.

Vegso, JJ, Harmon, LE (1982) Nonoperative management of athletic injuries of the ankle. *Clinics in Sports Medicine* **1** (1): 85–98.

Welford, AT (1976) *Skilled Performance: Perceptual and Motor Skills.* Scott, Foresman and Company, Glenview, Illinois.

Wickham, CAC, Walsh, K, Cooper, C, Barker, DJP, Margetts, BM, Morris, J, Bruce, SA (1989) Dietary calcium, physical activity, and the risk of hip fracture. *British Medical Journal* **299** (8): 89–892.

Wyke, B (1972) Articular neurology: a review. *Physiotherapy* **58** (3): 94–99.

13

Ergonomics

SUE HIGNETT

Introduction

This chapter provides an overview of the science and technology of ergonomics and its interrelationship with physiotherapy practice. These are two separate disciplines which have a degree of commonality in some areas of practice. The recognition that ergonomics is not merely a branch of rehabilitation or a therapy is important and the chapter will develop this point further.

Chapter Objectives

After reading this chapter, you should be able to:

- Define ergonomics and discuss where it can be applied in physiotherapy practice;
- Outline the overall approach and scope of ergonomics practice;
- Define anthropometry and discuss its use in the design of products, equipment and work stations;
- Outline the factors involved in a workplace assessment and discuss several different

methods of data collection for postural analysis;

- Discuss the use of functional capacity evaluation, work hardening and work conditioning with respect to industrial therapy;
- Discuss the potential overlap between occupational health physiotherapy and clinical ergonomics and how the skills of both disciplines can be used to optimize human physical performance.

What is Ergonomics?

Ergonomics is described as the study of human characteristics and the use of such knowledge to improve individuals' interactions with the things they use and with the environments in which they use them (Wilson and Corlett, 1995). In the USA ergonomics is generally known as 'Human Factors', however the two terms are considered to be synonymous with no difference in their practical applications (Sanders and McCormick, 1993).

In the 1990s the word 'ergonomic' became part of everyday language with many products advertised as being 'ergonomically designed'. What does this mean? Ergonomics is often described as 'designing for human beings'. This covers a wide scope of potential involvement from product design (cars, furniture, electrical goods etc.) to the design of industrial settings, with ergonomists working on the design of equipment, workplace layout and systems of work.

A comprehensive definition is given by Christensen *et al.* (1988, cited in Wilson and Corlett, 1995) which provides a good, simple, one sentence description of ergonomics.

Ergonomics is

that branch of science and technology that includes what is known and theorised about human behavioural and biological characteristics that can be validly applied to the specification, design, evaluation, operation and maintenance of products and systems to enhance safe, effective and satisfying use by individuals, groups and organisations.

Two simple objectives for ergonomics practice are:

1 To enhance the effectiveness and efficiency with which work and other activities are carried out;
2 To enhance certain desirable human values, including improved safety, reduced fatigue and stress, increased comfort, greater user acceptance, increased job satisfaction and improved quality of life (Sanders and McCormick, 1993).

It might be helpful here to consider a model (Figure 13.1) and a practical example (p. 460).

Development of Ergonomics

As with all disciplines, ergonomics is adapting to the changing world by modifying and extending its scope of practice. The interest in the relationship between people and their work is said to have

Figure 13.1 Ergonomics practice described by a simple model.

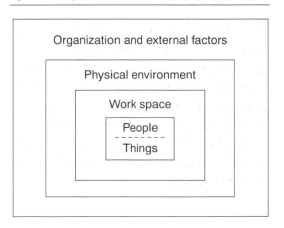

Practical Example

Most physiotherapists will be familiar with the task of giving treatment to a patient on a hospital bed, in a 'nightingale style' ward, in an acute hospital. Before treatment can be given the bed may require adjusting. The task of adjusting the bed will be used as an example to explain Figure 13.1.

At the centre of Figure 13.1 is the 'person–thing' interaction. The 'thing' is the hospital bed; some of the factors to consider in its design and usability are: is it height adjustable (hydraulic or electric)? Are the brakes accessible, their settings obvious (brake, steer or free) and do they work? Are the controls (pedals and/or hand set) labelled and the labels meaningful, i.e. the expected result occurs from activating a particular control?

Then there is the person, the physiotherapist, who will have particular physical (size, strength, dominant hand/foot etc.) and cognitive (recognition of symbols, previous experience, problem-solving etc.) personal characteristics.

The work space is a cubicle surrounded by curtains for patient privacy and dignity. This defines the dimensions of the available working space, and is likely to include a bed table, easy chair, locker, medical equipment (IV poles etc.) as well as the bed.

The personal work space exists within the larger physical environment of the ward so will be affected by noise, lighting, air flow, temperature, floor surface, and other external factors including the adjacent cubicles. The activity in neighbouring cubicles can often impinge on the work space.

How is the work organized? Does the physiotherapist carry out a number of tasks or treatments which may involve similar working positions or are a variety of different tasks planned to ensure job rotation throughout the working day?

External factors may include a number of issues, for example: (1) Legal – health and safety legislation, product liability law, British and European design standard etc. (2) Social – what are the patients' expectations on being admitted to hospital? The term 'pyjama paralysis' has been used to describe the phenomenon of a patient walking independently into the hospital, putting on pyjamas and then being pushed in a wheelchair when she/he is capable of walking. (3) Technological – advances in the design and technology will change the type of equipment being used and the type of treatment being offered. The work of a physiotherapist has changed over the years to reflect advances in medical and surgical knowledge and technology. (4) Financial – this is a very wide ranging factor which can impinge on issues about staffing levels, number of beds on the ward and availability or suitability of equipment.

started during the First World War when the drive for increased productivity in munitions factories created unexpected complications (Oborne, 1995). The term 'ergonomics' was first used in 1950, again following activity in the Second World War, when the ineffective use of equipment and systems designed to help the war effort was found to be due to lack of knowledge about people's performance capabilities and limitations. Since its initial inception ergonomics has developed from use solely in military engineering, through to space applications in the 1950s and on to wider industrial usage in the subsequent 30 years (pharmaceuticals, computers, cars and other consumer products). In the 1990s the role of ergonomics was recognized in human error prediction or post-disaster analysis, e.g. Chernobyl, Clapham rail crash and even the Grand National fiasco in 1993 (Reason, 1990; Sanders and McCormick, 1993; Wilson and Corlett, 1995). Many disasters are found to have a contributory factor of 'human error'. This is often due to a mismatch between the human capabilities and the task requirements.

In the UK there has been increased interest in ergonomics partly due to raised awareness of employers following the introduction of specific health and safety legislation, in particular Manual Handling Operations Regulations 1992 and Display Screen Equipment Regulations 1992. Ergonomics has also entered the legal world with ergonomists employed as consultants or expert witnesses for personal injury and product liability litigation.

Scope of Ergonomics Practice

Ergonomics is a science and a technology based on research, knowledge and skills from a multidisciplinary field. Oborne (1995) provides a grouped framework which identifies three branches as shown below.

1 Medicine: including physiology, anatomy and biomechanics. Providing information on physical capabilities and limitations.
2 Psychology: physiological and experimental. Physiological psychology looks at the nervous system and behaviour, whereas experimental psychology studies cognitive functions, e.g. perception, learning, memory.
3 Physics and engineering: studying the products, tools, equipment and environment with which people interact.

This multidisciplinary collaboration enables a wide scope of approaches and practical methods to be used. Figure 13.2 shows the integration of two of the branches. Medicine and psychology on one side bring a scientific structure, and on the other side technology represents the input of physics and engineering, looking at people as part of a system, interacting with tools, machinery,

Figure 13.2 Ergonomics as a science and a technology.

Science Medicine / Psychology	Ergonomics	Technology Physics and Engineering
Combined approach of anatomy, physiology, biomechanics and psychology	⟺	People as integral component of a working system
Assessment of workload and stress, usually in a laboratory		Allocation of function or tasks between people, machine and procedures

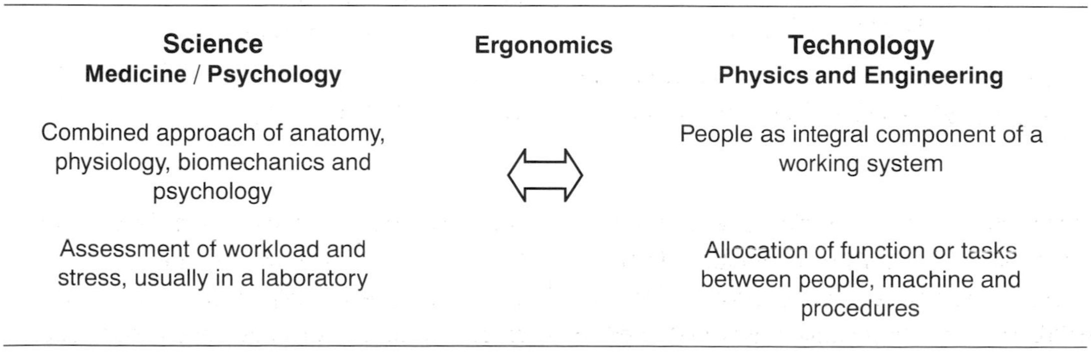

software, and other people. Wilson and Corlett (1995) provide a more detailed discussion on the definition of ergonomics as a science and a technology.

When considering the scope of practice of ergonomics there is also potential for input at an organizational level. The following three broad categories will be used to identify the specialist areas within ergonomics for the purpose of this chapter:

1 *Physical ergonomics.* The study and assessment of the physical design of the workplace and work tasks. This includes the identification of features which influence a person's performance at work and how the knowledge of structure and functioning of the human body is applied in the evaluation and design of work situations. This category effectively encompasses both the 'Medicine' and 'Physics and engineering' branches in Figure 13.2.

2 *Cognitive ergonomics.* This is very similar to the 'psychology' branch and studies how humans process information (perception, attention, memory) from a range of inputs including visual, auditory and tactile. It is beyond the scope of this chapter to cover this in detail and further reading is recommended at the end of the chapter.

3 *Organizational ergonomics.* This is a broader category than the branches defined above to

include the effectiveness and efficiency of an organization with respect to the management structure (e.g. vertical/horizontal), processes of work (including job design and analysis) and the attitude and behaviour of people in the organization as well as the implementation of change. Again, this is a specialist area and will not be taken any further here.

With such a large base for ergonomics practice there are many methodologies used. Individual ergonomists bring specialist skills, often related to a first degree or previous professional background (e.g. physiotherapy). Additionally, there are methods and techniques which have been developed within ergonomics. These often combine a range of approaches to give the 'full picture', including physical, cognitive and organizational factors. A detailed account of methodologies is given in Wilson and Corlett (1995). The area of physical ergonomics will be expanded in the next section, in particular with respect to anthropometry and postural analysis.

Table 13.1 gives a summary of the range of activities and interests of ergonomists which are used to deliver the full scope of ergonomics input. Grandjean (1988), Oborne (1995) and Pheasant (1991) provide useful further reading.

Table 13.1
Scope of ergonomics input

1	Collection and collation of data about people – abilities and limitations
2	Contribution to the design process
3	Evaluation of people–machine system performance
4	Evaluation of effects on people working in/with the system
5	Development of strategies and organization for ergonomics

Variety of Professional Backgrounds

The discipline of ergonomics is fairly unique compared with many other professions in that, for the most part, it is practised by people from a variety of related professional backgrounds with or without a formal education in ergonomics (Bullock, 1994) As suggested earlier this can be beneficial with additional skills and experience being brought into ergonomics, and it is possible to gain an insight into the practice of ergonomics by looking at the range of possible backgrounds of ergonomics practitioners (Table 13.2).

In the USA most of the members of 'The Human Factors Society' (the American equivalent to the British Ergonomics Society) have a background in psychology (45%) and engineering (19%) with only 3% coming from the medical field (Sanders and McCormick, 1993). This is believed to be a similar proportion to 'The Ergonomics Society' in the UK although the definitive figures are not known, and is in contrast to elsewhere in the world, for example, Norway, where most of the ergonomics practised in industrial settings is by ergonomists with a background in physiotherapy (Bullock, 1990). The professional backgrounds and specialist skills may be reflected in the approach or area of interest of the ergonomist,

e.g. a systems engineer may feel that the ability to carry through the design, development and implementation of a specific workstation, tool or piece of equipment is of particular importance, whereas a physiotherapist may be more concerned with a specific musculoskeletal risk factor and modifications to the workstation, task or tools to eliminate or reduce the risk of injury.

Ergonomics in Physiotherapy Practice

Ergonomics can be used in physiotherapy practice in a number of areas. The following three examples will be used to give some indication of the scope of ergonomic applications.

1 Risk of injury to the physiotherapist;
2 Advice given by physiotherapists to patients returning to manual activities (both work and leisure);
3 Physiotherapists and manual handling training.

Risk of Injury to the Physiotherapist

It has been suggested that physiotherapists can be under considerable physical loading due to the nature of their work (Hignett, 1995). Scholey and Hair published a study in 1989 which found

Table 13.2
Background qualifications and experience of ergonomists

- Psychology
- Engineering
- Ergonomics (undergraduate)
- Industrial design
- Education
- Physiology
- Medicine
- Paramedical (physiotherapy, occupational therapy)
- Business administration
- Computer science
- Occupational hygiene

that physiotherapists had a similar annual incidence, point and life-time prevalence and recurrence rate of low back pain (LBP) to a matched control group. Molumphy et al. (1985) found that the majority of physiotherapists tended to have their first attack of LBP within the first 4 years of working as a physiotherapist.

A criticism sometimes aimed at physiotherapy is the relatively limited research base for many of the methods and techniques used. With health and safety legislation in the European Community now focusing on the risk of injury from manual handling activities, the justification for many physiotherapy techniques must again be called into question when the safety and well-being of physiotherapists may be compromised. More information is given about health and safety legislation in the section on physiotherapists and manual handling training. Manual handling risks faced by physiotherapists may include the following.

Equipment This includes equipment such as wheelchairs, walking aids, standing frames and departmental furniture. The selection of equipment should be based primarily on treatment requirements but also on safety factors for both the patient and physiotherapist. Equipment design will be considered further in the section on anthropometry.

'Hands on' treatment One way of differentiating between care handling and treatment handling is in the definition of primary task. If a patient is being taken to the toilet (primary task) by a nurse then the safest possible transfer method should be used; this may require hoisting equipment. The actual transfer process is the secondary task, being carried out in order to achieve the primary task. If a patient is having walking practice with a physiotherapist, then the primary task is the rehabilitation of mobility skills. In order to deliver this

the physiotherapist will have to consider the selection of treatment technique as well as the safety of the patient and themselves. This may, on occasion, result in the physiotherapist being placed in a position of risk in order to advance the patient's ability (Hignett, 1994). Any foreseeable manual handling risks involving patient treatment are subject to the Manual Handling Operations (MHO) regulations (Manual Handling, 1992); advice should always be sought from a senior physiotherapist or manager and, if appropriate, a risk assessment carried out.

Working posture An area of concern which has been highlighted by the MHO regulations is working posture. One example is the working posture which may be required to provide respiratory therapy at a bedside. The issues raised earlier in the chapter with respect to the design of beds may be limiting factors. If the bed is not height adjustable (e.g. in a community setting) it may not be possible to 'fit the bed to the physiotherapist' and instead the physiotherapist may have to kneel, stoop or crouch to deliver the treatment. There will be other examples of this type of awkward working posture which the reader will be able to identify from personal experience.

HOW CAN THESE RISKS BE CONTROLLED?

Ergonomics has a role to play, using assessment techniques to evaluate the risk to the physiotherapist (Hignett, 1995), in the redesign of the workplace and working environment (Fenety and Kumar, 1992). The latter study identified that the use of mechanical aids was not always an option in rehabilitation where treatment handling was being performed and succeeded in identifying some simple ergonomic solutions to improve both the daily work organization and the physical environment.

As part of a MHO risk assessment, a survey of musculoskeletal discomfort was carried out amongst physiotherapists working with neurological patients at an acute hospital. It was found that over a 12-month period more than 70% had back pain and over 50% had neck pain. This led to the development of a minimum data set of questions to be asked before any treatment was undertaken (Hignett, 1996). This list is not exclusive and readers will probably be able to suggest modifications based on their own experience.

- What are the goals of treatment?
- What will the treatment make a difference to? Consider home circumstances, other treatment, support etc.
- Treatment should be selected or modified based on individual patient needs and the staffing levels available to assist.
- No treatment should be given on the floor unless appropriate equipment is available to safely raise the patient from the floor if they are unable to get up.
- Is the patient ready for standing transfers? If not, then only safe transfers (e.g. using a hoist) should be used until all the rehabilitation stages have been successfully completed prior to standing transfers.
- Can treatment be given in the wheelchair to avoid a transfer?
- Is the patient on a suitable bed for respiratory physiotherapy? If not, can alternative arrangements be made?
- Patients should be carefully selected for treatment. Pre-operative assessments should include an indication of the amount of post-operative mobility assistance which it is practicable to provide with respect to the equipment and number of staff available (e.g. bilateral total hip replacements).

Physiotherapy Advice

The second area is the advice that physiotherapists give to their patients when they are returning to a job or leisure activity, and it is in this area of occupational health that the physiotherapist has much to offer ergonomics. Physiotherapists are taught to be analytical about injury mechanism in order to be able to apply an appropriate treatment technique to alleviate symptoms, and a logical extension to this is the elimination of factors which contributed to the overuse of the bodily structures involved. For example, the design of a workstation contributing to the development of neck or back pain. There is potential for the physiotherapist to get involved in workplace and workstation assessments, using ergonomic techniques, to recommend improvements to eliminate or minimize the risk of re-injury.

Occupational health physiotherapists have a specialist role to play in workplace and workstation assessment and this role will be discussed further in the section on occupational health physiotherapy. Requests for input have been both proactive, via risk assessments and recommendations for improvements, and reactive in the management of a problem after an accident or incident has occurred.

BACK SCHOOLS

The back school approach for treatment is used in some areas of the UK for both acute and chronic sufferers of low back pain. As ergonomics is often a component part of the programme it is worth looking at the development of this approach and reviewing some of the research.

In the 1950s Hans Kraus devised a formalized education programme for back pain sufferers including exercise, relaxation and stretching, and strengthening. In the 1960s this trend continued with the development of the Californian Back School to include aspects of behaviours to reinforce health and ignore sick behaviours (Isernhagen, 1995). One of best known back school programmes is the Swedish Back School which gives instruction to low back pain sufferers in exercises, ergonomic techniques and the psychological aspects of low back pain. Zachrisson-Forssell (1980, 1981) reported that the Swedish Back School achieved a significant improvement in back pain sufferers with respect to length of sickness absence.

However, there have been a number of criticisms levelled at the back school approach, in particular focusing on the Swedish Back School (Berwick *et al.*, 1989). It was found in follow-up studies that longer term relapse rates remained unaffected. Additionally at least two controlled prospective studies (Lankhorst *et al.*, 1983; Lindquist *et al.*, 1984) found no effect of back school instruction on pain, function or sick leave at a one-year follow-up. These disappointing results contrast with anecdotal patient treatments and reports from uncontrolled trials. Klaber Moffett *et al.* (1986) carried out a study looking at the effectiveness of back school (based on the Swedish Back School) which found an improvement in both functional disability and pain levels for chronic low back pain sufferers. This programme has been developed further into a progressive rehabilitation exercise programme (Frost and Klaber Moffett, 1992) using a team approach (physiotherapists, occupational therapists, nurses, psychologists and medical staff) which is yet to be evaluated.

From an ergonomic perspective Buckle and Stubbs (1989) suggest that there is a fundamental divergence between the back school philosophy and an ergonomic approach. They suggest that many of the back school programmes have the same educational input on specific topics appertaining to ergonomics (e.g. biomechanics of the spine, lifting loads, and chair lumbar supports) but do not place them in the context of jobs and tasks or show that ergonomics is about the design of work and work systems to fit the capabilities of the user. So the cause of an injury may not be specifically addressed and the patient may return to work to be faced with the same injurious factors.

Physiotherapists and Manual Handling Training

In 1992 a series of *Guidance on Regulations* were published by the Health and Safety Executive. These aimed to assist employers in the implementation of health and safety directives from the European Commission. The framework directive, the *Management of Health and Safety at Work Regulations* (1992) extended the Health and Safety at Work Act, 1974 by setting out guidance for implementing a process of risk management. This process requires that a risk assessment be carried out to identify, assess and control risks to the health and safety of employees.

Manual handling operations are defined as 'any transportation or supporting of a load (including the lifting, putting down, pushing, pulling, carrying or moving thereof) by hand or by bodily force'. This covers a wide range of activities and the regulations have been a topic of much discussion in the physiotherapy profession. The Chartered Society of Physiotherapy (CSP) has a Moving and Handling Development Group which acts in an advisory role to the Professional Affairs Department. There is also a *Moving and*

Handling Pack available from the CSP which gives advice about a wide range of issues, from personal injury to acting as an expert witness in a training capacity.

There has been a tendency within the health care industry to use physiotherapists as a pool of in-house experts but without always providing the appropriate ergonomic training to enable them to deliver the service required. Frost and McCay (1990) described a cascade system used in an NHS Hospital Trust to provide lifting and handling training, which was quoted as including ergonomics and biomechanics. They used the hospital physiotherapists as part of The Prevention of Injury Group (TPIG) and found that one problem was the lack of formal ergonomics training within the group (although some members had limited knowledge).

In 1995 Crumpton carried out an extensive questionnaire survey of back care advisors in the UK. She found that of the physiotherapists employed in this role, 57% claimed to have had some training in ergonomics, but for 75% of these the training was limited to 1–3 day courses. She concluded that a greater awareness of the scope of ergonomics practice was needed in order to ensure that personal limitations were recognized. This topic will be discussed in more detail in the next section.

Occupational Health Physiotherapy

In the early days of physiotherapy, the fundamental intent was to 'assess, prevent and treat movement dysfunction and physical disability, with the overall goal of enhancing human movement and function' (Jacobs and Bettencourt, 1995). The scope of physiotherapy practice has extended well beyond this simple intention to include health promotion, fitness training, incontinence treatments etc., and also into the field of occupational health where physiotherapists may be required to have both proactive (preventative) and reactive (treatment) roles.

The Chartered Society of Physiotherapy (UK) has many specialist groups for both clinical interest and occupational practice. One of these is the Association of Chartered Physiotherapists in Occupational Health (ACPOH) which was founded in 1947 as the Association of Chartered Physiotherapists in Industry (ACPI) and renamed in 1985. As the title suggests this group was originally set up to provide a support network for physiotherapists working in industries other than the NHS. Richardson and Eastlake (1994) describe changes in the scope of practice of occupational health physiotherapy. This has increased over the last 50 years with the development of occupational health services and may now require knowledge and expertise in many specialist areas in addition to traditional physiotherapy skills.

The Chartered Society of Physiotherapy has produced a leaflet (*Physiotherapy and Occupational Health*) outlining the range of skills (Table 13.3) which they suggest should be available from a chartered occupational health physiotherapist.

Table 13.3
Skills of an occupational health physiotherapist

- Expert in human movement
- Advice to prevent further injury and help to speed recovery
- Evaluation of human–task–machine relationships (the study of ergonomics) and indentification of problem areas which could cause pain
- Specialized training in ergonomics and occupational health etc.

The scope of the occupational health physiotherapist in the UK has tended to be limited to an advisory role. Oldham (1988), for example, has recommended general fitness criteria for return to work after a major sickness absence, such that the worker should be able to:

1 Work a full normal day (8 hours) and work without undue fatigue and exhaustion or making the medical condition worse, or temporary part-time work may be needed.
2 Commute to and from work, and move around freely within the work environment.
3 Work safely and without creating a hazard to self, others or equipment.
4 Concentrate enough to function normally.

McPhee (1984) believes that many physiotherapeutic skills are wasted if only treatment services are provided. Worker rehabilitation should form a large part of the treatment. She states that if physiotherapists are to play a part in occupational health and ergonomics and develop the relevant skills they must first identify the areas where their expertise can be used most appropriately. McAtamney (1991) suggested that physiotherapists were well qualified to provide advice on aspects of physical ergonomics. They have expertise in and knowledge about the effect of loads and forces on the musculoskeletal system, of work physiology and in the prevention and treatment of musculoskeletal disorders.

So what level of knowledge in ergonomics is required by physiotherapists? How much detail is required? And how can this knowledge be obtained?

Knowledge in Ergonomics

Ferguson (1983) advocated three levels of education in ergonomics:

1 The level appropriate for all professionals to provide background knowledge. This can be gained as part of undergraduate physiotherapy education or a short 3–5 day course.
2 The level relevant to the professional person planning to apply ergonomics within their professional activity. A certificate or diploma in occupational health physiotherapy (approximately 6 months) would provide adequate training for ergonomic principles to be used by an occupational health physiotherapist.
3 The level needed by the professional working full-time in ergonomics. This would require postgraduate education (M.Sc. or Ph.D.), on a course recognized by the Ergonomics Society (UK), which provided the data set of core competencies suggested by Bullock (1994) and CREE (Appendix 1).

The interpretation of this role has already been seen in other countries, in particular in Scandinavia where ergonomics is a profession dominated by physiotherapists (Bullock, 1994). The preventive role includes job analysis, work posture monitoring, task design, personnel selection and placement, education, supervision of work methods, influencing motivation and attitudes, provision of activity breaks and physical fitness programmes. These topics will be discussed in more detail in the section on workplace assessment and postural analysis.

Physical Ergonomics

It is within the area of physical ergonomics that physiotherapists can bring much knowledge, experience and expertise. The scope of physical ergonomics includes anthropometry, postural analysis, biomechanics, work physiology and interface design. Many tools for both general workplace analysis and specific task analysis have been developed and a number of these will be mentioned.

Anthropometry

Anthropometry is the science of measuring and studying human body measurements (dimensions and composition). Once anthropometric measurements are known they can be used to design equipment and workstations to 'fit' a group or population of identified users (Pheasant, 1986).

ANTHROPOMETRIC DIMENSIONS

Anthropometric dimensions are available for a number of population groups giving ranges for age, sex and race. Figure 13.3 shows (a) a range of dimensions which have been measured, and (b) elbow height.

The variability of most bodily dimensions can be expressed as a normal distribution (Figure 13.4). The normal distribution is described by the mean (50th percentile) and the standard deviation (SD) or measure of dispersion. The standard deviation gives an indication of the extent to which a dimension might vary from the mean. An example of the gross application of this information in worker selection could be UK fire officers. There is a minimum height requirement of 5ft 6in. (Meikle, 1997) so this group or population would tend to have a mean height higher than the rest of the adult UK female population, but to have a narrower spread (or standard deviation).

The normal distribution curve (Figure 13.4) is symmetrical about the 50th percentile point, which is the most common value (highest frequency); the frequency then decreases on both sides of the curve to give dimensions only found, for example in 1:20 of the population (5th

Figure 13.3   (a) Anthropometric dimensions. (b) Elbow height. Reproduced from Peoplesize with permission of Friendly Systems Ltd.

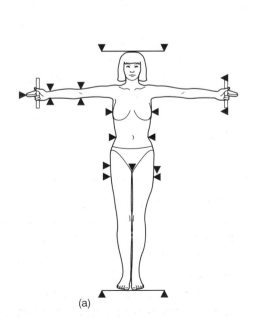
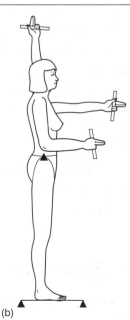

(a) (b)

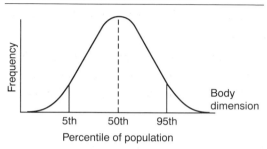

Figure 13.4 Example of normal distribution.

percentile/95th percentile). If the bodily dimension being considered is stature then for UK adult women (19–65 years) the 50th percentile height is 1610 mm (SD ± 62 mm), approximately 5ft 3in., with only 1:20 being above 1710 mm, 95th percentile approximately 5ft 5in., or below 1505 mm, 5th percentile approximately 4ft 7in. (Pheasant, 1996). Using the above example for fire officers, approximately 90% of UK adult women would be prevented from entering the fire brigade due to the height requirements (Meikle, 1997).

Pheasant (1986, 1996) provides extremely useful anthropometric data tables for population groups. The groups vary with respect to sex, age and race, and there are also dimensions for wheelchair users which are very useful when designing buildings and facilities for health care use and public access.

DESIGNING FOR DISABLED POPULATIONS

Hobson and Molenbroek (1990) describe a study which looked at the difference in anthropometric dimensions of disabled individuals compared with able-bodied. It aimed to develop anthropometric guidelines for designers concerned with the development and provision of improved specialized seating and mobility devices for a defined segment of non-ambulatory population. They found that disability type may markedly affect the dis-tributions of body dimensions, therefore there is a need for differentiation between disability types as well as age, race, sex etc. So, for example, in the cerebral palsy population there would need to be anthropometric information on body segment dimensions and ranges of spatial orientation of body segments. Jacobs and Bettencourt (1995) also identified the difficulties of designing for populations when few data exist on the anthropometric characteristics, capabilities and limitations of individuals with specific disabilities or elderly populations in varying climates and conditions. They concluded that until the abilities and restrictions of such populations are identified suitable products will not be developed on a consistent basis.

With the introduction of the Disability Discrimination Act (1995) there is an onus on the employer to ensure that appropriate facilities (access, equipment etc.) are provided for all employees. Physiotherapists and occupational therapists can offer considerable expertise in this area and will be able to apply their knowledge to the benefit of many employees.

EQUIPMENT DESIGN

Physiotherapists will use a range of different equipment throughout their working life. Some will be specifically designed for the task (often by or in conjunction with physiotherapists) but much will be general departmental, ward and clinic furniture. The design of this equipment can have a significant bearing on the risk of musculoskeletal injury to the physiotherapist.

Ergonomics can be used to help to ensure that mismatches do not occur between the equipment and the proposed users. It has often been said that equipment and furniture for the health care industry is 'manufacturer led' rather than being 'user led'. Ergonomics has considerable scope for input here throughout the design process and in the evaluation of products and equipment to ensure that they are 'fit for purpose'.

Before considering the design of a product or workstation there are a number of 'design fallacies' (Table 13.4) which have been coined by Pheasant (1986, 1996) with respect to the use of ergonomics in design.

Medical Equipment

The NHS is the largest purchaser of medical equipment in the UK (approximately 85% of the market). The changes in the structure of the NHS in the 1990s (with NHS Trusts and GP budget-holders) have resulted in more autonomy and should lead to greater competition for medical equipment sales. This will hopefully place the purchaser in a position of being able to lead the manufacturer with respect to product and equipment design.

An example of the use of ergonomics in product evaluation is given in the practical example on p. 472 looking at hospital transit wheelchairs.

THE DESIGN OF A WORK STATION

The expansion of information technology in the 1990s has led to a proliferation of display screen equipment, both with personal computers and via main frames, which has resulted in a transformation in many places of work. Many of the patients treated by physiotherapists will be returning to a desk-based job and will need basic information about the layout and location of their workstation.

Table 13.4
Design fallacies (based on Pheasant, 1986)

- *Designer as typical.* The designer assumes that they are a 'typical' person and designs for themselves. An example of this might be the height of mirrors in bathrooms, 'it must have been put up by a man' when the mirror is too high for the female users!

- *Design for average.* An average design is produced which does not reflect the wide range of shapes and sizes (and ages) of the user population. This would be like a one size T-shirt, much too large for some and much too small for others.

- *Too much human variability.* An excuse sometimes put forward for not incorporating ergonomics at the design stage is that the range of users would be too great and it would be impossible to design to 'fit' all. In this case a critical case limit can be set which identifies a specific user group likely to include all potential users. More detail about three constraints (reach, clearance and posture) is given in the section on display screen equipment.

- *The 'Procrustean' approach* assumes that humans are infinitely adaptable to any design or layout, they can stretch if something is too high, or bend if it is too low etc. Procrustes was a character from Greek mythology who could be likened to a modern day 'bed and breakfast' landlord where there is only one bed which is advertized to 'fit all'. Procrustes achieved the fit by stretching the traveller (on a rack) if they were too short or chopping off the excess leg length if they were too tall!

- *Some errors are design induced.* Errors which are likely and foreseeable should have been considered at the design stage and allowances made. This is a legal requirement under product liability and safety legislation. An example might be colour coding where red/green differentiation should not be used for important controls when a percentage of the male population is likely to be red/green colour blind.

Practical Example

In order to select a transit wheelchair for use in a large teaching hospital an ergonomic product evaluation was carried out. The initial stage was to ascertain the types of transit wheelchairs available and request samples of each to participate in the trial. Three types of chair were identified, two of which are shown in Figures 13.5(a) and (b).

A representative user population was defined to include portering and nursing staff, therapy assistants and outpatient assistants. Data were collected about the user group including: sex, and age (to identify the anthropometric population); grip diameter and elbow height (relevant anthropometric dimensions); job title (range of tasks normally undertaken); and years in job (experience). Although convenience sampling was used, a profile of the subjects showed an almost normal distribution with respect to sex; age and grip diameter. A slight skew was recorded with respect to elbow height, with a higher proportion below 50th percentile; and years in job with slightly more in the < 10 year group.

Four tests were carried out on each chair:

1 A data sheet was complied with engineering and maintenance information, and relevant ergonomic dimensions.
2 A user evaluation, where the user was the member of staff propelling the wheelchair. The chairs were presented to each user in a randomized order to eliminate bias. Data were collected using individual rating questionnaires, comparative ranking, rated perceived exertion (RPE), postural analysis (OWAS), speed for a 10-metre distance and total trial time. Photographs were taken to be used for postural analysis. It is interesting to note that a range of hand grips were used to propel the chairs (Figure 13.6(a)–(c)).
3 Client (sitter) evaluation was not a major objective of this trial. However, each chair was tested by experienced wheelchair users and rated with respect to comfort, arm rests, foot plates, transferring and overall impression.
4. Expert opinion was sought from therapists with respect to transfers and pressure care.

Findings included quality issues for the welding, brakes and finish, and safety issues about stability and spoke guards. The dimensions of the chairs were compared with respect to width, length and weight (overall and component parts). Interestingly there was found to be a wide variation in the height of handles, from 86.5 cm to 104 cm (floor to handle height) and this was reflected by the user rating results, preferring the mid-range handle height of approximately 95 cm. A particularly worrying finding was that none of the wheelchairs had operating instructions attached to the chair. As it was foreseeable that the chairs might be propelled by relatives or visitors this was felt to be essential for future transit wheelchairs.

The ergonomic evaluation resulted in the development of a product specification, which was used to order replacement transit wheelchairs.

Figures 13.5   Two types of wheelchair.

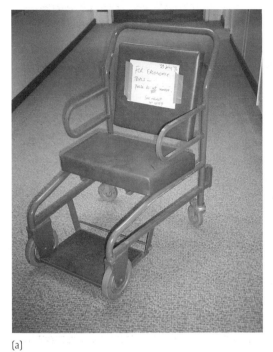

(a)

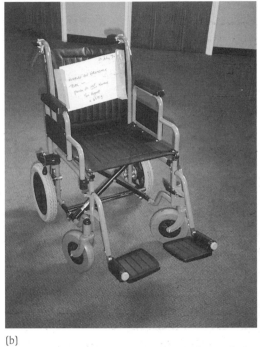

(b)

Figures 13.6   Different handgrips used to push the wheelchairs.

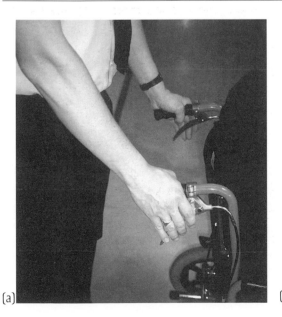

(a)

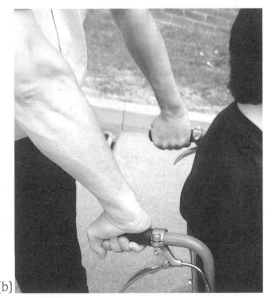

(b)

Figures 13.6   continued.

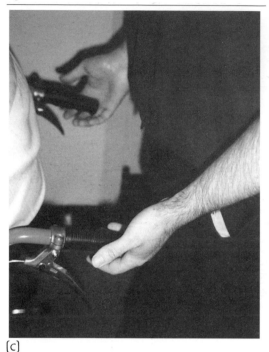

(c)

Display Screen Equipment (DSE)

Before looking at the workstation in detail, there are three anthropometric dimensions, commonly known as constraints, which are generally considered when designing a workstation. These are (1) clearance, (2) reach and (3) posture. Pheasant (1986, 1996) gives a detailed explanation of these constraints which has been summarized below. To design a work station using anthropometric data, the user population must first be defined and a range of 5th female–95th male percentile users is often used for the critical case limits.

- *Clearance* refers to the space required for head, knee and elbow room. This is used as a one-way constraint to accommodate the largest user. For example working at a reception counter in a seated posture, the largest user would be identified, possibly 95th percentile male, who would require a minimum leg space depth of about 470 mm to permit the receptionist to stretch their legs under the counter while seated.

- *Reach* is also a one-way constraint but in the opposite direction to accommodate the smallest user. For the reception counter the distance that the receptionist might have to reach across the counter to serve a client will be limited by the smallest user (probably 5th percentile female) which would give a maximum reach distance of about 650 mm. These two constraints give guidance on the depth of reception counter to the architect so that the maximum depth of the counter is 650 mm, and the minimum depth is 450 mm.

- *Posture* is the third anthropometric constraint which should be considered when designing a workstation. This is a two-way constraint to accommodate the largest and smallest users. In the above example the height of the reception counter would need to be specified on the basis of a defined range of potential users. So in a health care setting it would be appropriate to have more than one height of reception counter to allow for both standing and seated (e.g. wheelchair) users. If the counter was put at the correct working height for the tallest user the smallest users would be constantly stretching up, whereas if it was set for the smallest user the tallest users would be working stooped. A compromise must be chosen, preferably with the option of more than one height being available to fit as many users as possible.

Figure 13.7 shows basic dimensions which should be considered when assessing a DSE work station; the correct dimensions will depend on the worker. However, with the advent of 'hot desking' or 'hotelling' (shared work stations) there needs to be an element of adaptability built into all DSE work stations. This is achieved by having two out of the following three components adjustable:

Figure 13.7   Display screen equipment. Work station dimensions.

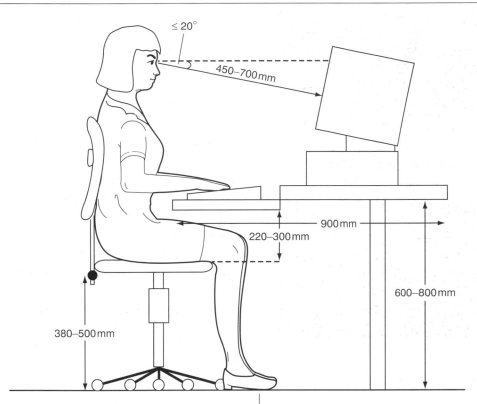

- Desk – adjustable height desks are available, but tend to be the most expensive option.
- Chair – adjustable height chairs are becoming standard for most DSE workstations. The range of height of the gas lift can be altered by having different length 'stems' fitted to the chair.
- Floor – this is easily adjusted by using either a foot rest on the floor or a foot ring around the chair stem.

There are additional considerations when assessing or designing a display screen workstation. The next section gives an example of some of the other factors which should be considered as part of a full ergonomic workplace assessment e.g. the work flow, rest pauses, layout of the rest of the workstation, lighting, air flow, temperature, noise etc.

Workplace Assessment and Postural Analysis

Traditional physiotherapy undergraduate courses teach physiotherapists how to assess and analyse human movement. To take this a stage further and assess the physical workplace and working postures there are a number of ergonomic techniques and methods which can be used. However, as with all methods of assessment, specialist training and practice is required before they can be used reliably. Before describing some of the different methods and techniques which are available it is appropriate to remember that all have a trade-off between the cost and the time required to perform the observation and analysis, the level of detail recorded and the type of occupation observed. The more complex the system of data collection used, the greater the limitation of the method for general applicability (Foreman et al., 1988).

WORKPLACE ASSESSMENT

Postural analysis should always take place as part of a wider ergonomic assessment and there are a number of multi-factor tools available (Wilson and Corlett, 1995). In this chapter only one tool will be discussed, ergonomic workplace analysis (EWA). This is an example of a multi-factor assessment method which can be used to screen a workplace and then followed up with more detailed analysis.

Ergonomic workplace analysis was developed by the Finnish Institute of Occupational Health (1989) to be used as a detailed analysis after initial identification of ergonomic problems had been carried out. The workplace is analysed according to 14 different items (Table 13.5) chosen to represent quantifiable factors which were important to the design and operation of a safe, healthy and productive workplace.

The scoring is done by both a worker and an ergonomist using assessments of the above factors. Areas of risk are identified by analysing the combined results. Following this initial screening more detailed assessment may be required and for factors 2, 3 and 4 there are a number of postural analysis methods which can be used.

On a more practical level, Corlett (1978) provided a list of basic principles for the design of workplaces to take account of human physical and cognitive needs.

1 The worker should be able to maintain an upright and forward facing posture during work.
2 Where vision is a requirement of the task, the necessary work points must be adequately visible with the head and trunk upright or with just the head inclined slightly forward.
3 All work activities should permit the worker to adopt several different, but equally healthy and

Table 13.5
Ergonomic work place analysis

---
1 Work site: horizontal work area, working height, viewing, leg space, seat, hand tools.
2 General physical activity: light, medium or heavy work, rest breaks, autonomy of worker.
3 Lifting: height, holding distance, weight.
4 Work posture and movement: position of neck–shoulders, elbow–wrist, back, hips–legs. Movement of body required by the work.
5 Accident risk: hazard analysis, possibility of accident occurring and severity.
6 Job content: number and quality of individual tasks included in the work.
7 Job restrictiveness: limitation to move and choose when and how the work is done.
8 Worker communication: opportunities for interacting with colleagues.
9 Decision-making: difficulty of decision-making, availability of information, risks involved in decision-making.
10 Repetitiveness of work: average length of repeated work cycle.
11 Attentiveness: attention and observation required by instruments, machines, displays, controls, processes etc.
12 Lighting: evaluated according to type of work.
13 Thermal environment: temperature, humidity, air velocity, thermal radiation, workload and clothing used.
14 Noise: assessed according to type of work done
---

safe, postures without reducing the capability to do the work.

4 Work should be arranged so that is may be done, at the worker's choice, in either a seated or standing position. When seated, the worker should be able to use the back rest of the chair at will, without necessitating a change of movements.

5 The weight of the body when standing should be carried equally on both feet, and foot pedals designed accordingly.

6 Work activities should be performed with the joints at about mid-point of their range of movement. This applies particularly to the head, trunk and upper limbs.

7 Where muscular force has to be exerted it should be by the largest appropriate muscle group available and in a direction colinear with the limbs concerned.

8 Work should not be performed consistently at or above the level of the heart; even the occasional performance where force is exerted above heart level should be avoided. Where light hand work must be performed above heart level, rests for the upper arms are a requirement.

9 Where a force has to be exerted repeatedly, it should be possible to exert it with either of the arms or either of the legs, without adjustment to the equipment.

10 Rest pauses should be allowed for all loads experienced at work, including environmental and informational loads, and the length of the work period between successive rest periods.

POSTURAL ANALYSIS

Colombini and Occhipinti (1985) reviewed the literature on posture analysis methods and identified two factors which they said were vital for a proper study of working postures. These were: (a) the description of the posture (spatial arrangement of individual body sections) with the collection and quantification of all factors and (b) an assessment of posture tolerability. They suggested that it was not the posture *per se* which was assessed but its tolerability in the particular spatial, temporal and operational conditions under which it occurred, so postures can be considered to be tolerable when they do not involve feelings of short-term discomfort (days) or cause long-term musculoskeletal disorders.

Postural data can be collected under laboratory conditions or in the field and, although laboratory data are likely to be more reliable as the activities can be more stringently controlled, there is a lack of realism and therefore validity is compromised. It is unlikely that many occupational health physiotherapists will have access to the resources (time, staff and equipment) required for laboratory data collection and so less detail is given.

Laboratory data collection

The methods available for laboratory data collection of postural information range from simple mechanical devices, for example tape measure, goniometer, inclinometer, stop watch, photography (Baty et al., 1986, 1987; Derkson et al., 1994), through to electromyography (EMG), biomechanical modelling, video analysis and physiological measurement of pressure changes. Electromyography is the most promising method of measuring muscular activity exerted in work situations; if calibrated correctly the data can be used in conjunction with biomechanical modelling tecniques to calculate the forces exerted. However, for EMG to be used the work being studied needs to be at a relatively slow pace with standard movements (Westgaard, 1988).

In biomechanical modelling the body is represented as a model with a set of articulated links in a kinetic chain with the articulations corresponding to the body joints and load moments calculated across body joints (Rohmert and Mainzer, 1986). Measurements can vary from the very simple, just allocating a range of movement, through to complex automated systems with three-dimensional tracking of a large number of motion segments, e.g. CODA (Cartesian Optoelectronic Dynamic Anthropometer, Wilson and Corlett, 1995). The latter is detailed in Chapter 8 on gait analysis.

Field Data Collection

The most commonly used field measures are questionnaires, rating scales, surveys and pictorial presentations (Kuorinka et al., 1987). Questionnaires can be used to gather epidemiological information. They tend to collect information about long-term musculoskeletal changes and aim to show statistical correlation between exposure to specific postures and the musculoskeletal change. One of the more frequently used self-reporting questionnaires is the Nordic questionnaire, where the subjects report information about musculoskeletal dysfunction based on a body map (Kuorinka et al., 1987; Wilson and Corlett, 1995). Interviews are also used to ascertain the level of musculoskeletal dysfunction.

An example of a useful work place survey is the Body Part Discomfort Survey (BPDS) which is used to provide information (from a body map) about cumulative discomfort over a period of time, e.g. 45 minute intervals over 3 hours (Corlett and Bishop, 1976). This survey combines rating scale methods and pictorial recording, with subjects rating their total discomfort and reporting the locality on a body map (Wilson and Corlett, 1995).

Table 13.6
Observational postural analysis methods

Event driven	Time driven
Benesh notation	Labanotation
Posture targeting	ARBAN
RULA)	OWAS
REBA	

A commonly used method for collecting data on posture tolerability is Rated Perceived Exertion (RPE). The Borg scale (Borg, 1970) gives a numerical value for RPE correlating to the heart rate (with a multiplication factor of 10).

Methods with more complex data analysis generally rely on videotaping the work in the field and then performing a detailed analysis in the laboratory with the ability to set the time sampling at an appropriate interval reflecting the type of work (Kember, 1976; Corlett and Manenica, 1980).

Observational postural analysis data collection methods can be classified as either time driven or event driven. Table 13.6 gives examples of both time and event-driven methods which will be outlined in more detail below. A time-driven method records the body posture at pre-set time intervals regardless of the activity taking place. This has obvious limitations as the extreme posture may not occur at the designated time interval and thus is not recorded. An event-driven system, in contrast, relies on the observer to record the posture when there is a specific pre-defined event occurring (or change in activity). This is a less stringent approach than the time-driven method and for that reason tends to be used more for repetitive work activities or single assessments.

Labanotation and Benesh Notation Labanotation and Benesh notation are both methods which have been used in physiotherapy practice. Labanotation records movement on a time basis whereas Benesh is event driven. Both methods have been described as requiring lengthy training to achieve proficiency (Kember, 1976).

ARBAN This is an observational method based on filming the work cycle, then freezing the film at intervals to allow detailed analysis of the posture. It codes the body as a 14-part functional unit for posture, and generation of force whilst handling external loads, vibration and static load. The computer calculates figures for the total ergonomic stress (based on the Borg scale, Borg, 1970) on the whole body as well as on separate parts of the body. This is represented as ergonomic stress/time curves, where the heavy load situations occur as peaks of the curve, producing a computerized 'trend' analysis which can be used to analyse different work methods and equipment (Wangenheim *et al.*, 1986; Holzman, 1982).

Posture Targeting Posture targeting notes the position of the limbs by ten marks on a chart and grades the postures in three to four degrees of severity for each limb position, considering each limb, trunk and head as linkages. On the diagram each link/part is provided with a set of segmented concentric circles, so when any of the body parts moves from the standard position a mark is made on the associated target (Corlett *et al.*, 1979). It gives a greater range for limb positions than OWAS, but takes several minutes to record each posture.

OWAS (Ovako Working Posture Analysis System) In its initial presentation, OWAS was described as a two-part method, an observation technique for evaluating work postures and a set of criteria for the redesign of working methods and places based on the evaluation of experienced workers and ergonomics experts (Karhu *et al.*, 1977). The current basic OWAS system has 84 basic posture types (4 back, 3 arm and 7 leg posture combinations), which is extended with the inclusion of 3 weight or resistance categories to give a 4-digit code and a total of 252 possible types of working postures (see Figure 13.8).

As with all time-driven techniques the data is collected by split-second observations that reveal the subject's postures at the very moment when the observer glances at the worker. The resultant postures are then

---

Figure 13.8   OWAS code.

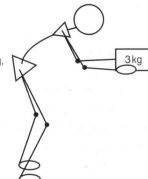

OWAS code = 2141

Back = 2 (flexion > 20°)
Arms = 1 (both below shoulder)
Legs = 4 (bilateral weight bearing, flexed > 30°)
Force = 1 (< 10 kg)

3 kg

Table 13.7
OWAS action categories

Action category	Action required
1	No actions required
2	Action required in the near future
3	Action required as soon as possible
4	Action required immediately

classified (from data tables) in the form of action categories (Table 13.7) giving an indication of the level of severity of the postural load (Louhevaara and Suurnäkki, 1992; Training publication no. 11, 1992, Wilson and Corlett, 1995).

The Institute for Occupational Health (Training publication no. 11, 1992) suggests that OWAS can be used: to assist in the development of a workplace or a work method to reduce its musculoskeletal load and to make it safer and more productive; to plan a new workplace or a work method; for ergonomic surveys, occupational health surveys and research and development.

OWAS is a simple, effective method of recording gross posture combinations in the field. One of its drawbacks is the sensitivity, which can be low due to the wide joint ranges in some of the codes, for example the knee position from 30° through to full flexion is in the same leg code.

RULA The Rapid Upper Limb Assessment is a method which was developed to assess the postures, forces and muscle activities known to contribute to upper limb disorders (ULD). The posture is recorded by observation and the severity of the posture (including information about muscle use and loads) is assessed using a series of tables which result in a posture score giving an indication of the urgency of action (McAtamney and Corlett, 1993; Wilson and Corlett, 1995). The RULA method was not designed to be used for entire body assessment but provides an excellent tool for tasks which involve repetitive upper limb, neck and head movement.

REBA The Rapid Entire Body Assessment method (REBA) (McAtamney and Hignett, 1995) records the exposure to risk factors associated with the development of musculoskeletal disorders. An action level is generated, on a 5-point scale of 0–4, which reflects the magnitude and severity of the exposure and therefore the priority upon which the implementing control measures can be based. The method was designed to evaluate tasks where postures are dynamic, static or where gross changes in position occur. It is suitable for use when assessing tasks for which basic OWAS is not sensitive enough and RULA was not designed.

In particular REBA has been designed to:

- Provide a postural analysis system which is sensitive to musculoskeletal risks in a variety of occupational and tasks;
- Divide the body into segments which are coded individually, but with reference to movement planes;
- Provide a scoring system for muscle activity caused by static, dynamic, rapid changing or unstable postures;
- Reflect that coupling is important in the handling of loads but may not always be via the hands;
- Give an action level with an indication of urgency;
- Require minimal equipment – pen and paper method.

Before using REBA, a general workplace assessment should have been carried out in order to place the results in context when presenting the report.

A specific task is identified and a posture selected. This is usually the most repeated or extreme working position. The posture is recorded photographically and field notes made about: activities preceding and following the snapshot; coupling; and the loads or forces. Also, REBA can be used to record postures in the field rather than retrospectively from photographs.

The body areas are divided into two groups (A and B) for the Trunk, Neck and Legs (GROUP A), and the Upper Arms, Lower Arms and Wrists (GROUP B) as shown in Figure 13.9.

The two following examples are given purely for illustrative purposes and are not intended as training material in the use of REBA. The REBA method should always be used, and therefore taught, as part of a full ergonomic workplace assessment.

Figure 13.9   Group A (below) and Group B (opposite page) diagrams. Copyright © Lynn McAtamney and Sue Hignett.

Group A

Trunk

Movement	Score	Change score:
Upright	1	
0°–20° flexion 0°–20° extension	2	+1 if twisting or side flexed
20°–60° flexion >20° extension	3	
>60° flexion	4	

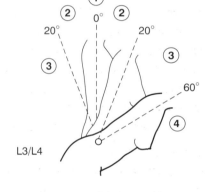

Neck

Movement	Score	Change score:
0°–20° flexion	1	+1 if twisting or side flexed
>20° flexion or in extension	2	

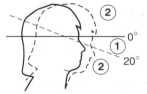

Legs

Position	Score	Change score:
Bilateral weight bearing, walking or sitting	1	+1 if knee(s) between 30° and 60° flexion
Unilateral weight bearing Feather weight bearing or an unstable posture	2	+2 if knee(s) are >60° flexion (n.b. Not for sitting)

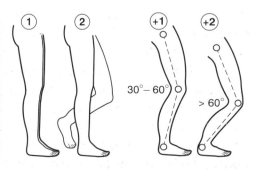

1 *Task of lifting a box from a table onto a chair (Figure 13.10)* The first example shows a box (10.3 kg) being lifted from a table onto a chair.

Using Group A diagrams and Table A (Figure 13.9) the REBA scoring sheet is competed as shown in Table 13.8.

Table A (Figure 13.11) is used by looking down the 'Trunk' column for score 2, then following along this line for Neck scores of 1. Within the 'Neck' scores there are 4 'Leg' categories, find leg score 2. This gives the Table A figure of 3.

The upper limb score was recorded for the right arm in Figure 13.10, the left is not visible. If both arms are visible, both should be scored and the

---

Figure 13.9   Continued

Group B

Upper arms

Position	Score	Change score:
20° extension to 20° flexion	1	+1 if arm is: • abducted • rotated
>20° extension 20°–45° flexion	2	+1 if shoulder is raised
45°–90° flexion	3	−1 if leaning, supporting weight of arm or if posture is gravity assisted
>90° flexion	4	

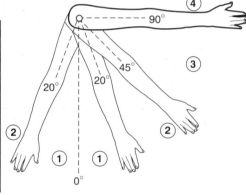

Lower arms

Movement	Score
60°–100° flexion	1
<60° flexion or >100° flexion	2

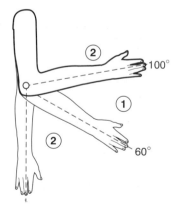

Wrists

Movement	Score	Change score:
0°–15° flexion/ extension	1	+1 if wrist is deviated or twisted
>15° flexion/ extension	2	

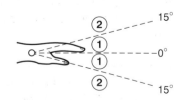

Figure 13.10(a) Task of lifting a box onto a chair. (b) Completed REBA score sheet. © Sue Hignett.

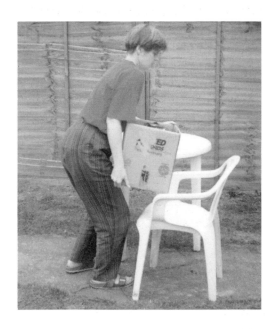

(a)

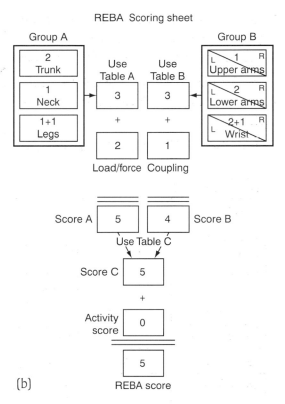

REBA Scoring sheet

(b)

Table 13.8

Completing the REBA scoring sheet using Group A diagrams and Table A

Body part	Movement or position	Score	Use Table A	Load	
Trunk	Flexion range 20°–60°,	2			
Neck	Flexion < 20°	1	= 3	= 2 (10.3 kg)	Score A = 5
Legs	Bilateral weight bearing knee flexion > 30°	1 + 1			

arm with the highest score used to complete the REBA scoring sheet.

Using Group B diagrams and Table B (Figure 13.12) the REBA scoring sheet was completed as shown in Table 13.9.

Table C (Figure 13.13) is used to obtain Score C from Score A (5) and Score B (4). The Activity score is zero, giving a REBA score of 5.

The action level is then looked up in the REBA action level table (Figure 13.14). A REBA score of 5 gives an action level of 2, 'medium' risk. This indicates that action (including further assessment) is necessary to decrease the risk of injury.

2 *Task of physiotherapist adjusting the foot position of a patient.* The following example is assessing the working posture of a

Figure 13.11   Table A and Load/force. Copyright © Lynn McAtamney and Sue Hignett.

Table A

Trunk		Neck												
		1♦				2				3				
	Legs	1	2♦	3	4	1	2	3	4	1	2	3	4	
1		1	2	3										
2♦		2	③	4	5									
3		2	4	5	6	4								
4		3	5	6	7	5	6							
5		4	6	7	8	6	7	8						

Load/force

0	1	2♦	+1
< 5 kg	5 – 10 kg	> 10 kg	Shock or rapid build up of force

Figure 13.12   Table B and Coupling. Copyright © Lynn McAtamney and Sue Hignett.

Table B

Upper arm		Lower arm					
		1			2♦		
	Wrist	1	2	3	1	2	3♦
1♦		1	2	2	1	2	③
2		1	2	3	2	3	
3		3	4	5	4		
4		4					
5							
6							

Coupling

0 Good	1♦ Fair	2 Poor	3 Unacceptable
Well fitting handle and a mid-range power grip	Hand hold acceptable but not ideal or coupling is acceptable via another part of the body	Hand hold not acceptable although possible	Awkward, unsafe grip, no handles

Coupling is unacceptable using other parts of the body |

Table 13.9

Completing REBA scoring sheet using Group B diagrams and Table B.

Body part	Movement or position	Score	Use Table B	Coupling	
Upper Arms	Flexion range 0°–20°,	1			
Lower Arms	Flexion 0°–60°	2	= 3	= 1 (Fair)	Score B = 4
Wrists	Extension > 15° Ulnar deviated	2 + 1			

Figure 13.13   Table C and Activity score. Copyright © Lynn McAtamney and Sue Hignett.

Table C

		1	2	3	4♦	5	6	7	8	9	10	11	12
S	1	1	1	1	2	3							
c	2	1	2	2	3	4							
o	3	2	3	3	3	4							
r	4	3	4	4	4	5							
e	5♦	4	4	4	(5)	6							
	6	6	6	6	7	8							
A	7	7	7	7	8	9							
	8	8	8	8	9	10							
	9	9	9	9	10								
	10	10	10	10									
	11												
	12												

(Score B across top)

Activity score

+1	• 1 or more body parts are static e.g. held for longer than 1 minute
+1	• Repeated small range actions e.g. repeated more than 4 times per minute (not including walking)
+1	• Action causes rapid large-range changes in posture or an unstable base

Figure 13.14   REBA action level.

Action level	REBA score	Risk level	Action (including further assessment)
0	1	Negligible	None necessary
1	2–3	Low	May be necessary
2♦	4–7	Medium	Necessary
3	8–10	High	Necessary soon
4	11–15	Very high	Necessary NOW

physiotherapist involved in treating a patient with a right hemiplegia (Figure 13.15). This posture is slightly more complicated so a few more details are needed in order to obtain the REBA score.

Group A. The trunk is flexed more than 60° and side flexed (4 + 1). The Neck is extended (2). The legs are both weight bearing and flexed more than

Figure 13.15 (a) Physiotherapist adjusting foot position, and (b) REBA completed scoring sheet.

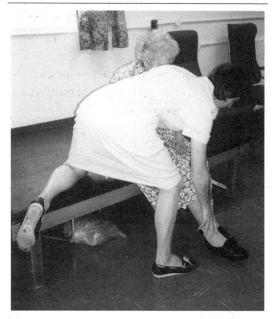

(a)

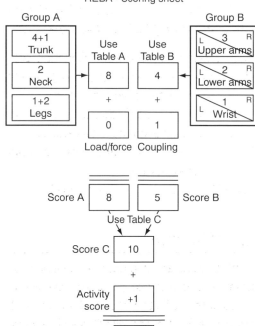

REBA - Scoring sheet

Group A

| 4+1 Trunk |
| 2 Neck |
| 1+2 Legs |

Use Table A → 8 → + → 0

Load/force

Use Table B → 4 → + → 1

Coupling

Group B

L	3	R	Upper arms
L	2	R	Lower arms
L	1	R	Wrist

Score A | 8 | | 5 | Score B

Use Table C

Score C | 10

+

Activity score | +1

| 11 |

(b) REBA score

60° (1 + 2). The patient has sitting balance so the Load/Force score is zero. Use Table A to find the subtotal and then add the Load/Force to get Score A.

Group B. Again only the right arm is fully visible and is flexed between 45° and 90° (3); however it is also abducted (+ 1) and gravity assisted (– 1) due to the position of the trunk. The lower arm is flexed less than 60° (2) and the wrist is between 0°–15° flexion/extension with no deviation or twist (1). The Coupling is fair (1). Use Table B to find the subtotal and then add the Coupling to get Score B.

Obtain Score C from Table C and add the Activity score. There has been a large range change in posture as the physiotherapist reaches forward to the floor to re-position the patient's foot (+ 1).

This gives a total REBA score of 11, with an action level of 4. There is a very high risk of injury to the physiotherapist and immediate action is necessary to further assess this task with the aim of reducing the risk level.

Industrial Therapy

Bullock (1994) proposed a model (outlined in Figure 13.16) which aims to optimize human performance by maximizing the expertise and input from both the physiotherapy and ergonomics professions in a combination of rehabilitation and therapeutic care together with design and prevention.

Ergonomic design and prevention of injury have been discussed earlier in this chapter. Rehabilitation of movement is the overall theme of this book, so let's consider functional capacity evalua-

Figure 13.16   Optimization of human physical performance (modified from Bullock, 1994).

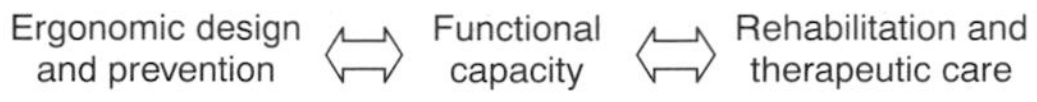

Ergonomic design and prevention ⟺ Functional capacity ⟺ Rehabilitation and therapeutic care

tion. In North America the advisory role of the occupational health physiotherapist has expanded into almost a new profession, with specialist skills, based in the application of work physiology and psychosocial research under the title of industrial therapy. Functional capacity evaluation is one of the core services of this speciality and so will be considered as part of the overall role of an industrial therapist.

Industrial therapy is a system which encompasses a wide spectrum of treatment based on the principle that a person working in industry, as anywhere else, has physical, emotional, vocational, educational, psychological and sociological needs which must be met to enable successful employment or, in the case of injury, rehabilitation and re-employment.

In the last 15 years it was noted (Bryan *et al.*, 1993) that industry physical therapists were moving away from the traditional role of treating injured workers in clinics and starting to provide services including injury prevention and rehabilitation as well as pursuing advanced work in related fields, e.g. engineering or ergonomics. In 1990 industrial physical therapy was recognized by the American Physical Therapy Association (APTA) and a joint committee was established to set standards for industrial rehabilitation therapy which was defined to include physical therapy, occupational therapy, vocational evaluation, work adjustment and industrial engineering (Hart *et al.*, 1994). The standards included a description of the objectives of services; a suggested knowledge base for clinicians; criteria for auditing quality of services; and

goals, admission criteria, contraindications and components of service. So the identity of an industrial therapist was born with the scope of providing functional capacity evaluations, work conditioning, work hardening within the practice of physical therapy, occupational therapy and certified vocational evaluators (as part of the physical or occupational therapy team).

There is an interesting distinction here in the difference in treatment goals between industrial physical therapy and traditional physical therapy. These are described by Wassell Twelves (1990):

- *Industrial therapy rehabilitation goal:* to return the worker to gainful employment (productivity enhancement);
- *Traditional physical therapy goal:* to return the patient to optimal functional level (symptom reduction).

The scope of the industrial therapist can include the following four areas of musculoskeletal vocational rehabilitation (Rippinen *et al.*, 1994):

1 Comprehensive vocational rehabilitation consisting of medical, social, psychological and vocational counselling and examination.
2 Intervention to alleviate chronic pain and to enhance working and functional capacity.
3 Therapy promoting functional capacity (including medical care).
4 Rehabilitation of severely handicapped.

Clinical Services

Clinical services are described as including an assessment of contributory work-related factors in terms of their effects of the condition on work performance. Treatment goals will then be recommended and discussed with the patient with the aim of maximizing work performance within a safe healing environment. In UK industries this includes the use of fitness gyms and there has been an increase in the number of organizations offering on-site facilities. In some organizations e.g. Rank Xerox and Marks & Spencer, these have been used to rehabilitate staff after heart attacks as well as improving the general fitness of staff. A number of indirect benefits have been claimed which include improved work performance, decreased absenteeism, increased job satisfaction, easier recruitment and improved company image (Richardson and Eastlake, 1994).

Functional Capacity Evaluation

Functional capacity evaluation (FCE) is used to determine the level of function of a client. The evaluation can take 4 to 8 hours over more than one day and will include a comprehensive neuro-muscular examination with measurement of physical impairment, worker behaviour and functional abilities. These will be compared with the physical demands of the job to ensure proper return-to-work decision-making or rehabilitation plan generation (Hart et al., 1994).

Lechner et al. (1991, 1994a) suggest that the interest in functional capacity evaluation has grown in response to the demand for quantitative measures of an individual's functional capacity from the insurance, legal, social security and workers' compensation industries. They claim that the use of FCE has been shown to be a cost effective evaluation procedure leading to savings in rehabilitation costs and earlier return to work. Unfortunately, as with many other areas of physiotherapy, there is relatively little research to establish either inter- or intra-reliability of the methods used in work conditioning/hardening programmes. It is this author's hope that future research will prove the valuable contribution that can be made by physiotherapists.

An FCE can have a number of objectives, each of which is distinctly different:

1 To determine a worker's physical abilities to perform the work;
2 To predict the potential ability to perform work after rehabilitation or a work hardening programme;
3 To determine areas of concentration for rehabilitation or a work hardening programme;
4 To document change after rehabilitation or a work hardening programme has been implemented.

Lechner et al. (1991) have identified 20 specific aspects of physical demands of work which can be tested in a functional capacity evaluation and then focused on in a work conditioning or work hardening programme as required. These demands include a range of activities, for example: lifting, walking, balancing, stooping, crawling, reaching and talking.

Lechner et al. (1994b) have further developed the use of functional capacity evaluation in a system designed to find workers' maximum physical functional capacity which is equivalent to the maximum that they can be expected to do at work (called the physical work performance evaluation, PWPE). The upsurge in the activity in this area in North America is connected to the Americans with Disability Act (1991) which stated that testing must be limited to only those tasks that are essential for the performance of the job. The limitation of PWPE and other similar assessment methods is that they only address physical activity and cannot be used to assess psychological factors which are important in motivation.

Work Conditioning

Work conditioning is the term used to describe a work-related, intensive goal-oriented treatment programme which is specifically designed to restore an individual's systemic, neuromuscular (strength, endurance, movement, flexibility and motor control) and cardiopulmonary functions. It is used for clients who are more than 6 weeks post-injury and aims to restore physical capacity and function for return to work (Hart et al., 1994). On the whole it tends to address the physical and functional needs that may be provided by one discipline (e.g. physical therapy or occupational therapy) and utilizes physical conditioning and functional activities related to work (Lechner, 1994a).

Work Hardening

Work hardening is the term used to describe a highly structured, goal-oriented, individualized treatment programme designed to return the person to work. It uses real or simulated work activities and is suitable for clients who are more than 12 weeks post-injury and are physically deconditioned but medically stable (Hart et al., 1994).

A work hardening programme addresses physical functions, and behavioural and vocational needs. In an evaluation of work hardening programmes (Lechner, 1994a) most were found to include some type of back school or patient education programme with instruction on body mechanics, lifting technique, back protection, anatomy and pathology of the spine, medications, surgical techniques and the theoretical basis for treatment. The success of work hardening is measured by a decrease in disability or speed of return to work, so there may be no change in symptoms but a major improvement in functional capacity with symptom-control strategies to maintain work productivity (Wassell Twelves, 1990).

Clinical Ergonomics

Most of this chapter has been looking at the role of ergonomics in physiotherapy; however, there is also some overlap from physiotherapy into ergonomics, in particular in the area of clinical ergonomics.

In the last few years the role of a clinical ergonomist has been suggested (Khalil et al., 1991) on the basis that the knowledge of human characteristics (anatomy, physiology and psychology) combined with strong scientific and engineering backgrounds might qualify ergonomists to make major contributions to treatment and rehabilitation of patients. The areas of clinical practice suggested include diagnostic electromyography, establishing diagnosis and treatment rationale based on biomechanical principles and functional capacity assessments.

This role has already been used in a study at the University of Miami which found that ergonomists working in a clinical setting were a valuable addition to the rehabilitation team (Abdel Moty et al., 1988). From reviewing the suggested areas of practice there seem to be many similarities to the activities of an occupational health physiotherapist. With such a potential cross-over or convergence there may be a need for interprofessional registration which acknowledges and requires appropriate recognized qualifications and experience.

Physiotherapy and Ergonomics: Converging and Diverging

Foster (1988) suggested that the disciplines of physiotherapy and ergonomics were divergent and convergent: divergent in that the scope of ergonomics covered all aspects of a person's interaction with their environment (physical, cognitive and organizational), whereas physiotherapy was concerned only with physical well-being; convergent in that both aimed to optimize human performance. He suggested that differing approaches were taken with physiotherapy achieving this aim by altering the person (e.g. work conditioning or musculoskeletal treatment), and ergonomics altering the task.

The divergence of the two disciplines is reinforced by Buckle and Stubbs (1989) looking from the ergonomics perspective. They suggested that there has been a polarization within ergonomics, with some ergonomists becoming more involved in information technology and the design of systems, and others remaining in the more traditional areas of job and equipment design. It is possible this polarization has, to some extent, limited the number of ergonomists who have the appropriate skills and knowledge base to work within a health care setting. This deficit may have left the onus on other professional groups to provide an ergonomic input. As discussed in the section on occupational health physiotherapy, there is an issue of qualifications and although physiotherapists, occupational therapists and other occupational health professionals may have background knowledge at the first level, few have received education in ergonomics.

For the physiotherapist intending to practice ergonomics as part of their full-time employment, Bullock (1994) advocated the definition of core ergonomic competencies (see Appendix) as a resource for educational planning, accreditation processes and certification processes. She suggested that among professionals practising ergonomics a common basic foundation of knowledge was required to ensure an adequate level of communication which would support the need for ergonomists to appreciate their own limitations and facilitate assistance being sought when required. These competencies would be met by most taught M.Sc. courses in the UK and form the foundation of the professional accreditation of the European Ergonomist (EurErg). The European Ergonomist (Centre for Registration of European Ergonomists, CREE) is an example of professional standardization which is not only found in the European Community but also in North America and Australia/New Zealand where common basic standards for professional practice have been agreed (see Appendix for CREE code of conduct).

There have also been a number of papers discussing the practice of ergonomics by physiotherapists (Bullock, 1991, 1994; Boyling, 1994; Foster, 1988). The general consensus seems to be that although physiotherapists have much to offer in the area of physical ergonomics, they need to know how best to use their expertise and to be able to recognize when an ergonomist with specialist knowledge should be consulted.

Summary

1 Ergonomics is 'that branch of science and technology that includes what is known and theorized about human behavioural and biological characteristics that can be validly applied to the specification, design, evaluation, operation and

maintenance of products and systems to enhance safe, effective and satisfying use by individuals, groups and organizations'.

2 Ergonomics can be used in physiotherapy practice to assess physiotherapy work, including treatment handling. Physiotherapists have considerable expertise to offer in the area of physical ergonomics especially with respect to postural analysis and anthropometry in product and equipment design.

3 Education in ergonomics is available at three levels:

- Background knowledge from a 3–5 day course;
- Using ergonomics as part of physiotherapy advice, certificate or diploma course (at least 6 months duration);
- Professional ergonomic advice following a full-time undergraduate or postgraduate course.

4 Anthropometry is the science of measuring and studying human body dimensions. Data are available for a wide range of populations by sex, age, race and for specialist populations, e.g. wheelchair users. Anthropometry data are widely used in product and workstation design.

5 An ergonomic workstation assessment takes account of physical, cognitive and organizational factors.

6 Postural analysis looks at the tolerability of a posture with respect to its spatial, temporal and operational conditions. There are a number of postural analysis tools which should be selected to best suit the task activities.

7 Industrial therapy is a specialist area of practice which includes functional capacity evaluation, work hardening and work conditioning as part of a team approach.

Further Reading

Mullins, LJ (1993) *Management and Organisational Behaviour* 3rd edition. Pitman Publishing

Singleton, WT (ed) (1982) *The Body at Work: Biological Ergonomics.* Cambridge University Press, Cambridge.

Wickens, CD (1992) *Engineering Psychology and Human Performance,* 2nd edition. Harper Collins.

Wilson, JR, Corlett, EN (1995) *Evaluation of Human Work: A Practical Ergonomics Methodology,* 2nd edn. Taylor & Francis, London.

References

Abdel-Moty, E, Khalil, TM, Asfour, SS, Rosomoff, RS, Rosomoff, HL (1988) Ergonomic considerations for the reduction of physical task demands of low back pain patients. In Aghazadeh, F (ed.) *Trends in Ergonomics/Human Factors V,* pp. 959–967. Elsevier Science Publishers, Amsterdam.

Baty, D, Stubbs, DA (1987) Postural stress in geriatric nursing. *International Journal of Nursing Studies* 24 (4): 339–344.

Baty, D, Buckle, PW, Stubbs, DA (1986) Posture recording by direct observation, questionnaire, assessment and instrumentation: a comparison based on a recent field study, in Corlett, EN, Wilson, JR, Manenica, I (eds) *The Ergonomics of Working Postures,* pp. 283–292. Taylor & Francis, London.

Berwick, DM, Budman, S, Feldstein, M (1989) No clinical effect of Back Schools in an HMO. A randomised prospective trial. *Spine* 14 (3): 338–344.

Borg, G (1970) Perceived exertion as an indicator of somatic stress. *Scandinavian Journal of Medical Rehabilitation* 2–3: 92–93.

Boyling, J (1994) Lightening the load: physiotherapy in industry. *Occupational Health* Oct: 342–345.

Bryan, SM, Geroy, GD, Isernhagen, SJ (1993) Non clinical competencies for physical therapists consulting with business and industry. *JOSPT* 18 (6): 673–681.

Buckle, P, Stubbs, D (1989) The contribution of Ergonomics to the rehabilitation of back pain. *Journal of the Society for Occupation Medicine* 39: 56–60.

Bullock, MI (ed.) (1990) Ergonomics. The Physiotherapist in the workplace. *International Perspectives in Physical Therapy* 6. Churchill Livingstone, Edinburgh.

Bullock, MI (1991) Harmonising professional standards in ergonomics while recognising diversity. *Ergonomics* 38 (8): 1558–1570.

Bullock, M (1994) Research to optimise human performance. *Australian Journal of Physiotherapy* 40th Jubilee issue, 5–17.

Christensen, JM, Topmiller, DA, Gill, RT (1988) Human Factors definitions revisited. *Human Factors Society Bulletin* 31: 7–8.

Colombini, D, Occhipinti, E (1985) Posture analysis. *Ergonomics* 28 (1): 275–285.

Corlett, EN (1978) The human body at work: new principles for designing workspaces and methods. *Management Services,* May: 20–52.

Corlett, EN, Bishop, RP (1976) A technique for assessing postural discomfort. *Ergonomics* 19 (2): 175–182.

Corlett, EN, Manenica, I (1980) The effects and measurements of working postures. *Applied Ergonomics* 11 (1): 7–16.

Corlett, EN, Madeley, SJ, Manenica, I (1979) Posture targeting – a technique for recording working postures. *Ergonomics* 22 (3): 357–366.

Crumpton, EJ (1995) *An investigation into the role of the back care advisor.* Unpublished M.Sc. dissertation, University of London.

Derkson, JCM, van Riel, MPJM, van Winerden, JP, Snijders, CJ (1994) A comparison of working postures of parcel sorters using three different working methods. *Ergonomics* 37 (2): 299–309.

Disability Discrimination Act (1995) Code of Practice – Rights of Access – Goods, Facilities, Services and Premises. HMSO, London.

Executive Health and Safety (1992) *Guidance for Regulations* L 26. Display Screen Equipment. HMSO Books, London.

Fenety, A, Kumar, S (1992) An ergonomic survey of a hospital physical therapy department. *International Journal of Industrial Ergonomics* 9: 161–170.

Ferguson, D (1983) *Ergonomics in Australia – past and future.* Proc 20th Annual Conference of the Ergonomics Society of Australia. Adelaide, Australia.

Finnish Institute of Occupational Health (1989) *Ergonomic Work Place Analysis.* Institute of Occupational Health, Helsinki, Finland.

Foreman, TK, Davies, JC, Troup, JDG (1988) A positive and activity classification system using a micro computer. *International Journal of Industrial Ergonomics* 2: 285–289.

Foster, M (1988) Ergonomics and the physiotherapist. *Physiotherapy* 74 (9): 484–489.

Frost, H, McCay, G (1990) Prevention of injury group initiative *Physiotherapy* 76 (12): 796–798.

Frost, H, Klaber Moffett, J (1992) Physiotherapy management of chronic low back pain. *Physiotherapy* 78 (10): 751–754.

Grandjean, E (1988) *Fitting the Task to the Man: A Textbook of Occupational Ergonomics,* 4th edn. Taylor & Francis.

Hart, DL, Berlin, S, Brager, PE, Caruso, M, Hejduk, JF, Hoular, JM, Snyder, KP, Susi, JL, Wah, MD (1994) Development of clinical standards in industrial rehabilitation. *JOSPT* 19 (5): 232–241.

Hignett, S (1994) Physiotherapists and the Manual Handling Operations Regulations. *Physiotherapy* 80 (7): 446–447.

Hignett, S (1995) Fitting the work to the physiotherapist. *Physiotherapy* 81 (9): 549–552.

Hignett, S (1996) *Physiotherapy treatment involving manual handling.* Internal document. Physiotherapy / Ergonomics departments, Nottingham City Hospital NHS Trust.

Hobson, DA, Molenbroek, JFM (1990) Anthropometry and design for the disabled: Experiences with seating design for the cerebral palsy population. *Applied Ergonomics* 21 (1): 43–54.

Holzman, P (1982) ARBAN – a new method for analysis of ergonomic effort. *Applied Ergonomics* 13 (2): 82–86.

Isernhagen, SJ (ed.) (1995) *The Comprehensive Guide to Work Injury Management.* Aspen Publishers, USA.

Jacobs, K, Bettencourt, CM (eds) (1995) *Ergonomics for Therapists.* Butterworth-Heinemann, Newton, USA.

Karhu, O, Kansi, P, Kuorinka, I (1977) Correcting working postures in industry: a practical method for analysis *Applied Ergonomics* 8 (4): 199–201.

Kember, P (1976) The Benesh movement notation used to study sitting behaviour. *Applied Ergonomics* 7 (3): 133–136.

Khalil, TM, Asfour, SS, Moty, EA, Rosomoff, R, Rosomoff, HL, (1991) *Clinical Ergonomics: Ergonomic Practice in Health Care Settings.* In Queinnec, Y, Daniellou, F, (eds), *Designing for Everyone Vol I,* Proc 11th Congress of IEA, Paris. pp. 314–316. Taylor & Francis, London.

Klaber Moffett, JA, Chase, SM, Portek, I, Ennis, JR (1986) A controlled prospective study to evaluate the effectiveness of a back school on the relief of chronic low back pain. *Spine* 11 (2): 120–122.

Kuorinka, I, Jonsson, B, Kilbom, A, Vinterberg, H, Biering-Sorenson, F, Andersson, G, Jorgenson, K (1987) Standardised Nordic Question-naires for the analysis of musculoskeletal symptoms. *Applied Ergonomics* 18 (3): 233–237.

Lankhorst, GJ, van de Stadt, RJ, Vogelaat, TW, van de Korst, JK, Prevo, AJH (1983) The effect of the Swedish back school in chronic idiopathic low back pain. *Scandinavian Journal Rehabilitative Medicine* 15: 141–145.

Lechner, DE (1994a) Work hardening and work conditioning interven-tions: Do they affect disability? *Physical Therapy* 74 (5): 471–493.

Lechner, D, Roth, K, Straaton, K (1991) Functional capacity evaluation in work disability Work. *Spine* 1 (3): 37–47.

Lechner, DE, Jackson, JR, Roth, DL, Straaton, K (1994b) Reliability and validity of a newly developed test of physical work performance *JOM* 36 (9): 997–1004.

Lindquist, S, Lundberg, B, Wikmark et al. (1984) Information and regime at low back pain. *Scan J Rehab Med* 16: 113–116.

Louhevaara, V, Suurnäkki, T (1992) OWAS – a method for the evalua-tion of postural load during work. Institute of Occupational Health, Centre for Occupational Safety, Helsinki, Finland.

McAtamney, L (1991) *Physiotherapy in Industry.* In Lovesey, EJ (ed.), *Contemporary Ergonomics.* Taylor & Francis, London.

McAtamney, L, Corlett, EN (1993) RULA: a survey method for the investigation of work-related upper limb disorders. *Applied Ergonomics* 24: 91–99.

McAtamney, L, Hignett, S (1995) REBA – A Rapid Entire Body Assess-ment method for investigating work-related musculoskeletal disorders. *Conference Proceedings Ergonomics Society of Australia, 31st Annual Conference* pp. 45–51. Adelaide, Australia.

McPhee, B (1984) Training and possible future trends in Occupational Physiotherapy. *NZ Journal of Physiotherapy,* Dec: 12–14.

Management of Health and Safety at Work Health and Safety Commis-sion (1992) *Management of Health and Safety at Work Regulations 1992.* Approved Code of Practice, L21. HMSO, London.

Manual Handling (1992) *Manual Handling Operations Regulations 1992.* Guidance for Regulations L23. HSE Books, London.

Molumphy, M, Unger, B, Jensen, GM, Lopopolo, RB (1985) Incidence of work-related low back pain in physical therapists. *Physical Therapy* 65 (4): 482–486.

Oborne, DJ (1995) *Ergonomics at Work* 3rd edn. John Wiley & Sons.

Oldham, G (1988) The Occupational Health Physiotherapist's role in assessing fitness for work. *Physiotherapy* 74 (9): 422–425.

Pheasant, S (1986) *Body Space: Anthropometry, Biomechanics and Design.* Taylor & Francis, London.

Pheasant, S (1991) *Ergonomics, Work and Health.* MacMillan, London.

Pheasant, S (1996) *Body Space: Anthropometry, Ergonomics and the Design of work*, 2nd edn. Taylor & Francis, London.

Reason, J (1990) *Human Error.* Cambridge University Press, Cambridge.

Richardson, B, Eastlake, A (eds) (1994) *Physiotherapy in Occupational Health. Management, Prevention and Health Promotion in the Work Place.* Butterworth-Heinemann Ltd, Oxford.

Riipinen, M, Hurri, H, Alaranta, H (1994) Evaluating the outcome of vocational rehabilitation. *Scandinavian Journal of Rehabilitation Medicine* 26: 103–112.

Rohmert, W, Mainzer, J (1986) Influence parameters and assessment methods for assessing body postures. In Corlett, EN, Wilson, JR, Manenica, I (eds), *The Ergonomics of Working Postures.* Taylor & Francis, London.

Sanders, MS, McCormick, EJ (1993) *Human Factors in Engineering and Industry*, 7th edn. McGraw-Hill Inc., USA.

Scholey, M, Hair, M (1989) Back pain in physiotherapists involved in back care education. *Ergonomics* 32 (2): 179–190.

Training Publication no. 11 (1992) *OWAS: a method for the evaluation of postural load during work.* Institute of Occupational Health, Centre for Occupational Safety, Helsinki, Finland.

Wangenheim, M, Wos, H, Samuelson, B (1986) ARBAN — a force ergonomic analysis method. In Corlett, EN, Wilson, JR, Manenica, I (eds), *The Ergonomics of Working Postures.* Taylor & Francis, London.

Wassell Twelves, J (1990) Physical therapy in Industry. *Clinical Management* 10 (5) Sept/Oct: 14–19.

Westgaard, RH (1988) Measurement and evaluation of postural load in occupational work situations. *European Journal of Applied Physiology* 57: 219–304.

Wilson, JR, Corlett, EN (eds) (1995) *Evaluation of Human Work. A practical ergonomics methodology*, 2nd edn. Taylor & Francis, London.

Zachrisson-Forssell, M (1980) The Swedish Back School. *Physiotherapy* 66 (4): 112–114.

Zachrisson-Forssell, M (1981) The Back School. *Spine* 6 (1): 104–106.

Appendix

CORE COMPETENCIES FOR ERGONOMISTS (BULLOCK, 1994)

1 Demonstrate an understanding of the theoretical basis for assessment of the workplace.

2 Demonstrate an understanding of the systems approach to human integrated design.

3 Demonstrate an understanding of the concepts and principles of computer modelling and simulation.

4 Communicate effectively with clients and professional colleagues.

5 Obtain information relevant to ergonomics from the client.

6 Collect supplementary information relevant to ergonomics relating to the history of the problem and current management.

7 Collect from the workplace, in an appropriate manner, quantitative and qualitative data relevant to the perceived problem and ergonomics.

8 Document ergonomic assessment findings.

9 Recognize the scope of ergonomic assessments.

CENTRE FOR REGISTRATION FOR EUROPEAN ERGONOMISTS (CREE)

Code of Conduct for those registered as European Ergonomists.

1 In the conduct of their profession they shall maintain high standards of integrity and respect for evidence, and maintain high ethical standards.

2 They shall present themselves as having expertise and abilities only in those areas in which they are competent.

3 They shall continually endeavour both to improve their competence in ergonomics and to contribute to the body of ergonomic knowledge.

4 They shall continually endeavour to safeguard the welfare and interests of all those affected by their work.

5 They shall protect the privacy of individuals or organizations about whom information is

collected and maintain the confidentiality of personal or commercially sensitive information.

6 They shall not allow their work to be affected by considerations of religion, sex, ethnic origin, age, nationality, class, politics or any other factors extraneous to the conduct of the work in which they are engaged.

7 They shall not accept any consideration from a client beyond that which was contractually agreed, neither shall they receive benefits from other sources for the same work without the agreement of all parties involved.

8 Where they perceive a question of professional misconduct which they cannot resolve with the individual concerned, they shall report it without malice to their national professional body or the board of CREE.

9 They shall ensure that all those working with them are aware of this code, and that those they supervise adhere to it.

February 1996 Centre for Registration for European Ergonomists (CREE)

National body: The Ergonomics Society, Devonshire House, Devonshire Square, Loughborough, Leicestershire LE11 3DW.

14

Health Education and Communication

KATE KERR AND MAUREEN MAXWELL

Introduction

The concepts of health education and health promotion have become more prominent in the public's consciousness over recent years, prompted by the Department of Health policy that individuals should take greater responsibility for their health (DHSS, 1976). There is a certain degree of confusion about the purposes and relationships between health education and health promotion;

Whitehead and Tones (1991) define health promotion as 'any planned measure which promotes health or prevents disease, disability and premature death'. They argue that this encompasses the two major components of health promotion, namely healthy public policy (which may include a range of measures such as legislation, environmental modification and various fiscal/economic interventions designed to make healthier choices easier) and health education.

Within the physiotherapy profession, concern for health education appears to have increased rapidly (Lyne, 1986), with physiotherapists commonly carrying out health education work with clients of all ages, and with their carers and teachers. Increasing numbers of physiotherapists working in the community may be provided with the opportunity to extend their health education role, by reaching and influencing people at an earlier stage than is usually possible (Leathley, 1988). Too often it seems that physiotherapists are prevented in their educational role by excessive pressure of clinical work, the general orientation of the NHS towards sickness rather than health, and lack of recognition by health authorities of the health education role of physiotherapy (Leathley, 1988).

In the present economic climate, where evidence of cost effectiveness is required before new initiatives can be implemented, it would appear that if the role of the physiotherapist as a health educator is to be accepted, some means of evaluating its effectiveness must be established. This in itself presents a problem, in that whether health education can be judged a success depends on one's perception of the purpose of that education (Whitehead and Tones, 1991). Furthermore, there is the view that when health education programmes are implemented, their effect is often impossible to evaluate by existing outcome measures (Baric, 1991).

If in its simplest form, health education can be regarded as a means of conveying a health message, the health educator requires certain knowledge and skills to ensure that the message is accepted and preferably acted upon. The educator needs:

- To be clear as to the purpose of the message (is it to inform, is it to persuade behavioural change, or is it to enhance personal choice and control?);
- To understand the personal, psychological and social reasons why the message may or may not be accepted;
- Adequate communication skills to assess the problems and convey the message.

This chapter will examine these three major requirements of the health educator, and apply them where appropriate to the role of the physiotherapist as a health educator.

Chapter Objectives

After reading this chapter, the student should be able to:

- Consider the purpose of health education;
- Identify the types of health education;
- Examine the practice of health education in physiotherapy:
  - the scope of health education,
  - the wider context of health education,
  - concerns regarding the practice of health education;
- Examine the social and psychological implications of health education;
- Review the factors influencing patient compliance:
  - views on illness causation,
  - health beliefs,
  - professional–patient relationship,
  - the nature of the illness / disability,
  - the nature of the treatment regimen,
  - knowledge,
  - social / situational;
- Identify the scope of communication;
- Explore the use of communication skills in physiotherapy practice:

- nonverbal communication,
- the therapeutic interview,
- history taking and physical examination,
- the conditions for effective interviewing,
- communication during therapeutic intervention.

The Purpose of Health Education

Before considering the specific purposes and theoretical models of health education, it is perhaps useful to explore more fully the general aims of health education, and its relationship and contribution to health promotion. Baric (1991) defined health education as

> the process of transmission and/or acquisition of knowledge and skills necessary for survival and the improvement of quality of life.

Baric (1991) admitted that this definition was much too general, and impossible to put into action, and proposed a more specific definition.

> The main aim of health education is [to influence the] health behaviour of individuals and groups. This includes routines as well as decisions about certain behaviour, and actions in terms of prevention and treatment of illnesses.

The methods used to achieve these aims will vary according to the perception and conceptualization of the problems related to health behaviours. It is in recognition of these different perceptions that a number of models of health education have been developed (Draper et al. 1980; Whitehead and Tones, 1991).

Health promotion has a much wider remit; this includes health education, but also encompasses other activities aimed at manipulating the physical and social environment of its target population. To bring about change in the social environment, the methods of health promotion may include legislation and lobbying of Members of Parliament, changing social norms, and influencing the provision and distribution of both financial and service resources.

At this stage, it appears that apart from those in managerial positions who can influence distribution of service resources, the majority of physiotherapists are engaged in health education rather than health promotion activities. This balance may well change in the future. For example, under their contract, general practitioners have responsibility not only for the medical treatment of those registered with their practices, but also for their health. Physiotherapists are well equipped to become involved in the health promotion clinics and health screening activities which are emerging as a result of this contract.

Types of Health Education

Draper et al. (1980) proposed that there were at least three types of health education.

The first type, and probably the most common, is education about the body, and how to look after it. Increased knowledge about the workings of the body should enhance appreciation of the benefits of healthy behaviours, and the possible consequences of unhealthy behaviours.

The second type of health education concerns the provision of information about available services and the sensible use of health resources. This should encourage the appropriate and timely use of health resources when required.

The third type concerns the wider environment, and approaches a social policy aspect of health promotion as defined by Baric (1991). This is concerned with education about national, regional and local policies, which, according to Draper *et al.* (1980) are too often devised and implemented without taking account of their consequences for health. Thus, while not directly influencing policy, this type of health education aims to increase public awareness of existing policies. There is also the possibility that this increased public awareness may, over a period of time, encourage the development of action groups to lobby for change.

Draper *et al.* (1980) use an example of cycling to illustrate the three types of health education, and how they interact. The first type of health education would be concerned with providing information about safe cycling practice and physical fitness, whereas the second type would offer advice on what to do in the case of an accident or injury, or whether the older cyclist should undergo periodic medical examination. The third type would be concerned with public understanding of how to create a safe and healthy environment for cycling; this might involve providing information on the relative costs (both health and economic) of providing safe cycle paths and using other forms of transport, on transport policy with regard to cycling, and on the practicalities of restricting motor vehicles on designated 'cycle routes'.

Draper *et al.* (1980) suggest that to implement the first two types of health education without the third amounts to social irresponsibility. This might be interpreted as implying that even when they have been provided with education and knowledge, people need support through social / public policy to implement and maintain changes in health behaviour.

This structural concept of health education could be applied by the physiotherapist in a number of situations. For example, in the overall management of back problems, the first type of health education would involve education about the anatomical structure of the back, the forces acting on it during a variety of functional activities, and advice on correct handling techniques. The second type would provide information on who to consult and what to do in the event of an exacerbation of the problem. The third type would be concerned with the creation of a 'safe' environment to lessen the risk of precipitating back problems, providing information on legislation and directives aimed at reducing the incidence of back pain in the workplace, and the organization of safe working practice.

To support Draper *et al.*'s conclusions about the importance of the balance between the three types of health education – to provide education about the back, and how to cope with exacerbations of the problem, but to allow the patient / client to return to a working environment which is ergonomically unsound seems at best to be counterproductive! Thus, to develop a comprehensive approach to the management of back pain in the working environment, working practice and the physical organization of the workplace needs to be considered. For example, a keyboard operator who sits on an uncomfortable chair, at a desk of the wrong height, will probably continue to have exacerbations of back pain until an ergonomically sound chair and desk have been provided.

Practical Task

It might be a useful exercise to consider how these three types of health education might be applied in other areas of physiotherapy which have been identified as demanding a health education input. Lyne (1986) included pregnant women, new mothers, children with asthma (and perhaps cystic fibrosis — author's suggestion), adults with hypertension and post-coronary, back care, and healthy clients involved in exercise leisure activities and sport, in a listing of areas in which physiotherapists consider they function as health educators. Select three areas, and apply the three types of health education as advocated by Draper et al. (1980).

Models of Health Education

Whitehead and Tones (1991) have identified four purposes or models of health education, and link them to the important issue of evaluating the success or effectiveness of health education intervention.

The Educational Model

The first purpose of health education (the *educational model*) is to provide information and create well-informed people. This information has the potential to raise awareness of the means by which they might prevent or reduce the impact of disease processes, make appropriate use of health services, and gain insight into the positive and negative influence of social and environmental factors on health. This level or aim of health education can be relatively simply evaluated by measuring the knowledge and understanding of a specific subject.

Thus, to follow up the earlier back care example, it should be possible to measure the patient's knowledge of the structure and function of the back, understanding of what to do in the event of an exacerbation, and how work and social environ-ment and practice can influence the health status of the back.

The Self-empowerment Model

The second purpose of health education is to facilitate genuine informed choice (the *self-empowerment model*). In addition to the provision of information, this model encourages people to have the confidence in their own ability to make decisions, and enhances the practical skills they need to implement those decisions. This can be evaluated not only by determining knowledge and understanding, but also by evidence of decision-making (which may involve healthy or unhealthy choices), and in the development of useful social skills.

In the back care example, in addition to evaluating the patient's knowledge, success might be demonstrated by the patient having the confidence to reject working practice which may be detrimental to healthy back function.

The Preventive Medical Model

The third function of health education can be viewed as persuading individuals to adopt what are generally (at least by the medical professions) regarded as healthy behaviours. This involves not only encouragement to adopt healthy behaviours, but also to make appropriate use of health services. To demonstrate the effectiveness of this approach, individuals should show that they have adopted a healthier lifestyle, or are making more effective and appropriate use of health services.

In the back care scenario, patients should demonstrate that they have adopted correct lifting and handling techniques, or perhaps have changed seating/workplace arrangements to avoid potentially damaging postures.

The Radico-political Model

Finally, the fourth view of the purpose of health education is to raise awareness of the need for healthy public policy (the *radico-political model*), so that people would be stimulated to tackle the various socioeconomic influences on health. This considers the remit of health education on a much wider scale, perhaps mirroring the third type of health education as suggested by Draper *et al*. (1980). Measures of success would be some indication of increased public awareness of health issues and, in the long term, that this awareness has ultimately produced change in public policy at local, regional or national level.

Recognition of the extent of the incidence of occupational back pain, and its economic consequences, has prompted many industries to review working practice to reduce the potential for damaging postures and work practice to result in back pain. This has been further regulated by legislation, originally emanating from the Health and Safety at Work Act (1974), and more recently by European Community Directives relevant to Health and Safety Law.

Practical Task

To what extent do you think you can apply each of the four views/purposes of health education as proposed by Whitehead and Tones (1991) to areas in which physiotherapists consider they function as health educators? Select the same three areas as previously.

Physiotherapy and Health Education

Having considered the different purposes and models of health education, and identified possible areas in which physiotherapists might function as health educators, let us now look at what evidence exists on the practice of health education within the physiotherapy profession.

In a study designed to investigate and promote health education in the practice of four of the professions allied to medicine (PAMs), members of all four professions (chiropody, dietetics, physiotherapy and occupational therapy) were shown to hold the view that the treatment they give is incomplete without an element of advice or education (Leathley and Stone, 1986). The type of advice/education identified included information on how the body works, detailed teaching about a specific medical condition, or discussion about independent living to assist patients in developing coping strategies. These three elements seem generally to fit in with the educational, self-empowerment and preventive medical models proposed by Whitehead and Tones (1991).

The Scope of the Health Education Role in Physiotherapy

The scope of the health education role in physiotherapy is wide. Leathley (1988) carried out a survey of all district/area physiotherapists in the UK, seeking to identify the whole range of activities which they saw as important for the health education aspect of physiotherapy. The most commonly cited areas of health education activities for physiotherapists were related to back care education (89% of all respondents) and ante- or post-natal care (47% of all respondents). In spite of the relatively small sample size (200), the concentration of 'mentions' into the two areas of back care and ante/post-natal, in comparison to the other areas which received considerably fewer mentions, appears to indicate either a narrow view of health education, or perhaps a misconception of what happens in practice. Perhaps if physiotherapists actively involved in clinical practice (as opposed to district/area physiotherapists, whose role is primarily administrative) had been targeted by the survey, or if the nature of health education had been defined, the results might have shown a more even distribution of areas. The entire range of health education activities can be seen in Table 14.1.

Other activities regarded as within the remit of health education included directing patients to other professionals or caring agencies, addressing small groups on specific medical conditions, preventive measures (for example in lifting and handling techniques) and describing the profession itself (Leathley and Stone, 1986).

Further evidence of the extent of the existing health education role within physiotherapy was provided in a study of the health education role of the PAMs (Lyne, 1986), in which both the target groups and the nature of the health education were identified. The target groups were categorized into women's health, children, and adults. For the women's health groups, education included relaxation training for pregnant women and pelvic floor care, methods of lifting and restoration of fitness for new mothers. Education on the use of medication and exercise was directed at asthmatic children. For handicapped and 'clumsy' children, education was in the form of everyday skills training, social behaviour training, and specialist work according to the degree and nature of the handicap. Health education for the adult group (which included stroke patients, hypertensive and post-coronary patients, and a broad classification of 'disabled') included relaxation training, rehabilitation, advice on diet and exercise resumption, and specialist work according to disability.

Perhaps one of the more interesting aspects of

Table 14.1
Most important health education activities (in order of frequency). (From Leathley, 1988, Physiotherapists and health education: report of a survey, *Physiotherapy 74* (5): 218–220.)

Health education activity	Number of mentions
Back care education	178
Ante-natal/post-natal education	102
Education concerning the elderly	24
Education concerning cardiac conditions	24
Relaxation/stress management techniques	20
Education to parents of asthmatic or handicapped children in the community	20
Education of carers/volunteers	18
General health education/advice (to staff, general public or patients)	16
Education involving stroke patients	13
Talks given to other disciplines about physiotherapy	13
Education on prevention of recurrence of soft tissue injury	10
Education on 'joint protection'	8
Prevention of incontinence	7
Management for patients with other chronic conditions	7

this study was the identification of a 'normal' classification in both the children's and adults' categories; here the health education role of the physiotherapist is seen more as a preventive role, rather than the training/teaching/treating role previously identified. The nature of health education in this situation included instruction in correct posture, movement, sports and training for children, advice on back care, posture and seating, relaxation, fitness training and avoidance of injury, and the preservation of mobility and independence by elderly people.

This represents a move towards 'proactive prevention' (which has been described as involving intervention, as in shutting the stable door before the horse escapes), from 'reactive prevention' (which is a secondary measure, as in shutting the stable door once the escaped horse has been recaptured and returned) (Hayne, 1988). Lyne (1986) noted that while physiotherapists expressed the desirability of working with healthy younger adults and children in a preventive role, they did not rate highly the actual possibility of this happening. However, physiotherapists' well established work in obstetrics can surely be regarded as proactive or primary prevention, and their increasing involvement in open access back care programmes, and in prophylactic work with at-risk, pre-retirement and health fitness groups illustrates the expanding role of the physiotherapist in health education.

It is interesting that one of the 'traditional' areas of health education was not mentioned in either of the studies by Leathley (1988) and Lyne (1986), namely that of smoking cessation. Prevention of smoking has been identified by the World Health Organization as the most potentially effective preventive health measure that developed countries can take (Silvestri and Flay, 1989), but the role of physiotherapists in promoting smoking cessa-

tion does not seem to have emerged (Balfour, 1993). Physiotherapists are in fact in an ideal situation to promote smoking cessation, partly because of their background knowledge of anatomy, physiology and pathology, and also because of the amount of time the therapist spends with the patient during a treatment session. However, in a study designed to investigate the sources and level of knowledge of senior physiotherapists on the effects of smoking, Balfour (1993) found that the level of knowledge was poor. This perhaps indicated that they did not consider this to be essential to effective treatment of the patient. It might be argued that if a treatment is regarded as incomplete without an element of advice or education, it is the responsibility of the physiotherapist to equip herself with the requisite knowledge to give that advice or education.

The actual methods used by physiotherapists in educating their patients were investigated by Sluijs et al. (1991), who recorded physiotherapy treatments on videotape, and analysed the educational input under the headings of (1) teaching and informing patients about their complaints or illness; (2) instructions for home exercises; (3) advice and information; (4) general health education; and (5) counselling on stress-related problems. He found that most information was given on exercises, and least on general health education, with most of the exercise information given on the first two sessions when compared with follow-up sessions. General health education and counselling remained fairly constant throughout the course of treatment.

Most studies seem to indicate that physiotherapists tend to limit their health education role to fairly specific areas — the structure of the body and how it works, information about specific medical conditions, description of exercises and instruction on correct techniques to avoid injury. However, there appears to be little reason why the informed physiotherapist should not extend the remit of the health education role to include such matters as smoking, blood vessel disease and diet. Payne (1986) offered a health education package to a 50-plus age group of women at a local sports centre, which incorporated relaxation and exercise, general information, specific individualized advice, and discussion. While not providing the type of measures of success as suggested by Whitehead and Tones (1991), the author felt a degree of success had been achieved by the apparent enjoyment of the group, the level of attendance, the amount and nature of interest and curiosity in the topics covered, and their participation in lively discussions.

Although the delivery of health education is time consuming, physiotherapists should be aware that, when successful, it is time well spent. The ability of patients to cope with their problems, and the reduction in recurrence rates should ultimately reduce demand for services, and consequently help to control waiting lists. The group setting is an ideal one in which to stimulate discussion and debate on health issues, and physiotherapists should perhaps make better use of this environment to deliver health education messages. Furthermore, by making contact with various health agencies, promotional literature can be obtained to supplement the verbal message.

Physiotherapy in the Wider Context of Health Education

The scope of physiotherapy education should equip physiotherapists to incorporate this wider notion of health education into their practice. Thow and Newton (1990) used their knowledge of exercise physiology, pathology and methods of exercise to embark on a programme of prevention using exercise as the basis of health promotion and positive lifestyle adaptations. The programme was aimed at cardiac rehabilitation patients and their families, hospital staff, high risk subjects and normal subjects (no pathology), and employed five strategies:

- Cardiac rehabilitation (phase I and II within the hospital environment);
- Progressive exercise programme for hospital staff;
- Community cardiac rehabilitation (phase III);
- Fitness testing and health promotion week, incorporating 'Good Hearted Glasgow', 'Glasgow 2000' and health exhibitions;
- A two-mile fun run, sponsored for the Chest, Heart and Stroke Association.

The programme was run within the limited resources of a busy physiotherapy department, and a number of physiological (predicted VO_{2max} heart rate) and psychological (Profile of Mood States rating scale which measures tension anxiety, depression, anger hostility, vigour, fatigue and confusion) outcome measures indicated improvement over the 3-month period of the programme for the staff group. Although it appears that no specific outcome measures were used, the patient groups progressed after 12 weeks from the hospital-based programme to a community-based programme. Finally, patient and staff groups teamed up with the health education department and the physiotherapy department to establish a mass media campaign to promote 'health and fitness', culminating in a week of activities. Using the resources of the group, hospital staff were targeted with the health and fitness message. Fitness testing was provided and individual exercise programmes developed, and a number of health initiatives established. The authors concluded that physiotherapists are skilled and well-situated to enhance health education.

Similarly, Shore (1986) evaluated the 'Look After Yourself' programme (incorporating the elements of exercise, relaxation and health topics) developed by the Health Education Council, and concluded that if physiotherapists are to be ready to meet the challenge of care in the community, the 'Look After Yourself' programme, which involves so much material already familiar to the physiotherapist, can provide a stepping stone for those interested in extending their health education role into the community. Other examples of physiotherapists' involvement in the wider context of health education include the supervision of occupational fitness programmes and involvement in group activity sessions for asthmatic children. The latter involvement included advice on medication taking, how to cope with exercise and participation in sports activities, all of which aim at preventing or minimizing the development of physical and psychological problems (Gemmell, 1986).

Concerns about Physiotherapy in Health Education

The increasing involvement of physiotherapists and other PAMs in the wider context of health education raises several issues. The potential for physiotherapy input into health education in its wider context far outweighs the actual provision of physiotherapists to deliver the service (Leathley and Stone, 1986). A degree of selectivity is therefore required to use their skills to their best advantage, and this may involve choices between the various levels at which these skills may be used. For example, effectiveness must be evaluated in a one-to-one setting, in group work,

or at a more strategic level in commercial organizations, local government or health service management. These choices will have to be made within the framework of existing resources, and may not reflect the 'ideal' mode of delivery of the service.

This leads on to well established problems regarding the evaluation of health education programmes (Baric, 1980; Leathley and Stone, 1986; Whitehead and Tones, 1991). Before new initiatives can be implemented, evidence of cost effectiveness is required by the budget controllers; health education is an element of physiotherapy practice which is accepted as being difficult to record, and consequently, it may not be acknowledged. Leathley and Stone (1986) suggest that there is an urgent need for all health professions to develop methods of recording and evaluating their practice according to their specific priorities. Physiotherapists may be assisted in developing these methods by making use of existing resources, including advice, from health education and health promotion units. They may also build on their knowledge of health education through educational courses designed to extend and develop existing qualifications and experience, which are considered to be insufficient in scope and application to enable people to fulfil the health education specialist's role (Norton, 1986).

Social and Psychological Implications

The change in government policy towards health as stated in the white paper 'Prevention and Health; Everybody's Business' (DHSS, 1976) represents a realignment of emphasis from the curative approach, dependent on the comprehensive provisions offered by the NHS after the war, to a preventive approach, in which the individual may be expected to hold the key to his/her own health (Pill and Stott, 1982).

The move towards a preventive approach is partly in response to the increasing morbidity and mortality resulting from degenerative disease, but also in response to the realization that curative medicine 'may be increasingly subject to the law of diminishing returns' (DHSS, 1976). Prevention is thus seen as providing a means of rationing the health care budget, by redistributing resources away from expensive hospital services, to cheaper community and primary care sources, and also directing the health care budget and resources into those areas where the benefits are likely to be greatest (Graham, 1978).

The major thrust of this shift in emphasis focuses on the concept that the 'greatest problem for preventive medicine now lies in changing behaviour and attitudes to health' (DHSS, 1976), and that it is in everybody's interest to adopt a healthier lifestyle. The success of this approach would appear to rely on three major assumptions: firstly, that the individual has the desire to change his/her lifestyle, secondly, that s/he has the knowledge and understanding about how to change; and thirdly, that s/he has the ability to control and then change behaviour and lifestyle.

Most physiotherapy treatment regimens involve active participation by the patient, not only during the time that the therapist is actually working with the patient, but also during the period following or between treatments, when the patient may be asked to carry out an individual 'treatment programme', either on his own or with the assistance of carers. The individual treatment programme should be tailored to meet the needs of the patient, and might involve exercise, relaxation, postural drainage, control of swelling, application of heat or cold, stretching and other health advice perhaps related to posture, ergonomics, lifting, diet and smoking. Thus, for a patient to adhere to a physiotherapeutic treatment regimen, that patient will be required to a greater or lesser extent to change behaviour and lifestyle.

Patient Compliance

The concept of patient compliance is a complex one, but one which must be understood if successful outcomes are to be achieved. This is so whether in the situation of a relatively short-term treatment regimen, in a longer-term approach in which the patient must take increasing responsibility for their own treatment and ultimate health destiny, or in the context of primary (proactive) or secondary (reactive) prevention. Various factors have been suggested as having an influence on the degree to which patients adhere to medical advice, take responsibility for their health destiny, and instigate change in their health behaviour.

Patient compliance is of considerable importance in physiotherapy, because treatment effects partly depend on it; the efficacy of therapeutic intervention can only be established when patients comply with the therapeutic regimen (Sluijs et al., 1991). Patient compliance is the extent to which patients do or do not follow their therapist's advice. The actual contact between the patient and the health professional is a manifestation of help-seeking behaviour, and consists of the individual deciding to do something about a symptom or distress. Help-seeking behaviour may be either medical, in which the patient makes contact with a doctor or other health professional (and a process whereby a health-care system forms around the patient), or nonmedical, where assistance is sought from nonmedical personnel, such as clergymen, friends and relatives (Leigh and Reiser, 1980).

'The Sick Role'

Society assigns specific expectations to the 'patient', by virtue of his being 'ill'. These expectations comprise what is known as the 'sick role' (Parsons, 1951, cited in Leigh and Reiser, 1980). In assuming the 'sick role', the patient expects to offer cooperation and compliance to the doctor or other health professional, in return for some assurance that attempts will be made to relieve the distress. It is therefore, perhaps, rather surprising to learn that compliance and cooperation do not always occur. Ley (1977) stated that irrespective of the advice given to patients, it is fairly certain that large numbers of patients will not follow it.

The *Oxford English Dictionary* defines compliance as 'action in accordance with request, demand etc; unworthy submission; yielding under applied force', implying a passive obedience, or obedience which does not necessarily reflect the beliefs, attitudes or perceptions of the individual involved. Thompson (1984) extended this view of compliance, stating that the term carries the 'unfortunate implication that patients are either passively obedient, or wilfully disobedient in the face of medical wisdom'. This same author argued that this view of patient response to medical advice reveals more about the inherent assumptions of medical practice, in that many doctors assume that patients will faithfully follow their advice.

Communication of Advice

It seems obvious that if a patient is expected to follow medical advice, the advice must be commu-nicated effectively. However, Ley (1977) stated that many doctors tend to ignore the problems of communication, either by assuming that if the will to communicate is there, all will be well, or they regard the ability to accurately diagnose, select appropriate treatment and manifest surgical skill as paramount, to the ultimate exclusion of consideration of communication skills.

This assumption of compliance by doctors has rarely been accompanied by any attempt to ascertain the degree of compliance (Thompson, 1984). The following information suggests that this assumption should be questioned!

- On average, 44% of patients *do not* follow advice (Ley, 1977).
- In a general medical clinic, 50% were complying with advice (Thompson, 1984), *but:*
  - only 11% of doctors estimated that only 50% complied;
  - 47% estimated that 75% were compliant;
  - 42% claimed that 'almost all' their patients followed advice given.

This state of ignorance has been blamed on the fact that most doctors did not question their patients on their adherence to medical advice. Lack of questioning tended to lead to non-compliance, and to the concealment of this fact; patients exhibiting this passive response may be assumed erroneously by the doctor to have accepted the advice given (Thompson, 1984). This tends to emphasize the concept of the authoritarian role of the doctor, and the passive, obedient, compliant role of the patient. It appears that when physicians check with patients about compliance, patients are more likely on follow-up to be found to comply (Thompson, 1984). Similarly, patients whose compliance is being monitored, and who receive feedback about their efforts and progress, comply better than patients without supervision (Dunbar *et al.*, 1979; Epstein and Cluss, 1982; Martin *et al.*, 1984; Knapp, 1988).

> ## Key Point
>
> *There is a message here for the physiotherapist. Do not assume that your patients are following your advice regarding, for example, home exercise programmes, rest, modification of work environment. Check with your patients specifically what they are doing, and identify any problems with their understanding/interpretation, and with their ability to follow the advice. Not only will they be more likely to comply, but they will feel that you are taking a real interest in their progress.*

Although most of the studies into patient compliance have investigated adherence to medical regimens, the indications are that non-compliance with physiotherapeutic, and more specifically exercise regimens, is as great as non-compliance with medical regimens (Sluijs *et al.*, 1991).

Sluijs *et al.* (1991) quote a number of reports of research into compliance with exercises, mostly concerned with cardiac rehabilitation programmes, preventive fitness programmes or back schools, which found that one-third to two-thirds of patients do not comply with exercise programmes, and that although in some cases early compliance was as high as 64% of patients, this dropped off to 23% in the long term. The difficulty of assessing compliance was acknowledged, as patients often do not admit non-compliance, and compliance is not an 'all or nothing' matter, but has many gradations.

The uptake of medical advice, and resultant behavioural change need not necessarily be based on the assumption of the obedient patient who changes behaviour, and in whom no attempt is made to change attitude. It appears that behavioural changes which occur without a concomitant change in attitude and/or beliefs are likely to be of short duration, as indicated by Sluijs and Kuijper (1990, cited in Sluijs *et al.*, 1991), whereas a change of attitude on the part of the patient might be expected to lead to more long-term behavioural changes (Thompson, 1984). A change of attitude requires some degree of decision making by the patient. Thus a patient may wish to emulate someone he admires, who, for example regards smoking as unattractive or unfashionable, and may wish to change his health-related behaviour to do so (identification); or he may change his behaviour and attitude based on a reasoned argument on the part of that individual (internalization). Both of these approaches to attitude and behavioural change imply active participation of the patient in the decision-making process related to the desired behavioural change.

Some of the factors influencing patient compliance are:

- Views on illness causation;
- Health beliefs;
- Professional–patient relationship;
- The nature of the illness/disability;
- The nature of the treatment regimen;
- Knowledge;
- Social/situational.

Views on Illness Causation

It has been claimed that the practice of western medicine has done considerable harm — side-effects of treatment, post-surgical complications, dependence on prescribed drugs — and that the introduction of the NHS has effectively removed the individual's control over health and illness

(Elwes and Simnett, 1985). People have become dependent on doctors and medicines, expecting a cure for every ill, and lost the ability to cope with sickness, disability and death. Thus people perceive that they have little control over their own health destiny (Townsend and Davidson, 1980), so exhortations to take responsibility for their own health may have little effect.

Helman (1981) cited Eisenberg (1977) and Kleinmann (1980) in attempting to explain the meaning of illness: illness refers to the subjective response of the patient being unwell; how he and those around him perceive the origin and significance of the event; how it affects his behaviour or relationships with other people; and the steps he takes to remedy this situation. These nuances of the meaning of illness to an individual, and the nature of his response are profoundly influenced by his social and cultural background, as well as his personality traits.

Melhuish (1982) observed that many people feel that they have no control over their own health — 'a bullet with their name on it which cannot be avoided'. Pill and Stott (1982) have argued that the readiness to accept responsibility for one's health depends partly on the beliefs held on the causation of illness. They explored beliefs of illness causation in a group of working class mothers, selected from socioeconomic group 9 (skilled manual workers). It emerged that about half the group were buying their own houses, and these women tended to have achieved a higher level of education than those who were not: this had implications for the findings of the study, which showed that the women who had a lower level of education, and were less likely to be buying their own homes, held somewhat fatalistic views on the causes of illness, mentioning germs, stress, environment and heredity as the principal causes.

These causes can generally be described as external causes, and seen as something beyond the control of the individual. In contrast, the group who were better educated, and more likely to be buying their own houses, referred to behavioural choices made by the individual when discussing the aetiology of illness.

Blaxter (1983) carried out a similar study involving middle-aged women, brought up in poor social circumstances, and again found that the most commonly perceived causes of illness were infection, heredity, familial tendency and environment (including working conditions and damp). These views underpin the assumption of many of the women in these studies that every illness has a single identifiable cause, and this view has been substantiated in other studies by Kendall (1975) and Cassell (1976). This view of illness causation seems to be one element in a cluster of attitudes, in which it is more acceptable to find an external/environmental cause of illness, than to admit personal responsibility; this creates a potential conflict with current official health policy in which greater emphasis in being placed on preventive rather than curative medicine, and places more responsibility on the patient.

CHOICE AND RESPONSIBILITY – A CONFLICT?

It is important to recognize the potential conflict created by ultimately placing responsibility for health on the patient. The concepts of accountability and responsibility imply an element of choice; people who hold these beliefs of external illness causation often live and work in circumstances which permit very little flexibility, and consequently they perceive that there is a lack of any real choice in their day-to-day existence (Cullen, 1979, cited in Pill and Stott, 1982; Blaxter,

1983). It can therefore be concluded that social circumstances influence both the perceptions of health and illness, and the practicalities of improving health status.

A large proportion of physiotherapy practice revolves around active participation of the patient in the treatment programme. This includes working with the therapist during treatment sessions, carrying out treatment techniques between patient–therapist treatment sessions, working semi-independently in rehabilitation programmes (circuits or group work within the rehabilitation setting), and carrying out home treatment programmes.

Patients' views of illness causation and their ability to influence its course will play a large part in determining the degree to which they actively participate in treatment. The patient with a fatalistic view will be much more likely to adopt a passive role, expecting the therapist to effect a 'cure'; assuming such a patient will work independently may be counterproductive, and alternative ways of achieving patient involvement in the treatment must be explored. Similarly, it may be unrealistic to expect, for example, a young mother, with a large demanding family, living in poor social circumstances and with little support, to carry out a complex and time-consuming home exercise programme, when she finds it difficult to see beyond 'getting through each day as it comes'.

Thus it is important that the therapist has a sound understanding of patients' views of their illnesses/problems, and their beliefs about how they may influence its course. With this understanding, the therapist and patient can then work out a strategy to make best use of available resources to encourage patient participation and compliance with treatment programmes.

Health Beliefs

Beliefs about the ultimate success, in terms of improved health, of changes in lifestyle will affect the individual's desire to change. Aizen and Fishbein (1980, cited in Thompson, 1984) stated that 'action is the reasoned outcome of cognitive beliefs, and emotional attitudes, conditioned by a group of subjective norms', proposing that for a change in behaviour to occur, there must be a concomitant change in beliefs. In health education terms, merely encouraging the individual to change behaviour will be unsuccessful, unless the individual believes in the desirability of a change in behaviour/lifestyle, and that it will result in a successful outcome in terms of improved health; it will also depend on the individual's belief in the value/benefits of improved health.

Becker (1974) put forward five prerequisites for patient compliance with health advice:

- The patient must possess some basic knowledge about health, and the motivation to achieve it, to provide a stimulus to action;
- S/he must believe him/herself to be vulnerable to illness/disability;
- S/he must believe that illness/disability has significant consequences;
- S/he must believe that the treatment will work;
- S/he must believe that this can be achieved at an acceptable cost.

This 'health belief model' can be applied to both curative medicine (adherence to treatment regimens) and preventive medicine (behavioural changes to reduce health risk), emphasizing the importance of patient perception. For example, an anti-smoking campaign which stresses health implications may not succeed in influencing young people, for whom the threat of eventual disease seems remote (Thompson, 1984). They may be more influenced by suggestions that smoking is unattractive, or unfashionable, and unless this is recognized, the exhortations may be fruitless.

Furthermore, the problem of perceived sacrifice cannot be ignored; a change in behaviour which involves loss of rewarding and enjoyable pursuits may be tolerated in the short term, but in certain circumstances, treatment procedures involve long-term or permanent alteration of accustomed habits and sources of pleasure (Bernstein and Bernstein, 1980). This is particularly relevant in preventive medicine, but may also apply in the case of treatment regimens directed at secondary prevention, as in the example of a runner sustaining a stress fracture of the lower limb, for which a prolonged period of rest is essential. It seems logical to assume that the amount of behavioural adjustment, particularly if it involves perceived self-sacrifice and loss of pleasure, will influence the success of treatment regimens or attempts to encourage a healthier lifestyle. It has been found that patients are less likely to do what they are told if the treatment involves considerable adjustment of lifestyle and perceived self-sacrifice (Thompson, 1984). This author notes that fear may assist compliance, but only when clear guidance and advice are given. In the example of the runner, explanations of the consequences of continued participation may provide this 'fear' factor, but compliance is much more likely to occur if advice and guidance is given on alternative physical/sporting activities in which the runner can participate during this period of enforced rest of the injured part. This is particularly important if the runner has become accustomed to a feeling of well-being associated with his running.

The 'health belief model' provides a neat framework within which explanations of a patient's compliance or non-compliance may be found, and which may also equip the health professional with the means of adopting a different approach to the delivery of health advice, resulting in improved compliance. However, the limitations of the model must be recognized, in that it tends to portray a rather simplistic picture, perhaps ignoring the complexity of external factors (family, environmental, economic) which can influence both the patient's perception of health, and his ability to exert control over it.

Professional–Patient Relationship

It might be argued that compliance with medical advice may be linked to the patient's perception of the doctor (or indeed any health professional), and to the doctor's perception of the patient. Most of the investigations in this area have concentrated on the 'doctor/patient' relationship, but information can readily be applied to physiotherapist's relationship with the patient. The physician who adopts an authoritarian role will prescribe a treatment regimen, assume that the patient will comply with this, and will see no necessity to monitor adherence. The patient, on the other hand, may see such a physician as showing little interest in his (the patient's) lifestyle or his reactions to illness, being solely concerned with the facts related to the diagnosis. He may feel intimidated and unable to give an adequate account of his symptoms; and he may not follow the treatment regimen (Bernstein and Bernstein, 1980). Lack of questioning on the part of the physician leads to concealment of non-compliance, and may erroneously transmit the impression to the patient, that the treatment is thought to be unimportant, or unlikely to work (Thompson, 1984).

This view of the professional–patient relationship in medical practice was conceptualized by Veatch

(1972, cited in Bernstein and Bernstein, 1980), who identified four models on which the relationship may be based.

1 The *'engineering model'* designates to the physician the role of the pure scientist, interested only in the facts, and therefore free from consideration of values in his interaction with patients.
2 The *'priestly model'* invests in the professional–patient relationship an almost religious aura, in which the physician's judgement on both medical and moral issues is pronounced in an authoritarian manner, and potentially removes from the patient freedom of choice, and the right to self-determination.

Both of these models would appear to operate on the assumption that the patient follows the physician's advice without question, and that his health-related behaviour will change in accordance with the advice.

Veatch suggested two further models of the professional–patient relationship, which involve a greater degree of active participation by the patient.

3 The *'collegial model'* requires that the professional and the patient become colleagues, 'pursuing the common goal of eliminating illness and preserving health'; while this model might be seen as 'preserving the values of trust, confidence, dignity and respect', Veatch sees it as unrealistic in view of differences in ethnic, class, social and economic values.
4 The *'contractual model'* is based on the recognition by the professional that the patient must maintain freedom of control over his own life and health destiny when significant choices are to be made, and means that relatively greater open discussion of the moral premises hiding in medical decisions is necessary, both before and as they are made.

'WORKING TOGETHER TO DEVELOP TREATMENT PROGRAMMES'

The latter two models represent a significant move away from the authoritarian view, to a more democratic approach in which the health professional and patient work in a mutually understanding relationship to prescribe and adhere to the most effective treatment regimen for the patient. This approach would seem desirable not only from an ethical point of view, but also when one considers the change in the nature of disease which has occurred during this century. Improvement in social conditions, medical and surgical practice and pharmacology have reduced the incidence of infectious diseases in which short-term compliance with relatively simple treatment regimens are effective.

These same factors are encouraging the elderly to live longer and healthier lives, improving survival rates for premature babies which may perpetuate the overall numbers of children with profound disabilities, and creating a greater demand on medical resources from the chronic, degenerative disease processes besetting the middle-aged and working population (Walker, 1995). The very nature of these disease processes dictates that a 'quick cure' is not possible; thus long-term management is required, necessitating behavioural change by the patient. This is more likely to occur if the patient has had greater involvement in the decisions relating to his treatment, and has an understanding of the nature and importance of his treatment regimen. Thompson (1984) noted that one-sided messages are very popular in the medical profession, but they are likely to be effective only with poorly educated subjects; others are more likely to respond to reasoned argument. This is supported by Walker (1995), who emphasized the importance of the thorough and systematic assessment which should inform the physiotherapist sufficiently to begin a dialogue with the patient on the intended plan of action, approximate time-scales, and in some cases an initial discussion on the intended outcome.

Walker (1995) also identified the links between the placebo effect and the patient–therapist relationship, emphasizing the importance of an empathetic rapport with patients, particularly when the intervention has a 'hands-on' emphasis. Peat (1981) quoted Basmajian (1975) in stating 'when one views the whole field of rehabilitation, including physical therapy, one is struck by the impression that rehabilitation's main virtue is *not* its scientific base. Rather its main virtue is the intensive relationship of the various professionals with individual patients'. Furthermore, Walker (1995) cited studies which support the notion that the patient's satisfaction and compliance are closely related to the doctor's or therapist's show of interest and concern (Bond *et al.*, 1976; Hulka *et al.*, 1976, cited in Walker, 1995).

> . . . time is the one thing that patients need *most* from those who treat them – time to be heard, time to have things explained, time to be reassured. Yet time is the thing health professionals find most difficult to manage (Peat, 1980)

The Nature of the Illness/ Disability

> Compliance should be viewed as a reflection of the experience of chronic illness (Alvin *et al.*, 1995)

Factors related to the nature of illness have been shown to influence compliance with treatment regimens.

- The nature of the illness has been shown to influence compliance: Alvin *et al.* (1995) investigated medical compliance in adolescents with chronic illness, and considered that the degree of compliance was a reflection of the total experience of chronic illnesss, including demographic factors, patient and family characteristics, aspects of the illness and treatment regimen, and the patient–doctor relationship.
- As illness passes from the acute stage, patients are less likely to adhere to a treatment regimen (Kent and Dalgleish, cited in Walker, 1995).
- Although coping is a dynamic process which plays a major role in a person's behaviour in responding in the best possible way to cope with his environment, it appears that in situations of chronic illness (e.g. asthma), behavioural modifications are often inappropriate (Deenen and Klip, 1993).
- Non-compliance appears in all therapies in which the patient is expected to administer his own medication, and this is particularly prevalent in chronic illness, where approximately 50% of patients do not take their medication, or do not take it in accordance with the prescription (Deenen and Klip, 1993).
- More than half of a sample of adult patients with cystic fibrosis claimed to take more than 80% of their treatments. Compliance with individual treatments varied according to their perceived unpleasantness and degree of infringement on daily activities (see Becker's health belief model above). The most common reason for omitting treatment was forgetfulness.

Palat (1994) considered the rehabilitation and education of the cardiac patient, arguing that the role of health education is not only to inform the patient, but to educate. He further argued that in the case of the chronic patient, providing the patient with a wider overall understanding of the nature of his disease (pathogenesis, intervention, rehabilitation and prophylaxis) may improve compliance with treatment regimens. Furthermore, increased understanding of the nature of the disease process may improve the ability of the patient to live with his disease; that is, it may provide the patient with coping strategies for his day-to-day existance. This is supported in a study by Blalock et al. (1995) who found in a group of 300 patients with osteoarthritis a variety of coping strategies, which included problem-solving, cognitive restructuring, social support, emotional expression, problem avoidance, turning to religion and information seeking.

This suggests a number of ways in which the physiotherapist may contribute to the coping strategies of patients with chronic disease — by providing information, problem solving with the patient, investigating and providing support networks, and encouraging the patient to develop new perspectives on their problems. Thus, the physiotherapist who is working with patients with chronic problems should have a comprehensive knowledge of the charities / support agencies associated with the problem area, which may help to provide, in particular, social support and advice.

A number of studies have investigated coping strategies of patients with chronic disease, and of their families / carers. Interestingly, two of these studies identified support from hospital staff as providing a means of coping. In a study involving 61 patients with Hodgkin's disease, the most commonly used strategies were compliance strategies and trust in doctors (Harrer et al., 1993). In another study investigating the stressors and coping strategies of families of children with chronic illness, the families relied on a number of coping strategies, of which securing information and obtaining support from hospital staff were most helpful (Horn et al., 1995). Different coping strategies may be used in different aspects of life — for example, Blalock et al. (1995) found that self-

criticism and social withdrawal were used more frequently for social relationship problems.

The nature of chronic disease perhaps demands different approaches to promote adherence to treatment regimens. In accepting that non-compliance with medication is one of the major factors in the failure of therapeutic programmes for patients with chronic disease, Guimon (1995) evaluated a group programme for schizophrenic patients which aimed at diminishing negative views on the use of medication. Positive results from this programme prompted the author to suggest that building up specific questionnaires might help in understanding the nature of prejudices towards the use of medication in patients with chronic diseases, and that the organization of group programmes could diminish patients' prejudices, thus improving compliance. Although physiotherapy programmes are of a different nature, it might be useful to identify the reasons for low compliance in patients with chronic disease, and to establish group programmes to involve the patients themselves in working out ways in which compliance might be improved.

The Nature of the Treatment Regimen

The nature of the treatment also influences the extent to which patients do what they are told. If a patient has strong expectations about the form of treatment he should receive, and a different treatment is prescribed, the patient is unlikely to comply (Thompson, 1984). Adherence to a prescribed treatment can be improved by recognizing the expectations of the patient, discussing these with the patient, and attempting to cater for them in the treatment regimen. Nowhere is this more apparent than in the treatment of sports injuries: adequate treatment of the injured jogger requires tolerance and understanding of the pressures which motivate a previously sedentary middle-aged office worker to become addicted to jogging. To prohibit further exercise, or to offer 'complete rest' as the only solution to the injury will result in non-compliance, and a search for alternative remedies (Piterman, 1983). Similarly, Kirby and Valmassy (1983) stated that insisting on complete rest, and effectively cutting out the injured runner's daily 'fix' will almost certainly result in low patient compliance with treatment.

Many treatment procedures lead to a temporary interference with daily pursuits which are rewarding and enjoyable. While the loss of such pursuits may be tolerated in the short term, in some circumstances treatment involves long-term or permanent alterations in accustomed habits and sources of pleasure (Bernstein and Bernstein, 1980). As stated above, the amount of behavioural adjustment will influence compliance; patients will be less likely to do what they are told if treatment involves considerable adjustment in lifestyle and perceived sacrifice. It has been found that when significant behavioural change is required, fear may assist compliance, but only when clear guidance and support are given (Thompson, 1984).

The perceived effectiveness of the treatment has an effect on the degree to which the patient will adhere to the treatment regimen, in that when treatment is perceived as being effective, compliance is higher (Hartman and Becker, 1978, cited in Thompson, 1984). Conversely, if the patient disagrees with the diagnosis, or the treatment regimen, compliance will probably be low (Thompson, 1984).

Similarly, if a patient is unprepared for the effects of treatment, which may include unpleasant side-effects, he will be less likely to adhere to the treatment. Most studies on the influence of giving patients adequate information about their treatment regimens have concentrated on the effects of pre-operative communication on the progress of surgical patients. Findings indicated that when patients are given prior information on what to expect, they adjust more readily during the post-operative period (Janis, 1971, cited in Ley, 1977).

Physiotherapists should therefore spend time with their patients in the pre-operative stage, explaining how the course of treatment will develop, and what the patient should expect. Practice of treatment techniques pre-operatively will also give the patient confidence in their ability to participate in the treatment, and will improve the likelihood of better cooperation post-operatively. This might also apply to the non-surgical situation, when prior knowledge of the possible effects of treatment may counteract the tendency for non-compliance with treatments which may have unpleasant side-effects, and premature termination of treatments which are perceived by the patient to have rapid success. A further extension of this may be in the physiotherapist giving patients (where possible) realistic short-term and long-term goals, which gives them a clear time-frame within which they can place their treatment programme. This can also give them clear 'markers' of progress, by which they can measure their return to normal functional activity.

Knowledge

'Being informed is not only a patient's right, it is also important in order to improve compliance and management' (Martin *et al.*, 1992). Many studies have been carried out to assess the effectiveness of patient education programmes, aimed at improving patient knowledge, in improving patient compliance, and other outcome measures such as patient satisfaction and health outcomes (Daltroy, 1993). Areas of investigation have included rheumatology (Daltroy, 1993), asthma (Deenen and Klip, 1993; Garret et al., 1994; Chmelik and Doughty, 1994, Allen et al., 1995; Sarma et al., 1995), women's health (Abrams and Berman, 1993; Evans et al., 1993; Blankson et al., 1994; Marshall, 1994; Kreher, 1995), cardiovascular risk (Carney et al, 1993; Landers et al., 1993; Peiss et al., 1995; Goodyer et al., 1995), and other less widely researched areas such as inflammatory bowel disease (Martin et al., 1992), and heart transplantation (Shapiro et al., 1995).

These studies have looked at different measures of compliance, namely attendance at clinics, taking of prescribed drugs / medication, and adherence to rehabilitation / prophylactic programmes; although the areas of investigation may not relate directly to physiotherapy practice, comparisons can be drawn, for example, attendance at physiotherapy clinics, application of treatment modalities such as ice, and adherence to exercise regimens.

Results from these studies indicate that the use of advice, counselling, education programmes and information pamphlets have inconsistent effects on compliance.

- Better information sharing leads to improved patient satisfaction, compliance and health outcomes in patients attending rheumatology clinics (Daltroy, 1993).
- Giving the patient more information does not always lead to better adherence to treatment regimen, as demonstrated in an asthma study in which, despite an extensive educational programme in the self-management of asthma,

compliance with the recommended treatment was only 40% (Chmelik and Doughty, 1994).

Some of the variation in outcomes from the studies may be explained by the observation that different measures of compliance were used; however other factors may contribute to the observed differences.

- The complexity of the treatment regimen may have an influence on the uptake of advice; a study of the impact of pharmacist counselling on medication knowledge and compliance, found that in all patients, medication knowledge and compliance decreased as the number of medications increased (Siguero et al., 1995). This may be due to patients' inability to retain a large body of information.
- An individualized reminder chart, which listed the patient's medications, and when they were to be taken, resulted in better compliance rates (Raynor et al., 1993).
- In a study on dietary advice in a coronary prevention programme, a second formal dietary consultation appeared beneficial in improving compliance and lipid control (Peiss et al., 1995).
- Patient information leaflets are used extensively to educate and inform patients; however, if the information pamphlets are beyond the reading and comprehension abilities of the target population, it should not be surprising if compliance rates with the information / advice contained in the pamphlets is low. A study on the comprehensibility of 50 Australian educational pamphlets for patients with asthma found that two-thirds of the pamphlets were written at or above the average reading level of 52% of Australians aged between 15 and 69 (Sarma et al., 1995). Thus, over half of the population could understand only one third of the pamphlets!

In addition to the provision of information of an inappropriate level, it has been suggested that informative material is often produced without prior analysis of what patients consider important to know (Martin et al., 1992). In an investigation into what patients want to know about their inflammatory bowel disease, 90% thought that educational material prepared according to their needs could be very useful, although 35% thought that knowledge of the possible severity of their disease might increase their anxiety. In a wider context, Feste and Anderson (1995) suggest that, particularly with respect to patients wirth chronic disease, health educators have a responsibility to address the physical, emotional, cognitive and spiritual needs of patients.

These studies provide much material which can be applied to many facets of physiotherapy practice in which the physiotherapist provides information for the patient; the physiotherapist needs to consider the amount and complexity of the information to be retained by the patient, the level of comprehension, and whether the information meets the needs of the individual patient. This may preclude the use of standardized sheets/pamphlets which are not tailored to the individual patient's needs. All this suggests that we should be consulting with our patients to ensure that the information we are giving them is appropriate and effective.

Social/Situational Factors

Researchers of health behaviour have concentrated on social, psychological and environmental factors instead of medical ones, and have identified the principal explanations of health behaviour as including:

1 Belief in the benefits of health behaviour and compliance with social norms;
2 The economic location of a person in determining opportunities to maintain a healthy lifestyle;
3 Lifestyle influences on the probability of having good health habits (Lock and Wister, 1992).

In a review of research on health care appointment breaking, Bean and Talaga (1992) found that demographic characteristics, psychosocial problems, previous appointment keeping, health beliefs and situational factors were predictors of non-attendance behaviour.

Social support has been cited as influencing compliance with treatment regimens; thus, patients who have a better family support network seem to adhere more closely to prescribed treatments. Patterson et al. (1993) found that 33% of the variance of an index of pulmonary health (FEV_1) in cystic fibrosis, over a period of 10 years, was explained by differences in family characteristics. Compliance with daily chest physiotherapy and with quarterly clinic visits was associated with a better FEV_1 trend, which in turn was associated with integrated family coping mechanisms and support; poor FEV_1 trends were associated with a more fragmented family environment, with family members spending more time outside the home. Lorenc and Branthwaite (1993) investigated compliance with prescribed medication in older and younger adults, and found that although age did not influence compliance, living with a relative was one of seven variables which were independently and significantly associated with better compliance.

This has implications for involving family and carers in the management of patients in the home environment, when greater understanding of the patient's problems, and the ability to give support in their management should improve compliance. Furthermore, Sutton *et al.* (1994) found that married or single women were more likely to attend a breast screening clinic than divorced, separated or widowed women, and that predictors of attendance included the attitudes of significant others (the women's husband/partner and children), again supporting the view that social support has a strong influence on health beliefs and behaviours.

Fishman (1995) noted that it is a well established fact that social support plays a key role in promoting health, decreasing susceptibility to disease, and facilitating recovery from illness. In the development of a programme of low to moderate intensity exercise designed to improve and control hypertension, physicians co-opted the support of family and friends.

- The patients are asked to identify who in their life loves or cares for them.
- In the presence of the physician, they phone the identified helper(s).
- The helper(s) then agree(s) to support the patient's treatment regimen.

This is an innovative approach, but the success of this particular programme has not yet been established. Social support was also found to be associated with perceived behavioural control, and exercise adherence during a 12-week exercise programme (Courneya and McAuley, 1995)

Key Points

Physiotherapists might usefully consider involving family/friends in treatment programmes; this could take the form of showing how they can help in the actual treatment, but additionally could include an educational element to improve their knowledge and understanding of the condition/problems, how it affects the patient, and how it might be mediated by the treatment.

Socioeconomic factors have also been implicated as an explanation for non-compliance. Griffiths *et al.* (1994) observed that attendance at health checks of patients already registered with a general practitioner is known to be poor, with those in greatest need being least likely to attend. In a survey of patients in seven east London practices aimed at determining characteristics of non-attenders it was found that non-attenders were significantly more likely than attenders to be of lower social class, unemployed, of African origin and to be heavy smokers. Non-attending mothers were significantly more likely than attending mothers to be single parents, a situation which may combine lower socioeconomic status and lack of social support. However, Sutton *et al.* (1994) found that although women living in rented accommodation were less likely to attend for breast screening, other indicators of education and social class were not predictors of attendance.

Cultural influences should also be taken into consideration; British Asians with type 2 diabetes have been shown to have poorer blood glucose control, awareness of diabetes management, and knowledge of complications (Hawthorne *et al.*, 1993). These authors suggest that understanding of dietary customs and health beliefs commonly held by Asian patients may help the physician understand why some patients appear to show poor compliance with accepted western medicine. Patients should always be approached as individuals with their own unique needs within the context of their own cultural backgrounds.

Summary of Compliance

There are many reasons why patients do or do not comply with treatment regimens; the interaction among these various facets makes the concept of compliance a complex one, and presents health professionals with a considerable challenge, if we are to ensure that our patients adhere to treatment programmes. Merril (1994) summarized the inherent difficulties in stating that compliance with programmes depends on behavioural change, and the support or barriers encountered in the behaviour change attempts.

In considering doctor–patient communication, Daltroy (1993) suggested that information sharing could be greatly improved, and that doctors and patients can be trained to improve information sharing, resulting in improved outcomes. He further suggested a number of techniques which could be usefully incorporated into the management of each patient:

- Encourage patients to write down their concerns before each visit.
- Address each concern specifically, however briefly.
- Ask patients what they think has caused their problems.
- Tailor treatment to patients' goals and preferences.
- Explain the purpose, dosage, side-effects and how to judge efficacy of treatment.
- Check patients' understanding.
- Anticipate problems with compliance, and discuss ways of coping with these.
- Write down diagnosis and treatment plan.
- Give patients available literature / pamphlets.
- Reinforce patients' confidence in their ability to manage their regimen.
- Use ancillary personnel in patient education.
- Refer patients to organized programmes in the community.

Many of these techniques are aimed at improving communication between the patient and the doctor; communication plays an important role in our everyday life, so much so that we perhaps take it for granted. In the clinical situation good communication between the therapist and patient is essential, but without a sound knowledge and understanding of the elements of communication which can maximize the patient–therapist relationship, efficacy of treatment may be compromised.

Communication

Communication is defined by the *Oxford English Dictionary* (1995) as 'the act or an instance of communicating, the imparting or exchange of information, ideas or feelings'.

Communication is a two-way process in the therapeutic setting and involves the physiotherapist and the patient interacting together to bring about a successful rehabilitation process. The physiotherapist has the professional knowledge to deliver information and ideas, regarding exercises for example, and the patient has the knowledge of their own painful problem and disability. Communication between the parties will include both verbal and nonverbal elements, and may not only be between therapist and patient but also with relatives / carers, and fellow members of the professional multidisciplinary team.

Thomquist (1990) pointed out that communication in some form or another is an integral part of any professional practice – there is a continuous exchange of messages containing a meaning. This meaning must be interpreted. Furthermore, communication takes place within a context and is crucially influenced by it.

The patient will be interpreting the context in their own way, dependent upon their own perceptions and fears of their pain / disability or indeed the alien environment of the hospital or surgery. As physiotherapists, we cannot assume that our clients are comfortable in the environment in which we work daily, or with our uniforms whether these be the classic 'white coat' or the popular sweatshirt with professional logo and trousers!

The First Meeting

The first face-to-face meeting is usually one in which the therapist will examine the patient in order to ascertain the exact nature of the problem. The most commonly used system is:

- *Phase 1*: subjective examination;
- *Phase 2*: objective examination;
- *Phase 3*: assessment of the findings; and
- *Phase 4*: plan of treatment
  (Grieve, 1982)

In *Phase 1* the physiotherapist will question the patient about various aspects of the condition including pain and disability and interference with activities of daily living. The patient will be watched closely throughout for gestures, such as a facial grimace.

In *Phase 2* the physiotherapist will perform various tests by palpating the area involved, measuring joint range of movement, finding out when pain is elicited by watching the patient's face or appreciating muscle spasm. Questions will also be asked regarding pain or symptoms elicited.

In *Phase 3* the physiotherapist will look back over the findings and record the most important on the patient's record chart prior to Phase 4.

In *Phase 4* the therapist will plan a treatment programme for the individual patient. During this phase various factors are taken into consideration — the present state of the pathological condition and the patient's perceived ability to cope with the disability.

These four phases should, of course, be followed by a fifth phase — *explanation to the patient!* The therapist should explain the findings of the examination of the patient and the aims and goals of the treatment plan. Together, therapist and patient will negotiate short-term and long-term goals in the rehabilitation process.

A range of communication skills have already been mentioned:

- Questioning;
- Nonverbal observation and interpretation;
- Touch;
- Empathy;
- Explanation.

Thornquist (1990) noted that the physiotherapist's approach and professional examination communicates to the patient what is relevant and what is irrelevant, what is important and what is unimportant, and at the same time the two parties are ascribed specific roles.

Verbal and nonverbal communication has occurred and impressions have been formed.

Classification of Communication Skills

A global classification would broadly be nonverbal and verbal skills. Examples of nonverbal skills would be physical contact (touch), gestures, posture, head nods, eye gaze, facial expression, physical characteristics and environmental factors. Examples of verbal skills would be questioning and explanation.

This broad classification would be inappropriate for physiotherapy practice as it is too broad and nonspecific (Hargie et al., 1994).

Saunders and Caves (1986) used analysis of videotaped therapy, in the professional context of speech therapy, in order to:

1 Identify effective/ineffective therapeutic behaviour;
2 Analyse and categorize effective/ineffective behaviour.

This research resulted in 20 categories of classified instances of communication skills — for example, positive reinforcement, physical contact, cueing, counselling, questioning. This study clearly attempted to identify the communication skills in speech therapy.

With regard to physiotherapy, a similar study was conducted in 1994 by Adams et al. The study recruited expert physiotherapists working in a range of adult specialities and paediatrics. The therapists were interviewed about their work and videotaped for 2 to 3 hours with patients; the findings were analysed and categorized using the Delphi technique (Duffield, 1990).

The resultant classification of the physiotherapists' communication skills was into two categories: instrumental and affective behaviours (see Table 14.2).

This classification (Adams et al., 1994), follows that of Rotor's Interaction Analysis System (RIAS), instrumental task clusters being identified as:

1 Information: all information statements related to medical condition, therapeutic regimen, lifestyle, feelings;
2 Questions: all open-ended and closed-ended

Table 14.2
Classification of physiotherapists' communication skills (From Adams et al., 1994.)

Instrumental behaviours	Affective behaviours
Verbal	*Verbal*
Questioning	Empathy/concern
Instructions	Encouragement/
Explaining/informing	motivation
Reinforcement	Rapport/social behaviour
Counselling	Quality of voice
Cueing	Praise
Emphasis	Reassurance
Use of language	
Identification/correction	
(of errors)	
Feedback	
Nonverbal	*Nonverbal*
Medical touch	Nonmedical touch
Demonstration	Listening

questions as well as asking for understanding, clarification or opinion;
3 Counselling: all persuasive statements related to medical condition, therapeutic regimen, lifestyle and feelings;
4 Directions: all statements that guide the patient through the consultation.

Affective behaviours on RIAS produced three factors.

1 Verbal attentiveness: showing agreement, paraphrasing and reflecting the patient's messages, legitimizing his behaviour or feelings and showing partnership;
2 Showing concern: showing worry and giving reassurance;
3 Social behaviour: personal remarks, jokes, showing approval (Bensing and Droukers, 1992).

It has been shown, therefore, that it is possible to classify the communication skills used by the physiotherapist in interaction with the patient.

Communication Skills in the Context of Physiotherapy Practice

The skills used have been identified, so when are they used? The professional role of the physiotherapist involves:

1 Observation of the patient and the recognition of 'stress' or difficulty;
2 Examination of the patient using careful questioning;
3 Teaching of exercises and home programmes;
4 Motivation and support for the patient, relatives and carer;
5 Social role.

The specific skills involved relate to:

1 Nonverbal communication (NVC);
2 Questioning Touch Listening;
3 Teaching skills — demonstration / explanation;
4 Counselling;
5 Social role / touch.

Nonverbal Communication

Nonverbal communication or behaviour refers not only to aspects of speaking, such as accent and intonation, but also to non-spoken aspects such as gestures and facial expressions. Even before we open our mouths to speak, messages are being sent to those we are communicating with, about our sex, age, status and occupation, especially if a uniform and a badge signifying seniority is worn.

Hargie *et al.* (1994) refer to kinesics — movements of the body such as gestures, limb movements, head nods, facial expressions, eye gaze and posture.

Para Language

Gestures are used frequently as para language — to support speech — imagine trying to describe a spiral staircase without using your hands! When giving directions to the Post Office or the physiotherapy department we would frequently use our hands to indicate right or left. Lecturers frequently use gestures, and larger limb movements, to illustrate a point and keep the attention of students and one only has to observe a group of people in conversation to appreciate the use of hand movements to animate speech.

In the physiotherapy context, the patient uses gestures to explain where the pain is located — if the patient points to one spot, the therapist can be reasonably sure that the pain is localized; if a larger gesture is used — for example from the shoulder to the fingers covering the whole of the upper limb, the therapist will be considering the possibility of referred pain in the upper limb.

Smaller movements of the hands such as fiddling with one or two fingers can alert us to situations in which the person feels uneasy or nervous.

Hargie *et al.* (1994) noted that hand gestures can also reveal other emotional dispositions such as embarrassment (hand over the mouth), anger (knuckles showing white), aggression (fist clenching), shame (hands covering the eyes), nervousness (nail and finger biting). The physiotherapist should be aware of these signs and act accordingly to ameliorate the situation for the patient.

Posture

As therapists we are aware of the basic starting positions and their modification for the purpose of exercise therapy and rehabilitation. We are also aware of abnormal postures caused by physical disability, from low back pain to stroke.

Posture can also send important information regarding a person's inner feelings. The depressed patient is more likely to have a slouched, rounded shoulder posture with the arms hanging limply by the sides whereas the patient racked with pain or fear will exhibit the same posture but with the arms held tightly across the chest – thus protecting themselves from intrusion.

Head Nods

These are important and signify agreement or understanding. In physiotherapy these are used in the therapeutic interview to show understanding, and when used discreetly encourage the patient to talk on and explain more. The use of head nods by the physiotherapist and a forward leaning posture during interaction with the patient signify interest and concern.

Eye Gaze and Facial Expression

As students of anatomy and the muscles of facial expression, physiotherapists are aware of the combination of eye movements and the muscles around the orbit to convey fear, surprise, disdain and pleasure. It is very annoying if the person you are talking to is not looking at you – this shows a lack of interest in you and the message you are trying to send and it is imperative therefore that the therapist maintains eye contact to be aware of messages coming from the patient. Eye gaze can also be used successfully by the therapist to control a talkative patient – the tactic here is simply to drop the eyes and break contact, thus discouraging the patient from talking.

Eye gaze *from* the patient is also very important and can often be the only means of communication with a neurologically impaired patient. In cases where patients are suspicious of a life-threatening diagnosis it is often the physiotherapist who will be available to listen – appreciation of eye gaze as a two-way communication system is imperative, as *your* eyes will also be sending a message when the professional knows the diagnosis and prognosis, and the patient only suspects!

Due to the in-depth study of anatomy in undergraduate courses in physiotherapy, we are very aware of the use of the muscles of facial expression in communication.

Proxemics

This refers to the positions adopted by the persons in communication. During the patient interview it is more conducive for communication to take up a position at right angles to, as opposed to opposite, the patient. Not *all* interviews will be conducted at a table or the side of a treatment couch, but if the patient is lying on the couch or in bed, it is more appropriate for the therapist to sit beside them rather than assuming the more dominant standing position.

In conclusion, therefore, it should be noted that therapists need to be fully aware of the nonvocal and nonverbal aspects of communication.

Touch

Touch is one of the most important factors involved in nonverbal communication. Touch has various significant functions and meanings in medical settings. It is accepted as being normal to console a pet or child by touching them, but such an approach is less acceptable towards distressed adults (Buis *et al.*, 1991).

Various researchers have considered the use of touch in social and medical settings. In work with infants (Montagu, 1971) and Morris (1973, cited in Fisher *et al.*, 1976) indicated that tactile stimulation is important for emotional, intellectual and physiological development. This may be true in the physiotherapy rehabilitation of the neurologically impaired patient, but there is a paucity of research into touch in the physiotherapeutic relationship. Fisher *et al.* (1976) noted, however, that touch implies that a communication is intended, but the content of the communication may not be clear.

It has been noted that the body's largest organ is the skin and that one of its most important functions is as a human communication organ. One of the functions of the skin is that is embodies the sense of touch – and yet the concept of 'therapeutic touch' has elicited little attention (Schulte, 1991).

Touch in the therapeutic relationship may be in the form of palpation of a body part, used by the doctor and / or the therapist with the aim of identifying the correct anatomical site of the lesion. Many patients expect to be touched in this professional advice seeking session.

Professional persons also use touch as a form of social greeting or social helping. Social greeting may be in the form of a hand shake or social helping – taking a patient's arm, a hand on the back, or an arm around the waist – to assist the patient to the treatment area.

But how does the patient interpret this? Is it helping and facilitating? Or an invasion of their personal space?

As Cashar and Dixson (1967) noted, touch may convey either physical or psychological intimacy, as in a feeling of warmth and friendliness, or it may convey physical or psychological assault such as an invasion of one's privacy. Touch can take various forms and as physiotherapists we must be aware of the use made of touch in the many and varied situations associated with therapeutic practice. *Touch cannot be taken for granted.*

As pointed out by Schulte (1991), the importance of touch has been recognized by the nursing profession and it would be well if the therapeutic benefits of touch were similarly understood by all those in the health care community.

For example, Cashar and Dixson (1967) ask:

'How many patients have you touched today?'

'Can you identify your reasons for touching them?'

These questions should be given careful consideration by the physiotherapist as one would expect to have touched every patient treated.

We need to make it clear to the patient *why* we are touching them, whether this be palpation in the objective examination of the patient, or the use of touch to facilitate one exercise and maximize patient performance.

Cashar and Dixson (1967) have categorized therapeutic touch into three broad stages:

1 Reality orientating: defined as promoting an awareness of the existing situation, with reference to time, place and identity of persons including the self – this would relate to the objective examination of the patient and the use of touch in proprioceptive neuromuscular facilitation, for example.
2 Support: defined as meeting the patient's unmet needs while allowing him to remain as independent as possible – a pat on the back to reassure the patient, or holding the patient's hand during a test, for example.
3 Physical protection: defined as defending oneself or others from injury or destruction by the use of manual restraint – this is important in the aggressive or confused patient and especially in certain client groups. It may simply involve holding the patient's arm firmly until the aggression phase ceases.

Cashar and Dixson (1967) found through their research study that touch was frequently used without conscious planning in the nursing environment. This may be only partially true in the therapeutic environment of physiotherapy. Adams *et al.* (1994) found that the physiotherapist generally only touches for therapeutic reasons. The therapist spends little time on social routines and general conversation with the patient in comparison with treatment orientated conversation.

Nevertheless, the physiotherapist needs to consider the characteristics of the audience, i.e. the patients – research has shown that less intelligent patients will respond better with a simpler, more direct approach (Wagstaff, 1982).

Patients need to have explained to them what will happen next – not only during treatment but also during the initial meeting or encounter, or the patient interview, to ascertain the nature of the problem.

The Therapeutic Interview

The therapeutic interview is probably the first objective meeting between therapist and patient. Like the doctor–patient interview, this is where verbal communication is used by both parties to obtain and give information (Bain, 1976).

Bain (1976) tape recorded interviews with patients in a health centre and found that the doctor did more talking than the patients and that the largest verbal contribution made by the patients was in 'symptom presentation'. However, in physiotherapy it has been noted that relatively extensive and intensive contact with the physiotherapist, coupled with the fact that the physiotherapist is frequently regarded as not being a member of the regular ward staff, make it more likely that the concerns of patients will be discussed and their

suppressed anxieties ventilated (Dickson and Maxwell, 1985).

It is possible to identify two kinds of therapeutic interview – history taking and physical examination (Thomquist, 1990) – and the counselling interview (Croft, 1980).

History Taking and Physical Examination

This is the consultation interview. Havelock (1991) has identified seven tasks for the consultation interview:

1 To define the reasons for the patient's attendance, including:
  – the nature and history of the problems,
  – the aetiology,
  – the patient's ideas, concerns and expectations,
  – the effects of the problem.
2 To consider other problems:
  – continuing problems,
  – at-risk factors.
3 To choose an appropriate action with the patient for each problem.
4 To achieve a shared understanding of the problem via the patient.
5 To involve the patient in the management of the condition and to encourage acceptance of appropriate responsibility.
6 To use time and resources appropriately:
  – in the consultation (short term),
  – in the long term.
7 To establish or maintain a relationship with the patient which helps achieve the other tasks.

This relates closely to the SOAP (Subjective Objective Assessment Plan) and the use of the Problem Oriented Medical Records (POMR) system used in physiotherapeutic practice.

Apart from an awareness of nonverbal communication, noted throughout the interview by observation, the two main skills involved are *questioning* and *listening*.

Questioning

A simple definition of a question is: *a statement phrased in such a way that it evokes a response from another.*

However there are different types of questions:

Closed questions These are usually recall questions where the patient is expected to recall a date of injury for example. Closed questions could also relate to questions requiring a Yes or No answer, for example:

'Have you ever had any physiotherapy treatment before?'

'Do you live in a bungalow?'

Open questions These are questions where the physiotherapist will encourage the patient to elaborate on their symptoms or feelings or expectations, for example:

'Tell me about your pain.'

'How do you feel today?'

Probing and prompting questions Probing questions direct the patient to think more deeply about the initial answer and to express themselves more clearly, for example:

Therapist: 'You had physiotherapy treatment previously – what did you think about it?'

Patient: 'It was nice.'

Therapist: 'What was nice about it?' (probe)

The use of prompting questions consists of giving hints to help the patient.

A series of prompts followed by encouragement can help the patient gain confidence in giving replies and open up the interview:

Therapist: 'Tell me about your pain.'

Patient: 'It is inside my knee.'

Therapist: 'Can you describe it?'

Patient: 'Well . . . No!'

Therapist: 'Have you ever had this type of pain before?' (pause) 'Is it like toothache?' (pause) 'Does it throb?'

Patient: 'Yes – it's like toothache – it pulses all the time!'

As in social interaction, if we as therapists can manage to get the person we are talking to, or interviewing, to talk about themselves, the task of questioning becomes easier. An extremely talkative patient can be halted by the physiotherapist removing eye contact.

There are several ways of improving the use of questions:

1 Clarity and coherence: the language used must be understandable, we must not use medical terminology but return to the colloquial – such as shoulder blade and collar bone. If by any chance you find yourself using complicated language, stop and start again.
2 Pausing and pacing: pausing allows the patient time to think and put their answer in a logical order, especially with regard to a response to an open question. Pacing, on the other hand, allows for variety in the interview and this is achieved through a mix of closed questions and open questions and contributes to the structure of the interview.

Remember, a poorly conducted interview leaves the patient dissatisfied (Heavey, 1988).

Listening

Listening in the history-taking interview serves mainly to:

1 Focus specifically upon the messages being communicated by the other person;
2 Gain a full, accurate understanding of the other person's communication;
3 Convey interest, concern and attention;
4 Encourage full, open and honest expression (Hargie *et al.*, 1994).

The therapist can display listening and interest by adopting a forward-leaning posture (thus conveying interest), using head nods to convey understanding and to prompt the patient to talk, and facial expression to convey empathy.

THE CONDITIONS FOR EFFECTIVE INTERVIEWING

These conditions relate principally to the *setting* and the *structure* of the interview.

The Setting
Croft (1980) pointed out that the ideal setting for an interview is a private room or one not overwhelming, noisy or distracting. This may not always be possible as patients are interviewed in many different settings, such as hospital wards, busy physiotherapy outpatient departments, and their own homes.

However, the therapist can use skills of nonverbal communication, such as eye contact and posture, to create a relaxing atmosphere for the patient.

The Structure
The initial contact interview may be viewed by some as a fact finding mission – the danger here being that the interview is turned into an inter-

rogation as the therapist sets about the work of the detective in the rehabilitation process.

Initially the health professional requires some demographic data regarding the patient's age, sex, marital status etc. and most of this can be obtained from the medical records or the source of referral. Initial questions regarding any gaps in the demographic data required can be easily obtained using closed questions, but these should be kept to a minimum.

The patient wants to tell you about their problem and wants you to help sort it out; as the therapist, the health professional needs to find out about their symptoms prior to embarking upon objective testing, but you do have specific mandatory questions to ask regarding contraindications and any medical or laboratory tests.

Clinical Example

The patient interview may commence with an open question such as, 'Tell me about your pain'.

The therpaist continually probes throughout the interview with the occasional prompt in order to achieve a picture of the exact nature and behaviour of the patient's symptoms and personal difficulties.

The most appropriate structure for this interview is the funnel sequence (see Table 14.3) (Hargie *et al.*, 1994). In this structure an interaction starts with an open question, the level of openness is gradually reduced and a focus develops.

Table 14.3
Example of a funnel sequence of questions

Question	Strategy	Question
Open	Prompt	Tell me about your pain/problem
Open	Prompt	How does it affect you every day?
Open	Probe	What is it like in the morning?
	Probe	. . . the afternoon?
	Probe	. . . the evening?
Closed		Have you had it before?
Closed		Did you have treatment?
	Probe	What was it?
Closed		Did that help
	Probe	How?

Communication During Therapeutic Intervention

Following the patient examination, and assessment of the subjective and objective findings, the physiotherapist designs a rehabilitation programme for each specific patient. This programme must take into account the person's physical state and frequently the psychological state. The 'psychological state' of the patient is often a subjective perception on the part of the physiotherapist and should this perceived state be considered an addition to the problem list, then the advice and consultation of the clinical psychologists in the multidisciplinary team should be sought.

The physiotherapist has, therefore, an initial responsibility to design an individual treatment programme for each patient and must carefully plan the programme of exercise or other therapeutic interventions to be delivered to the patient.

The specific communication skills involved include explanation and demonstration of the programme and exercises plus the global skill areas of *stimulus variation* and *reinforcement, set induction and closure.*

STIMULUS VARIATION

Stimulus variation is the means whereby a physiotherapist retains and directs the interest of the patient using, for example, vocal tone, gestures, direction of the exercises and alterations in position. This skill is widely used in social interaction and communication.

People often supplement their speech with gestures to emphasize the verbal component, and the result is a reduction in boredom and monotony as we all respond to a certain level of change or variety.

In the rehabilitation programme the physiotherapist must plan for stimulus variation through different exercises and changes in focus:

1 Changes in body position can be used to perform the same exercise, or to make an exercise easier or more difficult.
2 The therapist may use demonstration as a change in focus as well as audio/visual aids

such as videotape to provide feedback in the analysis and recording of performance and progress.

3 Vocal tone can be altered for the sake of emphasis and reinforcement. This is important in the performance of proprioceptive neuro-muscular facilitation techniques where the tone of the voice would be increased, but equally important in relaxation where the tone of the voice would be lowered gradually to induce relaxation and tranquillity and gradually raised to signify the end of the relaxation session and return to the 'real' world.

4 In rehabilitation, the major stimulus may tend to be the therapist but the patient should be involved totally. Stimulus variation as a communication skill involves the change of sensory focus – from listening to talking; from talking to feeling; from feeling to doing – thus switching the focus from one sense organ to another and achieving the rehabilitation goal of movement.

5 The use of a change in vocal pattern by the physiotherapist is particularly useful. The use of the change of tone, volume and speed of the vocal pattern are all conducive to the rehabilitation of the patient. The use of accelerated speech and a loud voice facilitates performance of exercise using proprioceptive neuromuscular facilitation techniques whereas a slower, quiet vocal tone would facilitate relaxation.

In planning a treatment schedule it is important to remember that boredom and monotony produce problems with compliance, and planned variety reduces these problems.

While variety may be important in life – so too, is reward!

REINFORCEMENT

Reinforcement is the process whereby the likelihood of the occurrence of behaviours or events is increased or decreased.

Reinforcement can be positive or negative. Positive reinforcement results in a reward of some kind and implies that you would wish that event to occur again – a reward for performing an exercise well. Negative reinforcement would most commonly be referred to as 'punishment' – the physiotherapist would wish to decrease the likelihood of that behaviour occurring again given a similar situation.

Most of the theoretical background on reinforcement stems from the work of Skinner on operant conditioning (Argyle, 1983).

There are two broad categories of reinforcement:

1 Primary reinforcers – food, water, shelter.
2 Secondary reinforcers – these are *learnt*.

In the second category, 'learnt' reinforcers are evident in the social communication environment, for example:

- Verbal and non-verbal reinforcers: e.g. praise, attention, acknowledgement, approval, affection;
- Tokens: e.g. stars, charts of achievement, enjoyable activity, holidays.

In the therapeutic enviromnent, it is advisable to use positive reinforcement (reward) early on in the rehabilitation process, followed by more unpredictable intermittent rewards to facilitate achievement and motivation (Argyle, 1983).

The most commonly used forms of reinforcement in the therapeutic environment are:

1 Delayed reinforcement: Here it is better to use the most relevant reward component, as soon as possible following the desired response, in

order to ensure that the connection between the reward and the response is strengthened, e.g. 'Well now, you did that exercise well, let's try again – and push harder this time!'

2 Partial reinforcement: This refers to partially accepting the performance of the patient during an exercise – it is closely related to avoiding negative reinforcement and criticism while emphasizing the positive approach (give the good news first!), e.g. 'Well done! Next time, at the end of the movement you will need to push harder, you lost interest half-way through!'

It is important to draw attention to the positive aspects of the response to the exercise first and follow this comment with the critical comment or comments afterwards. This ensures that the patient has been initially rewarded, but will make more note of the criticisms for future performance.

The advantage of the use of reinforcement is that a relationship can be built up between therapist and patient; it is recognized that people work better if encouraged and that the frequent use of reinforcement builds the patient's confidence (Argyle, 1983; Adams et al., 1994). A disadvantage would, of course, be over-confidence if reinforcement is used too frequently.

Stimulus variation and reinforcement are two global skill areas to be considered in the delivery of a therapeutic programme. Planning of the therapeutic programme of exercise by the therapist must therefore include an awareness of the global communication skills of stimulus variation and reinforcement. These are important skills in order to provide feedback to the patient on performance and progress. Further explanations of the effects of reinforcement are offered in Chapter 15.

Equally important are the skills of *explanation* and

demonstration. The therapist must be able to explain the rehabilitation programme to the patient and, if necessary, demonstrate exercises to supplement the verbal explanation.

Explanation

The definition of explaining, or to explain, is to give understanding to another. But also, having given that explanation the sender of the message is looking for feedback to ensure that the message has been received and understood (Argyle, 1983).

The skill of explaining is based on the work of Piaget (Argyle, 1983); the perceived adequacy of an explanation is related to the patient's cognitive state, or indeed stage of cognitive development. An explanation must be relevant and adequate to the age, experience and background of the patient. Two types of explanation have been identified:

- planned
- unplanned

Planned Explanation
A planned explanation is usually carried out in the preparation phase prior to the therapeutic episode.

This could be an examination of the patient. The therapist may prefer to explain to the patient that various questions will be asked regarding the symptoms and, following this, various tests will be carried out in a number of positions in order to find out exactly what the patient's problem is. In this way therapist and patient work together to ascertain the problem and find a possible therapeutic solution or intervention strategy.

Unplanned Explanation
An unplanned explanation would be in response to the patient's questions regarding various

examination procedures, or the desired effects of exercise for example. An unplanned explanation may need to be given to members of the multi-disciplinary team, to home carers or relatives.

There are three specific skills to be employed when planning an explanation. While the explanation itself may be 'pre-planned', these skills should also be considered mentally by the physiotherapist in the 'unplanned' explanation.

In providing an explanation it is important to consider:

1 Presentation skills;
2 Linking;
3 Feedback

PRESENTATION SKILLS

Clarity can be achieved by pausing prior to proceeding to the next phase of the explanation.

Fluency in speech is also an important consideration and sentences must be kept short and the person explaining should avoid the use of 'ums' and 'ers'. Examples should be used in order to relate new and unfamiliar concepts, facts or ideas to situations which are being experienced by the patient.

Examples can be of three different types:

- verbal: an analogy, own description, the experience of friends or acquaintances;
- diagrammatic: a drawing, chart or anatomical model;
- actual: a working model or demonstration (a skill considered later).

LINKING

The pattern in which examples are linked to the overall explanation, whether verbal or written, is also important. There are in fact three distinct patterns for clear explanations:

1 Rule — example — rule

Clinical Example		
RULE	Therapist:	'This exercise has been shown to relieve back pain.'
EXAMPLE		'Now, lie on your tummy and push up on your arms'.
RULE		'Now, did you find that relieved your pain?'

2 Example — then rule or general principles: Here we would introduce the patient to the known (known from past experience of symptom behaviour for example) or previous life experiences, and proceed to the unknown, or not yet experienced in the rehabilitation programme.

Clinical Example		
EXAMPLE	Therapist:	'Do you remember when you went to swim? The water held you up and you floated.'
RULE		'Well we are going to use water and floating in your treatment — you are going to have hydrotherapy.'

3 Alternatively, an explanation could begin with a generalization — such as walking, and the general gait pattern of the arm swinging while the opposite leg is striding forwards for heel strike.

Clinical Example

GENERALIZATION	*Therapist:*
	'Look at the way I walk
	. . . my right arm swings
	forward with my left leg
	going forward
RULE	*'Now, let's look more*
	closely at walking.'

It is here that the use of demonstration would supplement and support the verbal explanation.

EMPHASIS

This is an important part of explanation and is where the physiotherapist calls attention to the important and essential information whilst paying less attention to non-essential details.

Emphasis can be provided successfully by variation in your behaviour — such as variation in vocal tone, movement around the treatment area and/ or the use of gesture, and the use of audio and visual aids.

Further emphasis can be provided by summarizing the main points and paraphrasing the patient's questions and your responses as the explanation progresses.

FEEDBACK

It is not sufficient to accept that your explanation has been understood or absorbed by the patient.

It is important to determine if the patient has understood what is required of him and what the consequences of poor performance of an exercise or lack of compliance in a health education or rehabilitation programme may be.

There are a number of ways in which the physiotherapist can check on the patient's understanding and give more information if necessary. One obvious method would simply be to ask the patient if they have any questions, or questions could be asked of the patient to find out if they have understood your message. Once again the questions should be carefully worded and patients would probably relate more to open-ended questions as opposed to closed questions where overuse may seem more like a form of interrogation — the 'third degree'!

Therapists need to be aware of the skill of explanation. The best advice is to proceed from the known to the unknown and the simple to the complex — even if unplanned.

The explanation should be tailored to the rehabilitative stage of the patient and their level of intelligence and life experiences. It is better to cover a small amount of material in depth and with precision rather than to proceed rapidly. Otherwise the quality of the rehabilitation process will suffer.

In physiotherapy rehabilitation an explanation can often be usefully supplemented by a demonstration.

Demonstration

The skill of demonstration is closely allied to explanation. A long explanation is really not called for in physiotherapeutic practice where movement should be the outcome. It may be appropriate to use yourself as a model in order to break up a lengthy monologue and also add stimulus variation. This helps to motivate patients – they want to be able to do the exercise or movement.

A demonstration must, like an explanation, be planned and this should be done by the physiotherapist prior to the patient's appointment time, thus allowing the therapist to plan 'talk' time. The demonstration must include an introduction, some form of therapist activity and patient activity, perhaps some form of enabling activity with the therapist and patient working together, and a concluding statement.

The introduction to the explanation / demonstration, essentially, contains two parts – the introduction, and the qualifying statement.

1 *The introduction*

e.g. 'I want you to watch me walk.'
      'I want you to watch me stand up.'

2 *A qualifying statement* This is given in order to show a reason, or reasons, for the correct sequencing of a movement – or indeed reasons for the use of the demonstration.

e.g. 'You must do this so you do not fall.'
      'Watch my feet, and where they are, before I stand up.'

It is possible to go through the complete demonstration without talking, but it may be more appropriate in the rehabilitation situation to talk through the demonstration and explain and emphasize throughout.

Any rehabilitation skill will be viewed by your patient as complex, and it is necessary to break this skill down into smaller *achievable* parts and to work through these parts slowly, giving positive or partial reinforcement appropriately, according to level of achievement.

It goes without saying, therefore, that it is neces-

sary to talk the patient through the actions of the exercise as he is doing them.

Clinical Example

'I want you to watch me stand up.'

'You must do this so you do not fall.'

'Watch my feet and the position before I stand up.'

. . . .

'Yes, that's right! Good! Well done!'

'Now, let's try that together – you get your feet right and I will help you stand up.'

On the conclusion of the performance of the exercise, the physiotherapist can ask the patient for their views on the activity, what were the difficulties (if any) and what they need to work on next. This is the concluding statement.

Demonstrations can be very reinforcing in physiotherapy practice. While we would not expect the patient to perform perfectly the exercise that has been demonstrated, we must use the skill of reinforcement to encourage the patient, particularly if perfection in performance is only partially achieved given their physical ability and psychological state.

It is important not to use negative models of demonstration as this could really be seen as a threat to the patient and compliance with the rehabilitation programme.

The skill of demonstration can be used successfully to supplement therapist / patient interaction and also to support carers, relatives and professionals in the multidisciplinary rehabilitation team. The physiotherapist may be required to teach others involved in the health care process basic skills regarding walking practice and maintenance exercises, and in community care situations knowledge of the components of the skill of demonstration is invaluable.

Set Induction

Set induction is that event which occurs when an organism is usually prepared at any moment for the stimuli it is going to receive and the response it is going to make. It is important that the physiotherapist prepares the patient for all that they are going to do in the treatment session (Argyle, 1983). Three kinds of set have been recognized:

- Social set
- Perceptual set
- Cognitive set (Hargie et al., 1994)

SOCIAL SET

With regard to social set, Adams et al. (1994) recognized nine components relating to social behaviour by the physiotherapist. These components are identified as:

- Social greeting;
- Social interaction to establish rapport;
- Use of patient's forename for familiarity;
- Social interaction to reassure;
- Social interaction to distract from pain;
- Use of patient's surname to maintain formality;
- Use of humour to defuse a tense situation;
- Use of humour to relax the patient;
- Personal remarks about patient's hair/clothes.

Social set is very important in the physiotherapist's efforts to establish rapport with the patient. As a component, social greeting should be friendly and may involve a handshake or social touch and certainly involves nonverbal communication in the form of facial expression – wide eyes and a smile – plus questioning such as 'How do you feel today?' If the patient replies 'Not so good,' then the facial expression must change to one of empathy or concern.

Touch is also considered to be a component of social set induction as opposed to therapeutic touch. Touch in this instance can be used as a social greeting or reassurance that 'You are in good hands,' and 'Welcome to our department'.

Adams et al. (1994) do not identify the specific communication skills associated with social greeting and social interaction in order to establish rapport with the patient. While many patients prefer to be referred to by their Christian names, it would seem inappropriate for the professional physiotherapist to assume that patients wish to be referred to as 'Joe' or 'Alice'. It is preferable professional practice to adopt the formal approach of use of the patient's surname and title prior to building a rapport with the patient – the only person who can give you permission to use a familiar term is the patient.

The term the patient uses to address you is your choice – your name badge may include your preferred first name and your surname. One must respect the patient's wish to address you by your first name or title and surname.

PERCEPTUAL SET

Perceptual set arouses curiosity and/or stimulates attention. As a physiotherapist you may have planned a move from the gymnasium to the hydrotherapy pool, or vice versa. The main purpose would be:

1 To induce in the patient a state of readiness appropriate for the immediate rehabilitation process through gaining attention and arousing motivation;

2 To indicate to the patient realistic limits for the current rehabilitation goal and to suggest what might be a reasonable achievement in the treatment session;

3 To establish links between what the patient has already achieved and experienced and the new phase in the rehabilitation process to be achieved.

This is in order to show that the patient understands the process of progression of rehabilitation. The physiotherapist can explain part of the content or progression and ask questions to ascertain that the progress has been understood. These questions may also be asked of the carers, parents or relatives who support the rehabilitation process in the more formal confines of the physiotherapy department.

TECHNIQUES OF SET INDUCTION

Various techniques can be employed, the most common of which, in the rehabilitation process, is a change of focus from the enclosed 'clinical' cubicle to the more wide open environment of the gymnasium or the hydrotherapy pool.

Visual aids can be used in the form of wall charts, videotapes of previous patients or demonstration. Surprise and curiosity are also useful devices, where the physiotherapist can show or introduce the patient to the new environment several days before this is actually planned in the progression of treatment, thus promoting arousal and motivation to proceed to the next phase of treatment.

Set induction can be used successfully in the initial stages of treatment, from day 1 when the patient first meets the physiotherapist, during planning of any explanation and demonstration to the patient in any phase of the rehabilitation, through to conclusion of physiotherapeutic input.

Closure

Closure may be considered to be the natural follow-on from set induction. A rehabilitation interaction would naturally begin with preparation for the event about to occur but this event must also come to an end and the closure of the treatment session. However, closure could also happen at various phases throughout a rehabilitation session, as the therapist changes the focus of the session, from strengthening exercises to balance exercises for example. Closure is used to reiterate major points in a sequence thus providing a link between exercises learnt in the past and new exercises which have been introduced as part of treatment progression. If at any time during the planned treatment session, treatment needs to be cut short and abandoned, closure can be used to draw the patient's attention to what has been achieved during the session.

Closure serves a useful purpose. It focuses attention on what has been learnt and achieved and thus provides the patient with feedback and a sense of achievement.

PERCEPTUAL CLOSURE

This may simply be the ambulance man calling for the patient, or the receptionist or physiotherapy assistant announcing that the therapist's next patient has arrived.

COGNITIVE CLOSURE

This is summing up the treatment, or part of treatment, which has just concluded — or it may be providing a link firom the strengthening exercises to the balance exercises.

SOCIAL CLOSURE

This is usually some statement which we know closes the communication phase, e.g. 'Don't forget! I'll see you tomorrow!'

In physiotherapy practice it could be making, or checking, that a further appointment has been made. The techniques of closure may also include a recap by questioning about what the rehabilitation session has included, especially in relation to ante-natal and post-natal classes and back schools. It also allows the patients to clarify any vague points or problems they have, remembering exercises or postures, or why they have to practise. One of the main functions of closure in the rehabilitation session would be the provision of home exercises including a clearly planned explanation of why it is necessary to practise at home. In this way a future link may be given by the therapist to the next session and the next level of achievement.

Summary

Physiotherapists should become more actively involved in the wider context of health education. To do this effectively, the physiotherapist needs to know the purposes of health education and to understand its links with health promotion, and to have a sound grasp of models of health, and the reasons why patients do or do not heed health advice. Finally, it is essential that the physiotherapist uses appropriate communication skills in the delivery of the health message.

- Health education is one of the two components of health promotion; the other component is public health policy.
- The three types of health education include education about the body and how to look after it, information about health services, and education about national, regional and local health policies.
- Models of health education include educational, self-empowerment, preventive and radico-political models.
- The most commonly cited areas of health education activities for physiotherapists are back care and ante- and post-natal care.
- Patient compliance is the extent to which patients do or do not follow their therapist's advice.
- Factors influencing compliance include views on illness causation, health beliefs, professional–patient relationship, the nature of the illness/disability, the nature of the treatment regimen, knowledge and social/situational factors.
- Communication is a two-way process in the therapeutic setting, with the patient and therapist interacting to bring about a successful rehabilitative process.
- The broadest classification of communication skills is into verbal and nonverbal skills.
- Physiotherapists' communication skills have been classified into instrumental behaviours and affective behaviours.
- Nonverbal skills include posture, head nods, eye gaze and facial expression, proxemics (positions), and touch.
- Verbal skills include questioning and explaining.
- Skills commonly used in treatment sessions include explanation and demonstration, which in turn incorporate the global skills of stimulus variation, reinforcement, set induction and set closure.

Further reading

Bartlett, EE, Grayson, M, Barker, R, Levine, DM, Golden, A, Libber, S (1984) The effects of physician communications skills on patient satisfaction: recall and adherence. *Journal of Chronic Disorders* **37**: 755–764.

Brody, DS (1980) An analysis of patient recall of their therapeutic regimens. *Journal of Chronic Disorders* **33**: 57–63.

DHSS (1974) Health and Safety at Work Act, HMSO, London.

Dickson, D, Maxwell, RM (1987) A comparative study of physiotherapy students' attitudes to social skills training undertaken before and after clinical placement. *Physiotherapy* **73**: 60–64.

Dickson, D, Hargie, O, Morrow, NC (1991) *Communication Skills Training for Health Professionals*. Chapman and Hall, London.

Dockrell, S (1988) An investigation of the use of verbal and non-verbal communication skills by final year physiotherapy students. *Physiotherapy* **74**: 52–55.

Francis, V, Korsch, BM, Morris, MJ (1969) Gaps in doctor-patient communication. *The New England Journal of Medicine* **280**: 535–540.

Gartland, GJ (1984) Teaching the therapeutic relationship. *Physiotherapy Canada* **36**: 24–28.

Gartland, GJ (1984) Communication skills instruction in Canadian physical therapy schools: a report. *Physiotherapy Canada* **36**: 29–35.

Grant, D (1979) The physiotherapist as patient counsellor. *Physiotherapy* **65**: 218–220.

Hamilton-Ducken, P, Kidd, L (1985) Counselling skills and the physiotherapist. *Physiotherapy* **71**: 179–180.

Hulme, JB, Bach, BW, Lwis, JW (1988) Communication between physicians and physical therapists. *Physical Therapy* **68**: 26–31.

Korsch, BM, Gozzi, EK, Francis, V (1968) Gaps in doctor-patient conununication: doctor-patient interaction and patient satisfaction. *Pediatrics* **42**: 855–871.

Lubbock, G (1985) Using video-tape in clinical practice. *Physiotherapy* **71**: 53–54.

Payton, O (1983) Effects of instruction in basic communication skills on physical therapists and physical therapy student. *Physical Therapy* **63**: 1292–1297.

Saunders, C, Maxwell, RM (1988) The case for counselling in physiotherapy. *Physiotherapy* **74**: 592–596.

Schultz, CL, Wellard, R, Swerissen, H (1988) Communication and interpersonal helping skills: an essential component in physiotherapy education? *Australian Journal of Physiotherapy* **34**: 75–79.

References

Abrams, B, Berman, C (1993) Women, nutrition and health. *Current Problems in Obstetrics, Gynaecology and Fertility* **16** (1): 5–49.

Adams, N, Bell, Saunders, C, Dickson, D (1994) *Communication Skills in Physiotherapist – Patient Interactions*. Centre for Health and Social Research, University of Ulster.

Allen, RM, Jones, MP, Oldenburg, B (1995) Randomised trial of an asthma self-management programme for adults. *Thorax* **50**: 731–738.

Alvin, P, Rey, C, Frappier, JY (1995) Medical compliance in adolescents with chronic illness. *Archives de Paediatrie* **2**: 847–882.

Argyle, M (1983) *The Psychology of Interpersonal Behaviour*. Penguin, Harmondsworth, Middlesex.

Bain, D (1976) Doctor–patient communication in general practice consultations. *Medical Education* **10**: 125–131

Balfour, C (1993) Physiotherapists and smoking cessation. *Physiotherapy* **79**: 247–250.

Baric, L (1991) *Health Promotion and Education*, 2nd edition. Barns Publications, Altrincham, England.

Bean, AG, Talaga, J (1992) Appointment breaking: causes and solutions. *Journal of Health Care Marketing* **12**: 14–25.

Becker, MH (1974) The health belief model and sick role behaviours. *Health Education Monograph* **2**: 409–419.

Belgrave, FZ, Lewis, DM (1994) The role of social support in compliance and other health behaviours for African Americans with chronic diseases. *Journal of Health and Social Policy* **5**: 55–68.

Bensing, JM, Dronkers, J (1992) Instrumental and affective aspects of physician behaviour. *Medical Care* **10**: 283–298.

Bernstein, L, Bernstein, R (1980) *Interviewing: A Guide for Health Promotion*, 3rd edn. Appleton-Century-Crofts.

Blalock, SJ, DeVellis, BM, Giorgino, KB (1995) The relationship between coping and psychological well-being among people with osteoarthritis: a problem-solving approach. *Annals of Behavioural Medicine* **17**: 107–115.

Blankson, ML, Goldenberg, RL, Keith, B (1994) Noncompliance of high-risk pregnant women in keeping appointments at an obstetric complications clinic. *Southern Medical Journal* **87**: 634–638.

Blaxter, M (1983) The cause of disease: women talking. *Social Science and Medicine* **17**: 59–69.

Brown, G, Atkins, M (1988) *Effective Teaching in Higher Education*. Welnen and Company, London

Buis, C, De Boo, T, Hull, R (1991) Touch and breaking bad news. *Family Practice* **8**: 303–304.

Carney, S, Gillies, A, Smith, A, Taylor, M (1993) Hypertension education: patient knowlwedge and satisfaction. *Journal of Human Hypertension* **7**: 505–508.

Cashar, L, Dixson, BK (1967) The therapeutic use of touch. *Journal of Psychiatric Nursing* 442–451.

Cassell, EJ (1976) Disease as 'it': concepts of disease revealed by patients' presentation of symptoms. *Social Science and Medicine* **10**: 143–146.

Chmelik, F, Doughty, A (1994) Objective measures of compliance in asthma treatment. *Annals of Allergy* **73**: 527–532.

Conway, SP, Pond, MN, Hamnett, T, Watson, A (1996) Compliance with treatment in adult patients with cyctic fibrosis. *Thorax* **51**: 29–33.

Courneya, KS, McAuley, E (1995) Cognitive mediators of the social influence-exercise adherence relationship: a test of the theory of planned behaviour. *Journal of Behavioural Medicine* **18**: 499–515.

Croft, J (1980) Interviewing in physical therapy. *Physical Therapy* **60**: 1033–1036.

Daltroy, LH (1993) Doctor-patient communication in rheumatological disorders. *Baillier's Clinical Rheumatology* **7**(2): 221–239.

Deenen, TAM, Klip, EC (1993) Coping with asthma. *Respiratory Medicine* **87**: 67–70.

DHSS (1976) *Prevention and Health: Everybody's Business*. HMSO, London.

Dickson, D, Maxwell, RM (1985) The interpersonal dimension of physiotherapy: implications for training. *Physiotherapy* **71**: 306–310.

Draper, P, Griffiths, J, Dennis, J, Popay, J (1980) Three types of health education. *British Medical Journal* (August): 493–495.

Duffield, C (1989) The Delphi technique. *Australian Journal of Advanced Nursing* **6**: 41–45.

Dunbar, JM, Marshall, GD, Howell, MF (1979) Behavioural strategies for improving compliance, in: Haynes, RB, Taylor, DW, Sackett, DL (eds), *Compliance in Health Care*. The Johns Hopkins University Press, Baltimore, MD.

Elwes, L, Simnett, I (1985) *Promoting Health: A Practical Guide to Health Education*. J Wiley, Chichester..

Epstein, LH, Cluss, PA (1982) A behavioural medicine perspective on adherence to long-term medical regimens. *Journal Consult Clinical Psychology* **50**: 950–971.

Evans, V, Foley, M, Pagan, L, Mason, J (1993) Patient education: bridging the gap between inpatient and ambulatory care. *Journal of Community Health Nursing* **10**: 171–178.

Feste, C, Anderson, RM (1995) Empowerment: from philosophy to practice. *Patient Education and Counselling* **26**: 139–144.

Fisher, J, Rytting, M, Heslin, R (1976) Hands touching hands: affective and evaluative effects of an interpersonal touch. *Sociometry* **39**: 416–421.

Fishman, T (1995) The 90–second intervention: a patient compliance mediated technique to improve and control hypertension. *Public Health Reports* **110**: 173–178.

Garrett, JE, Fenwick, JM, Taylor, G, Mitchell, E, Stewart, A, Rea, H (1994) Prospective controlled evaluation of the effect of a community based asthma education centre in a multiracial working class neighbourhood. *Thorax* **49**: 976–983.

Gemmell, J (1986) Physiotherapy for asthmatic children in sports centres. *Physiotherapy* **72**: 52–53.

Graham, H (1978) Prevention and health: every mother's business: a comment on child health policies in the 1970s, in: Harris, C (ed.), *Sociology and the Family*. Social Review Monograph.

Grieve, GP (1984) *Mobilisation of the Spine*, 4th edn. Churchill Livingstone, Edinburgh.

Griffiths, C, Cooke, S, Toon, P (1994) Registration health checks: inverse care in the inner city? *British Journal of General Practice* **44**: 201–204.

Goodyer, L, Miskelly, F, Milligan, P (1995) Does encouraging good compliance improve patients' clinical condition in heart failure? *British Journal of General Practice* **49**: 173–176.

Guimon, J (1995) The use of group programmes to improve medication compliance in patients with chronic diseases. *Patient Education and Counselling* **26**: 189–193.

Hargie, O, Saunders, C, Dickson, D (1994) *Social Skills in Interpersonal Communication*, 3rd edn. Routiedge, London and New York.

Harrer, ME, Mosheim, R, Richter, R, Walter, MH, Kemmler, G (1993) Coping and quality of life of Hodgkin's disease survivors. A contribution to the problem of adaptivity of coping. *Psychotherapie Psychosomatik Medizinische Psychologie* **43**: 121–132.

Havelock, P (1991) Improving consultation skills. *The Practitioner* **23** (5): 495–498.

Hawthorne, K, Mello, M, Tomlinson, S (1993) Cultural and religious influences in diabetes care in Great Britain. *Diabetic Medicine* **10**: 8–12.

Hayne, CR (1988) The preventive role of physiotherapy in the National Health Service and industry. *Physiotherapy* **74**: 2–3.

Heavey, A (1988) Learning to talk with patients. *British Journal of Hospital Medicine* **39**: 433–439.

Helman, C (1981) Disease versus illness in general practice. *Journal of the Royal College of General Practitioners* **31**: 548–552.

Horn, JD, Feldman, HM, Ploof, DL (1995) Parent and professional perceptions about stress and coping. *Social Work in Health Care* **21**: 107–127.

Kendall, RE (1975) The concept of disease and it implications for psychiatry. *British Journal of Psychiatry* **127**: 305–315.

Kirby, K, Valmassy, RL (1983) The runner patient history: what to ask and why. *Journal of the American Podiatry Association* **73** (1): 15–21.

Knapp, DN (1988) Behavioural management techniques and exercise promotion, in Dishman, RK (ed.), *Exercise Adherence: Its Impact on Public Health*. Human Kinetics Pub Inc., Champaign, IL.

Kreher, NE, Hickner, JM, Ruffin, MT, Chen Sheng Lin, IV (1995) Effect of distance and travel time on rural women's compliance with screening mammography. *Journal of Family Practice* **40**: 143–147.

Landers, R, Riccobene, A, Beyreuther, M, Neusy, AJ (1993) Predictors of long-term compliance in attending a worksite hypertension programme. *Journal of Human Hypertension* **7**: 577–579.

Leathley, M (1988) Physiotherapists and health education: report of a survey. *Physiotherapy* **74**: 218–220.

Leathley, M, Stone, S (1986) Shared concerns: reflections on some health education issues which are common to four of the professions allied to medicine. *Physiotherapy* **72**: 12–13.

Leigh, H, Reiser, MF (1980) The patient: biological, psychological and social dimensions of medical practice. Plenum Medical.

Ley, P (1977) Communicating with the patient. In Coleman, J (ed.) *Introductory Psychology*. Routledge and Kegan Paul.

Lock, JQ, Wister, AV (1992) Intentions and changes in exercise and behaviours. *Health Promotion International* **7**: 195–207.

Lorenc, L, Branthwaite, A (1993) Are older adults less compliant with prescribed medication than younger adults? *British Journal of Clinical Psychology* **32**: 485–492.

Lyne, P (1986) The professions allied to medicine – their potential contribution to health education. *Physiotherapy* **72**: 8–10.

Lyne, PA, Phillipson, C (1986) The barriers to health education. *Physiotherapy* **72**: 10–12.

Marshall, G (1994) A comparative study of re-attenders and non-attenders for second triennial national breast screening programme appointments. *Journal of Public Health Medicine* **16**: 79–86.

Martin, JE, Dubbert, PH, Katell, AD (1984) Behavioural control of exercise in sedentary adults: studies 1–6. *Journal Consult Clinical Psychology* **52**: 795–811.

Martin, A, Leone, L, Castagliuolo, I, Di Mario, F, Naccarato, R (1992)

What do patients know about their inflammatory bowel disease? *Italian Journal of Gastroenterology* 24 (9): 477–480.

Melhuish, A (1982) *Work and Health*. Penguin, Harmondsworth.

Merrill, BA (1994) A global look at compliance in health/safety and rehabilitation. *Journal of Orthopaedic and Sports Physical Therapy* 19: 242–248.

Norton, S (1986) Support for physiotherapists in health education. *Physiotherapy* 72: 5–7.

Palat, M (1994) Rehabilitation and education of the cardiac patient. *Eurorehab* 4:221–224.

Patterson, JM, Budd, J, Goetz, D, Warwick, WJ (1993) Family correlates of a 10-year pulmonary health trend in cystic fibrosis. *Pediatrics* 91: 383–389.

Payne, R (1986) Health education for small groups. *Physiotherapy* 72: 56–57.

Peat, M (1981) Physiotherapy: art or science? *Physiotherapy Canada* 33: 170–176.

Peiss, B, Kurleto, B, Rubenfire, M (1995) Physicians and nurses can be effective educators in coronary risk reduction. *Journal of General Internal Medicine* 10: 77–81.

Pill, R, Stott, NCH (1982) Concepts of illness causation and responsibility: some preliminary data from a sample of working class mothers. *Social Science and Medicine* 16: 43–52.

Piterman, L (1983) The hazards of running and jogging. *Australian Family Physician* 12: 943–948.

Raynor, DK, Booth, TG, Blenkinsopp, A (1993) Effects of computer generated reminder charts on patients' compliance with drug regimens. *British Medical Journal* 306: 1158–1161.

Sarma, M, Alpers, JH, Prideaux, DJ, Kroemer, DJ (1995) The comprehensibility of Australian educational liytreature for patients with asthma. *Medical Journal of Australia* 162: 360–363.

Saunders, C, Caves, R (1986) An empirical approach to the identification of communication skills with reference to speech therapy. *Journal of Further and Higher Education* 10: 29–44.

Schulte, MAB (1991) Self care activating support: therapeutic touch and chronic skin disease. *Dermatology Nursing* 3: 335–339.

Shapiro, PA, Williams, DL, Foray, AT, Gelman, IS, Wukich, N, Sciacca, R (1995) Psychosocial evaluation and prediction of compliance problems and morbidity after heart transplantation. *Transplantation* 12: 1462–1466.

Shore, M (1986) The Health Education Council 'look after yourself' programme. *Physiotherapy* 72: 14–16.

Siguero, JPL, Aedo, MJM, Moreno, MDL, Valverde, AM (1995) Treatment with growth hormone – what do children know and how do they accept it? *Hormone Research* 44: 18–25.

Silvestri, B, Flay, BR (1989) Smoking education: comparison of practice and state-of-the-art. *Preventive Medicine* 18: 257–266.

Sluijs, EM, Kok, GJ, Van der Zee, J, Turk, DC, Riolo, L (1991) Correlates of exercise compliance in physical therapy. *Physical Therapy* 73: 771–786.

Sutton, S, Bickler, G, Sancho-Aldridge, J, Saidi, G (1994) Prospective study of predictors for breast screening in inner London. *Journal of Epidemiology and Community Health* 48: 65–73.

Thompson, J (1984) Compliance. In Fitzpatrick, R, Hinton, J, Newman, S, Scambler, G, Thompson, J (eds), *The Experience of Illness*. Tavistock Pub.

Thomquist, E (1990) Communication: what happens during the first encounter between patient and physiotherapist. *Scandinavian Joumal of Primary Health Care* 8: 133–138.

Thow, M, Newton, M (1990) The Gartnaval experience in health promotion 1986. *Physiotherapy* 76: 2–7.

Townsend, P, Davidson, N (1980) Inequalities in health (the Black Report). DHSS.

Wagstaff, GF (1982) A small dose of commonsense – communication, persuasion and physiotherapy. *Physiotherapy* 68: 327–329.

Walker, A (1995) Patient compliance and the placebo effect. *Physiotherapy* 81: 120–126.

Whitehead, M, Tones, K (1991) Avoiding the pitfalls. Health Education Authority.

15

Application of the Cognitive–Behavioural Approach

VICKI HARDING

Chapter Objectives
•
Definitions of Terms
•
Introduction
•
Major Models Operating in Medicine and Rehabilitation
•
Treatment Components of the C–B Approach
•
Prevention of Chronicity
•
Delivery
•
The Challenge of the C–B Approach
•
Conclusions
•
Key Points

This chapter will describe the cognitive–behavioural (C–B) model and approach to rehabilitation, contrasting it with the more traditional disease models. Discussion and review of its application will use examples drawn from the chronic pain field. This is an area that has been relatively well developed and tested compared to other areas (Williams and Erskine, 1995). Pain associated with musculoskeletal disorders causes more days off work than any other physical condition. It accounts for 15% of all GP consultations (Hackett et al., 1993) and forms the majority of the workload in most outpatient physiotherapy departments. The principles of the C–B approach can be usefully applied in the management of these disorders, and indeed in all spheres of physiotherapy rehabilitation.

Chapter Objectives

After reading this chapter you should be able to:

- Understand the basic models of disability and pain operating in rehabilitation;
- Appreciate the development and theoretical and scientific principles of the C–B model, and contrast it to simple medical disease models;
- Understand how C–B principles can be utilized to enhance physiotherapeutic treatment, particularly that of chronic pain;
- Promote the acquisition of skills and self-management by patients, and demonstrate an awareness of the importance of encouraging independence rather than dependence;
- Understand the factors important for initiating and maintaining behaviour change and for preventing chronicity;
- Discuss how the C–B approach may help physiotherapists to be more critical of traditional practices and take a broad evidence-based approach to the whole patient. Appreciate how it provides some directions for successful development of the physiotherapy profession.

Definitions of Terms

Cognition: Thought or belief.

Cognitive: Concerning thoughts and beliefs, and in this context the emotions associated with them.

Behavioural: Concerning observable actions, including 'body language'.

Cognitive–behavioural (C–B): Concerning cognitive aspects of a person's behaviour. Behaviour associated with a person's thoughts, beliefs and emotions.

Modelling: Observational learning, e.g. showing a patient how to do an exercise.

Operant learning: The control of behaviour by its consequences.

Affective: Concerning emotions (affect).

Generalization: The application of new behaviours, habits and skills learned in one setting, e.g. therapy, to all other environments, e.g. work, home.

Introduction

Physiotherapy has its roots in rehabilitation and is still one of the main health professions helping patients take an active part in their return to function. Rehabilitation has its 'ups' and 'downs' for both patient and therapist. For example, physiotherapists find it more challenging when patients' expectations, or those of their medical carers, are distinctly lower than their own. It is also harder when patients fear taking an active role or seem to prefer medical 'fix it' approaches, interpreting symptoms and difficulties as indications of pathology requiring medical intervention.

Applying psychological models and principles of change can bridge these gaps. It can make sense of patients' predicaments, and provide possibilities for change and improved function (Harding and Williams, 1995). This is much more than the application of 'common sense'. It is applying tested theory in a systematic way to observable and measurable patient behaviour, in the patients' setting. This is instead of following therapists' hunches or guesses about what the patients are experiencing or what they need. It also addresses patients' cognitions. These are the thoughts or 'self-statements' they have. It will especially be those associated with patients' beliefs and perspectives of their situation, and the feelings these thoughts produce in them.

Psychological factors have been found to be the most powerful for determining function and outcome. Jensen *et al.* (1991) reviewed 62 studies looking at the relationships between beliefs, coping and adjustment to pain and disability for chronic pain, back pain, rheumatoid and osteoarthritis patients. They showed disability level to be more strongly linked to unhelpful cognitions, self-efficacy beliefs (confidence), outcome expectations, pain beliefs, coping style and perceived control, than to either intensity of pain, chronicity or degree of pathology. One cannot overemphasize the need for the physiotherapist to consider psychological factors when treating patients.

Major Models Operating in Medicine and Rehabilitation

A model pulls together the reasoning and the process behind methods of practice. This chapter focuses on psychological models operating in the chronic pain field, in particular the C—B model. First, to distinguish the C—B model from other models operating in medicine and rehabilitation, the evolution of these main models will be briefly examined. Since patients' models influence the way they experience interaction with health professionals, their models will be included too.

Evolution of Medical / Disease Models of Ill Health

The medical model or disease model was postulated by Hippocrates in the fourth century BC. Waddell (1987) describes how modern medicine traces its roots to the European Renaissance of the sixteenth and seventeenth centuries. The scientific method of careful observation, systematic collection of information, and mathematical reasoning, enabled people to unlock nature's secrets uninfluenced by religious or traditional dogma. Studies of human anatomy and physiology were used to apply reason to the understanding of illness. After the discovery that infection was caused by microbes, and Virchow (1821–1902) proposed the concept of cellular disease, a medical model was established: patterns of symptoms and signs are recognized, a diagnosis is inferred, and physical treatment aimed at the underlying pathology. With the practice of increasingly technological medicine this has meant that the focus has been on physical aspects of disease rather than on psychological and social aspects. In pain management, medical / disease models encourage a tireless search for the cause of pain, and a therapy that will eliminate it from the tissue 'at fault'.

Unfortunately chronic conditions do not conform well to disease / pathology models. Much of the variability found in chronic disease is due to psychological and social factors (Payer, 1990) and at the end of the twentieth century it is not only disease that accounts for ill health (Black *et al.*, 1990, 'The Black report'; Whitehead, 1990, 'The health divide'). To an extent disease variability is accounted for by habit, e.g. smoking and exercise, but further factors include a sense of control at work and living conditions. Some of these factors can be influenced or changed by the individual, but some not. These psychosocial factors are not always critical to health, but medical explanations of disease are clearly just not enough. A further complication is that medical intervention is not necessarily related to cause. Diseases like cancer have many causes at many levels, none of which are related to chemotherapy. It is interesting that despite the acceptance of medical supremacy in matters of health, all the main risk factors mentioned in the UK government's *The Health of the Nation* document can be influenced by changes in behaviour (Secretary of State for Health, 1992).

Psychosomatic, Psychogenic and Personality Models of Ill Health

As mentioned above, simple disease models that match severity of pathology with severity of patients' symptoms, complaints and disability do not appear to fit the bill for the majority of patients with chronic conditions such as chronic pain. Trying to account for supposed discrepancies between pathology and disability by proposing other 'pathogenic' factors, i.e. emotional or personality-based factors, compounds the problem (Gamsa, 1994a, b). Where patients don't 'fit' the expected level of disability, they may be described as showing 'functional overlay', hypochondriasis, or even psychogenic pain – that is to say psychopathology. This development of the disease model is fraught with difficulties and open to biases since it requires behaviour to have set norms. This does not allow, for example, for cultural differences: some cultures may encourage people to want to say 'Yes' and not to complain, while other cultures may encourage loud complaining. Another development of the medical model occurs if, when a 'cause' cannot be found that explains things, e.g. a broken bone

on X-ray, tumour on a scan or a 'positive' blood test, the patient is blamed: 'they don't have a REAL illness', i.e. it's 'in their head', rather than blaming this on the limitations of modern medicine.

Personality diagnoses do not strictly fall into a disease model – they are more about abnormality. They are acceptable to psychiatry, but run alongside psychiatry's models of pathology rather than within them. According to psychiatric theorists, maladaptive behaviours (exhibited by for instance a chronic pain patient) provide a vehicle by which patients communicate their distress and unmet emotional needs (Keefe, 1989). This assumes much more limited and more enduring ways of behaving than people in fact show, and underestimates environment. People at a football match on Saturday will behave quite differently amongst their few colleagues at work on Monday. People have enormous ranges of behaviour. There are some preferences, but to say that people have an inner drive to behave in a certain way, e.g. as hypochondriacs, seems odd and there is no evidence that this is so. Since personality traits[1] are by definition unchangeable, these labels can seem advantageous: it is the patient's fault, so this takes away the therapist's responsibility. Attempts to test psychiatric or psychoanalytical models have failed to provide evidence for them (Gamsa, 1994a, b). It is easy for therapists to make value judgements masquerading as clinical opinion.

Psychoanalytical treatment is long and drawn out, is not accessible to physiotherapists, and nothing has been shown to be effective as yet, especially in the chronic pain field, so it will not be discussed further in this chapter.

---

[1] Trait is a theoretical *enduring* characteristic of a person that serves to explain observed regularities and consistencies in behaviour.

In summary, Sternbach (1969) understood chronic pain to be poorly served by the models and methods of orthodox medicine, indicating the need for other models:

> Our current approaches leave us much to be desired with respect to patient care ... approaches based on the assumption that the duality exists in the process, so that the pain is either mental or physical, penalise the patient in pain. If it is decided that the pain is 'mental', then the treatment is usually exclusively psychiatric, and the patient is forced to endure much suffering while attention is focused, for weeks or months, on the underlying conflicts. If it is decided that the pain is physical, then one somatic treatment follows another: thinking is dulled by drugs, and surgical assaults become more desperate. It is not pain which is mental or physical, functional or organic, psychic or somatic, but our ways of thinking about pain and the systems of terms we use to describe pain which may be so dichotomized. All pain can be described in both languages, the psychological and the physiological. Pain itself is not one or the other. (pp. 147–148)

The Rehabilitation Model of Disability and Impairment

Since the orthodox medical model can be such a poor fit for some patients, especially those with chronic conditions, medicine has nevertheless accepted that not all patients can be returned to full health and wholeness. A different direction was needed and so a branch of medicine termed *Rehabilitation* developed, particularly at times of war when larger numbers of people required rehabilitation for the disabilities brought about by traumatic injuries. Awareness of the limitations of the hospital ward as the setting for change and adaptation have meant that rehabilitation centres such as Stoke Mandeville have developed where the patient is moved away from the hospital ward environment as soon as his/her medical condition has stabilized. The patient can then be empowered to make change, with social attention from staff tending to reinforce *increases* in activity, rather than drug use and *withdrawal* from activity as can occur on the hospital ward. The environment is also much closer to the home environment and the outside world to which the patient is being returned (Bromley, 1991).

From the rehabilitation viewpoint, the Prince of Wales Advisory Group on Disability (1985) included as a key principle: 'Recognition that disability is not synonymous with illness and that the medical model of care is rarely appropriate'. This statement not only applies to the relatively small number of disabled with congenital or hereditary conditions, but also to the huge number of people who are disabled by degenerative conditions and inappropriate lifestyles (Martin *et al.*, 1988; Bennett *et al.*, 1996). These 'diseases' are principally found in western cultures and include the respiratory, circulatory, cardiac and autoimmune diseases, cancers, arthritides, allergies and digestive problems. They are caused by a multitude of problems that include lack of sufficient activity, over-refined and processed low nutrient diet of limited variety, cigarette smoking, pollution of food, air, water and soil, and worker exploitation. To these need to be added the medical iatrogenic diseases due to overprescription of bed rest (Waddell *et al.*, 1997), drugs (Pither and Nicholas, 1991; McTaggart, 1996) and surgery (Waddell *et al.*, 1979, 1997; French, 1992b).

The World Health Organization (1980) has defined impairment as: 'any loss or abnormality of psychological, physiological, or anatomical structure or function', and disability as: 'any restriction or lack (resulting from an impairment) of the ability to perform an activity in the manner or within the range considered normal'. The Task

543

Force on Pain in the Workplace (1995) suggest these definitions are too narrow, for example not including environmental context. They explore them further, particularly in relation to current approaches to disability management.

Models of Ill Health and Disability Operating in Physiotherapy

Physiotherapists have generally been trained in the traditional medical and rehabilitation models. Apart from those physiotherapists who work in mental health, until recently most physiotherapists have generally had little *practical* training in psychiatry or in psychology or learning.

One particular model that physiotherapists have more recently evolved is to use a descriptive diagnostic or neuro-biomechanical approach to a problem. This is a more useful, practical approach than the medical model. It helps patients understand the rehabilitation model. 'Lumbar spondylitis' provides a poorer working model for the therapist and the patient, than a concept of the patient's individual complex of tightness, weakness, stiffness and spasm, with reference to the postural forces and abnormal movement patterns helping to generate or perpetuate these signs. It is important though, that in working with signs and symptoms to determine treatment, rather than with pigeon-hole diagnoses or Latin or Greek diagnostic labels, the physiotherapist realizes that this does not explain everything, and that psychological or learning processes also play a part in illness and disability. Plenty of people function well with atrocious biomechanics, others have pain and disability with very few objective signs.

Watson, a physiotherapist, in 1996 gave his definition of rehabilitation as 'a problem-solving and educational process aimed at restoring a state of health or well-being . . . and . . . independence . . . Self-responsibility and self-management are the cornerstones of rehabilitation'. He stated that diagnosis should 'remain sufficiently broad-based to encompass psychosocial factors and maladaptive pain mechanisms'. He also added words of warning: 'Unfortunately . . . for many people it has become synonymous with the automatic dispensing of 'therapies' . . . A critical review of the literature fails to demonstrate why we have been seduced by the technology [of electrotherapy] . . . We must promote ourselves as specialists in rehabilitation, not simply as experts in palliative care.'

DIFFICULTIES THAT INDICATE THE NEED FOR A PSYCHOLOGICAL COMPONENT TO PHYSIOTHERAPY AND REHABILITATION MODELS

There are several difficulties that physiotherapists encounter indicating the need for a psychological component to their models. Physiotherapists probably remember working alongside health professions who assume that they have to resort to coercion or bullying in order to achieve improved function in patients who are unwilling. Patients may assume this too when they believe the physiotherapist's expectations are more than they can cope with. The undoubted effectiveness of physiotherapy is testimony to physiotherapists' abilities to teach, to improve patients' confidence, as well as to their treatment skills and knowledge. However, some patients require special handling. Problems can arise with the very anxious patient and those who appear to have little 'motivation' for making changes. Other problems are plateauing or dropping off in improvement after discharge from rehabilitation, and seeking further referral. Unshakeable faith in the power of a machine poses difficulties when the more chronic patient keeps returning for a 'top-up', especially when it substitutes for changing old unhelpful habits. Other difficulties can arise with the patient who continues to attend with an implicit 'do something!', yet reports every time that therapy, especially any requiring movement or exercise, made the pain worse or unbearable.

Psychology *practice* has been sparse in physiotherapy training, and most physiotherapists would have difficulty defining their skills in understanding and helping more challenging patients, or knowing what went wrong when problems continue. Nicholas *et al.* (1991) found that subjects in combined psychological/physiotherapy treatment conditions improved significantly more than subjects in physiotherapy-only conditions, indicating that physiotherapists ideally need to have access to psychologists, and certainly to integrate psychological skills into their treatment programmes.

Lay Models of Disability and Pain or 'How the Patient Sees it'

If you hope to help patients make changes in behaviour, it is necessary to look at patient models as well as theorists' models in order to understand things from their perspective. Patients generally believe that pain is a warning sign of damage or injury – certainly something wrong. Cleeland, Williams and Erskine very clearly describe how persisting pain can challenge lay models of pain and lead to self-doubt and confusion.

Patients' response to pain may be:

to seek medical help to identify the problem, in the belief that this in turn will lead to a cure (or to confirmation of the patient's worst fears, of some sinister disease). In this frame of mind, the patient is unlikely to find reassurance in repeated negative findings on investigation . . . Furthermore, many patients believe that the X-ray or more expensive investigation is only ordered if the [doctor] is seriously worried that a sinister finding will emerge. . . . Whatever the course of failed treatments, negative investigations or waiting and hoping in vain, . . . months since the initial injury or emergence of pain problem . . . the patient has often felt confused, dismissed, disbelieved, abandoned, and ultimately blamed for the pain. It is not unusual for medical and nursing personnel to treat X-rays and other imaging results as 'hard' data, and the patient's experience as 'soft' data. Nor is it unusual for clinicians to feel that they can estimate the pain better than the patients themselves on the basis of those data. (Cleeland, 1989)

The patient's concern about the involvement of psychological factors in his or her problems usually increases as successive medical interventions fail to relieve the pain. Patients may also begin to observe how their pain varies in relation to states such as fatigue, feeling stressed, boredom or pleasant distraction. One acceptable lay model of persistent pain not associated with damage, and influenced by psychological factors ('stress'), is that of recurrent headache. However, at the point where investigations are leading nowhere, most patients feel very vulnerable about the possible role of psychological factors. Phrases such as 'all in the mind' and 'mind over matter' (as an intervention) offer little practical guidance, and imply that the patient lacks the will to get rid of the pain problem. Not surprisingly, in order to counter such suspicions, many patients emphasize their determination, both verbally and in heroic overactivity; they usually suffer considerably from the resulting exertion. (Williams and Erskine, 1995)

> ### Key Point
>
> *If rehabilitation is attempted without understanding how the patient sees their predicament or giving them a more helpful rehabilitation model, this self-doubt and confusion will contribute to poor maintenance of any improvement they make.*

Psychological / Social Models of Disability

Whereas medical models are based on theories of causation and cure, psychological models have arisen from learning theory and are based on a normal rather than a disease model of human behaviour. They address the successful and unsuccessful attempts by the person to adapt to various circumstances such as illness, major life change, loss of valued activities and roles, and repeated failed treatments. The knowledge of how humans learn and unlearn habits can be applied to the physical, practical and psychological habits associated with chronic conditions, and to their accompanying fears, depression and other emotions. The focus is on what can be described, defined and measured, both of behaviour and the circumstances in which it occurs, and of beliefs.

HISTORICAL BACKGROUND TO THE DEVELOPMENT OF C–B APPLICATIONS

A brief description of some theories that relate to the development of C–B applications in chronic pain follows to place it in historical and therefore developmental context (more fully described in Atkinson *et al.*, 1987).

Behavioural science and theories about learning grew at the beginning of the twentieth century after a time of introspection when researchers had attempted to gain enlightenment through contemplation and writing down all their thoughts. A sense of impatience had developed with this, especially as it was proving completely unproductive. So, at a time of optimism when it was thought that science would provide the answer to everything, a behavioural science that made recordable observations was understandably more acceptable than what had gone before.

Classical Conditioning

Classical conditioning was first reported by Ivan Pavlov in 1902 and described more fully in 1927 (Pavlov, 1927). He demonstrated in certain circumstances that it was possible to pair a previously irrelevant stimulus to a relevant stimulus for animals (sound of a bell to salivation in dogs). Particular behaviours are more conditionable to some things than others, e.g. ringing of a bell can condition salivation but not vomiting, pigeons can be trained to peck for some things but not others, and pecking cannot be conditioned out. When a response has been conditioned in animals it is usually already prepared with pathways in the brain set up to be conditioned. No human experiment has ever been able to demonstrate classical conditioning, except at organ level, e.g. the immune system (Spector, 1990; Weinman, 1987, pp. 76–77). It is supposition that a patient's limp may be paired to a doctor's white coat – again this has never been demonstrated.

Pavlov and other Russian researchers found that it was also possible to condition emotional responses such as fear. An animal will respond to an electric shock with increased heart rate and a fear response, but not to a red light. If however the red light is paired to the electric shock, the animal will, after several pairings, respond to the red light with a conditioned fear response. It is thought that this may be relevant in human fear responses, e.g. chemotherapy patients vomiting in response to a doctor's white coat, but in pain it has again never been demonstrated, and it is likely that any pairing of patient muscle tension or limping with a doctor's white coat is by association with painful examinations via cognitive processes (patient's thoughts, beliefs and assumptions). People are not much affected by paired stimulation unless they recognize that the events are linked (Dawson and Furedy, 1976). Cognitive processes are thus much more important factors than classical conditioning is likely to be.

Patients who 'make a fuss' or 'don't try' in response to your requests may be associating physiotherapists with painful exercise or manipulation. They may dislike being pushed or not feeling fully in control, or think the intensity of their pain or their predicament has been dismissed or not believed by a physiotherapist in the past. Although it may appear that the patient has been conditioned to respond this way, change in this behaviour is more effectively brought about on a cognitive level: helping patients question their beliefs or find alternative ways of evaluating the situation.

Learning theory therefore was originally built on these relatively simple and reductionist models of conditioning derived from animal experimentation. It was never regarded as a comprehensive explanation of human behaviour and experience but just the beginning. Classical conditioning is historically important, and generated research in learning mechanisms, but is unlikely to be useful in everyday clinical practice.

Operant Learning

Operant learning (also called operant conditioning) was refined by Skinner (1959) whose work

demonstrated in animals the learning of complex patterns of behaviour through manipulation of reinforcers. He defined a reinforcer by the effect it has on a behaviour, not as a reward or a punishment. Positive reinforcers increase the frequency of required behaviours, negative reinforcers increase the frequency of unwanted behaviours.

Example 1: Operant Learning

On Monday you go into a shop, wait politely, but don't get served.

On Tuesday you go into a shop, bang on the counter and get served straight away.

Which behaviour will you tend to use when you go to the shop on Wednesday?

If a patient finishes a physiotherapy session with a sense of achievement and that the physiotherapist is pleased, he is likely to do his home programme, look forward to the next session and attend well.

If a patient, however, finishes a physiotherapy session in severe pain and the physiotherapist appears indifferent to how hard he has tried, he is likely to leave with a sense of hopelessness and is unlikely to return.

Operant learning does not explain all learning however. For example, infants of all species are wired up to walk and humans to talk, and will do so without reinforcement. Children produce novel sentences and systematic errors that indicate they are applying rules and working things out for themselves, not merely responding to a system of linked rewards.

Fordyce *et al.* (1973, 1976, 1986) has shown that operant learning has practical relevance for chronic pain – one can think in operant terms with patients (see Examples 1 and 14 and case histories in Roberts, 1986).

Operant learning is therefore important but is still not enough to fully explain patients' behaviour. It has therefore been amalgamated into the C–B approach, giving a range of applications that more fully cover the learning methods and difficulties experienced by patients.

Social Learning Theory

This theory was proposed amongst others by Rotter (1954) and developed by Bandura (1977a) as a means of understanding the origins of various patterns of personal and interpersonal behaviour. Bandura observed that humans require a social environment to learn, learn fairly rapidly – more rapidly than could have occurred through operant learning – and learn things they have not done before. He proposed the concept of modelling, or learning by watching – observational learning.

Observational learning is said to be important in acquisition of information and skills that are relevant for avoiding physical danger and minimizing pain, although it appears to be the primary mode of acquiring most patterns of behaviour (Bandura, 1977a). The odds of survival would be greatly reduced if learning about harm required personal experience. Observing someone else in pain can provide the necessary instruction without the damaging effects of direct experience. Explicit teaching however also has an important role here, with subjects instructed in what to do in certain circumstances. Trying something out is then refined by steadily making further corrections based on feedback on your performance from others or yourself. Cognitive mechanisms are also important in social learning. Individuals will interpret and evaluate normal and strange/abnormal sensations from their bodies with information obtained from the family, friends, the community and now the media, as well as from their own experience. A patient whose father died of heart disease may well feel anxious when an extra strong curry gives indigestion pain, or running for the bus produces some fast heart beats and unaccustomed breathlessness.

The individual can readily learn what is likely to generate pain, what sensations should be experienced as alarming or not, how one is likely to feel as a result of various injuries and diseases, and the cognitive, behavioural and social skills useful in minimizing personal distress. Crosscultural studies effectively demonstrate the variability that has emerged in different societies for recognizing and caring for states of disease and injury (Craig, 1978). Craig (1979) describes the social and observational learning that may occur between parent and child. Inadequate training in self-care may increase the risk of illness through life. Craig's (1979) studies have indicated that chronic low back pain patients who did not gain improvement from surgical care tended to construe both themselves and their children as tending towards ill health.

The Cognitive Model

This model links the thoughts that patients have about their situation with their feelings. Cognitions include pre-existing beliefs, assumptions, expectations and perspectives, in other words the patients' 'way of seeing things'. They are self-statements patients think to themselves, often quite fleetingly, and are reflected in what patients say to others.

Example 2: Unhelpful Cognitions or Habits of Thinking

- *All or nothing thinking:* 'If I don't get finished in time, I'm a complete failure' *(feel hopeless)*
- *Mental filter (believing that one negative feature of a situation characterizes it all):* 'The bus conductor annoyed me, it's ruined the whole day' *(feel angry)*
- *Mind-reading (believing yourself to be thought of negatively by others):* 'The physiotherapist must be thinking I'm not trying' *(feeling anxious)*
- *Catastrophizing (believing things to be worse than they are):* 'My shoulder's hurting again, I must have really injured it, I won't be able to manage work for weeks, I may lose my job' *(feel worried, desperate)*
- *'Should' statements (believing that your standards expressed as should, ought to, must and have to, are fixed absolutes — also called 'musturbation'!):* 'I should be able to manage lifting that weight / I must finish all my typing today / the physiotherapist ought to be helping me more' *(feel exasperated, desperate, angry)*
- *Labelling (believing yourself or others to be defined by one or more acts):* 'It's really pathetic I can't lift my leg, I'm a real wimp' *(feel annoyed, a failure)*

Key Point

Cognitive therapy aims to help patients to monitor for and capture these thoughts and link them to their feelings. Patients are then taught how to replace patterns of thoughts associated with feelings such as distress, frustration, anger, depression or confusion with more helpful styles of thought.

Bandura developed the concept of self-efficacy (Bandura, 1977b); that is, all voluntary behaviour change is regulated by a person's perception of their ability to do the activity and to make the change. This work was thus particularly important in drawing attention to cognitive factors. Self-efficacy can influence behaviour: for example, the self-efficacious person will be more likely to engage in coping behaviours because success is anticipated. In contrast, a person with low levels of self-efficacy will be less likely to use adaptive or helpful coping behaviours because of the beliefs that these behaviours may not be effective (Williams and Keefe, 1991). Low self-efficacy, in conjunction with poor physical performance, predicted dropout from treatment on a C–B pain management programme (Coughlan *et al.*, 1995). Patients understand self-efficacy as confidence, and, recognizing the important role of confidence, usually wish to work on building confidence.

It is suggested therapeutically, that confidence is most successfully helped with practice of tasks in a graded way using pacing and helping patients challenge unhelpful thoughts that lead to low self-efficacy.

Example 3: Self-Efficacy and Confidence

When a patient says, 'I feel safe to walk without my stick here, but I couldn't go to the shops without my husband and my stick', *and they have a wish to go shopping alone, then it can be identified that it is confidence that needs working on. Phrases like* 'If I thought I wouldn't fall I'd do . . . XYZ' 'I don't know if I can manage' 'I don't dare . . .' *or indications that patients feel fragile, mean confidence is an important factor.*

The C–B Model

The C–B model evolved from a merging of behavioural and cognitive approaches. It recognizes that there are complex interactions among cognitive, affective and behavioural change. Positive change in one of these areas may promote positive change in the others. This is particularly important because change may be more readily and effectively accomplished in one area than another. Learning to deliver assertive statements convincingly, cope with pain, inject insulin etc., through modelling, role playing, or practice with coaching and feedback is almost certain to help patients think of themselves as better able to deal with problems. This self-perception of increased resourcefulness heightens a sense of control and self-confidence (Bandura, 1977b). These cognitive and affective changes, coupled with the patient's newly established behavioural skills, increase the probability he or she will respond differently in problem situations.

The evolving literature on C–B modification is *not merely* suggesting a host of new treatment procedures. More important, C–B modification is evolving as a perspective, a model, or a theoretical account of behaviour change. The C–B approach uses environmental manipulations, as does the behavioural approach. For the former, however, such manipulations represent informational feedback trials, which provide an opportunity for the patient to question, reappraise, and acquire self-control over maladaptive cognitions, feelings and behaviours.

Example 4: Cognitions in a Social Setting – Alternative Cognitions and Problem Solving

The patient has stopped having friends round. She thinks to do this she:

- *has to cook a meal*
- *has to be hospitable and remain so for a certain length of time*
- *her home has to be spotless* (should statements)

She feels she has to be pain-free / have a lot of time to do all this, and so it becomes 'impossible' (all or nothing thinking).

Patients would be encouraged to look at what their friends expect, considering their circumstances, and whether their friends would rather want to see them or just taste their cooking (more helpful cognitions). *Alternatives to cooking a major dinner party and cleaning the house from top to bottom can be investigated* (problem solving):

- *buying ready prepared food*
- *having friends round for coffee*
- *seeing friends somewhere else*
- *doing something other than cooking, e.g. listening to music together, watching a video*
- *organizing a picnic where everyone brings something*

It is obvious how helping patients do this exercise will help change behaviour, but importantly it has been found to be very effective for depression (Fennell, 1989, p. 209) and also in sport (Example 5).

Example 5: Helpful Cognitive Strategies from Sport

Just before competing:

NOT focusing on

- *how well the other person may have won last time*
- *that he has won three out of the last four matches*

Focusing on:

- *your achievements during training*
- *times when you have won and focusing on the strategies that helped this*

The major components of the C–B approach can be found in Kanfer and Goldstein (1991), Bellack and Hersen (1985) and Beck (1989). In chronic pain management they are those of operant learning (Fordyce, 1976; Roberts, 1986), the goal-setting approach with its emphasis on systematically paced activity (Fordyce, 1976; Gil *et al.*, 1988), the application of practical coping strategies such as relaxation (Linton and Melin, 1983), and cognitive change (Turk *et al.*, 1983). The aims of the approach are not to find the elusive cause for the patient's problem or a magic cure, nor even the perfect exercise programme, but to help the patient cope better with problems.

Treatment Components of the C–B Approach

This section looks at both theory and application of the various treatment components of the C–B approach.

Information

Patients need relevant and understandable information to help them make choices and change behaviour (Ley and Llewelyn, 1995). In general patients are given oversimple explanations. 'Trapped nerves' and 'slipped disc' do not explain complex pain/dysfunction states many years down the road. It is more helpful to give more complete information, and this requires an unthreatening relationship so that patients feel able to ask when they don't understand. Patients may also need guidance to filter information down from all sources (including their own experience) to that which helps them make change. You also cannot explain or inform until you know what the patient understands already, so it is helpful to ask them what they know or think about their condition first. Unless misunderstandings are corrected early on, it is possible for your plausible but conflicting explanation to seem complete nonsense to them (Example 6).

Not all people absorb information in the same way, so providing visual and written, as well as spoken information is helpful, not forgetting the value of observational learning through modelling. Patients often understand and recall information when it has been presented in the form of a case history or 'real life' situation. People usually retain a fairly small proportion of the information they are presented with, so written back-up

> Example 6: Misunderstandings or Conflicting Beliefs
>
> Physiotherapist: *You have pulled a muscle in your back so it needs exercise to help it heal up.*
>
> Patient (thinks): *But the trapped nerve in my bottom is pinched when I exercise, the pain is really sharp — it's excruciating — I can't possibly do that, I might cause severe damage to the nerve.*

should be given, especially as many patients say it is helpful and that they want it (Ley and Llewelyn, 1995).

Information alone is not sufficient for behaviour change. Patients need help to make the practical behaviour changes that are necessary. Moser (1990) demonstrated this in patients who showed significant improvement in their *knowledge* of back protection and ergonomics after attending back school over patients who did not attend. However, they did not improve their *practice* post-back school as measured by a videoed obstacle course.

When patients are keen to learn and are pleased that someone is providing them with useful information, they can get really excited and want to know more. This is great, but it is also important that the therapist does not fall into the trap of delaying progress by substituting information and theoretical understanding for actually 'giving something a go.' Information is not a substitute for gathering hard evidence from trying things out and seeing what happens. Therapists should be aware of the risks of reinforcing avoidance by continuing to provide information well beyond where behaviour change might be expected to

have begun. For example, you may become aware that whenever it is time to do a particular exercise or activity, a patient asks lots of questions, leaving little or no time for exercising. He may not show unhelpful pain behaviour — in fact may look extremely interested and complement you on your knowledge and skill. When this pattern is noticed, you need to stop repeating information, or giving information that might be for a stage more advanced than the patient's. The patient needs to be encouraged to use the knowledge they already have:

Physiotherapist (gently): *'Try that out.'*

Patient: *'I don't know how to do it/I won't be able to do it properly.'*

Physiotherapist: *'See what you can manage, then we'll go from there.'*

Operant Learning: Reinforcing Behaviour Helpful for Rehabilitation

Learning new skills or re-learning old skills is most rapidly brought about by being systematic according to learning theory.

> Learning can occur through trial and error and is established through practice. It is also possible to influence the learning process by providing people with rewards and punishments which 'shape' their behaviour in a different direction. Human beings are very sensitive to subtle signals of approval and disapproval from others and in this way we affect each others' behaviour and learning patterns. Sally French (1992a)

Fordyce described the use of operant learning in the treatment of pain and has clearly described use of the approach with patients (Fordyce *et al.*, 1973). This section explains its theoretical basis then looks at its practical application in physiotherapy.

REINFORCER

Any consequence (stimulus or event) of a given behaviour which is associated with an increase in the frequency of that behaviour or its maintenance is a reinforcer. A reinforcer is often thought of as something 'pleasant', but can be anything. A child's naughtiness can actually be reinforced by smacking if this produces the attention for which the child is craving. A reinforcer thus is identified *only* by its apparent effect on the behaviour it follows. It should follow the behaviour it is reinforcing as immediately as possible.

Activities that patients learn to do should eventually be reinforcing in themselves, giving a sense of enjoyment, satisfaction or achievement. Until this occurs, patients need reinforcement from other sources to bridge the gap.

Cairns and Pasino (1977) studied the effects of reinforcement on patients with low back pain receiving daily measurement of walking distance and exercycle. Significant increases in performance were obtained when patients were reinforced verbally (praise and engaging in desirable conversation only if walking or bike riding distance increased over its previous level) with or without giving feedback by plotting progress on a graph. There were no significant increases in the activities for the control patients or patients under the graph-feedback only condition. They also discovered that operant learning could be effective 'regardless of the presence of so called psychogenic factors' and state that 'patients such as these have typically been labelled "unmotivated," by the treatment staff when, in fact, the absence of reinforcement for attempts to increase

physical function may contribute to the failure of rehabilitative efforts'.

Information and Reinforcement

To be useful for behaviour change, reinforcement should be the means for learning. For example, rather than general praise such as 'Well done!' it is helpful if what you want is included in your praise: 'Your shoulder muscles look so much more relaxed and looser now, that's a really good improvement'. This will usually result in further and more frequent relaxation that will continue far beyond the effect produced by 'try to relax your shoulders, they are very tense'. Thus information has been provided about what is *right*, and the patient is pleased. Curiosity is a powerful drive, so providing information is also itself a form of reinforcement.

Independence from External Reinforcers: Self-Reinforcement

Patients may respond well in an environment where all staff carefully only reinforce well behaviours, but revert to their original behaviours once back in the environment that reinforces pain and passive behaviours. It is thus very important that patients do not become dependent on *therapists'* reinforcement.

From the start of treatment patients should be encouraged in self-reinforcement, that is to reinforce themselves (Kratochwill, 1989). This is an important skill to help them carry over new skills to their environment after discharge. If this is not done, patients are likely to think the therapist was responsible for change and will expect neither further improvement nor the need to practise their new skills. With absence of therapist reinforcement for achievement, there will be no alternative to the old reinforcers for unhelpful behaviours, so it is likely that these return.

Reinforcement is necessary until the patient receives enough satisfaction from the activity for this to be reinforcing in itself. Patients can learn to praise themselves, choose a range of treats for keeping going with their exercise plan, and learn to generate reinforcement from their family and friends. Old reinforcers for previously unhelpful behaviours can be re-used. If a patient previously rested in response to pain (focus on pain reinforced by rest), he can now use 20 minutes rest as reinforcement for a new behaviour. It is just a case of changing the connections (contingencies).

Social Reinforcement

Many activities, especially social ones, eventually become reinforcing in themselves. More naturally reinforcing social goals should therefore be given priority. Joining a dance or yoga group for certain patients will strongly help the patient maintain activity levels.

Intermittent Reinforcement

When learning a new behaviour, immediate, regular and frequent reinforcement is usually most effective. However, once the behaviour has been learned its frequency will usually be greatest if intermittent reinforcements are given, the reinforcers being thinned out (Atkinson et al., 1987, p. 228; Deitz, 1989). Intermittent reinforcers are the most powerful, an example being gambling. Once gambling has been taught, it is the hope of winning next time that keeps the gambler hooked — they hardly ever have to win anything. If however they won every time, boredom would set in and the behaviour would diminish. When a behaviour such as being on time, or weight bearing through a limb, has been established through frequent reinforcement, it is suggested that the behaviour will occur more frequently or strongly if reinfor-cement is thinned out, e.g. every fourth time the person is on time or seen to be weight bearing. Again, intermittent reinforcement need not be external. Provided the patient sees/feels and recognizes some improvement himself, from time to time, this is a powerful reinforcer for continued work at the new behaviour.

Shaping

Shaping is the process of gradually changing the quality of a response through reinforcement of successive levels of a target behaviour until the target behaviour occurs (Atkinson et al., 1987, pp. 226–227). For example, when first learning a language, a person should be reinforced (i.e. with praise) whenever s/he makes anything remotely like the right sound. Gradually, reinforcement should be provided only when sounds closer and closer to the desired sound are made. In other words, the criteria for reinforcement are gradually raised as the responses get more like the desired ones, until reinforcement is given only when the desired or correct responses are made. Shaping can be aided by demonstrating the new level of skill to be learned before shifting the reinforcement.

Extinction

This is reduction in behaviour frequency to zero, i.e. the behaviour stops occurring. This may be achieved by completely removing reinforcers (Poling, 1989). When extinction starts, the response rate is likely to increase for a period before declining, i.e. leaving babies to cry when putting them to bed rather than going back and picking them up and rocking them, will initially result in louder crying. This is know as an extinction phenomenon. This behaviour will eventually stop however, provided the reinforcer (picking up and cuddling/rocking) is not given again.

Speed of extinction is mainly determined by the previous use of reinforcers. Rapid extinction follows where the behaviour was reinforced regularly and frequently. More gradual extinction will follow where reinforcers for the behaviour have been more intermittent and therefore more powerful.

Reducing Unhelpful Habits

A number of unhelpful habits in chronic problems may be adaptive in the acute stage, e.g. limping, but create problems when they continue beyond healing. Stopping or reducing these habits is thus helped by removing reinforcements that maintain them, and by teaching and reinforcing competing or incompatible behaviours. Paying no attention to patient's wincing and tensing may mean the habit is repeated a few times, but provided no reinforcement is given, it will eventually stop. As mentioned before, this will occur faster if it has been regularly reinforced in the past, perhaps by 'over-caring' health professionals who have provided a model for the family to pick up. 'Paying no attention' or 'ignoring' can become punishing, however, if it is the patient that is ignored rather than the behaviour. Patients' responses and states should be perceived as habits or behaviours in a value-free way rather than as wrong. Patients do not do unhelpful things deliberately, or because they are neurotic, hysterical or wicked, but because those behaviours have been reinforced by consequences or others' responses.

These 'behaviours' also have powerful cognitive elements to them. For example, patients who seem to be groaning and exhibiting a lot of pain behaviour, are often discovered to believe that they or their pain are not believed – often with very good past evidence. If when they groan the only strategy is to ignore them, it is not discussed with them, and they are not reinforced for achievements, this will confirm their beliefs and is unlikely to lead to extinction of the groaning.

PUNISHMENT

A punisher is something given or occurring after a behaviour that results in a reduction in frequency of the behaviour. A punisher is often thought of as aversive, but may be anything. As with a reinforcer, the identification of a punisher is *not* based on its perceived qualities of aversiveness or pleasantness, but rather on its effect on the response it follows. Thus if caning a child is not followed by a decrease in the child's unruly behaviour, it (the caning) is not acting as a punisher for that behaviour. Similarly, if praising a child for doing something is not followed by an increase in the frequency of that behaviour, praise is not acting as a reinforcer for that behaviour. Punishment is far less effective than reinforcement. Generally, if patients are punished they do something else. If this is also punished, then the therapist becomes the aversive consequence and a therapeutic alliance is destroyed.

PRACTICAL APPLICATION: MAKING CHANGES, LEARNING NEW BEHAVIOURS, TAKING AN ACTIVE ROLE IN REHABILITATION

Operant principles are directly applicable to some aspects of patients' behaviour. If a patient only stops an exercise at the point where he is in increased pain, and is frightened, this makes for an aversive experience. Providing positive consequences for learning a new behaviour such as walking without aid or increasing knee flexion through use and exercise is likely to reinforce it, particularly when the reinforcements are provided immediately and frequently for small achievements in the early stages. It is likely that patients will improve faster and be less anxious in a physiotherapy setting where they observe reinforcement being used with other patients. The focus is moved away from unhelpful behaviours, and shaping is used later to achieve the finally desired exercise or posture rather than criticism. Pain is not denied, it is just the pain behaviour that is not reinforced.

The aim is then for the patients to take over reinforcement with a system of rewards or, ideally, by their own sense of enjoyment or achievement. It is helpful to introduce a new behaviour that competes with unhelpful behaviour, e.g. pacing an activity is incompatible with overactivity, regular bouts of activity are incompatible with prolonged resting.

In busy physiotherapy departments it can seem more sensible to leave patients who are improving to 'get on with it themselves', i.e. tend to ignore them, while focusing attention on those with 'difficulties' and 'problems'. It is much easier to dodge between those who stop at the first difficulty: 'I can't do it', 'What can I do?' and 'Can you help me?', their eyes following you round the room, rather than giving systematic reinforcement to those who are getting on with things.

Instead of criticizing the quality of a patient's attempts, unrelieved by reinforcement:

'Higher with that leg and keep your weight on that buttock, don't let it lift up, that's making you use the wrong muscles and your back twist.'

reinforcing the patient for what he is doing will result in more rapid and secure improvement:

'Great, that leg's coming up higher now, you're putting more weight through your right buttock which makes your back straighter when you do it. I'm pleased as you're coming on really well with that. I think you're ready for the next stage. Try putting your arm out at the same time — you'll find this helps you to lean even further to the right and feel the weight more through here — that's it, you've got it, brilliant!'

If absolutely nothing in the way of improvement can be discerned, reinforcement can still be given that helps confidence and aids progression:

'That's a difficult exercise for you, you're doing very well to keep trying and I noticed you're still remembering to keep your left arm relaxed as you do it, great.'

Body language and touch can be used to good effect. Physiotherapy is a very 'hands on' profession, but we can use our hands in different ways: instead of 'controlling', prodding, pushing and firmness, we can use touch at the same time and in the same anatomical places yet convey praise, warmth, fun and reassurance that patients are on the right track. Physiotherapists have potentially very varied ways of reinforcing patients.

Empowering patients and providing them with opportunities to problem-solve and discover solutions is vital if patients are to take an active role. It helps patients to gain confidence and make it more likely they will continue with what they have learned after discharge. Rather than the physiotherapist always coming up with solutions to problems, it is better to encourage patients to use and develop their knowledge and experience.

Example 7: Encouraging Self-Attribution and Problem Solving

A: *Physiotherapist solves the problem/ tells patient what to do:*

Physiotherapist: *Hi, nice to see you. You look looser and straighter, your head's moving more freely.*

Patient: *Oh, is it? I feel much more sore than last week.*

Physiotherapist: *That's because you're moving more. Show me how the exercises are going (patient does neck rotation, but with tension in the neck and shoulders and some wincing).*

Physiotherapist: *That looks pretty tense, try relaxing, do it slower, keep breathing.*

Patient: *(continues as above) Yes, I'm trying to relax, but I can't.*

Physiotherapist: *Try letting your shoulders sink down, breathe in, then as you breathe out, gently turn your neck.*

Patient: *Like this?*

Physiotherapist: *Yes good, but you need to let your shoulders relax down more.*

B: *Patient encouraged to recognize HIS achievements and problem-solve:*

Physiotherapist: *Hi, nice to see you. You look looser and straighter, your head's moving more freely.*

Patient: *Oh, is it? I feel much more sore than last week.*

Physiotherapist: *So, you're moving better, but it's much more painful. Why do you think that might be?*

Patient: *Well, I don't know, that's why I asked you!*

Physiotherapist: *What makes it particularly sore?*

Patient: *I think it's some of the exercises. I know they're helping, I'm freer, so I don't want to stop them, but whenever I do the turning exercise it seems to set off that awful muscle spasm.*

Physiotherapist: *That's a good link to have made. What do you think could help?*

Patient: *Well, I'm trying to relax, but it's not easy.*

Physiotherapist: *Great, and relaxing isn't easy to start with. Show me how they are going (patient does neck rotation, but with tension in the neck and slightly in the shoulders).*

Physiotherapist: *What are you feeling?*

Patient: *Well I'm trying to relax my shoulders.*

Physiotherapist: *Yes, I can see that, that's good. Anything else?*

Patient: *It's tight round here (touches right CI area) and actually that's where it's really sore.*

Physiotherapist: *Yes, it's really hard to relax where it's really sore. Is there anything else you've tried to help relax up there?*

Patient: *Well maybe I could do a smaller exercise to that spot to loosen it up, like the nodding exercise.*

Physiotherapist: *'Mmmm Good! I think you're on the right track there. Keep going like that, it will come eventually. Are you pleased with how it's going?*

Patient: *Yes, it's been stiff a long time, so I suppose that's pretty good!*

N.B. *Notice how both physiotherapists*

- *acknowledged the pain without reinforcing the pain talk*
- *reinforced achievement*

The physiotherapist in the second example

- *didn't always come up with the answers*
- *encouraged the patient to think 'why', 'what' and problem solve*
- *encouraged the patient to reinforce himself*

FUNCTIONAL ANALYSIS

It is not always easy to find what functions as a reinforcer for a particular patient, nor sometimes to immediately make the links between a patient's behaviour and the cues and reinforcers in the environment. It is helpful in these situations to establish what is happening by doing a functional analysis. This is described in Groden (1989), though for aggressive behaviour rather than for the situations that occur on hospital wards or physiotherapy outpatient departments and suggests a rather complex format.

A simple way to approach functional analysis is via the acronym ABC (see Table 15.1) (Sturmey, 1996; Fordyce et al., 1973):

Unhelpful cues and behaviours that may occur in rehabilitation are shown in Table 15.2.

It can be helpful as an exercise to do a functional analysis on particular behaviours to understand the mechanisms involved, as in Example 8.

It is not always necessary to do a full analysis. Sometimes just looking at cues and reminders for instance is sufficient. Behaviours can require constant reminders to change them. If a physiotherapist is the only cue to new habits, e.g. the patient who sits up straight every time he

---

Example 8 Functional Analysis of Patient Behaviour

Behaviour: Tensing and straining while doing an exercise, grimacing with pain and effort.

External cue/setting: Exercise sheet with feared exercise, physiotherapist.

Internal cue: Pain with exercise, muscles feel weak and shake with effort.

Cognitive cues/beliefs: 'I must try harder', 'the pain is so bad I need to get this over quickly', 'The physio might make me do more if I don't try', 'God that was pathetic, how did I let myself deteriorate so much?'

Reinforcer: Physiotherapist notices effort.

Functional analysis of changes the patient may make with guidance

Alternative behaviour: Trying active relaxation and breathing while exercising, stopping frequently to loosen and relax.

Challenge to external cue: 'I did manage the exercise yesterday, it wasn't easy but my exercise chart shows that I'm improving', 'This physiotherapist wants me to learn not to push, she'll be pleased if I don't.'

Challenge to internal cue: 'I'll have pain but it will be less if I learn not to tense and push', 'If I relax, the muscles won't shake so much and I won't get so tired, — the exercise will still get done.'

Reinforcer to alternative behaviour: Friends and staff notice patient is more relaxed and comment on improving flexibility and looseness.

Cognitive summary: 'It's not easy to unlearn old habits when I had to drive myself to get things done before, but I've made a start, I'm having a go at relaxing and doing less to begin with, and I'm noticing it's working a bit. If I keep going I'll probably get better at it.' Feel more confident and in control.

Table 15.1
Functional analysis: antecedent, behaviour, consequence (ABC)

Antecedent (cue)	Behaviour	Consequence
Setting		Reinforcer
• Place		
• Beliefs:		
— previous information		
— personal evidence		
Trigger		
• other's behaviour		
• thoughts		
• feelings		

Table 15.2
Unhelpful cues and behaviours that may occur in rehabilitation

ANTECEDENTS/CUES
Setting/place
Scene of previous aversive experience, e.g. DSS doctor's office
No handholds/support
Pain
Something going wrong
Difficult task
Aversive task

Beliefs
Causal, e.g. 'The bones have worn away and the nerves are trapped' or 'Pain is damage'
About activity, e.g. 'Rest is best; if it hurts — stop'
(more examples can be found in Harding and Williams, 1995)

Behaviour of others
TOLD to do task, with 'sergeant major' or strident tone of voice
Leaning towards the person to express sympathy
Hands on hips (can seem emphatic or authoritarian)

Cognitive or internal cues
Thinking others expect too much, are critical of you, think you are stupid not to be able to do it easily (mind reading)
Fear of damage
Feel disbelieved
Feel pressurized
Feel helpless

BEHAVIOURS
Poor posture
Reduced level of activity, e.g. work, household chores, social activities, sport
Poor gait, limping, avoiding full weight-bearing through a leg (motor behaviours)
Increased levels of complaints about pain and other somatic symptoms (verbal pain behaviour)
Use of aids, e.g. walking sticks, braces, collars, corsets
Increasing frequency of passive and catastrophizing thoughts e.g. 'I can't go on', 'Why won't somebody help me?'

Example 9: Cues for New Behaviour

For the person who sits hunched over their knitting, shoulders tensed and raised

New behaviour	Cue for new behaviour
Sit upright, leaning back against the chair	*Sight of newly firmed up chair with appropriate lumbar support*
Knitting raised up with thick cushion on lap	*Knitting bag left on top of cushion*
Shoulders relaxed down	*At end of every row stretch shoulders down then relax*
Frequent regular breaks for arm and neck stretches	*Keep wool in knitting bag, so need to regularly pull out 3 arm lengths of wool: cue to put knitting down and do brief stretch routine*
Regular breaks every 20–30 minutes to get up and walk about for at least 2 minutes	*Get up in TV commercial breaks or set kitchen timer as a reminder, and go and make a cup of tea*

This is also an example of how introducing a behaviour that competes with the old behaviour is helpful.

sees her, but doesn't the rest of the time, then he needs guidance to think of cues in his environment that will occur sufficiently frequently to securely establish the new behaviour / habit.

Inappropriate Interpretation of the Operant Approach

There are various considerations to be taken when using the operant approach.

Taking Care with Terms and Explanations — is the Operant Approach about 'Controlling Behaviour'?
Simple everyday occurrences can attain unhelpful connotations merely by using certain words.

'Conditioning' can have an association with experiments and animals like laboratory rats or performing dogs, or with things that are not under patients' control. Operant learning is a kinder term to use and can be applied in day-to-day physiotherapy as will be seen from the examples that follow. The word 'behaviour' also needs to be used with caution since it can be used to imply bad behaviour, 'in the mind', faking, putting it on etc. 'Habit' can be a more useful, less loaded word.

Some therapists may baulk at using the operant approach, disapproving of using something that appears to manipulate people's behaviour. It has to be remembered though that we all work, partake in hobbies, sport and social occasions or perform tasks in response to reinforcement, and that we are constantly positively (or negatively) reinforcing others' behaviour. All that the operant approach in physiotherapy does is to take more care in observing behaviour change and what reinforces it, so that our responses and behaviour can be more helpful to patients' learning rather than punishing it inadvertently. Importantly it must be remembered that it is easier to increase behaviour you want by reinforcement, than withold reinforcement to attempt to extinguish behaviour you don't want. When helpful behaviours are learned through reinforcement they are generally incompatible with and supercede the unhelpful behaviours.

Treating Patients with Respect

When operant learning is viewed merely as ignoring 'unacceptable behaviour' — in the chronic pain field this might be seen to mean never talking about pain — operant learning can seem rigid and bleak. It is difficult to pinpoint exactly how this impression has come about, but operant learning carries with it the risk that it is applied in a mechanistic way. This does not fit with treating patients as human beings.

There have been a number of ways in which operant learning theory has been used to justify bad practices such as:

- Focusing only on withholding reinforcement for undesirable behaviours (especially ignoring);
- Taking away rights such as going home for the weekend with the idea that they are privileges in the gift of the staff;
- Labelling patients as malingering on the assumption that their behaviour is under concious control.

Control of Behaviour — Conscious or Not Conscious, Real or Fake?

Being able to interfere with a behaviour consciously does not mean that its production is consciously controlled. People with no pain can fake a limp, but find it hard to maintain for long, as concentration turns to other activities. A patient with a long established limp will maintain that limp long past their (or anyone else's) concentration span, indicating that nonconscious mechanisms are involved. The notion that someone is consciously controlling or 'faking' a limp across all contexts and across time is far fetched.

Attention is not infinite — one cannot cram more and more into attention, unlike memory where there is no clear limit or sense of finite. During intense distraction for instance, pain can appear to go, though it returns when the distraction is stopped. If one walks down a corridor with a patient who limps, and distracts him by talking to him, telling jokes, laughing, pointing out things etc., his limp will change. This patient is not faking. Many factors are involved in the causes, cuing and reinforcement of a limp. These are so complex and on so many levels, it is simplistic and crude to take changes in behaviour such as limping as evidence that the limp is somehow not 'real'.

Awareness

Some behaviours are particularly resistant to change. These are often the ones that are not under conscious control, or ones where it is very difficult for people to be aware of their own quality of performance, e.g. posture, tension in muscles, limps etc.

Patients are also not aware of the extent of their behaviours and how they affect other people. Videoing patients while they walk provides feedback for them on their improvements and achievements, and also helps them to problem-solve with their physiotherapist as to the next thing to work on – the next advance. What is astonishing is how most patients are really surprised to see themselves, are unaware of limps, postures, tension and other visible physical habits. Patients who exhibit a lot of pain behaviour will nevertheless also report that they don't talk about their pain and go to a lot of effort to hide that they have pain. They are quite unaware of how they appear or come over to others.

This experience further demonstrates that behaviours are not generally consciously controlled. Patients are unaware of the link between reinforcement, cues and pain behaviours. They do not generally make the link between their feelings and how they think about themselves or what they think others think of them. Since feelings can also influence behaviour, this can complete the circle with little awareness on the patient's part of their role in any of this.

Patients have to know what they need to change, so therapists must be specific in their guidance. One of the most important and unique skills that physiotherapists can bring to pain management is their skill of observation and problem solving for physical behaviours and difficulties. Raising the level of awareness about behaviours such as tension, avoidance or abnormal movement / gait patterns, can be extremely helpful provided it is broached in a non-blaming way, and is also coupled with helping patients look at the consequences of the behaviours and look at ways of reducing or changing them.

Adherence or Compliance?

Rather than using terms like 'compliance with treatment', the C–B approach looks at 'how to establish new habits in place of unhelpful ones'

and tends to think in terms of treatment adherence. One sometimes wishes patients had been less compliant and passive where certain medical interventions have led to poor outcome (Pither and Nicholas, 1991; French, 1992b). Compliance is about following instructions. It assumes that the treatment on offer is unquestionably beneficial, and suggests obedience with no implied choice. Adherence is about using advice and is a term that implies partnership, and choice on the patient's part. Patients need to make informed decisions, sharing and eventually shouldering responsibility for management in their own environment (Ley and Llewelyn, 1995).

Promoting Self-Management: Can the Physiotherapist Ever Help the Patient?

Helping patients by giving physical support, being the sole source of information and always coming up with solutions for their problems results in patients being disempowered and unlikely to maintain improvement once they have left treatment. What patients achieve with the safety of the therapist present and in the hospital setting may also be much harder at home on their own. This needs to be addressed from the very beginning (Marlatt and Gordon, 1980) with patients taught to take a realistic look at generalizing the skills they are learning to activities at home where appropriate help is unlikely to be available.

It is obviously a main aim to ensure that the physiotherapist does nothing that can be construed as 'help', and that the patient is always encouraged to take an active part in chronic pain management and in the learning of skills. However, very occasionally, the fear of an activity, combined with very little or no skill in performing the new behaviour means the therapist needs to give more directive and even physically supportive help initially. Provided this is done in such a way

Example 10: Therapist Support as Part of Graded Exposure

Weaning a patient off crutches or support from another person while walking can get stuck. The patient may get off one or both crutches, but still be walking hanging onto walls. He may even be willing to try a few steps into a room away from the walls, but can seem to be unable to coordinate (1) swinging the arms, which gives him balance, with (2) relaxing and (3) an even right—left gait, despite showing him how to (modelling). Provided you know what is a meaningful reinforcer for him, it is quite OK to start by taking his hand.

Begin by holding his hand:

- *swing the arms while standing, then*
- *walk on the spot swinging the arms, then*
- *set off at an easy rhythmical pace into the room swinging the arms with him.*

Provide constant reinforcement in addition to the reinforcement of your help, then move up the hierarchy of difficulty:

- *walk as before with your hand on his back, still modelling a rhythmical relaxed pace with your other arm swinging, then*
- *walk with him without touching him but staying close, then*
- *gradually move further away, until he walks across on his own.*

All the time provide meaningful reinforcement. At the end make sure he is pleased with HIS achievement, and drum up praise and acknowledgement of the achievement from others, especially relatives or friends.

that the patient is still able to attribute improvement to himself, there is no harm in this at all. The principles of graded exposure (see later) are being used, from mild exposure with the therapist helping, to exposure with the therapist present, to finally strong exposure without the therapist present.

Rapid exposure as in Example 10 to a feared activity is very very effective, even though 'help' was given. Because it provides the patient with a lot of evidence of his success it is likely to maintain well, though of course it needs frequent practice in the early stages to 'set' the new behaviour, and it is necessary to ensure the patient goes on to practise his new skills at home and when going out.

Social Learning

The effects of modelling on pain and illness behaviour are apparent with therapeutic interventions for patients with excessive avoidance and fears of medical or dental procedures. An effective way of reducing fear and helping cooperation is to model realistic coping reactions to the procedures (on film: Pinto and Hollandsworth (1989) or with other patients: Faust et al. (1991)) though it is important that the model's response should be realistic and believable (Vernon, 1974). People withstand painful medical procedures better when they know what to expect and believe they can control the procedure (Melamed, 1977). Physiotherapists may aid modelling by inviting a patient undergoing rehabilitation to talk to another patient who has undergone similar rehabilitation without experiencing untoward effects. Conversely it may be unhelpful to meet another patient who describes their experience in dramatically negative terms (Klaber-Moffett and Richardson, 1995).

Certain people appear to have unfortunately misunderstood the concept of social learning, believing it to be merely a matter of common sense, with the implication that patients who have unhelpful behaviours lack common sense. If a patient's behaviour is not seen by a therapist in the context of his learning history, circumstances and environmental influences, that therapist is less likely to be able to help the patient make changes. Another problem is that people tend to search for meaning and quick solutions, so if something seems to be very obvious, we tend to overestimate its contribution or influence. It is thus important not to make rapid judgements about a person ('they're just like so and so' 'no wonder they've got pain when they're so tense' etc.) but make sure the whole picture has been seen and understood from the patient's perspective. Factors like the way their family views pain or the role of medicine may be having undue influence, so their beliefs need to be checked out.

Goal Setting and Pacing

Chronic pain can lead to changes in people's activity levels.

Common changes that some people with chronic pain report include:

- Not working;
- Reduced level of housework or DIY;
- Pushing oneself to do things — not easy any more;
- Decreased pleasurable activity;
- Decreased social activities;
- Not trying new activities;
- Avoiding people or certain activities;
- Rest or reclining frequently during the day;
- Taking pain medication *prn* or escalating;
- Sleep problems.

GOAL SETTING

Goal setting involves agreeing with the patient detailed, specific goals for each of the problem areas which are going to be worked on (Kirk,

Table 15.3
The SMARTER principle

SPECIFIC and MEASURABLE	'What' and 'how much' will help to clarify what is being aimed for.
AGREED	Having a stated, written and agreed goal helps focus the patient towards goal achievement; approval from the therapist helps the patient realize he is on the right track.
REALISTIC	Within financial means, appropriate for age, family situation etc. not necessarily immediately achievable but gradually, as capabilities improve.
TIME-PLANNED	Establish 'when' it is expected short and long-term goals are to be achieved and the time of reviews.
EXCITING	It is most important that goals should include pleasurable and exciting activities that provide reinforcement for the patient's effort, as well as being relevant to the quality of life changes he really wants to work on.
RE-EVALUATED	Rather than just checking or auditing goal achievement, re-evaluation helps problem solving and refinement of the skill, e.g. 'I managed well, but I put myself at risk of doing too much: next time I need to plan more time for breaks and negotiate a back up to look after the children'. Having a flare-up plan is also important here, ready for when evaluation points to the need for this.

1989). Often people give up hobbies and interests, and social activities as well as work and chores. It is important that these 'quality of life' activities are included in both short and long-term goals on which to be worked. Goals can be based on the SMARTER principle shown in Table 15.3.

Once a range of goals have been identified, patients need to think about what is stopping them achieve them. It may be inability to sit or walk for long enough, insufficient information for goals like work, courses etc., fear of the activity, e.g. the jarring involved travelling in a bumpy bus, or finding it hard to say 'No' or to stop, and causing a flare-up. They will then try to work out the steps needed to achieve their goals, breaking them down into their constituent parts or 'building blocks'. Outcome goals should always be set in combination with performance goals, e.g. exercise and building blocks, providing the mechanism by which to achieve the outcome.

Using the goal-setting approach links behaviour change and treatment goals to the patient's longer term goals by means of pacing, a systematic approach which provides graded exposure (see later) for feared activities (Kanfer and Goldstein, 1991). Cott and Finch (1991) suggest that active participation by the patient in the goal-setting process is of primary importance. They found that factors identified in the literature as improving goal achievement include setting specific and measurable goals, the degree of goal difficulty depending on patient expectations, goal acceptance and access to feedback. Schmitz et al. (1996) showed that being able to adjust personal goals flexibly reduced the effect of pain intensity and pain-related disability on mood (depression). Additionally, they found that reduction in disability due to the use of pain-related coping strategies only occurred when accompanied by a high degree of flexible goal adjustment. Patients thus need to be able to be flexible in the way they set goals, learning how to alter their expectations and adjust their goals, or to look at other options according to changing circumstances.

The Overactivity/Underactivity Cycle

Patients often have a tendency to cycle from over-doing activity or pushing hard, to underdoing activity or resting/avoiding when the overactivity has resulted in pain flare-ups and they are unable to keep going. The danger times are when the pain is easier or the patient feels better, since this is when they do too much and initiate the cycle that ends in rest. An example is the back pain patient who goes shopping on a 'good' day, only to find that this infrequent and too strenuous activity causes a flare-up in pain requiring 2 or 3 days in bed to settle it down. Physiotherapy patients can do this by trying too hard with their exercises or having them set too high. They barely manage the journey home, then have to rest up or stop exercising until their next appointment. Although many chronic pain patients are very unfit and have rested too much, it is the overactivity that is at the root of the problem. Patients cannot improve their fitness unless they first prevent the tendency to push themselves. Setting targets as 'bulls' eyes, i.e. target to hit exactly, avoiding 'as far/as much as you can' type targets is a good guide. Shooting an arrow past the target scores no points, whereas points are scored for being near the bull's eye. It also helps prevent patients using how they feel to decide on the target.

PACING

Pacing makes an activity or behaviour time- or quota-dependent rather than symptom-dependent. Since pain is not a helpful guide as to when to stop – often informing patients to stop far too late, or hurting before they have hardly started – patients learn what their body can manage, then stick to those quotas. It is after all physiological sense to work to muscle, bone, ligament and circulatory capabilities than rely on sensation that is fickle and influenced by so many different physical and cognitive factors.

Principles of Pacing Activities

- Make a plan. Prioritize what has to be done on a daily basis.
- Start activities with realistically low baselines, then build up tolerance to the activities gradually and systematically.
- Take regular rests in between activities.
- Change position regularly while performing activities.
- Do small amounts often, rather than doing everything at once.
- Avoid long unbroken periods of either activity or rest.

Pacing from modest baselines is incompatible with overactivity/underactivity cycles so helps change this habit. A good rule is for patients to make two or three measurements of the activity, ideally at different times of the day, then they are taught to average these measurements and start at 80% of the average. This prevents any risk that they may be starting too high. It is helpful to explain to chronic pain patients that a baseline cannot be set too low since the amount will build up with pacing, but that if they start too high, they will not be able to maintain it on bad days and will not have learnt to break the habit of overdoing or pushing. If a patient has had a problem for many years there is no need to rush towards achieving high levels of activity or fitness. It is more important that patients learn *how* to do it, since they

can then continue the process themselves over a more realistic time span.

Example 11: Pacing a Complex Activity

COOKING A MEAL

For back pain patient with:

10 minutes standing tolerance and 10 minutes sitting tolerance.

PLAN   menu   ingredients
             utensils   time required
             pacing

PREPARE *(5 min standing/walking)*
             Brief rest

PREPARE *(10 min sitting, chopping/
             peeling etc)*
             Brief rest

COOK *First half (stand 10 min)*
         Brief rest

COOK *Second half (stand 10 min)*
         *Brief rest while dish finishing
         off in the oven, then*

LAY THE TABLE

DISH OUT AND EAT

Pacing Exercises

Pacing is also applied to exercises (Fordyce, 1976). Rather than starting with the maximum possible or stopping when it starts to hurt or the pain increases, patients are taught to begin with 'an easily manageable amount, unlikely to cause a pain flare-up later in the day'. It can help to first discuss with patients their pain experience without evidence of damage, and reassure them that they are not being given an exercise that will harm them. Establishing with patients the uselessness of using pain as a guide, e.g. 'sometimes it tells you to stop too early, sometimes much too late' helps break the link. Patients then just set a baseline for each exercise that is an easily manageable amount with less close monitoring of the pain. On less painful days they should be encouraged to set baselines 'bearing in mind days with more pain'.

As with activity, two or three baselines are taken to encourage a gentle 'trial and error' approach; these are averaged and patients start at 80% of this average. Patients are then taught to build up or 'pace up' their exercises, first with the guidance of the physiotherapist, then gradually learning to do it for themselves until they can do it without any supervision.

SET-BACK PLANS

All chronic conditions fluctuate and sooner or later patients need to cope with a set-back. Pain flare-ups can often be managed with a flare-up plan which reminds patients to utilize helpful coping strategies (see later) for a difficult day. Sometimes, however, patients may feel they cannot continue despite coping strategies: perhaps the flare-up is lasting more than a day or two, or they have a heavy cold and are finding it difficult to continue. Having a set-back plan keeps them in control and on target without the feeling that pain has begun to take over again by making the decisions on what can be managed. The set-back plan will include a systematic cut-back then re-build back up to the previous quota in a set time, e.g. cut exercises and building block tolerances by half and build back up in 5 days. Patients will learn to recognize a 3-day, 5-day, week set-back etc. and whether to cut back by half, a third etc.

OVERCOMING AVOIDANCE AND FEARS WHICH LIMIT ACTIVITY: THE BEHAVIOURAL APPROACH

Avoidance of an activity previously linked to a strongly aversive stimulus such as severe pain can be extremely resistant to extinction, and continue long after the stimulus has become harmless (Solomon and Wynn, 1954). The avoidance of or relief from distressing emotion is frequently an immediate effect and reinforcer of a problem behaviour, and is often the most potent maintaining factor (Kirk, 1989). Fear of keyboards can continue long after healing of tenosynovitis; fear of weight bearing can continue long after healing of a knee injury. In these cases there is also the double bind: avoidance can lead to pain and stiffness due to disuse or to hypersensitivity. It then appears that the fear of the harmless stimulus — typing a few words or weight bearing evenly — is justified, since the activity is still painful, as well as frightening. Avoidance in chronic pain patients is often more than just of painful movement, frequently including avoidance of social activities and leisure pursuits or even work (Philips, 1987).

Treatment: Graded Exposure

Treatment for avoidance of activity is the same as that for phobias, which was developed particularly from the work of Wolpe on systematic desensitization. Graded exposure requires facing something previously avoided because it provoked feelings of anxiety, in a systematic graded way. First, the person identifies all the things that are avoided, and orders them according to difficulty in a 'graded hierarchy'. The feared activity or situation is then introduced at a level where the person feels capable of attempting it, but sufficient to provoke a small amount of anxiety. The task is repeated frequently and regularly until anxiety starts to subside. Next the person moves up the graded hierarchy of difficulty. An example of graded exposure applied to spider phobia is described in Butler (1989), but it can be applied to avoidance of feared activities in just the same way (see Example 10). By approaching rather than avoiding, the patient has the opportunity to learn that the situation is not in fact dangerous. The child who never goes near a dog again may remain fearful, while the one who approaches them is likely to regain confidence. Treatment therefore requires that patients repeatedly make contact with the things that they fear, and remain in contact with them until the fear subsides.

The cognitive approach to fear avoidance will be covered later but the reader will already be observing how behavioural and cognitive elements interact.

Relaxation as a Coping Strategy

Relaxation was used successfully in the treatment of chronic pain patients in the community by Seers (1993): compared to a control group who received equal attention from the therapist, the relaxation group showed small but significant changes in pain rating, anxiety, disability and sleep scores, at the end of treatment and up to 4-month follow-up. James et al. (1993) showed with headache patients that subjects using explicit time goals for using coping strategies (including relaxation) reported lower pain levels and medication usage compared to waiting list controls and subjects told to use strategies for as long as possible. This suggests that setting goals with patients for using coping strategies such as relaxation at specific frequencies and times can enhance the general efficacy of C–B therapy for chronic headache pain.

A more detailed review of relaxation therapy in different contexts is given in Chapter 10, Neuromuscular Techniques, but the following applies to pain patients.

RELAXATION FOR MUSCLE TENSION

There is a basic assumption that some people have chronically increased muscle tension, but this has not been demonstrated. Specific muscle tension is associated more with movement — particular patterns of muscle tension where muscles do not relax when the next group take over. This failure to relax is related to psychological variables of fear of activity and self-efficacy rather than to pain or range of movement (Watson et al., 1995).

Relaxation can be taught in an attempt to reduce either general or specific muscle tension affecting pain, despite lack of evidence for such a mechanism (Keefe and Gil, 1986; Gamsa, 1994a). The connections between tension and pain appear to be more complex, in relation to static and dynamic muscle use and relationship with muscle use in pain-free areas (Kravitz et al., 1981). Ahern et al. (1988) found chronic low back pain patients and non-pain controls manifested differences in lumbar paravertebral EMG on movement but not at rest. Differences were not only in tension of the muscles required to make a particular movement (pain sufferers showed more muscle activity than normals in achieving half the lumbar flexion), but also in the failure to relax muscles which were not required. Kravitz et al. (1981) found only occasional pain subjects showed elevated resting tension, rather than this being the norm. However, Flor et al. (1985) demonstrated that while low back pain patients, in comparison with non-back-pain and non-pain controls, had no higher resting EMG, they showed elevated tension in lumbar musculature in relation to personal stressful stimuli (e.g.

a row at home) but not to general (e.g. a maths test), with slower than normal return to baseline.

Relaxation training for reducing muscle tension while moving requires a physiotherapist; someone with ingenuity who can take information from the patient and observe and intervene, to teach patients to apply relaxation skills appropriately.

RELAXATION TO REDUCE ANXIETY

Elton and Stanley (1987) describe the use of imagery for those who find creating a blank mind difficult due to anxious thoughts that intrude.

Images need to:

- Be meaningful and relevant to the patient (personal);
- Be interesting and stimulating;
- Have pleasant associations;
- Be free of disturbing or unhappy associations;
- Contain an element of change to hold the attention.

When patients can master this they can progress towards images without change, gaining control over intruding thoughts.

ENHANCING THE EFFECTS OF GRADED EXPOSURE

Relaxation can also enhance the effects of graded exposure to feared situations (Borkovec and Sides, 1979a). In the physiotherapy setting these might include fear of falling when climbing stairs or walking without a walking aid, or fear of getting down on the floor (fear of not being able to get up). This use of relaxation is part of systematic desensitization that is described in Wolpe (1989). It aims to weaken anxiety response habits by using responses competitive with anxiety. Deep muscle relaxation and diaphragmatic rather than apical breathing are examples of this. Patients can use these skills to help themselves regain a sense of control in feared situations. They can rehearse graded exposure to, for instance, climbing stairs with even weight-bearing and without a walking aid.

SENSE OF CONTROL

Holroyd et al. (1984) demonstrated that it is a sense of control that is important in relaxation. Headache patients using EMG biofeedback reported fewer headaches whether they were in a group where the biofeedback was given for decreasing or for increasing frontal EMG activity. This demonstrates the importance of cognitive elements in skills training. Linton and Melin (1983) showed that it is applied relaxation that is important in pain patients. Patients can do this by either practising relaxation in real situations that are difficult for them or if this is not possible to do or mock up, relax in the presence of a painful stimulus.

Other Coping Strategies

FLARE-UP PLANS

The use of a flare-up plan is one of the most important coping strategies. It helps patients cope with times of high risk for giving up or going back to unhelpful strategies. Patients are taught to recognize their personal coping strategies, e.g. regular 10-minute relaxation breaks, using loose and rhythmical movement, ice for muscle spasm, stretch for tight muscles, local relaxation etc., then to work out a plan for the first hour so they can follow it when concentration is difficult rather than ploughing on regardless or panicking. 'Forewarned is forearmed' so teaching patients to prepare and use a flare-up plan gives them a sense of remaining in control, as well as having something practical and useful to do.

SUMMARY

A range of relaxation techniques is available but it is important that whichever technique is taught, relaxation should be presented as a skill to be learned by repeated practice. It should be practised not just in comfortable pleasant surroundings but also as an applicable skill for times of increased mental or muscle tension, e.g. in a traffic jam, when facing a feared situation or at moments of increased pain. A method of applied relaxation can be found in Clark (1989) though the first stage of tensing muscles prior to relaxation is generally avoided in pain patients since it usually provokes pain. It is important that patients are taught relaxation and rehearse it, and are not just handed a 'how to' tape. Studies indicate that audio-tapes alone are rarely effective (Borkovec and Sides, 1979b). Telling patients what to do is not enough — relaxation is a learned skill not a passive instruction.

Cognitive Principles

Beck's cognitive approach (Beck, 1989) is the main cognitive approach adopted in C–B pain management. Beck applied it principally to depression at first, but later extended his approach to a wide range of emotional disorders such as anxiety and phobias. In contrast to the traditional psychiatric view of depression, Beck suggested that the pronounced negative thinking in depression is not just a symptom, but actually has a central role in maintaining it. Treatment was therefore aimed at helping patients to identify and challenge or modify their unhelpful thoughts. Beck suggests that unhelpful cognitions or beliefs that occur (such as in depression), are learnt as early on in life as the

pre-verbal stage. This emphasizes the close link between social learning and cognitive models. Beck's approach appears valid but there is no evidence for, and some against, his hypotheses. It is still not clear if there are general frameworks for thinking that are triggered by life events. Examples include the hopeless, depressed thoughts that can occur at times such as around exams. Many will recognize in themselves and others self-statements such as 'I'm a hopeless failure, nothing will work out, I can't do it'.

> Cognitive restructuring is designed to help patients 1) to appreciate that there is a relationship between thoughts and feelings and their behaviors and 2) to identify faulty, self-defeating, pain-engendering thoughts, and then to replace these cognitions with coping thoughts, feelings and behaviors. For example, patients who report thoughts that they are incompetent and helpless in controlling the pain they experience would be guided to appreciate how such thoughts may exacerbate the intensity and increase the duration of their pain, thus acting as self-fulfilling prophecies. (Turk et al., 1983)

Basic behavioural skills can easily become a part of mainstream physiotherapy practice. Cognitive skills are less easy to acquire and more complex cognitive problems need the expertise of a clinical psychologist. There are three main areas however that physiotherapists can recognize, and by helping patients identify and challenge their more unhelpful thoughts and beliefs, can bring about changes in patient's feelings and associated behaviours.

1 Unhelpful beliefs commonly encountered in physiotherapy are typically about pathology and images of the body: for example, 'wear and tear' (thoughts associated with exercise wearing them out further and rest being essential); 'trapped nerves' (worrying thoughts / images of raw nerves which require

surgical untrapping) and degenerative joint/disc disease or 'arthritis' (images of crumbling bones or joints with dire implications for the future).

Jensen *et al.* (1994) found that the belief that one is disabled and that activity should be avoided because pain signifies damage was associated positively with physical disability. Physiotherapists know of the plasticity of the nervous system, the ability of the body tissues to strengthen and toughen, and how best to enhance this. Patients need to know this too. They need information; they may also require help to challenge unhelpful beliefs by looking at the evidence for and against them. Worry from one or two falls, an article in the newspaper etc., is laid against other evidence that counters it, including the patient's own experience.

Williams and Thorne (1989) found that physical therapy compliance was diminished by a strongly held belief that pain will be enduring, and belief in the mysterious nature of pain. They suggest that patients who lack a framework for understanding their pain may view the sore muscles resulting from some physical therapy treatments as time ill-spent or even counterproductive given their understanding of pain. Belief in pain as mysterious is also associated with little improvement post-treatment in psychological distress.

2 Fears and anxious thoughts, such as beliefs that the patient is unable to manage without the therapist, cannot always be resolved easily by reassurance. Repeated reassurance by health professionals can lead to *raised* anxiety and behaviours that are sometimes unhelpfully labelled hypochondriasis (Salkovskis and Warwick, 1986). Reassurance is only reassuring if the patient (not just the therapist) feels reassured! Patients need to reassure themselves using good quality information and experience. Relief of anxiety by avoiding a feared activity perpetuates avoidance. If a patient thinks pain signals deterioration, he is likely to avoid activities that increase that pain, even if it will bring about improvement, since this also relieves anxiety. A desired behaviour that is absent cannot be reinforced, so the cause of the anxiety needs to be tackled. The physiotherapist can help the patient do this with information, and by teaching relaxation skills and graded exposure (see above).

3 Depressed mood is common in chronic conditions and can also be present in more acute illness or post trauma. Patients' thoughts focus on feeling like not doing anything, that doing anything does not feel worth it, or even that they themselves are not worth it. They tend to focus on personal failure and difficulties, setting themselves unrealistic and unreasonable targets with which to measure success, construing even achievements as failures or as chance events. Depression can be mistaken for 'poor motivation', a hypothetical construct of little practical use. Factors that improve mood include aerobic exercise, having a range of worthwhile and pleasurable goals to work towards, and interrupting the downward spiral into depression with challenging meaningful thoughts: 'I've coped before, I can do it again', 'The doctor/physiotherapist said I will improve, it's slow and I'm feeling down, but I'm further on than last week'.

THE COGNITIVE MODEL OF ANXIETY / PANIC

In this model (Clark, 1989) patients misinterpret a range of body sensations such as breathlessness, aches, pains, pins and needles, palpitations and dizziness, in a catastrophic way. They may perceive them as signs of imminent physical or mental danger or disaster. As patients often take the absence of any obvious triggers for these attacks as evidence that they are due to serious physical disorder, identifying the antecedents of a spontaneous attack can be a helpful way of challenging patients' catastrophic interpretations. These could be being angry or excited, drinking coffee, getting up quickly etc.

Avoidance prevents learning and expanding personal experience as can be seen in Example 12 from Clarke (1989).

It is understandable that patients who have actually had a heart attack can also get into this bind since they have some medical back-up for their personal evidence.

Some patients attribute the onset of their pain to a relatively innocuous routine activity such as bending lifting or twisting. They may appraise the experience as 'my back just gave out', or 'I felt it snap', or 'something seemed to pop out of place'. Their experience seems to be that fairly minor physical trauma produces quite frightening 'pathology'.

This is compounded when the chiropractor tells them they have 'put the disc back in', the doctor tells them they have 'wear and tear' and to rest (it will obviously wear out if you don't) or the physiotherapist tells them to *never* bend over or do sit-ups. A traditional medical myth is that the back is a delicate structure, to be protected care-

---

Example 12: Avoidance Preventing Learning

A patient who was preoccupied with the idea he might be suffering from cardiac disease avoided exercise (such as digging in the garden) or sex whenever he noticed palpitations. He believed that this avoidance helped to prevent him from having a heart attack. However, as he had no cardiac disease, the real effect of the avoidance was to prevent him from learning that the symptoms he was experiencing were innocuous. Instead his avoidance tended to reinforce his negative interpretation because he took the reduction in symptoms which followed avoidance as evidence that he really would have had a heart attack if he hadn't stopped what he was doing.

Another anxious patient sat down or leaned against solid objects whenever she felt faint. She believed this prevented her from collapsing. Instead it prevented her from learning that the feeling of faintness which she got when anxious would not lead to collapse.

From Clark, DM (1989) Cognitive Behaviour Therapy for Psychiatric Problems: A Practical Guide, Hawton, K, Salkovskis, PM, Kirk, J, Clark, DM (eds). By permission of Oxford University Press)

---

fully from strain or damage. In fact the opposite is true — constant use strengthens it while disuse leads to weakening (Twomey, 1991). In their efforts to explain the cause of recurrent back pain, doctors and physiotherapists often point to various structural defects. Terms like degeneration, spondylosis etc. are used despite the lack of evidence relating them to pain or disability (Waddell, 1987). Patients report being told they have crumbling spines / discs / bones, slipped discs, pinched nerves, trapped nerves, that they will end up in a wheelchair etc. The horrors and mystique that has built up around arachnoiditis, RSI, irritable bowel, ME etc. are not entirely the patients' fault.

Studer and Yeager (1994) argue that even basic bed mobility requires the concurrent use of cognitive skills and motor skills. Why, then, should the cognitive and the motor be separated in the delivery of therapy?

This section is merely a pointer to cognitive principles and the physiotherapist needs to remember her limitations. A few helpful comments cannot sort out depression for example, and it is easy to get into contradictions that become a barrier to further improvement. Cognitive intervention is best left to clinical psychologists who have the expertise and experience to recognize patients in more serious states of distress, and who know what to do.

Generalizing Gains

The main advantage of the C–B approach is that it gives the patient a tool kit – a set of skills that have application to a range of difficulties, some for frequent use, others for emergencies. It teaches a different way of thinking things through and behaving so that skills will maintain and generalize to other environments. Generalization skills can be cued intitially, followed by gradual withdrawal of prompts to reinforce self-generalization to other environments, as shown in Example 13.

Example 13: Teaching Patients to Generalize Skills to Their Environment

Physiotherapist: 'What did you do there to help you manage it?'
'What did you find effective / helped you stop doing it the old way?'

Patient: 'I did stop.'

Physiotherapist: 'Right, so you paced it.'
'How did you find it went compared to before?'
'Have you found pacing useful for anything else?'
'Where does it seem difficult to pace?'
'How might you tackle that?'

Principles:

- *Look for specific skills that they have used in their daily life similar to ones they have used in interactions with you.*
- *Reinforce them for using skills.*
- *Help them see the generalization.*
- *Help them self-reinforce / recognize their achievements.*
- *Finally, once the skill has generalized, leave the patient to tell you of any new generalizing skills, making them independent of your cues (questions).*

Maintenance

What patients take with them into real life may be more important than what they accomplish during physiotherapy sessions (Hall and Vaiarello, 1994). Maintenance is vital, and is aided by:

- Making links between new behaviours and a patient's beliefs – incompatibility between them will result in decline once patients are away from therapist reinforcement and influence;

- Encouraging patients to work towards independence from the start using self-reinforcement, finding reinforcements in their own environments and using behaviour cues and reminders;
- Patients attributing improvements to their own efforts, not entirely to the will or skill of the physiotherapist. Rather than accepting compliments from the patient, 'You are so wonderful, I couldn't do it without you, such healing hands!' etc., it is important that therapists gently hand these back to the patient, and while acknowledging their role in guidance, place the responsibility for improvement back with the patient.

Self-attribution is taught from the very beginning.

Acceptance of responsibility for their body and health means acknowledging that patients' hard work and the healing capabilities of their bodies brought about change. Physiotherapists can be catalysts and guides, but it is important they do not take credit for what belongs to the patient. Nicholas (1992) has examined the use of C–B therapy for relapse prevention in more detail, going into factors associated with relapse, patient beliefs, improving adherence to treatment strategies and relapse prevention.

And the Whole Package?

Utilizing all the C–B principles mentioned may seem daunting, but the range of principles do give a natural direction in practice, as can be seen in Example 14.

Example 14: Using a Range of C–B Principles

Teaching passive lumbar extension in prone lying to a patient who experiences severe spasm on extension, and has previously been told to stop if it hurts.

Stage 1

- *Show him how to do the exercise (modelling);*
- *Describe the exercise simply, explaining how to do it without pushing or tension, and reassuring him that the exercise cannot harm him (information / modelling); and*
- *Describe how to start with a very slight approximation of the final exercise (graded exposure / graded hierarchy), explaining the need to start with a low baseline followed by a steady build-up (pacing) rather than going for it and ending up with a pain flare-up (overactivity / underactivity cycling);*

- *Show immediately that you are interested and pleased with the patient's efforts at each stage of tackling the exercise: decide to begin, get down on the floor, turn prone, place his hands, start to push himself up, remember not to force the exercise, decide that he has gone far enough and to stop before he sets off major muscle spasm (reinforcement of helpful behaviours) for example, asking if he thinks he has done enough before he shows effort behaviour, rather than when he puffs and pants, sighs, grimaces, looks tired etc., implying that you think his efforts are acceptable, and rewarding his efforts with permission to stop;*

- *Don't react in a concerned way, and appear neutral rather than interested when the patient refuses, does not make any attempt to start, or exhibits pain behaviour, vocal or in his body language* (non-reinforcement of unwanted behaviours);
- *If the patient does absolutely nothing that warrants reinforcement, remind him you want it to be up to him what he does, but your advice is to do it very very gently* (repeat information clearly) *then leave him to try it alone* (avoid reinforcing passive behaviour), *testing to see if you are a cue for pain behaviour – pain behaviour reduces – or if being left alone is more of a reinforcement for that individual than being paid attention – exercise behaviour increases* (functional analysis);
- *Importantly, avoid letting the patient off an exercise altogether after several failed attempts* (avoid intermittent reinforcement of unhelpful behaviour) *rather direct him to be satisfied with a small achievement, 'That's a really good start, especially in view of the problems you've had with it before'* (setting a manageable baseline to begin graded exposure – pacing – for a feared activity);
- *Encourage the patient to review his achievements: 'Are you pleased with how that went?'* (self-reinforcement training); *'Why do you think that went better than before?'* (problem-solving skills training);
- *Encourage the patient to practise little and often* (establishing repeated contact with feared activity) *getting him to fill out a chart* (planning) *and think of cues to remind him to do it* (establishing behaviour in their own environment).

Stage 2

- *Thin out your attention or whatever reinforces the patient's exercise behaviour* (intermittent reinforcement);
- *Set targets of gradually increasing difficulty for the provision of your reinforcement, e.g. (1) hands placed correctly, head up, (2) chest off the floor, (3) chest further off the floor, glutei relaxed, (4) lumbar hyperextension, (5) lumbar hyperextension with relaxed erector spinae* (behaviour shaping), *letting your reinforcement contain the clues to what the next step is, 'There, your back muscles relaxed, that's great!'* (information within reinforcement) *rather than being directive* (avoid making the patient passive) *or telling the patient what you don't want 'don't tense your back muscles'* (avoid punishment);
- *Review the patient's beliefs now he has experienced new behaviour and help him challenge his old beliefs with the new evidence, 'I thought pain meant damage and that I shouldn't bend my back backwards. I can see now that if I do it gently, it doesn't spasm so much or flare the pain up badly'* (cognitive challenging), *'Maybe if I continue, I'll be able to reach up to high shelves again and get some control over this back'* (generalization of skills to patient's environment).

Prevention of Chronicity

Most acute conditions clear in time, only some patients go on to become chronic (Clinical Standards Advisory Group, 1994). Cognitive–behavioural management for chronic pain is well established, but for many years practitioners have been interested in prevention. What might be important in the acute phase for the prevention of chronicity?

Fordyce et al. (1986) performed a randomized study of acute back pain patients attending casualty, comparing traditional with behavioural management. The traditional group were given exercises with the advice 'Let pain be your guide', and given pain killers to be taken 'as needed', with a repeat prescription if asked for. The behavioural group were given a preset number of exercises on a preset incremental schedule, and unrenewable analgesia prescriptions for fixed time intervals. No group differences were found on activity-level measures. Traditional group subjects, however, showed significant increases in chronicity and how impaired they said they were from pre-onset to 9 months follow-up. The behavioural group subjects had returned at follow-up to pre-onset levels. Fordyce thus showed that the method of presentation of acute therapy is important in the prevention of chronicity.

Linton et al. in 1993 suggested that current concepts of chronic pain clearly indicate that proper care at the acute stage should prevent the development of chronic problems. He demonstrated that relatively simple changes in treatment for pain appeared to be crucial in his study of 198 patients seeking health care or sick leave for acute musculoskeletal pain. Both the early intervention group (average wait for doctor 2.8 days and three physical therapy meetings, underscoring return to function and emphasizing 'well' behaviour) and the control groups ('treatment as usual', average wait for doctor 8.8 days) demonstrated significant improvement for pain intensity and activity levels. However, for patients who had not had time off work for pain before, the early active intervention group resulted in significantly less sickness absenteeism than the delayed, treatment as usual group. The risk of developing chronic (>200 sick days) pain was also 8 times lower for the early active intervention group.

McKinney (1989) demonstrated in his study of acute neck sprains that a single session of advice from a physiotherapist was more beneficial than 10 tailor-made treatment sessions of physiotherapy, these results being of greater significance at 2 year follow-up. He concluded that information and advice on posture, controlled movement and early mobilization contributed to patient self-sufficiency for managing acute minor episodes, and that there may be psychological advantages in making people responsible for their treatment rather than victims of their pain.

Lindstrom et al. (1992) compared a graded activity programme with a control group receiving traditional care recommended by their physicians (including time off work, rest, analgesics and 'available physical therapy'). Patients on the graded activity progamme returned to work significantly faster, and significantly reduced long-term sick leave (mean of 12.1 weeks in the second follow-up year compared to 19.6 weeks for the controls).

Physiotherapists are in an ideal position to take this work further and to record and analyse the contribution of immediate (e.g. casualty department and general practice surgery) over early and late physiotherapy intervention, passive (electrical) over movement therapies, and behavioural over traditional approaches.

Delivery

Individual or Team, Single Profession or Interdisciplinary?

A chronic condition such as intractable pain, with its intrinsic set of complex psychological, social, legal and physical problems has led to calls for multidisciplinary teams as the most desirable approach for comprehensive treatment (Bonica, 1974). Turk and Steig (1987) argue that teams described as multidisciplinary often consist of professionals who have little direct communication or common philosophy, providing the services. 'Multidisciplinary team' tells nothing of the nature of team interactions, the mechanics of team operation, the delegation of responsibility, the quality of communication among team members, or even the composition of the team. They go on to describe the construction and workings of a team described as 'interdisciplinary' and although they provide no evidence, they suggest, based on good practical reasons, that:

> All team members need to be committed to a perspective that views psychosocial, behavioral, and physical factors as critical in successful rehabilitation. For example, a physical therapist who disavows the importance of psychosocial and behavioral factors in the maintenance of chronic pain syndrome and who gears his or her treatment plan entirely to the physical aspects of the problem will sabotage the team's efforts by denigrating the importance of these factors in the patient's own conceptualization of the problem. Such a physical therapist (who is probably locked in his or her thinking in the acute medical model) is also likely to deliver passive treatment modalities to dependent patients (e.g. ultrasound and/ or hot packs) rather than the active therapies (such as education and/or reconditioning) that are so critical to successful rehabilitation.

Single Therapist C–B Practice

Although interdisciplinary teams appear to be the ideal treatment approach, and there are increasing numbers of programmes starting up, there are insufficient clinical psychologists, resources or opportunity to have this luxury in every district general hospital at present. Some physiotherapists, however, are developing their management of the less severely distressed chronic pain patients, seeing them individually or in groups. As yet there is no literature on outcome but the method seems to be providing exciting opportunities for patient change.

The more complex patient requires so much and multifactorial input that a physiotherapist cannot cope alone. She will need mutual support from:

- A *psychologist* for more complex cognitive and behavioural problems related or not to the pain problem and requiring skilled management and patient training;
- An *occupational therapist* for goal setting and work rehabilitation;
- A *nurse* or *doctor* for drug reduction.

Nevertheless, a physiotherapist may be able to start the patient on simple tasks while awaiting referral to a multidisciplinary programme or other agency, without fear of causing iatrogenic problems. This is provided she remains in the C–B rather than the medical model and clearly explains to the patient what is possible and what is beyond a physiotherapist's remit or skills. The physiotherapist can also have a valuable role for the patient who is wary of seeing a psychologist or attending a programme with a psychologist on the staff — 'so you think it's in my mind'.

Explaining that psychologists are educators not pill prescribers, and that psychology treatment is about learning skills for coping, will help allay the patient's fears, as will reaffirmation that they do have a real physical problem, even if that problem is getting them down.

Insufficient Skills?

Although physiotherapists can utilize basic psychological principles to enhance treatment effectiveness for patients who do not follow the usual course of recovery, it can be helpful to discuss management with a clinical psychologist or refer on to an interdisciplinary C–B programme. These also exist for the head injured, spinal injury, chronic pain, coronary rehabilitation and chronic fatigue, and are becoming more widespread. Some patients, although they have very real physical problems, may also have a background of psychological problems or psychological difficulties that are beyond the skill of even an experienced physiotherapist. These patients require the expertise and experience of a clinical psychologist in this field. It can be helpful though for the physiotherapist to continue to contribute to the patient's rehabilitation through assessment and advice in conjunction with the treatment of the clinical psychologist. It cannot be overemphasized how worthwhile and fulfilling these therapeutic alliances can be.

The Challenge of the C–B Approach

By learning the C–B approach and integrating it with their own skills, physiotherapists are making further major contributions to rehabilitation and interdisciplinary management programmes. This is an exciting and also very satisfying area of work, and the more widespread adoption of the approach into physiotherapy generally should contribute to enhancing practice and outcome.

An integrated C–B approach, however, raises some questions about the validity and appropriateness of certain current treatment approaches.

Physiotherapists need to seriously reconsider:

- Aids that undermine confidence in weight bearing and movement.
- Re-assessment and re-treatment when the problem is the same as before – is it bolstering the medical model rather than an active coping approach?
- Repeated reassurance by the therapist: is anxiety increasing, and should the patient learn to reassure themselves?
- The power of placebo elements in any treatment, affected (among other variables) by the patient's and therapist's expectations (Richardson, 1995; Hashish et al., 1986; Hashish, 1986).
- Using other than evidence-based treatments with clinically significant benefit over placebo in double blind, randomized controlled trials. It can be argued that most of the electrotherapy literature that compares genuine with sham treatment should also be comparing an active approach to the modality being investigated, as has been done for chronic lateral epicondylitis (Pienimaki et al., 1996).[2]

[2] Wyper et al. in 1978 produced an average 9% increase in blood circulation during ultrasound, but an average 1600% increase with simple quadriceps contractions performed to confirm the blood flow measurement method was working as it should! If it were possible to measure, one suspects that the degree of mobilization of fibroblasts by ultrasound in the laboratory would pale into clinical insignificance if compared to continuous passive motion or regular gentle active motion at 5-minute intervals.

- Providing treatment or modifying behaviour based on hunches rather than on evidence. Common sense provides contradictory guidelines (Sutherland, 1994).
- Oversimple explanations of a problem which suggest high risk, e.g. 'crumbling bones' seen on X-ray, or encourage expectations of a technological 'fix-it', e.g. untrapping a 'trapped' nerve.
- Expecting information alone to change well-established maladaptive habits, when the patient does not have the required skill in his repertoire, or confidence in using it. Back school should not just inform, it should provide opportunities for patients to practise the skills they are meant to acquire with access to guidance. Handouts should not replace the therapist's supervision of the patient's practice, but back it up.

Conclusions

The C–B approach looks at the way people adapt to illness, disability or changed circumstances. Rather than taking a conventional disease model of cause and cure, it examines the interaction between behaviours, circumstances and beliefs. Treatment or management is aimed at successfully teaching the patient skills for making changes and maintaining their use into the future. Physiotherapists can utilize the approach, applying it practically to facilitate patient treatment or management.

Summary of Behavioural Factors that Help Patients Make Changes

Physiotherapy rehabilitation has three main aims for behavioural change: initiating and increasing desired behaviours, maintaining these behaviours, and decreasing and/or stopping undesired behaviours. The principles of the behavioural approach include various practical strategies to help patients make changes:

- *The provision of clear information* to help patients make informed choices;
- *Operant learning* of behaviour by selective reinforcement;
- *Goal setting* to ensure intended behaviour change results in meaningful achievements for the patient;
- *Systematic pacing* rather than pain controlled activities or overactivity/underactivity cycling;
- *Use of coping strategies* such as relaxation and set-back or flare-up plans;
- *Use of cues, reminders, plans and timetables* to facilitate learning and maintenance;

The following factors help patients bring about behaviour change:

- Having a sense of being listened to and taken seriously (to counter fears that others think they are malingering, and don't believe them);
- Recognition of personal achievements, i.e. self-reinforcement;
- Working towards meaningful personal goals, e.g. knitting a jacket for the new grandchild, visiting friends abroad, etc.;
- Having a sense of coping, 'I managed last time it was difficult: I can do it again';
- Experiences of success that are incompatible with pain behaviour and of more value than unhelpful reinforcers, e.g. enjoying going out for a walk in the park with the dog or visiting the pub with friends, is more reinforcing than being brought meals in bed;
- Having a sense of control through good planning and problem-solving skills;
- Having a range of coping skills for the inevitable

difficult times with prepared and practised plans for set-backs.

This chapter has outlined a significant section of psychological theory and practice that is of immense relevance to physiotherapy practice.

Key Points

1 The traditional medical model of disease does not explain the discrepancies between pathology, test findings, disability and response to treatment. Psychological models can explain many of these discrepancies without resorting to simplistic labels or blaming patients. They provide both a theoretical framework and practical solutions for patients' difficulties that are measureable and testable.

2 The patient needs to be seen as a whole. Not only the local injury or problem, but its effect on the whole physical body. This includes:

- General levels of activity or disuse with their secondary physical effects;
- Previous learned habits;
- The patient's beliefs about their situation and experience;
- The role of their environment in terms of the cues, reinforcers and social learning for behaviours that has been occurring;
- Secondary effects on the patient's mood, led by their thoughts.

3 Patient rehabilitation needs to focus on the prevention of chronicity, teaching patients self-management and maintenance skills, with the ultimate goals of treatment being closely related to the patient's own goals.

4 Cognitive–behavioural skills can be integrated into physiotherapy practice and enhance outcome. The approach is different from the conventional approach, but is straightforward and rewarding.

Further Reading

Broome, A, Llewelyn, S (eds) (1995) *Health Psychology: Processes and Applications'*. Chapman and Hall, London.

Gatchel, RJ and Turk, DC (eds) (1996) *Psychological Approaches to Pain Management*. Guilford Press, New York.

Hawton, K, Salkovskis, PM, Kirk, J, Clark, DM (eds) (1989) *Cognitive Behaviour Therapy for Psychiatric Problems: A Practical Guide*. Oxford Medical Publications, Oxford.

Schone, N (1995) *Coping Successfully with Pain*, 2nd edn. Sheldon Press, London.

Wilson, PH, (ed) (1992) *Principles and Practice of Relapse Prevention*. Guilford Press, New York.

References

Ahern, DK, Follick, MJ, Council, JR, Laser-Wolston, N, Litchman, H (1988) Comparison of lumbar paravertebral EMG patterns in chronic low back pain patients and non-patient controls. *Pain* 34: 153–160.

Atkinson, RL, Atkinson, RC, Smith, EE, Hilgard, ER (1987) *Introduction to Psychology*, 9th edition. Harcourt Brace Jovanovich, Florida.

Bandura, A (1977a) *Social Learning Theory*. Prentice-Hall, Englewood Cliffs, New Jersey.

Bandura, A (1977b) Self-efficacy: towards a unifying theory of behaviour. *Psychological Review* 84(2): 191–215.

Beck, AT (1989) *Cognitive Therapy and the Emotion Disorders*. Pelican.

Bellack, AS, Hersen, M (1985) *Dictionary of Behaviour Therapy Techniques*. Pergamon Press, New York.

Bennett, N, Jarvis, L, Rowlands, O, Singleton, N, Haselden, L (1996) Living in Britain: Results from the 1994 General Household Survey. Office of Population Censuses and Surveys.

Black, D, Morris, JN, Smith, C, Townsend, P (1990) The Black Report, in Townsend, P, Davidson, N (eds) *Inequalities in Health*. Penguin, Harmondsworth.

Bonica, JJ (1974) Preface, in Bonica, JJ (ed) *Advances in Neurology*, vol. 4. Raven Press, New York.

Borkovec, TD, Sides, JK (1979a) The contribution of relaxation and expectancy to fear reduction via graded, imaginal exposure to feared stimuli. *Behaviour Research and Therapy*. 17: 529–540.

Borkovec, TD, Sides, JK (1979b) Critical procedural variables related to the physiological effects of progressive relaxation: a review. *Behaviour Research and Therapy*. 17: 119–125.

Bromley, I (1991) *Tetraplegia and Paraplegia: a Guide for Physiotherapists*, 4th edn. Churchill Livingstone, Edinburgh.

Butler, G (1989) Phobic disorders. In Hawton, K, Salkovskis, PM, Kirk, J, Clark, DM (eds) *Cognitive Behaviour Therapy for Psychiatric Problems: A Practical Guide*. Oxford Medical Publications, Oxford.

Cairns, D, Pasino, JA (1977) Comparison of verbal reinforcement and feedback in the operant treatment of disability due to chronic low back pain. *Behavior Therapy.* 8: 621–630.

Clark, DM (1989) Anxiety states: Panic and generalized anxiety. In Hawton, K, Salkovskis, PM, Kirk, J, Clark, DM (eds) *Cognitive Behaviour Therapy for Psychiatric Problems: A Practical Guide.* Oxford Medical Publications, Oxford.

Clinical Standards Advisory Group (1994) Epidemiology Review: the epidemiology and cost of back pain. Annex to the CSAG report on back pain. HMSO, London.

Cleeland, CS (1989) Pain control: public and physician's attitudes. In Hill, CS, Fields, WS (eds) *Advances in Pain Research and Therapy,* vol. 11. pp. 81–89. Raven Press, New York.

Cott, C, Finch, E (1991) Goal-setting in physical therapy practice. *Physiotherapy Canada* 43(1): 19–22.

Coughlan, GM, Ridout, KL, Williams, CdeC, Richardson, PH (1995) Attrition from a pain management programme. *British Journal of Clinical Psychology* 34: 471–479.

Craig, KD (1978) Social modelling influences on pain. In Sternbach, RA (ed.) *The Psychology of Pain* pp. 73–110. Raven Press, New York.

Craig, KD (1979) A social learning perspective on pain. In *Research in Psychology and Medicine,* vol. 1. pp. 27–34. Academic Press, London.

Dawson, ME, Furedy, JJ (1976) The role of awareness in human differential autonomic classical conditioning: The necessary-gate hypothesis. *Psychophysiology* 13: 50–53.

Deitz, SM (1989) Schedules of reinforcement. In Bellack, AS, Hersen, M (eds) *Dictionary of Behaviour Therapy Techniques,* pp. 189–190. Pergamon Press, New York.

Elton, D, Stanley, GV (1987) The psychologist and management of chronic pain. In Burrows, GD, Elton, D, Stanley, GV (eds) *Handbook of Chronic Pain Management.* Elsevier Science, Amsterdam.

Faust, J, Olson, R, Rodriguez, H (1991) Same-day surgery preparation: Reduction of pediatric arousal and distress through participant modelling. *Journal of Consulting and Clinical Psychology* 59: 475–478.

Fennell, MJV (1989) Depression. In Hawton, K, Salkovskis, PM, Kirk, J, Clark, DM (eds) *Cognitive Behaviour Therapy for Psychiatric Problems: A Practical Guide.* Oxford Medical Publications, Oxford.

Flor, H, Turk, DC, Birbaumer, N (1985) Assessment of stress-related psychophysiological responses in chronic back pain patients. *Journal of Consulting and Clinical Psychology.* 53: 354–364

Fordyce, WE (1976) *Behavioral Methods for Chronic Pain and Illness.* CV Mosby, St Louis.

Fordyce, WE, Fowler, RS, Lehmann, JF, DeLateur, BJ, Sand, PL, Trieschmann, RB (1973) Operant conditioning in the treatment of chronic pain. *Archives of Physical and Medical Rehabilitation.* 54: 399–408.

Fordyce, WE, Brockway, JA, Bergman, JA, Spengler, D (1986) Acute back pain: a control-group comparison of behavioral vs traditional management methods. *Journal of Behavioral Medicine.* 9(2): 127–140.

French, S (1992a) Teaching and learning in the clinical setting. In French, S (ed.) *Physiotherapy: A Psychosocial Approach.* Butterworth Heinemann, Oxford.

French, S (1992b) Society and the changing nature of illness and disease. In French, S (ed.) *Physiotherapy: A Psychosocial Approach.* Butterworth Heinmann, Oxford.

Gamsa, A (1994a) The role of psychological factors in chronic pain. I. A half century of study. *Pain* 57: 5–15.

Gamsa, A (1994b) The role of psychological factors in chronic pain. II. A critical appraisal. *Pain* 57: 17–29.

Gil, KM, Ross, SL, Keefe, FJ (1988) Behavioral treatment of chronic pain: four pain management protocols. In: France, RD, Krishnan, KDD (eds) *Chronic pain,* pp. 376–413. American Psychiatric Press, Washington.

Groden, G (1989) A guide for conducting a comprehensive behavioral analysis of a target behaviour. *Journal of Behaviour Therapy and Experimental Psychology.* 20(2): 163–169.

Hackett, G, Bundred, P, Hutton, JL, O'Brien, J, Stanley, IM (1993) Management of joint and soft tissue injuries in three general practices: Value of on-site physiotherapy. *British Journal of General Practice.* 43: 61–64.

Hall, KG, Vaiarello, LM (1994) Transfer-appropriate processing: low back. *PT – Magazine of Physical Therapy.* 2(6): 57–8, 64.

Harding, VR, Williams, ACdeC (1995) Extending physiotherapy skills using a psychological approach: Managing chronic pain in a cognitive—behavioural multidisciplinary team. *Physiotherapy* 81(11): 681–688.

Hashish, I, Harvey, W, Harris, M (1986) Anti-inflammatory effects of ultrasound therapy: evidence for a major placebo effect. *British Journal of Rheumatology* 25: 111–116.

Hashish, I (1986) The effects of US therapy on post-operative inflammation. PhD thesis, Institute of Dental Studies, University of London.

Holroyd, KA, Penzien, DB, Hursey, KG, Tobin, DL, Rogers, L, Holm, JE, Marcille, PJ (1984) Change mechanisms in EMG biofeedback training: Cognitive changes underlying improvements in tension headache. *Journal of Consulting and Clinical Psychology* 52(6): 1039–1053.

James, LD, Thorn, BE, Williams, DA (1993) Goal specification in cognitive-behavioral therapy for chronic headache pain. *Behaviour Therapy* 24(2): 305–320.

Jensen, MP, Turner, JA, Romano, JM, Karoly, P (1991) Coping with chronic pain: a critical review of the literature. *Pain* 47(3): 249–283.

Jensen, MP, Turner, JA, Romano, JM, Lawler, BK (1994) Relationship of pain-specific beliefs to chronic pain adjustment. *Pain* 57(3) 301–309.

Kanfer, FH, Goldstein, AP (1991) *Helping People Change: A textbook of methods,* 4th edn. Pergamon Press, New York.

Keefe, FJ (1989) Behavioral measurement of pain. In Chapman, CR, Loeser, JD (eds) *Advances in Pain Research and Therapy, Vol. 12: Issues in Pain Measurement.* Raven Press, New York.

Keefe, FJ, Gil, KM (1986) Behavioral concepts in the analysis of chronic pain syndromes. *Journal of Consulting and Clinical Psychology.* 54(6): 776–783.

Kirk, J (1989) Cognitive-behavioural assessment. In Hawton, K, Salkovskis, PM, Kirk, J, Clark DM (eds) *Cognitive Behaviour Therapy for Psychiatric Problems: A Practical Guide.* Oxford Medical Publications, Oxford.

Klaber-Moffett, JA, Richardson, PH (1995) The influence of psychological variables on the development and perception of musculoskeletal pain. *Physiotherapy Theory and Practice.* 11: 3 11.

Kratochwill, TR (1989) Self-reinforcement. In Bellack, AS, Hersen, M, (eds) *Dictionary of Behaviour Therapy Techniques,* pp. 199–200. Pergamon Press, New York.

Kravitz, E, Moore, ME, Glaros, A (1981) Paralumbar muscle activity in chronic low back pain. *Archives Physical Medicine and Rehabilitation.* **62**: 172–176 .

Ley, P, Llewelyn, S (1995) Improving patients' understanding, recall, satisfaction and compliance. In Broome, A, Llewelyn, S (eds) *Health Psychology: Processes and Applications*, pp. 75–98. Chapman and Hall, London.

Lindstrom, I, Ohlund, C, Eek, C, Wallin, L, Peterson, L, Fordyce, WE, Nachemson, AL (1992) The effect of graded activity on patients with subacute low back pain: a randomized prospective clinical study with an operant-conditioning behavioral approach. *Physical Therapy.* **72**(4): 279–93.

Linton, SJ, Melin, L (1983) Applied relaxation in the management of chronic pain. *Behavioural Psychology* **11**: 337–350.

Linton, SJ, Hellsing, A-L, Andersson, D (1993) A controlled study of the effects of an early intervention on acute musculoskeletal pain problems. *Pain* **54**(3): 353–359.

Marlatt, GA, Gordon, JR (1980) Determinants of relapse: implications for the maintenance of behaviour change. In Davidson, PO, Davidson, SM (eds) *Behavioral Medicine: Changing Health Lifestyles*, pp. 410–452. Brunner/Mazel, New York.

Martin, J, Meltzer, H, Elliot, D (1988) The prevalence of disability among adults. Report 1. Office of Population Censuses and Surveys, HMSO, London.

McKinney, LA (1989) Early mobilisation and outcome in acute sprains of the neck. *BMJ.* **299**: 1006–1008.

McTaggart, L (1996) What doctors don't tell you. Thorsons, London.

Melamed, BG (1977) Psychological preparation for hospitalisation. In Rachman, S (ed.) *Contributions to Medical Psychology*, vol. 1. pp. 43–74. Pergamon Press, Oxford.

Moser, J (1990) An investigation into changes in knowledge and behaviour following attendence at a back school. MSc thesis, Southampton University.

Nicholas, MK (1992) Chronic pain. In Wilson, PH (ed.) Principles and Practice of Relapse Prevention, pp. 255–289. Guilford Press, New York.

Nicholas, MK, Wilson, PH, Goyen, J (1991) Operant-behavioural and cognitive–behavioural treatment for chronic low back pain. *Behaviour Research & Therapy* **29**(3): 225–238.

Pavlov, IP (1927) *Conditioned Reflexes.* Oxford University Press, New York.

Payer, L (1990) *Medicine and Culture: Notions of Sickness and Health in Britain, the US, France and West Germany.* Victor Gollancz Ltd, London.

Philips, HC (1987) Avoidance behaviour and its role in sustaining chronic pain. *Behaviour Research and Therapy.* **25**(4): 273–279.

Pienimaki, TT, Tarvainen, TK, Siira, PT, Vanharanta, H (1996) Progressive strengthening and stretching exercises and ultrasound for chronic lateral epicondylitis. *Physiotherapy* **82**(9): 522–530.

Pinto, RP, Hollandsworth, JG (1989) Using videotape modelling to prepare children psychologically for surgery: Influence of parents and costs versus benefits of providing preparation services. *Health Psychology* **8**: 79–95.

Pither, CE, Nicholas, MK (1991) The identification of iatrogenic factors in the development of chronic pain syndromes: abnormal treatment behaviour? In Bond, MR, Charlton, JE, Woolf, CJ (eds) *Proceedings of the VIth World Congress on Pain*, pp. 429–434. Elsevier, Amsterdam.

Poling, A (1989) Extinction. In Bellack, AS, Hersen, M (eds) *Dictionary of Behaviour Therapy Techniques.* Pergamon Press, New York.

Prince of Wales Advisory Group on Disability (1985) *Living Options: Guidelines for those planning services for people with severe physical disabilities.* London.

Richardson, P (1995) Placebos: their effectiveness and modes of action. In Broome, A, Llewelyn, S (eds) *Health Psychology: Processes and Applications*, pp. 75–98. Chapman and Hall, London.

Roberts, AH (1986) The operant approach to the management of pain and excess disability. In Holzman, AD, Turk, DC (eds) *Pain Management: A Handbook of Treatment Approaches*, pp. 10–30. Pergamon Press, New York.

Rotter, J (1954) *Social Learning and Clinical Psychology.* Prentice Hall, Englewood Cliffs, New Jersey.

Salkovskis, PM, Warwick, HMC (1986) Morbid preoccupations, health anxiety and reassurance: a cognitive–behavioural approach to hypochondriasis. *Behaviour Research Therapy* **24**: 597–602.

Schmitz, U, Saile, H, Nilges, P (1996) Coping with chronic pain: flexible goal adjustment as an interactive buffer against pain-related distress. *Pain* **67**(1): 41–51.

Secretary of State for Health (1992) *The Health of the Nation: A Strategy for Health in England.* HMSO, London.

Seers, K (1993) Maintaining people with chronic non-malignant pain in the community: teaching relaxation as a coping skill. Report submitted to Department of Health.

Skinner, BF (1959) *Cumulative Record*, pp. 430. Appleton-Century-Crofts, New York.

Solomon, RL, Wynn, LC (1954) Traumatic avoidance learning: the principles of anxiety conservation and partial irreversibility. *Psychological Review* **61**: 353–385.

Spector, NH (1990) Behavioral aspects of the modulation of immunity. In Schmidt, LR et al. (eds) *Theoretical and Applied Aspects of Health Psychology.* Harwood, Switzerland.

Sternbach, RA (1969) *Pain: A Psychophysical Analysis.* Academic Press, New York.

Studer, M, Yeager, KK (1994) The cognitive and the motor: inseparable. A transdisciplinary approach. *PT – Magazine of Physical Therapy* **2**(6): 52–6.

Sturmey, P (1996) *Functional Analysis in Clinical Psychology.* Wiley Press.

Sutherland, S (1994) *Irrationality: The Enemy Within.* Penguin, London.

Task Force on Pain in the Workplace (1995) *Back Pain in the Workplace: Management of Disability in Nonspecific Conditions.* Fordyce, WE (ed.) IASP Press, Seattle.

Turk, DC, Steig, RL (1987) Chronic pain: the necessity of interdisciplinary communication. *Clinical Journal of Pain.* **3**: 163–167.

Turk, DC, Meichenbaum, D, Genest, M (1983) *Pain and Behavioral Medicine.* Guilford Press, New York.

Twomey, LT (1991) Musculo-skeletal physiotherapy: the age of reason. *Proceedings, World Confederation for Physical Therapy 11th International Congress.* **1**: 343–347.

Vernon, D (1974) Modelling and birth order in response to painful stimuli. *Journal of Personality and Social Psychology.* **29**: 794–799.

Waddell, G (1987) A new clinical model for the treatment of low-back pain. *Spine.* **12**(7): 632–643.

Waddell, G, Kummel, EG, Lotto, WN, Graham, JD, Hall, H, McCulloch, JA (1979) Failed lumbar disc surgery and repeat surgery following industrial injuries. *JBJS.* **61**A(2): 201–207.

Waddell, G, Feder, G, McIntosh, A, Lewis, M, Hutchinson, A (1997) *Low back pain evidence review. British Journal of General Practitioners,* in press.

Watson, G (1996) Neuromusculoskeletal physiotherapy: Encouraging self-management. *Physiotherapy.* **82**(6): 352–357.

Watson, PJ, Booker, CK, Chen, ACN, Main, CJ (1995) Surface electromyography in the identification of patients with chronic low back pain and assessment of treatment outcome. *Physiotherapy.* **81**(8): 452 [Abstract].

Weinman, J (1987) *An Outline of Psychology as Applied to Medicine,* 2nd edn. Wright, Bristol.

Whitehead, M (1990) The health divide. In Townsend, P, Davidson, N (eds) *Inequalities in Health.* Penguin, Harmondsworth.

Williams, CdeC, Erskine, A (1995) Chronic pain. In Broome, A, Llewelyn S (eds) *Health Psychology: Processes and Applications,* 2nd edn. Chapman & Hall, London.

Williams, DA, Keefe, FJ (1991) Pain beliefs and the use of cognitive–behavioural coping strategies. *Pain.* **46**(2): 185–190.

Williams, DA, Thorne, BE (1989) An empirical assessment of pain beliefs. *Pain.* **36**: 351–358.

Wolpe, J (1989) Systematic desensitization. In Bellack, AS, Hersen, M (eds) *Dictionary of Behaviour Therapy Techniques,* pp. 215–219. Pergamon Press, New York.

World Health Organisation (1980) *International Classification of Impairments, Disabilities and Handicaps.* World Health Organisation, Geneva.

Wyper, DJ, McNiven, DR, Donnelly, TJ (1978) Therapeutic ultrasound and muscle blood flow. *Physiotherapy* **64**(10): 321–322.

Index